MW00835351

Emerging Topics and Controversies in Neonatology

Elaine M. Boyle • Jonathan Cusack

Editors

Emerging Topics and Controversies in Neonatology

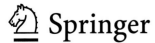 Springer

Editors
Elaine M. Boyle
Department of Health Sciences
George Davies Centre for Medicine
University of Leicester
Leicester
UK

Jonathan Cusack
Department of Health Sciences
George Davies Centre for Medicine
University of Leicester
Leicester
UK

Department of Neonatology
University Hospitals of Leicester NHS Trust
Leicester
UK

Department of Neonatology
University Hospitals of Leicester NHS Trust
Leicester
UK

ISBN 978-3-030-28828-0   ISBN 978-3-030-28829-7   (eBook)
https://doi.org/10.1007/978-3-030-28829-7

This Springer imprint is published by the registered company Springer Nature Switzerland AG
The registered company address is: Gewerbestrasse 11, 6330 Cham, Switzerland

Contents

Part I
The Fetus

Chapter 1
Pregnancy–Related Complications and Preterm Delivery

Suzanna Dunkerton and Penny C. McParland

Topics for Discussion in This Chapter
- Prematurity prevention including identifying those at high risk and interventions such as cerclage, progesterone and cervical pessaries.
- Intrapartum interventions to improve the outcome for the preterm neonate.
- Delivery at the limits of viability.
- Mode of delivery of the preterm breech baby.
- International strategy on stillbirth prevention and the increase in iatrogenic prematurity.
- Identification of fetal growth restriction.

Introduction

It is inevitable that complications of pregnancy and their obstetric management will impact on the wellbeing of the newborn infant and the care provided by neonatologists. Almost all aspects of obstetrics will be encompassed by this principle. However, in this chapter we have endeavoured to focus on the aspects of obstetrics that are undergoing the greatest change at present and also have the greatest potential to impact on the newborn baby and its wellbeing. Although many of these changes are occurring internationally, particularly in the developed world, there is inevitably a focus on changes to practice within the UK. We have therefore focussed on prematurity (both prevention and intrapartum care) and prevention of stillbirth. Although the latter would seem intuitively to be less relevant to neonatal outcomes, the consequences of the changes in practice that have occurred will impact on the care of neonates especially with a potential increase in iatrogenic prematurity.

S. Dunkerton · P. C. McParland (✉)
University Hospitals of Leicester NHS Trust, Leicester Royal Infirmary, Leicester, UK
e-mail: penelope.mcparland@uhl-tr.nhs.uk

© Springer Nature Switzerland AG 2020
E. M. Boyle, J. Cusack (eds.), *Emerging Topics and Controversies in Neonatology*, https://doi.org/10.1007/978-3-030-28829-7_1

Prematurity

Preterm birth is the leading cause of perinatal morbidity and mortality in developed countries [1, 2]. 7.8% of babies in the UK in 2016 were born at less than 37 weeks of gestation [3]. Approximately one third of preterm births are 'iatrogenic' (e.g. due to conditions such as pre-eclampsia or fetal growth restriction). The remaining preterm births are spontaneous and may occur because of preterm labour with intact membranes or following preterm prelabour rupture of the membranes (PPROM).

The majority of preterm births will arise in the apparently low-risk obstetric population. Whilst there are lifestyle changes that will impact on preterm birth risk for the population (such as smoking cessation and pregnancy spacing) there are as yet no reliable screening methods or interventions to offer to women in this group. Interventions are therefore usually targeted at women who are recognised as being at high risk of preterm birth [4]. Many major hospitals will have a specialist preterm birth antenatal clinic; however there is significant heterogeneity in practice between them in terms of investigations undertaken and interventions provided [5].

Risk Factors for Prematurity

Risk factors for preterm birth include previous preterm birth, multiple pregnancy, congenital uterine anomaly and maternal smoking. Previous cervical surgery for cervical intraepithelial neoplasia, such as large loop excision of the transition zone and cone biopsy, is also now established as a risk factor for preterm birth. Hopefully with the introduction of the human papillomavirus (HPV) vaccine this will reduce the number of HPV positive cervical smear changes and reduce the number of cervical loop excisions undertaken. These risk factors are routinely screened for at the antenatal booking visit to allow appropriate targeted antenatal care. More recently, previous second stage Caesarean section has been identified as a risk factor for early preterm birth and late miscarriage [6–9] and is associated with a threefold increase in risk in delivery at less than 30 weeks gestation [7]. It has been suggested that this is caused by the interruption of the sphincteric muscle fibres around the cervix either due to unintentional surgical laceration of the cervix at the time of uterine incision or by the passage of the surgeon's hand into the pelvis to disimpact the fetal head [7, 10]. This risk factor may gain greater importance in antenatal care as the rate of second stage Caesarean sections increases and that of mid-cavity and rotational instrumental deliveries decreases [11]. Novel systems such as the fetal pillow (Fig. 1.1) have been developed to aid disimpaction at second stage Caesarean section. These have been shown to reduce trauma to the fetal head and to reduce complex uterine extensions that can include the cervix [12]. However, it has yet to be demonstrated whether this will impact on the subsequent risk of prematurity in the next pregnancy.

Fig. 1.1 This shows the positioning of the Fetal Pillow beneath the head of the baby, elevating the head within the maternal pelvis. (Figure from Safe Obstetric Systems, reproduced with permission)

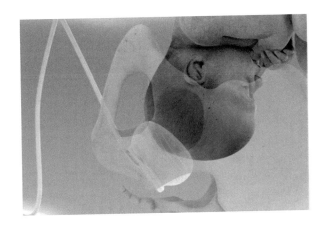

Cervical Length Screening

Women at high risk of preterm birth are typically offered cervical length assessment by transvaginal ultrasound in the second trimester. The exact timing and frequency of these assessments is not standardised. There is an established link between a short cervical length and subsequent preterm birth, with cervical length of less than 25mm in the second trimester being associated with an increased risk of preterm birth before 35 weeks [13]. The temporal relationship between the shortened cervix and subsequent delivery is not, however, reliably predictable.

Cervical Cerclage

The purpose of assessment of cervical length in women at high risk of preterm birth is clearly to identify those in whom intervention can be offered to reduce the risk of preterm birth. The concept of the 'incompetent' cervix has now been refined and replaced with a model of a preterm parturition 'syndrome'; with interaction between cervical function, vaginal flora, and the maternal immune system and inflammatory response [14]. Hence, the previous commonly used intervention of cervical cerclage has been challenged. Cervical cerclage is an intervention that has been widely used with a limited evidence base. The only previous randomised trial of cerclage carried out over 30 years ago indicated that its use conferred a reduction in risk of preterm birth before 33 weeks from 18 to 13% [15].

Further studies since then support a reduction in preterm birth risk for cerclage insertion in high risk women [16]. Cerclage insertion is now commonly used either as an elective procedure in women with multiple previous early preterm births, as an ultrasound-indicated procedure due to shortened cervix on scan, or as a 'rescue' procedure in women with a dilated cervix.

Vaginal Progesterone

It is, however, now clear that alternative interventions may have similar efficacy to cerclage in the prevention of preterm birth in the high risk population, most notably progesterone treatment and the use of the Arabin pessary. Progesterone has been used to reduce the risk of preterm birth in high risk women since 2003 [17, 18], particularly women with a short cervix on scan [19]. However, its use is controversial and clinical trials have given conflicting results regarding the benefit conferred. The largest, most recent UK trial suggested that it is of no benefit [20], although meta-analysis that includes this trial still favours proges- terone use [21]. Internationally, guidelines differ, with advice from the American College of Obstetrics and Gynecology that states 'a woman with a singleton gestation and a prior spontaneous preterm singleton birth should be offered pro- gesterone supplementation starting at 16–24 weeks of gestation, regardless of transvaginal ultrasound cervical length, to reduce the risk of recurrent spontane- ous preterm birth' [22] and UK advice which recommends it only in selected women with a cervix length of less than 25 mm [23]. It is commonly used as an alternative to cervical cerclage in women with a short cervix. A number of stud- ies are now trying to compare the efficacy of progesterone with cervical cerclage and the Arabin pessary in order to identify the best treatment option [24]. The Arabin pessary is more commonly used in Europe and has the advantage of being inserted and removed in the outpatient setting without the need for anaesthesia (see Fig. 1.2).

Abnormal vaginal flora, as indicated by a diagnosis of bacterial vaginosis especially in the first half of pregnancy, is recognised to have an association with preterm birth [25]. The role of routine screening and treatment with antibiotics remains controversial [26] and there is wide variation in the assessment and treatment of abnormal vaginal flora in the setting of the prematurity antenatal clinic [27].

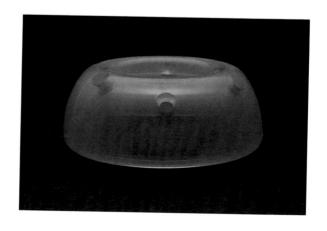

Fig. 1.2 The Arabin pessary is a flexible silicone ring that sits within the vagina and supports the cervix. (Figure supplied by Dr. Birgit Arabin, reproduced with permission)

Preterm Birth: Intrapartum Care

The intrapartum management of preterm labour is focused on optimising the condition of the preterm neonate. Whilst tocolysis is an attractive option, there is no evidence that it reduces the chance of preterm birth [28, 29]. Instead the aim is to delay the inevitable preterm birth by a few days to permit interventions that may benefit the baby. There is limited evidence that this strategy improves neonatal outcome; however that may be due to the age and limitations of the trials that have been carried out. All trials of tocolysis have limited power to demonstrate any benefit to the baby, as the majority of women presenting with threatened preterm labour will deliver at term irrespective of interventions undertaken. Tocolytics in current UK use include the oxytocin receptor antagonist atosiban, and nifedipine [23]. They should only be used where there is no evidence of fetal or maternal compromise, and where delay in delivery may be of benefit to the baby. Commonly this time delay would be used for administration of corticosteroids, magnesium sulfate, and for consideration of transfer to a tertiary unit if needed.

Corticosteroid administration prior to preterm deliveries is now routine practice to reduce risk of respiratory distress and its consequences. However maximal benefit is conferred if delivery is within a week of administration. If there is a significant time delay before preterm birth, then the risks of repeated course of steroids needs to be weighed up against the potential benefit. Current guidance is not to routinely give a second course of steroids but to consider it on an individual patient basis if there has been a significant time interval since the original course [23]. This is a horizon for future research.

Magnesium Sulfate

Intrapartum magnesium sulfate administration improves neurodevelopmental outcome in preterm infants [30] but the timing, as with steroids, can be difficult to optimise. Consensus is that administration should occur within 24 h of delivery and it should therefore be given to those women diagnosed as being in established preterm labour, or those in whom prelabour delivery is planned within 24 h. Although different regimes have been used in clinical trials, it appears that its administration confers approximately 30% reduction in risk of cerebral palsy in the surviving preterm baby [30, 31]. In the UK, administration is recommended prior to all births at less than 30 weeks of gestation, and consideration of administration up to 34 weeks [23].

Threshold of Viability

The greatest challenges for both the obstetric and neonatal teams are in dealing with babies born at the threshold of viability (22–25 weeks). Active resuscitation is attempted for 84% of those born between 23 + 0 and 23 + 6 weeks of gestation [32].

When in labour at the limits of viability fetal monitoring is challenging. Continuous cardiotocogram (CTG) may be technically impossible and cannot be interpreted using the same criteria used at term. A frank discussion, including the neonatal team, is required with women at high risk of delivering at the limits of viability. This discussion should include information on likely neonatal outcomes, and the limitation of monitoring and intervention. There is no evidence that delivery by Caesarean section at this gestation will improve the fetal/neonatal survival, but it may impact significantly on maternal morbidity in both the current and future pregnancies. It should then be questioned that if intervention is not to be carried out, there may be no value in monitoring of the fetal heartbeat continuously or even intermittently.

However the potential consequence of an intrapartum fetal death should be explained and discussed explicitly. This decision making should be individualised and cannot be standardised by a guideline [33].

Non-cephalic Presentation

In spontaneous preterm labour there is a higher incidence of breech presentation compared to at term, making decision making more difficult. A recent large systematic review has shown Caesarean section reduced severe intraventricular haemorrhage by 41% and death by 49% in the extreme preterm breech. The study was limited to those actively resuscitated and born at less than 28 weeks of gestation and the advantages were more apparent at earlier gestations [34]. The EPIPAGE-2 study looked at preterm breech births from 26 to 34 weeks of gestation and showed no improved outcomes, including survival without associated morbidity, by delivering by Caesarean section [35]. Unfortunately, at earlier gestations there is an increased risk of the need for upper segment Caesarean section which comes with higher maternal morbidity for this and subsequent pregnancies. This includes increased rates of post-partum haemorrhage, need for caesarean hysterectomy and greater risk of uterine scar dehiscence in future pregnancies [36].

Group B Streptococcus

Management of any preterm labour should also include consideration of antibiotic administration. Infection is a major underlying aetiology of preterm labour, especially at extreme preterm gestations. The ORACLE trial suggested that routine administration of broad spectrum antibiotics in preterm labour with intact membranes did not improve neonatal outcomes [37]. In the UK there is now a recommendation to give antibiotics for prophylaxis against Group B Streptococcus (GBS) to all women in established preterm labour, as the sequelae of GBS infection are more severe in the preterm neonate [38].

Stillbirth Prevention and Fetal Growth Surveillance

There are many new obstetric initiatives aiming to reduce rates of stillbirth. This has been highlighted as a major international priority. Reducing stillbirths will ultimately involve increasing iatrogenic preterm delivery and must be supported by the neonatal facilities to deal with this consequence.

International: 'Ending Preventable Stillbirth'

The Lancet 'Ending Preventable Stillbirth' series in 2016, highlighted the annual estimated stillbirth incidence of 2.6 million and noted that half of these occur during labour and birth [39]. Ninety percent of stillbirths occur in countries with lower incomes; they can often be associated with maternal infection, notably syphilis and malaria, and poor access to care. With appropriate resources and recognition many of these stillbirths can be prevented. The availability of worldwide stillbirth data has increased significantly. Sixty-eight countries had no available data in 2009 and this has dropped to 38 countries in 2015. It is noted that global leadership and responsibility is key to improving outcomes. The United Nations inter-agency group for Child Mortality Estimation has now taken overall responsibility for reporting rates and it is hoped this will improve data available for assessment. The Every Newborn Action Plan aims to reduce stillbirth in all countries, to less than 12 per 1000 births by 2030 [39]. Considering the international impact of stillbirth, it is proportionally underfunded.

The Lancet review recommends cohesive care, starting prenatally with health optimisation and access to contraception. Access to antenatal care, with adequate infection recognition and treatment and fetal surveillance, is required. Intrapartum care should include fetal monitoring and access to obstetric intervention if needed. It also recommends the de-stigmatisation of stillbirth with worldwide education and postnatal support for those affected. The burden is both psychological and financial, with many families struggling to return to work after such a traumatising event. Clearly the above ideology is sound, but implementing internationally in countries with poor resources and conflict or natural disaster will be complex.

It is important to recognise the shift may see stillbirth rates drop but an increase in neonatal deaths if neonatal support in a country is inadequate to deal with neonates with complications.

UK: Saving Babies' Lives

The above recommendations are already being implemented in most developed countries.

In the UK the 'Saving Babies Lives' care bundle, launched in 2016, and updated in 2019, aims to halve stillbirths by 2025. The care bundle includes improving smoking cessation, risk assessment and surveillance for fetal growth restriction, raising awareness of reduced fetal movements and effective fetal monitoring during labour [40]. In high income countries the stillbirth is often antenatal rather than intrapartum and may be associated with modifiable lifestyle factors such as obesity and smoking [41]. Smoking cessation can be improved with routine carbon monoxide (CO) testing at booking and cessation education given. Initial evaluation of the Saving Babies Lives care bundle has demonstrated good uptake of the themes outlined. CO testing was almost universally undertaken, and an increased proportion of small-for-gestational-age babies was identified antenatally (up from 33.8% to 53.7%). The stillbirth rates in the earlier adopter trusts fell by 20% [42].

Each Baby Counts

Running in parallel with 'Saving Babies Lives', 'Each Baby Counts' is a 5-year programme launched by the Royal College of Obstetricians and Gynaecologists in 2015 to reduce the rate of term intrapartum related stillbirths, neonatal deaths and brain injuries. It collects data and implements local reviews on all term intrapartum stillbirths, hypoxic ischaemic encephalopathy grade 3 and neonatal deaths, reviewing whether the event was avoidable and assesses the quality of the local review undertaken.

Obstetrics needs to strive to achieve safety levels that other industries such as aviation accomplish. Human factors training, popular in the aeronautical industry, is being implemented in many hospitals to improve situational awareness and reduce serious incidents [43, 44].

Fetal Growth Restriction

'Saving babies lives' highlights the need to monitor fetal growth as fetal growth restriction (FGR) is a major risk factor for stillbirth [44, 45]. Careful assessment of risk factors for FGR should be undertaken at booking for antenatal care (Fig. 1.3).

Women who are assessed to have no risk factors can then have growth surveillance with midwifery symphysis-fundal height assessments from 26 to 28 weeks of pregnancy, with growth scans only carried out if triggered by abnormal measurements or growth velocity. If major risk factors for FGR are identified at booking, then serial ultrasound growth assessments from either 28 weeks (if abnormal uterine artery Doppler) or 32 weeks are recommended [54].

If multiple minor risk factors are identified then the Royal College of Obstetricians and Gynaecologists currently recommend uterine artery Dopplers at the 20 week anomaly scan, with serial growth scans if these are abnormal. Clearly,

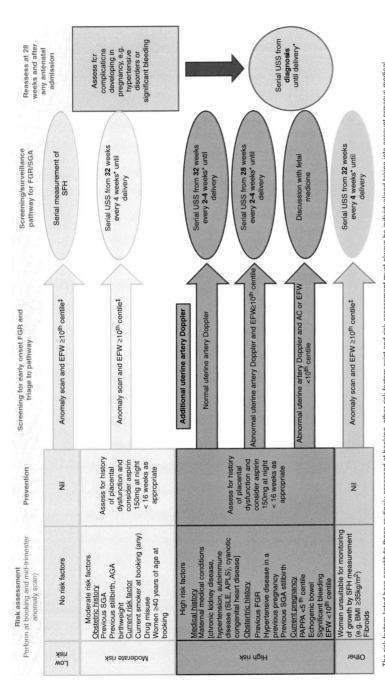

Fig. 1.3 Saving Babies Lives Version 2 suggests this algorithm to stratify the type of fetal growth assessment used in singleton pregnancy. (From Saving Babies Lives Version 2, with permission [54])

this is dependent on risk factors being identified at booking and being reassessed at each contact with a healthcare professional.

Customised Growth Charts

There is a division of opinion, especially in the UK, regarding which growth charts should be used. Currently, the charts favoured by many UK hospitals are Gestational Related Optimum Weight (GROW) charts, which are also being used internationally [46]. They offer a customised chart showing the tenth and 90th centiles for a given woman, based on her height, weight, parity and ethnicity. An alternative system used is INTERGROWTH 21st (IG21) which uses a universal standard created from an apparent multi-ethnic population and is based on the premise that fetal growth should not differ by ethnicity in a well-nourished population [47]. Studies comparing both INTERGROWTH 21st and GROW have shown neither to be a perfect solution but IG21 highlighted 20% of babies were large for gestational age babies and only 4.4% SGA and this could be due to it being based on a much smaller cohort of countries.

GROW is based on a much larger multi-ethnic population and picks up more SGA babies and this cohort had a higher stillbirth rate. Those not picked up by IG21 as SGA still had a relative risk of stillbirth of 1.9 (95% CI 1.6–2.2). The highest relative risk for stillbirth (3.5; 95% CI, 3.1–4.1) was observed for babies identified as SGA by both IG21 and GROW although using both methods is clearly impractical [48].

Fetal Dopplers

Fetal growth scans are used to estimate fetal weight and undertake Doppler studies. The umbilical artery Dopplers are looked at in combination with fetal growth.

Early Onset, Small for Gestational Age

Early onset, severe small-for-gestational-age (SGA) fetuses need very careful assessment including fetal medicine review, with possible genetic investigation such as karyotyping and microarray analysis if available.

Infection screening for toxoplasmosis and cytomegalovirus is also required for this group, and for some high risk populations testing for maternal malaria and syphilis are performed.

Prior to 32 weeks, if the umbilical artery Dopplers demonstrate an increased pulsatility index (PI) or resistive index (RI), then increased surveillance is appropriate. If end diastolic umbilical artery blood flow is absent or reversed, then the ductus venosus wave form is analysed. Decisions about delivery in the early onset SGA baby should be made after careful joint counselling with the neonatal team, and the prognosis offered should take into account not only gestation, but the estimated fetal weight. It would be unusual to offer delivery with an estimated fetal weight of less than 500 g, due to the very poor prognosis.

Antenatal corticosteroids should be considered when preterm delivery appears likely, and magnesium sulfate should be administered once the decision for delivery is made.

Late Onset SGA

Later onset SGA is more likely to be due to placental dysfunction. In the UK, NICE recommends use of aspirin to be commenced prior to 16 weeks of gestation for those at risk of pre-eclampsia to reduce risk of pre-eclampsia and improve SGA incidence in this cohort [49]. In addition to umbilical artery Doppler studies, in the third trimester, the middle cerebral artery (MCA) Doppler study can be undertaken to look for redistribution and cerebral sparing secondary to hypoxia. A reduced MCA PI of below 5% would suggest an increased cerebral blood flow and in combination with increased umbilical PI would be a sign of growth restriction. The cerebro-placental ratio less than 1 has been shown to be a predictor of stillbirth and of need for emergent intrapartum delivery following CTG concerns [50, 51].

Dawes Redman CTG

Abnormal growth and Dopplers at earlier preterm gestations can necessitate inpatient stays and frequent Doppler assessments until delivery. The midwife can use the Dawes Redman CTG to provide additional information in-between ultrasound Doppler assessments. Dawes Redman CTGs electronically assess non-labouring fetuses [52]. This computerised model has learned from a bank of 100,000 CTGs and can more quickly conclude the CTG as being normal ('meeting the Dawes Redman criteria'). It is important to also incorporate clinical history and ongoing concerns when deciding to take off and stop the electronic CTG. The output it creates is complex and can be poorly understood by all labour ward staff, if criteria is not met at 60 min. However, if used correctly it can function to pick up potentially hypoxic babies that could be missed with conventional CTG and visual human interpretation.

Impact on Neonates

Increasing fetal surveillance techniques and timed use of corticosteroids has allowed the obstetrician to opt to deliver to try to avoid stillbirth and has also improved neonatal morbidity and mortality within the iatrogenic preterm birth group. Subsequently, iatrogenic preterm birth has increased over recent years.

A large population review in the USA showed an increase in iatrogenic preterm birth from 2.2 in 1995 to 3.7 per 100 live births in 2005 (odds ratio = 1.77, 95%CI:1.76–1.79), whereas spontaneous preterm rates are fairly stable [53].

Ultimately, regardless of the choice of pathway followed, the ultrasonography resource requirement to improve detection of the SGA baby and reduce stillbirth risk will be significantly increased. They will also need to postnatally review any false negatives and false positives created by their programme and adapt to improve accuracy. Those that have been shown as falsely SGA by these methods may have been subjected to unnecessary intervention whether that be induction or Caesarean. Those that are not correctly identified as SGA will not have been induced or delivered in a timely manner and will therefore inadvertently been subjected to an increased risk of stillbirth.

Conclusion

The care of the preterm infant has improved dramatically, due to advances in both obstetric and neonatal management. The identification of those at high risk of preterm birth needs more research, to enable treatments such as pessaries, cerclage or progesterone to be targeted. When preterm birth is threatened or occurring, obstetric antenatal care can include interventions to improve lung maturation, neurodevelopment and to reduce risk of neonatal sepsis. This aims to reduce neonatal admissions and long term follow up.

The increased international drive to reduce stillbirth will identify more small-for-gestational-age babies, which are likely to require iatrogenic preterm delivery. This may cause additional strain on neonatal services but with the reduction in stillbirth and its devastating sequelae for the families, this may be a small price to pay.

References

1. Saigal S, Doyle L. Preterm birth 3. An overview of mortality and sequelae of preterm birth from infancy to adulthood. Lancet. 2008;371:261–9.
2. Goldenberg R, Culhane J, Iams J, Romero R. Preterm birth 1. Epidemiology and causes of preterm birth. Lancet. 2008;371:75–84.
3. Haines N. Office of national statistics. Birth summary tables England and Wales 2016. Updated 2016. https://www.ons.gov.uk/peoplepopulationandcommunity/birthsdeathsandmarriages/livebirths/bulletins/birthsummarytablesenglandandwales/2017. Accessed 19 Oct 2019.

4. Iams J, Romero R, Culhane J, Goldenberg R. Preterm birth 2. Primary, secondary and tertiary interventions to reduce the morbidity and mortality of preterm birth. Lancet. 2008;371:164–75.
5. Sharp N, Alfivirec Z. Provision and practice of specialist preterm labour clinics: a UK survey of practice. BJOG. 2014;121:417–21.
6. Berghella V, Gimovsky A, Levine L, Vink J. Cesarean in the second stage: a possible risk factor for subsequent spontaneous preterm birth. Am J Obstet Gynecol. 2017;217:1–3.
7. Watson H, Carter J, David A, Seed P, Shennan A. Full dilatation caesarean section: a risk factor for recurrent second-trimester loss and preterm birth. Acta Obstet Gynecol Scand. 2017;96:1100–5.
8. Wood S, Tang S, Crawford S. Cesarean delivery in the second stage of labor and the risk of subsequent premature birth. Am J Obstet Gynecol. 2017;217(63):e1–10.
9. Cong A, De Vries B, Ludlow J. Does previous caesarean section at full dilatation increase the likelihood of subsequent spontaneous preterm birth? Aust N Z J Obstet Gynaecol. 2018;58:267–73.
10. Nott J, Pervolaraki E, Benson A, et al. Diffusion tension imaging determines three-dimensional architecture of human cervix: a cross-sectional study. BJOG. 2018;125:812–8.
11. Corry E, Ramphul M, Rowan A, Segurado R, Mahony R, Keane D. Exploring full cervical dilatation caesarean sections—a retrospective cohort study. Eur J Obstet Gynecol Reprod Biol. 2018;224:188–91.
12. Seal S, Dey A, Barman S, Kamilya G, Mukherji J, Onwude J. Randomized controlled trial of elevation of the fetal head with a fetal pillow during caesarean delivery at full cervical dilatation. Int J Gynaecol Obstet. 2016;133:178–82.
13. Crane J. Use of transvaginal ultrasonography to predict preterm birth in women with a history of preterm birth. Ultrasound Obstet Gynecol. 2008;32(5):640–5.
14. Gotsch F, Romero R, Erez O. The preterm parturition syndrome and its implications for understanding the biology, risk assessment, diagnosis, treatment and prevention of preterm birth. J Matern Fetal Neonatal Med. 2009;22:5–23.
15. MRC/RCOG Working Party on Cervical Cerclage. Interim report of the medical research council/royal college of obstetricians and gynaecologists multicentre randomized trial of cervical cerclage. Br J Obstet Gynaecol. 1988;95:437–45.
16. Alfirevic Z, Stampalia T, Medley N. Cervical stitch (cerclage) for preventing preterm birth in singleton pregnancy. Cochrane Database Syst Rev. 2017;6:CD008991. https://doi.org/10.1002/14651858.CD008991.pub3.
17. Meis P, Klebanoff M, Thom E. Prevention of recurrent preterm delivery by 17 alpha-hydroxyprogesterone caproate. N Engl J Med. 2003;348:2379–85.
18. Da Fonseca E, Bittar R, Carvalho M, Zugaib M. Prophylactic administration of progesterone by vaginal suppository to reduce the incidence of spontaneous preterm birth in women at increased risk: a randomized placebo-controlled double-blind study. Am J Obstet Gynecol. 2003;188:419–24.
19. Fonseca E, Celik E, Parra M, Singh M, Nicolaides K. Progesterone and the risk of preterm birth among women with a short cervix. N Engl J Med. 2007;357:462–9.
20. Norman J, Marlow N, Messow C, Shennan A, Bennett P, Thornton S. Vaginal progesterone prophylaxis for preterm birth (the OPPTIMUM study): a multicentre, randomised, double-blind trial. Lancet. 2016;387(10033):2106–16.
21. Romero R, Nicolaides K, Conde-Agudelo A. Vaginal progesterone decreases preterm birth ≤34 weeks of gestation in women with a singleton pregnancy and a short cervix: an updated meta-analysis including data from the OPPTIMUM study. Ultrasound Obstet Gynecol. 2016;48:308–17.
22. ACOG. Prediction and prevention of preterm birth. Practice bulletin 130. Obstet Gynecol. 2012;120:964–73.
23. National Institute for Health and Care Excellence. Preterm labour and birth. NICE guideline NG25. Updated 2015. https://www.nice.org.uk/guidance/ng25.
24. Hezelgrave N, Watson H, Ridout A. Rationale and design of SuPPoRT: a multi-centre randomised controlled trial to compare three treatments: cervical cerclage, cervical pessary and

vaginal progesterone, for the prevention of preterm birth in women who develop a short cervix. BMC Pregnancy Childbirth. 2016;16:358.

25. Hay P, Lamont R, Taylor-Robinson D, Morgan D, Ison C, Pearson J. Abnormal colonisation of the genital tract and subsequent preterm delivery and late miscarriage. BMJ. 1994;308:295–8.

26. Haahr T, Ersboll A, Karlsen M. Treatment of bacterial vaginosis in pregnancy in order to reduce the risk of spontaneous preterm delivery—a clinical recommendation. Acta Obstet Gynecol Scand. 2016;95:850–60.

27. Brocklehurst P, Jordon A, Heatley E, Milan S. Antibiotics for treating bacterial vaginosis in pregnancy. Cochrane Database Syst Rev. 2013;(1):CD000262.

28. Gyetvai K, Hannah M, Hodnett E, Ohisson A. Tocolytics for preterm labour: a systematic review. Obstet Gynacol. 1999;94(869):877.

29. Flenady V, Reinebrant H, Liley H, Tambimuttu E, Papatosonis-Dimitri N. Oxytocin receptor antagonists for inhibiting preterm birth. Cochrane Database Syst Rev. 2014;(7):CD006169.

30. Peebles D, Kenyon A. Magneisum sulphate to prevent cerebral palsy following preterm birth. Scientific impact paper 29. Magnesium sulphate to prevent cerebral palsy following preterm birth scientific impact paper no. 29. RCOG. 2011.

31. Rouse D, Hirtz D, Thom E, Varner M, Spong C, Mercer B. A randomized, controlled trial of magnesium sulfate for the prevention of cerebral palsy. N Engl J Med. 2008;359:895–905.

32. Costeloe K, Hennessy E, Haide S, Stacey F, Marlow N, Draper E. Short term outcomes after extreme preterm birth in england: comparison of two birth cohorts in 1995 and 2006 (the EPICURE studies). BMJ. 2012;345:7976.

33. David A, Soe A. Extreme prematurity and perinatal management. Obstetr Gynaecol. 2018;20(109):117.

34. Grabovac M, Karim J, Isayama T, Liyanage S, McDonald S. What is the safest mode of birth for extremely preterm breech singleton infants who are actively resuscitated? A systematic review. BJOG. 2018;125(6):652–63.

35. Lorth E, Sentilhes M, Quere M, et al. Planned delivery route of preterm breech singletons and neonatal and 2-year outcomes: a population-based cohort study. BJOG. 2019;126:73–82. https://doi.org/10.1111/1471-0528.15466.

36. Greene R, Fitzpatrick C, Turner M. What are the maternal implications of a classical caesarean section? J Obstet Gynaecol. 1998;18:345–7.

37. Kenyon S, Taylor D, Tarnow-Mordi W. Broad-spectrum antibiotics for spontaneous preterm labour: the ORACLE II randomised trial. ORACLE collaborative group. Lancet. 2001;357(9261):989–94.

38. Royal College of Obstetricians and Gynaecologists. Prevention of early-onset neonatal group B streptococcal disease. BJOG. 2017;124(12):e280–305.

39. De Bernis L, Kinney M, Stones W. The lancet ending preventable stillbirths series study group with the lancet ending preventable stillbirths series advisory group. stillbirths: Ending preventable deaths by 2030. Lancet. 2016;387:703–16.

40. O'Connor D. Saving babies lives. A care bundle for reducing stillbirths. NHS England 26th. Updated 2016. https://www.england.nhs.uk/wp-content/uploads/2016/03/saving-babies-lives-car-bundl.pdf. Accessed 19 Oct 2018.

41. Flenady V, Wojcieszek A, Middleton P. The lancet ending preventable stillbirths study group and the lancet stillbirths in high income countries investigator group. Stillbirths: recall to action in high-income countries. Lancet. 2016;387:691–702.

42. Widdows K, Roberts S, Camacho E, Heazell A. Saving babies' lives project impact and results evaluation (SPiRE): a mixed methodology study. BMC Pregnancy Childbirth. 2018;30(1):43.

43. Jackson K, Hayes K, Hinshaw K. The relevance of non-technical skills in obstetrics and gynaecology. Obstetr Gynaecol. 2013;15(4):269–74.

44. National Quality Board. Never? Appendix 2, Department of Health Human Factors Reference Group interim report. Updated 2012. http://www.england.nhs.uk/wp-content/uploads/2013/11/DH-2.pdf. Accessed 30 Jul 2018.

45. Gardosi J, Madurasinghe V, Williams M, Malik A, Francis F. Maternal and fetal risk factors for stillbirth: population based study. http://www.bmj.com/content/346/bmj.f108.
46. Gardosi J, Francis A, Turner S, Williams M. Customized growth charts: rationale, validation and clinical benefits. Am J Obstet Gynecol. 2018;218:S609–18.
47. Papageorghiou A, Ohuma E, Altman D. International standards for fetal growth based on serial ultrasound measurements: the fetal growth longitudinal study of the INTERGROWTH-21st project. Lancet. 2014;384:869–79.
48. Francis A. Customized vs INTERGROWTH-21st standards for the assessment of birthweight and stillbirth risk at term. Am J Obstet Gynecol. 2018;218(2):S692–9.
49. NICE. Hypertension in pregnancy guideline. https://www.nice.org.uk/guidance/cg107/resources/hypertension-in-pregnancy-diagnosis-and-management-pdf-35109334011877. Accessed 19 Oct 2018.
50. DeVore G. The importance of the cerebroplacental ratio in the evaluation of fetal well-being in SGA and AGA fetuses. Am J Obstet Gynecol. 2015;213(1):5–15.
51. Khalil A, Morales-Roselló J, Townsend R, et al. Value of third-trimester cerebroplacental ratio and uterine artery doppler indices as predictors of stillbirth and perinatal loss. Ultrasound Obstet Gynecol. 2016;47(1):74–80.
52. Dawes G, Lobb M, Moulden M, Redman C, Wheeler T. Antenatal cardiotocogram quality and interpretation using computers. BJOG. 1992;99:791–7.
53. Lisonkova S, Hutcheon J, Joseph K, et al. BMC Pregnancy Childbirth. 2011;11:39. https://doi.org/10.1186/1471-2393-11-39.
54. NHS England. Saving Babies Lives Version 2. A care bundle for reducing perinatal mortality. Updated 2019. https://www.england.nhs.uk/wp-content/uploads/2019/05/saving-babies-lives-care-bundle-version-two.pdf. Accessed 26 Jun 2019.

Chapter 2
Maternal Chronic Conditions and the Fetus

Kate Jones, Abigail Anness, and Farah Siddiqui

Pre-conception Care

Pre-conception care (PCC) is the provision of interventions to women prior to conception. It aims to improve their health status and change behaviours that contribute towards poor maternal and child outcomes [1]. PCC provides the opportunity to review a woman's disease status, change medication regimes to avoid teratogens and perform baseline investigations (for example, retinopathy and renal function screening for those with diabetes). Women with suboptimal disease control may be advised to defer pregnancy until their disease has been stabilised in order to lower the risk of adverse maternal or fetal outcomes. Women at a higher risk of neural tube defects will be advised to take 5 mg (rather than the standard 400 µg supplement) of folic acid daily. The pre-conception counselling should also include a frank discussion regarding a healthy diet, target body mass index and smoking cessation.

Pre-conception care is associated with decreased rates of congenital malformations [2] in women with epilepsy and pre-existing diabetes. It is also associated with improved glycaemic control in the first trimester and decreased perinatal mortality in women with pre-existing diabetes [2]. Ideally PCC should be provided to all women with chronic medical conditions.

Epilepsy

Annually there are approximately 2500 pregnancies in the UK in women with epilepsy [3]. Most pregnancies have a good outcome; however epilepsy had the highest maternal mortality rate for any medical condition in the 2015 Mothers and Babies;

K. Jones · A. Anness · F. Siddiqui (✉)
Department of Fetal and Maternal Medicine, Leicester Royal Infirmary,
University Hospitals of Leicester NHS Trust, Leicester, UK
e-mail: farah.siddiqui@uhl-tr.nhs.uk

© Springer Nature Switzerland AG 2020
E. M. Boyle, J. Cusack (eds.), *Emerging Topics and Controversies in Neonatology*, https://doi.org/10.1007/978-3-030-28829-7_2

Reducing Risk through Audits and Confidential Enquiries across the UK (MBRRACE-UK) report [3, 4] so it is important that these patients are carefully managed in the multidisciplinary clinic.

Preconception Advice

Pre-conception counselling aims to achieve seizure control with the lowest dose of antiepileptic drug (AED), avoiding polytherapy where possible. Women with epilepsy should take 5 mg of folic acid pre-conceptually and throughout the pregnancy to reduce the risk of neural tube defects and long-term cognitive deficits [5].

Maternal and Fetal Implications

Antenatal care seeks to achieve seizure control whilst minimising the potential teratogenic effects of AEDs. Seizures in pregnancy are associated with a risk of cerebral palsy and fetal death, and sudden unexpected death in epilepsy (SUDEP) is more common in poorly controlled disease [5]. The physiological increase in plasma volume associated with pregnancy can alter serum AED levels so dose adjustments may be required during pregnancy. AEDs are associated with an increased risk of congenital malformations (mainly cardiac defects, facial clefts and neural tube defects) and cognitive deficits [4, 5]. This risk is dose dependent and increases with polytherapy [4]. Carbamzepine, lamotrigine, levetiracetam and phenytoin carry the lowest risks (1–5%). Sodium valproate carries the highest risk (6–10%) and its use in women of childbearing age is restricted by Medicines and Healthcare products Regulation Authority (MHRA) regulations whose guidance about Valproate use in pregnancy has recently been updated [6].

Delivery and Postnatal

Epilepsy is not usually an indication for induction of labour or Caesarean section. The risk of maternal seizures is greatest around the time of delivery and immediately post-partum. Seizures in labour should be treated promptly with intravenous or rectal medication, usually a benzodiazepine, as they may lead to fetal hypoxia or injury if a fall is sustained [5].

Babies born to women with epilepsy taking enzyme inducing AEDs should be offered 1 mg of intramuscular vitamin K to prevent haemorrhagic disease of the newborn [5]. Whilst this is offered to all infants in the UK, its importance for this group of patients should be emphasised. Most AEDs are secreted into breast milk but only low levels are absorbed by the neonate, so women should be encouraged to breast feed. There is a theoretical risk of withdrawal in the neonate if the mother is taking AEDs antenatally—breast feeding may reduce this risk due to the small doses in the milk [7]. Women with epilepsy and their families should be advised of safety measures such as sitting on the floor to feed, avoiding co-sleeping and not bathing the baby alone.

Cardiovascular Disease

Advances in surgical techniques for the management of congenital heart disease, mean that children with these conditions are increasingly surviving into adulthood, allowing them to have children of their own. The details and outcomes of congenital heart disease surgery in children are discussed elsewhere in this book; here we discuss the management of pregnancy in women with corrected congenital heart disease.

Preconception Advice

Cardiac disease is the leading cause of indirect maternal deaths, with a rate of 2.34 per 100,000 maternities [3]. Women with known complex cardiac disease of reproductive age should be offered contraception; those considering embarking on a pregnancy should be assessed in a pre-conception clinic. Pregnancy is relatively contraindicated in the presence of pulmonary hypertension (25–40% mortality rate [7]), severe aortic or mitral stenosis, cyanotic heart disease or in the presence of poor left ventricular function [8]. Women with cyanotic heart disease have an increased risk of congenital malformation, miscarriage, fetal death and fetal growth restriction [9].

Maternal and Fetal Implications

Antenatal care is usually based around symptom control, such as management of arrhythmias, or reduction in cardiac pre-load. Medications most commonly used in pregnancy for cardiac disorders include beta-blockers, flecainide and digoxin. Women taking warfarin pre-pregnancy will usually be changed to a low molecular weight heparin, with haematological advice. Beta-blockers can cross the placental barrier and may be associated with growth restriction, respiratory depression, neonatal bradycardia and hypoglycaemia [8, 10]. These effects are more pronounced if the drugs are commenced in the first trimester. Women with complex disease and those on medication should be offered serial ultrasound assessments of fetal growth and wellbeing. If a maternal arrhythmia is refractory to medical treatment or there is cardiogenic shock, electrical cardioversion may be required. Case reports suggest that electrical cardioversion should be considered safe in pregnancy; it should ideally be carried out with facilities available for continuous fetal monitoring and emergency caesarean although maternal health is the main consideration [11, 12]. Patients in cardiac failure may require extracorporeal membrane oxygenation (ECMO) which is discussed later in this chapter. Congenital cardiac conditions in either parent increase the risk of a fetal cardiac defect by 2–5% (background risk 1%), so a fetal echocardiogram may be offered.

Delivery and Postnatal

The timing, location and mode of delivery in a patient with cardiac disease will vary depending on the severity of the maternal condition and the resources in the booking hospital. Complex disorders, such as aortic root dilatation or a history of life-threatening arrhythmia, may require transfer to a specialist centre for delivery. Severe or deteriorating disease is likely to result in a preterm delivery, often by caesarean section. Where a vaginal birth is planned, shortening the second stage should be considered (for example by performing an instrumental delivery) and care with uterotonic medication such as ergometrine and syntocinon. Unless contra-indicated, epidural anaesthesia is often advised as it helps to maintain stability in blood pressure, but this is assessed on an individual basis by the multidisciplinary team.

Infants of women taking antenatal beta-blockers may require neonatal assessment for respiratory depression, bradycardia and hypoglycaemia [8, 10].

Hypertension

Hypertension in pregnancy may be pre-existing, pregnancy induced hypertension (PIH) or a component of pre-eclampsia (PET) [7]. Hypertension is the most common medical problem in pregnancy, affecting 10–15% of all pregnancies [7] and 8–10% of all preterm births result from hypertensive disorders [13]; PET is the most common cause of iatrogenic prematurity.

Preconception Advice

Pre-conception counselling should include an assessment of end organ damage, evaluation for secondary causes, weight loss if obese and optimisation of drug treatment.

Maternal and Fetal Implications

Women with hypertension require 75 mg aspirin from 12 weeks of gestation as prophylaxis for PET. In the UK, all pregnant women have their blood pressure measured and urine checked for protein at every antenatal visit in order to screen for PET. If detected they will undergo investigations to assess severity, including quantification of proteinuria, renal and liver function tests and platelet counts. They may require anti-hypertensive treatment, usually methyldopa, labetalol or nifedipine. Women with pre-existing hypertension or PET are at risk of fetal growth restriction and should have serial ultrasound scans for fetal growth. Severe pre-eclampsia carries maternal risks of eclampsia, intracranial haemorrhage, pulmonary oedema and placental abruption. It should be managed in a high-dependency setting—intravenous magnesium sulphate is used for maternal seizure prophylaxis.

Delivery and Postnatal

Delivery is the only cure for PET and in severe disease preterm delivery is often needed. Regional anaesthesia is encouraged unless there is thrombocytopenia with platelet counts less than $60–80 \times 10^9/l$[13].

Respiratory Disease

Asthma

Asthma affects up to 7% of women of reproductive age and is regularly encountered in pregnancy [7, 14].

Maternal and Fetal Implications

Women with mild asthma are unlikely to encounter problems but those with severe disease are at risk of deterioration of their asthma as well as an increased risk of fetal growth restriction and pre-eclampsia [14, 15]. These women should be offered fetal surveillance accordingly. Reducing or stopping medication is a common cause of symptom deterioration in pregnancy. Women should be encouraged to continue treatment and seek help promptly if unwell. In addition to common environmental triggers, maternal smoking, maternal obesity and antenatal exposure to respiratory viral infections are particularly significant risk factors for severe exacerbation of asthma [15]. Acute severe exacerbations should be treated aggressively using the stepwise approach of the British Thoracic Society/Scottish Intercollegiate Guidelines Network guidelines or equivalent that are also used in non-pregnant patients [16]. Close liaison with respiratory physicians can aid management strategies for women with complex or brittle asthma, particularly during the third trimester. Most medications used to treat asthma appear to be safe in pregnancy and during lactation [7, 14].

Tuberculosis

The UK national incidence of tuberculosis was 4.2 per 100,000 pregnancies in 2008 [17]. It is most prevalent in women of ethnic minorities.

Maternal and Fetal Implications

Pregnancy is not an independent risk factor for tuberculosis (TB) and does not affect the clinical course of the disease [18]. Effective treatment usually results in normal pregnancy outcomes but delayed diagnosis, ineffective treatment or disseminated disease increases the risk of pre-eclampsia, maternal respiratory failure, fetal growth restriction and preterm delivery [18]. Treatment regimens are similar to those used outside pregnancy, although streptomycin should be avoided as it can cause fetal ototoxicity [19]. A typical treatment regimen may last 6–12 months and include isoniazid, rifampicin and ethambutol together with pyridoxine to reduce the risk of isoniazid-induced neuropathy.

Postnatal

All drugs are considered to be safe for breast feeding. Neonates should be treated with prophylactic isoniazid for 3 months if the mother is sputum positive [7]. The Bacillus-Calmette-Guerin (BCG) vaccine is offered to neonates at risk of TB exposure (based on family history or geographical location) [20].

Congenital TB, caused by vertical transmission, is rare [18]. It may occur where there has been delayed diagnosis or ineffective treatment of maternal TB. Infants present with symptoms at 2 or 3 weeks of age.

Cystic Fibrosis

The improving survival rates of women with cystic fibrosis (CF) mean there are increasing numbers of pregnancies in this high-risk population.

Preconception Advice

CF is the most common autosomal recessive disorder in the United Kingdom. Pre-conception genetic counselling and partner screening should be offered to all women who are known to be carriers of a CF gene or who have a relative with CF. In cases where the partner is also carrier or unavailable for testing, the choice of a chorionic villus sampling or amniocentesis should be offered, as some women may choose to discontinue their pregnancy if the fetus is affected.

Maternal and Fetal Implications

Pregnancy outcomes are related to pre-pregnancy lung function and disease status, and many women will tolerate pregnancy well. Outcomes are worse in women with FEV1 less than 60% predicted and pregnancy is contraindicated in the presence of cor pulmonale or pulmonary hypertension [7, 21]. The mainstay of antenatal care is physiotherapy, nutritional support and aggressive treatment of pulmonary infections, as well as regular assessment of fetal growth [22]. Maternal complications may include weight loss, infective exacerbations, unpredictable loss of lung function and congestive cardiac failure. The most common pregnancy complications are prematurity (25% [21, 22]) and fetal growth restriction. Poor maternal weight gain is predictive of preterm delivery and stillbirth. There is also a risk of maternal gestational diabetes and its associated complications.

Gastro-Intestinal Disorders

Inflammatory Bowel Disease

Quiescent inflammatory bowel disease (IBD) is not associated with adverse pregnancy outcomes; however, active Crohn's disease or ulcerative colitis at the time of conception is associated with a higher risk of complications. These include miscarriage, stillbirth, preterm delivery and growth restriction [23, 24]. Children of parents with inflammatory bowel disease have an increased risk of developing IBD.

Maternal and Fetal Implications

Antenatal care focuses on maternal disease control. Azathioprine, sulphasalazine and mesalazine are safe in pregnancy and breast feeding. Sulphasalazine interferes with folate absorption, therefore women should take 5 mg of folic acid. Corticosteroids can be used to manage flares—transplacental passage of steroids does occur, but rapid metabolism by the fetus leads to low fetal blood concentration.

Long term use increases the risk of gestational diabetes and parenteral steroid cover may be required in labour. Biologic anti-TNF agents can be used in pregnancy but should be discontinued around 26–28 weeks of gestation to minimise neonatal risk of impaired immunity. There is no known association with birth defects or teratogenicity [7, 24]. Methotrexate and thalidomide are contra-indicated during pregnancy and should be discontinued at least 3–6 months prior to conception.

Maternal antenatal care also seeks to optimise maternal nutrition and avoid anaemia, as this is also a risk factor for preterm delivery and fetal growth restriction.

Delivery and Postnatal

The mode of delivery is usually determined by obstetric indication unless the woman has perianal disease or has an ileal pouch, in which case elective Caesarean section may be recommended. Caesarean section will be more complex in the presence of active disease or a history of extensive abdominal surgery and may require collaboration with bowel surgeons. Live vaccines should be avoided for the first 6 months of life in infants exposed to anti-TNF medication in utero because anti-TNF levels are detectable during the first 6 months of life [7, 24].

Obstetric Cholestasis

Obstetric cholestasis (OC) is a pregnancy-specific disorder, in which reduced flow within the maternal bile ducts cause leakage of bile acids into the blood stream, causing pruritis and/or deranged liver function in the mother.

Maternal and Fetal Implications

OC is associated with increased risks of spontaneous preterm labour, intrauterine passage of meconium and stillbirth [25, 26]. Stillbirth in OC occurs without placental insufficiency or growth restriction [27] and the mechanism is unknown. It is hypothesised that acute anoxia occurs due to bile acid deposition in the fetal heart causing an arrhythmia, or in the placenta causing acute vasoconstriction [27]. Fetuses born to mothers with bile acid levels greater than 40 μmol/L [25, 26] have previously been considered most at risk, although more recent evidence suggests that the risk is not significantly elevated until maternal bile acid levels are greater than 100 μmol/L [28].

In the United Kingdom guidance produced by the Royal College of Obstetrics and Gynaecology recommends the use of ursodeoxycholic acid (UDCA) to alleviate the symptoms of pruritis and reduce derangement of liver function in the mother, but it is uncertain whether UDCA offers any improvement in perinatal outcomes [29]. Five to 10 mg of vitamin K daily is recommended where maternal clotting function is deranged, although this is associated with a small increased risk of haemolytic anaemia, jaundice and kernicterus in the neonate [30].

Delivery and Postnatal

Current guidance suggests elective delivery of the fetus after 37 weeks of gestation to reduce the risk of stillbirth. However, this should be balanced against the increased risks of admission to the neonatal unit, particularly if delivery occurs by caesarean section [29]. The universal application of this guidance is becoming contentious, particularly for women with bile acid levels under 40, but delayed delivery has not yet been the subject of randomised controlled trials.

Chronic Renal Disease

Maternal and Fetal Implications

Chronic renal disease (CRD) is associated with increased rates of miscarriage, preterm delivery, fetal growth restriction and pre-eclampsia. The extent of the association appears to depend primarily on the severity of renal impairment at the start of pregnancy [31]. Those with mild CRD can generally expect a good pregnancy outcome, but the prognosis deteriorates with worsening renal function, as the Table 2.1 below shows.

Other predictors of adverse pregnancy outcomes are the aetiology of the renal disease, with active lupus nephritis and polyarteritis nodosum [32, 33] affecting pregnancy particularly severely, and the presence of hypertension and proteinuria at the onset of pregnancy.

All women with CRD should take aspirin from 12 weeks of gestation to reduce the risk of pre-eclampsia, and should have increased monitoring of their blood pressure. Fetal wellbeing should be monitored with serial growth scans [33].

Outcomes in pregnancy following renal transplantation also correlate to baseline renal function, proteinuria and hypertension. Most pregnancies result in a live birth, but the incidence of PET and fetal growth restriction is high [34]. Transplant recipients should defer pregnancy for at least a year after transplantation to allow stabilisation on their immunosuppressant regime [35]. Prednisolone, azathioprine, ciclosporin and tacrolimus are safe in pregnancy, but mycophenolate mofetil is teratogenic and should be avoided if possible [33].

Table 2.1 Incidence of pregnancy complications according to baseline renal function [7, 32]

	PET	FGR	Perinatal mortality
Creatinine <125 µmol/L (mild CRD) (%)	22	25	1
Severe CRD requiring dialysis (%)	75	>90	50

Delivery and Postnatal

Delivery is timed according to maternal renal function and fetal wellbeing but will be preterm in 30% of women with mild CRD, rising to more than 90% in women on dialysis [7, 32].

Connective Tissue Disorders

Systemic Lupus Erythematosus

Preconception Advice

Systemic lupus erythematosus (SLE) is associated with an increased risk of miscarriage, pre-eclampsia, preterm delivery, growth restriction and intrauterine fetal death [7, 36]. Active disease at the time of conception, the presence of antiphospholipid antibodies, lupus nephritis and hypertension are associated with worse pregnancy outcomes [36, 37]. Women with quiescent disease without these complications have pregnancy risks similar to the background rates in the general population. The risk of disease flare during pregnancy is up 60% [7].

Maternal and Fetal Implications

Antenatal management includes close observation of disease activity and surveillance for complications such as pre-eclampsia and fetal growth restriction. Anti-Ro/La antibodies are present in up to 30% of patients with SLE [7]. Women with these antibodies should be offered a fetal echocardiogram at 18–20 weeks of gestation because of the associated risk of congenital heart block [36] and the fetal heart rate should be auscultated every 2–4 weeks. Evidence of an arrhythmia will require referral to a fetal medicine centre for assessment. Corticosteroids can be continued although long term use increases the risk of gestational diabetes and parenteral steroid cover may be required in labour. Hydroxychloroquine and azathioprine can be continued through pregnancy [38]. Non-steroidal anti-inflammatory drugs can be used with caution during the second trimester but are associated with fetal renal complications and premature closure of the ductus arteriosus when used beyond 32 weeks of gestation [39]. Methotrexate, mycophenylate mofetil and cyclophosphamide should be discontinued at least 3–6 months prior to conception as they are teratogenic. Ciclosporin can be used with care.

Delivery and Postnatal

Transplacental passage of maternal autoantibodies can cause neonatal lupus syndrome, which may be characterised by cutaneous lesions, thrombocytopenia, neutropenia, elevated liver enzymes or congenital heart block (CHB). Infants of mothers with anti-Ro/La antibodies have a 5% risk of cutaneous lupus and 2–3% risk of CHB [7, 40]. The risk of neonatal lupus increases in subsequent pregnancies—16–20% with one previously affected child and up to 50% with two [7, 40]. Cutaneous lesions usually appear in the first 2 weeks of life and regress spontaneously by 6 months of age, as maternal antibodies are cleared from the infant circulation. Haematologic and hepatic abnormalities also resolve at this age. Cardiac complications do not resolve spontaneously. CHB carries a 15–30% mortality rate and most surviving infants require a pacemaker [7, 40]. It may be associated with cardiomyopathy, structural abnormality, myocarditis, pericardial effusion and heart failure. There have been trials of antenatal steroids and intravenous immunoglobulins to treat CHB but these have not yet shown benefit [40].

Rheumatoid Arthritis

Maternal and Fetal Implications

Up to 50% of women with rheumatoid arthritis (RA) experience symptom improvement during pregnancy, but 90% will suffer a postpartum flare [7, 37, 41]. Well controlled RA has no adverse effects on pregnancy, but severe disease is associated with growth restriction and preterm delivery. Women with RA should be screened for anti-Ro/La antibodies as infants of women with these antibodies are at risk of neonatal lupus (see SLE section). Management of RA involves analgesia and control of joint swelling and stiffness. Non-steroidal anti-inflammatory medications (NSAIDS) can be used with caution in the second trimester [39]. They should be avoided during early pregnancy as they can interfere with implantation, and they should be avoided after 32 weeks because of the risk of oligohydramnios and premature closure of the ductus arteriosus. Corticosteroids can be continued during pregnancy although long term use increases the risk of gestational diabetes and parenteral steroid cover may be required in labour. Azathioprine, sulfasalazine and hydroxychloroquine are safe in pregnancy and lactation. Biologic agents can be continued until 26–28 weeks of gestation, at which point they should be discontinued due to the risks of fetal immunosuppression. Methotrexate is contraindicated in pregnancy [38].

Antiphospholipid Syndrome

Antiphospholipid syndrome (APS) is strongly associated with adverse maternal and fetal outcomes but, with careful management, successful pregnancy outcomes can be achieved in more than 80% of patients [42]. Adverse pregnancy outcomes include recurrent early miscarriage, miscarriage/fetal death beyond 10 weeks of gestation or preterm delivery before 34 weeks of gestation due to severe PET (often early onset) or features of placental insufficiency, such as intrauterine growth restriction [7]. The risks of these complications vary according to maternal antibody status and disease severity.

Maternal and Fetal Implications

Women with APS require close antenatal monitoring, tailored to their disease history. Antenatal care aims to improve fetal outcomes and reduce the risk of maternal thrombosis and PET. Women will usually be offered aspirin to prevent pre-eclampsia and anti-thrombotic therapy, usually low molecular weight heparin (LMWH) [42]. Women with previous thromboembolic disease are at high risk of further events in pregnancy and will require higher doses of LMWH. They will need serial ultrasound scans for surveillance of fetal growth and wellbeing. Women with anti-Ro/La antibodies will also require fetal echocardiogram scanning (see discussion in SLE section). Transplacental transfer of antiphospholipid antibodies may result in neonatal APS, although this is rare [43].

Metabolic and Endocrine Disorders

Diabetes

Diabetes affects between 2 and 5% of pregnancies, making it the most common medical disorder encountered. The majority of these pregnancies are affected with gestational diabetes (87.5%). The remainder have pre-existing type 1 or type 2 diabetes [44].

Preconception Advice

Pre-existing diabetes confers a higher risk of fetal congenital abnormalities, directly related to glycaemic control at the time of conception and early pregnancy. In particular the fetus is at risk of neural tube defects and cardiac anomalies [7]. Fetal sacral agenesis is pathognomic of maternal diabetes, but is very rare. Women with pre-existing diabetes should therefore aim for a glycosylated haemoglobin (HbA1c) level of less than 48 mmol/L before falling pregnant and those with a level greater than 86 mmol/L should be advised against pregnancy as the risk of congenital abnormalities may be as high as 25% [45]. All pregnant women with pre-existing diabetes should be prescribed high dose (5 mg) folic acid from pre-conception to protect against neural tube defects [44].

Maternal and Fetal Implications

Women with pre-existing diabetes should be prescribed aspirin from 12 weeks of gestation for the prevention of pre-eclampsia. Both pre-existing and, to a lesser extent, gestational diabetes, are associated with increased perinatal mortality and morbidity. Since glucose can cross the placenta, maternal hyperglycaemia, in turn, causes hyperglycaemia, pancreatic beta-cell hyperplasia and hyperinsulinaemia in the fetus. This sequence of events causes fetal macrosomia (since insulin is an anabolic hormone), and polyhydramnios (due to fetal polyuria) [7]. Monitoring of fetal growth with serial ultrasound scans is recommended. After delivery, the neonate is at risk of hypoglycaemia, due to loss of the glucose supply from the maternal blood, as well as respiratory distress syndrome, polycythaemia and jaundice.

Pre-existing and gestational diabetes are both associated with sudden unexplained intrauterine stillbirth. The risk is increased in macrosomic fetuses, but in more than 50% of stillbirths the precise cause is unknown [46].

Since the risk of all complications is decreased (although not eliminated) with good glycaemic control, this is the focus of antenatal care. Metformin, glibenclamide and short and intermediate acting insulin analogues can be used safely in pregnancy. Those with pre-existing diabetes may be managed on insulin pumps [47].

Delivery and Postnatal

Delivery is aimed at 37 + 0 to 38 + 6 weeks of gestation in those with pre-existing diabetes, or gestational diabetes requiring medication, and at 40 + 6 weeks of gestation in diet controlled gestational diabetes. However, delivery may be offered at earlier, and even preterm gestations if there are any fetal or maternal complications. Decisions about mode of delivery will take into consideration the estimated fetal weight and other obstetric risk factors. Elective caesarean section is recommended if the estimated fetal weight is more than 4500 g due to an increased risk of shoulder dystocia during delivery of a macrosomic baby [44].

Endocrinology

Hyperthyroidism

Maternal and Fetal Implications

Undertreated hyperthyroidism is associated with increased rates of miscarriage, fetal growth restriction, preterm labour and increased perinatal mortality, so biochemical euthyroidism is therefore the aim of antenatal care. Carbimazole can be used in pregnancy, but in rare cases is associated with fetal aplasia cutis. Propylthiouracil (PTU) is therefore generally considered to be first line management in the first trimester of pregnancy but can be changed to carbimazole in the second trimester due to the small risk of maternal liver failure associate with PTU [48].

Fetal thyrotoxicosis due to transplacental passage of thyroid stimulating antibodies occurs in 1% of women with previous or current Graves disease, but is more common in those with uncontrolled disease in the third trimester [7]. It is associated with fetal tachycardia, growth restriction and a fetal goitre, which may restrict the flexion of the fetal head necessary to achieve vaginal delivery. Stillbirth occurs in up to 15% of cases [49]. High maternal antibody titres should prompt serial ultrasound surveillance for fetal heart rate, morphology and growth [48].

Hypothroidism

Maternal and Fetal Implications

The fetal thyroid becomes active at 12 weeks of gestation, and until this point, the fetus is dependent on the maternal supply of thyroxine. Undertreated hypothyroidism is associated with miscarriage, preterm delivery, fetal growth restriction, pre-eclampsia and stillbirth. There is increased risk of neurodevelopmental delay (independent of iodine deficiency) for the offspring [48]. Thyroid stimulating hormone (TSH) receptor–blocking antibodies can cross the placenta causing neonatal hypothyroidism, but this is very rare [50]. Management is with levothyroxine, as for a non-pregnant woman, with a TSH level less than 2.5 mU/L the target [48].

Pituitary Disease

Maternal and Fetal Implications

Hypopituitarism can cause subfertility. When pregnancy does occur, under-treated hypopituitarism is associated with miscarriage and stillbirth [51]. Acromegaly increases the risk of GDM and PIH [49], and may case fetal macrosomia [7]. Somatostatin analogues are not known to cause any fetal malformations, but there is a lack of safety data regarding their use in pregnancy. Diabetes insipidus is not known to have any significant fetal effects, but may occur in association with PET [52].

Prolactinomas do not cause and fetal complications [7]. Due to a lack of safety data, dopamine antagonists (DA) are usually stopped in pregnant women, except in cases of invasive macroprolactinomas or prolactinomas which increase in size during the pregnancy [53]. A theoretical risk of fetal cardiac valve fibrosis exists with cabergoline, but no studies have confirmed this association [49].

Postnatal Care

DAs are safe to use while breastfeeding, but may interfere with milk production [49], so that top-up formula feeds are required.

Adrenal Disease

Maternal and Fetal Implications

Cushing's disease is associated with increased rates of pre-term delivery, PET, GDM and perinatal mortality. High maternal cortisol levels can suppress fetal corticosteroid production, leading to neonatal adrenal insufficiency [7]. Live birth rates are improved if treatment is initiated prior to 20 weeks of gestation [54], but ketoconazole should be avoided in pregnancy as it is potentially teratogenic [49].

Well controlled Addison's disease has no fetal effects [7]. Adrenal antibodies do cross the placenta, but neonatal disease is rare [49]. Congenital adrenal hyperplasia (CAH) may cause subfertility, but where pregnancy does occur it is associated with PIH and GDM. If a CAH affected woman's partner is a carrier of CAH, there is a risk of virilisation of a female fetus. If the carrier status of the partner is known, this can be avoided by commencing steroid replacement therapy before 9 weeks of gestation. Non Invasive prenatal testing (NIPT) from 10 weeks can be used the extract fetal DNA from a maternal blood sample to identify the sex of the fetus, and if female, steroid replacement should be continued [49].

Both Conn's syndrome and phaeochromocytoma can cause hypertension in pregnancy, with associated risks of placental abruption and preterm delivery. Undiagnosed phaechromocytoma is associated with fetal death in 26% of cases [49].

Haematological Disorders

Thrombocytopenia

Maternal platelet disorders may cause abnormalities with fetal platelets. Five to ten percent of pregnant women may have thrombocytopenia at term, but most of these will have 'gestational' thrombocytopenia [7].

Maternal and Fetal Implications

Gestational thrombocytopenia has no adverse effects for the fetus, however it may be clinically indistinguishable from idiopathic thrombocytopenia (ITP), particularly if first detected on maternal bloods at booking. ITP can be associated with fetal thrombocytopenia due to transplacental passage of antiplatelet antibodies. The diagnosis of ITP may become more evident if maternal platelet levels drop below 80, or if there is a history of heavy bleeding pre-pregnancy (for example menorrhagia or with dental procedures).

Delivery and Postnatal

Most clinicians would assume there will be a degree of fetal thrombocytopenia in women with thrombocytopenia and plan delivery accordingly, with avoidance of fetal scalp electrodes, fetal blood sampling and ventouse delivery, as these carry a risk of fetal bleeding. A baby born to a mother with thrombocytopenia should have a cord blood sample obtained at delivery to determine full blood count. Vitamin K should be administered orally unless platelet levels are known. There is very low neonatal morbidity with current management in the UK [55].

Anaemia

Anaemia is commonly encountered in pregnant women and should be actively treated. The most common cause is iron deficiency, often caused by the dilutional effect of the physiological increase in plasma volume seen in pregnancy.

Maternal and Fetal Implications

Iron deficiency is associated with preterm delivery, low birth weight and placental abruption. It is also associated with increased maternal morbidity through infections, poor performance and cognitive disturbances and increased risk of postpartum haemorrhage [56].

Postnatal

There may be an increased risk of neonatal iron deficiency in the first 3 months of life [56].

Sickle Cell Disease

Preconception Advice

Sickle cell disease and the thalasseamias are disorders with autosomal recessive inheritance and, as such, women should be offered pre-conception genetic counselling and partner screening. In cases where the partner is a carrier or unavailable for testing, the option of chorionic villus sampling or amniocentesis should be offered, as some women may choose to discontinue their pregnancy if the fetus is affected.

Maternal and Fetal Implications

Women with sickle cell disease have an increased risk of disease complications during pregnancy and up to 50% of pregnancies in these patients will be complicated by a crisis [57]. There is a significantly increased perinatal mortality rate. There is an increased incidence of miscarriage, fetal growth restriction, preterm labour, pre-eclampsia, placental abruption, fetal distress and Caesarean section. Women also have an increased risk of infection [7].

Maternal Mental Health

Psychiatric illnesses may occur as pre-existing or de novo disorders. They are common, affecting around 1 in 4 pregnancies, and can have significant maternal consequences [58]. Between 2013 and 2015, 27% of maternal deaths occurring between 6 weeks and 1 year postpartum were due to suicide or other psychiatric causes [3].

Maternal and Fetal Implications

Mental illnesses themselves have no direct effect on the fetus, but some medications used to treat the disorders are associated with an increased risk of congenital abnormality or withdrawal symptoms in the neonate. However, given the serious implications and risk of mortality conveyed by poorly controlled disease, maternal mental wellbeing should remain the priority during the antenatal and postpartum periods. As such, no medication should be withdrawn abruptly or without the supervision of a medical professional, and the use of medications associated with fetal or neonatal effects are accepted if they are necessary to maintain the emotional wellbeing of the mother (Table 2.2).

Dermatological Disorders

Maternal and Fetal Implications

Most pre-existing skin diseases have no direct effect on the fetus, and can be managed as in a non-pregnant patient. Topical emollients and steroids, ultraviolet therapies, and immunologic agents such as ciclosporin and anti-TNFα therapies can all

Table 2.2 Fetal and neonatal effects of drugs used in the management of mental health disorders [59]

	Fetal effects?	Neonatal effects?	Fetal/neonatal management
Lithium	Possible increased risk of cardiac abnormalities. Estimated risk of Ebstein's abnormality 1 in 1500 [60]	Risk of neonatal toxicity	Fetal echocardiography; neonatal serum levels shortly after delivery; avoid breast feeding
Selective serotonin reuptake inhibitors (SSRI)	No proven teratogenic effect of fluoxetine, sertraline, citalopram Possible increased risk of cardiac abnormalities with paroxetine	Dose dependant withdrawal symptoms; slight increased risk of persistent pulmonary hypertension of the neonate (PPHN)	Observation of neonate postnatally, but currently no nationally accepted guideline to recommend duration [61]
Tricyclic antidepressants (TCA)	No known increased risk of congenital abnormality (but limited data) Possible association with miscarriage, preterm labour, preeclampsia	Possible risk of withdrawal symptoms; poor neonatal adaptation syndrome (PNAS)	Observation of neonate postnatally, but currently no nationally accepted guideline to recommend duration
Typical antipsychotics (Haloperidol)	No known effects, but extremely limited data	Withdrawal symptoms; PNAS	Observation of neonate postnatally, but currently no nationally accepted guideline to recommend duration
Atypical antipsychotics	No known increased risk of congenital abnormality (more data for quetiapine, olanzapine and risperidone, less data for clozapine and amisulpride) Increased risk of large for gestational age fetus and GDM	Withdrawal symptoms; PNAS	Maternal GTT; serial growth scans; observation of neonate, but currently no nationally accepted guideline to recommend duration Breastfeeding contraindicated on clozapine (risk of neonatal agranulocytosis and seizures) [62]
Benzodiazepines	No recent studies suggest an increased risk of congenital malformation	Withdrawal symptoms	Observation of neonate, but currently no nationally accepted guideline to recommend duration

be used safely in pregnancy. The exceptions are methotrexate, tetracylines and retinoids, which are all teratogenic and ideally should be stopped pre-conception [19].

There are several pregnancy-specific dermatoses, however only two are of any significance to the fetus. Impetigo herpetiformis is a generalised pustular form of psoriasis originating in the skin flexures [63], and is associated with maternal fever and hypocalcaemia and fetal growth restriction [7, 64]. Pemphigoid gestationis, is an autoimmune condition in which itchy papules and plaques involving the umbilicus precede the appearance of bullous lesions [65]. Fetal outcomes include growth restriction [7, 66], spontaneous preterm labour [7, 66] and stillbirth [7], correlating with disease severity [66]. A neonatal bullous eruption occurs in 10% [67] due to transplacental passage of the antibodies. Both conditions require increased fetal monitoring [7, 64, 66].

Maternal Life Saving Therapies

Extra-Corporeal Membrane Oxygenation (ECMO)

In cases of severe respiratory disease that is refractory to conventional ventilation, ECMO has been used to improve maternal survival. Adult Respiratory Distress Syndrome secondary to influenza is a common indication [68, 69]. A multidisciplinary discussion should occur prior to starting ECMO as to whether expedited delivery would improve maternal ventilatory status however delivery is not always required. Pregnant women have been managed on ECMO, decannulated once their respiratory status has improved and have continued to carry the pregnancy to term. Maternal complications with ECMO mainly result from the patient being fully anticoagulated; this is particularly challenging around delivery and in a recently postnatal patient. Maternal and fetal survival rates with maternal ECMO are around 78% and 65% respectively [68].

Peri-Mortem Caesarean Section (Resuscitative Hysterotomy)

Cardiac arrest is a rare event in pregnancy, occurring in 1 in 12,500 women [70]. Due to aortocaval compression from the gravid uterus, the efficacy of chest compressions is reduced and in women more than 20 weeks of gestation, peri-mortem caesarean section should therefore be commenced after 4 min of ineffective cardiopulmonary resuscitation [71]. The procedure is performed for the benefit of the mother, and as such, delivery of the fetus is accepted at extremes of prematurity or even pre-viability.

Summary

The number of pregnancies in women with pre-existing medical conditions is rising. Diabetes, asthma, hypertension, mental health disorders and epilepsy are encountered most frequently by the obstetrician, but women with increasingly complex chronic medical disorders are also being seen, such as adult survivors of corrected congenital heart disease. Maternal health can affect the fetus via several mechanisms, including the predisposition to congenital malformations, the effect of maternal disease on placental function and fetal growth or as a result of long-term medication. All women with pre-existing medical conditions should have pre-conception care, to optimise maternal health and review medication regimes prior to pregnancy. Antenatal care takes a multidisciplinary approach, focusing on maternal disease control, fetal surveillance and planning for safe delivery.

References

1. World Health Organisation. Preconception care to reduce maternal and childhood mortality and morbidity. Geneva: WHO; 2012.
2. Lassi Z, Imam A, Dean S, Bhutta Z. Preconception care: screening and management of chronic diseases and promoting psychological health. Reprod Health. 2014;11(Suppl 3):S5.
3. MBRRACE-UK. Saving lives, improving mothers' care; 2017.
4. Bhatia M, Adcock JE, Mackillop L. The management of pregnant women with epilepsy: a multidisciplinary collaborative approach to care. Obstet. Gynaecol. 2017;19:279–88. https://doi.org/10.1111/tog.12413.
5. Royal College of Obstetricians and Gynaecologists. Green-top guideline no. 68: epilepsy in pregnancy. London: Royal College of Obstetricians and Gynaecologists; 2016. https://doi.org/10.1016/S0957-5847(05)80054-X.
6. Medicines and Healthcare Products Regulatory Agency (MHRA). Guide for health professionals: information on the risks of valproate use in girls (of any age) and women of childbearing potential; 2018.
7. Nelson-Piercy C. Handbook of obstetric medicine. 5th ed. Boca Raton: CRC Press; 2015.
8. Regitz-Zagrosek V, Blomstrom Lundqvist C, Borghi C, et al. ESC Guidelines on the management of cardiovascular diseases during pregnancy. Eur Heart J. 2011;32(24):3147–97. https://doi.org/10.1093/eurheartj/ehr218.
9. Thorne SA. Pregnancy in heart disease. Heart. 2004;90(4):450–6. https://doi.org/10.1136/hrt.2003.027888.
10. Merino JL, Perez-Silva A. Tachyarrhythmias and pregnancy. E J Cardiol Pract. 2011;9(31):1–7.
11. Tromp CHN, Nanne ACM, Pernet PJM, Bolte R, Tukkie AC. Electrical cardioversion during pregnancy: safe or not? Neth Hear J. 2011;19:134–6. https://doi.org/10.1007/s12471-011-0077-5.
12. Barnes EJ, Eben F, Patterson D. Direct current cardioversion during pregnancy should be performed with facilities available for fetal monitoring and emergency caesarean section. BJOG. 2002;109:1406–7.
13. NICE. Hypertension in pregnancy: the management of hypertensive disorders during pregnancy the management of hypertensive disorders. London: RCOG Press; 2010.
14. Goldie MH, Brightling C. Asthma in pregnancy. Obstet Gynaecol. 2013;15:241–5. https://doi.org/10.1111/tog.12048.
15. Vanders R, Murphy VE. Maternal complications and the management of asthma in pregnancy. Womens Heal. 2015;11:183–91. https://doi.org/10.2217/WHE.14.69.
16. British Thoracic Society, Scottish Intercollegiate Guidelines Network. British guideline on the management of asthma: a national clinical guideline; 2016.
17. Knight M, Kurinczuk J, Nelson-Piercy C. Tuberculosis in pregnancy in the UK. BJOG. 2009;116:584–8.
18. Mahendru A, Gajjar K, Eddy J. Diagnosis and management of tuberculosis in pregnancy. Obstet Gynaecol. 2010;12:163–71.

19. UK Teratology Information Service. Use of aminoglycoside antibiotics in pregnancy; 2018. http://www.uktis.org.
20. NICE. Tuberculosis—NG33; 2016.
21. Goddard J, Bourke SJ. Cystic fibrosis and pregnancy. Obstet Gynaecol. 2009;11:19–24.
22. Edenborough FP, Borgo G, Knoop C, et al. Guidelines for the management of pregnancy in women with cystic fibrosis. J Cyst Fibros. 2008;7:S2–32. https://doi.org/10.1016/j.jcf.2007.10.001.
23. Nguyen GC, Seow CH, Maxwell C, et al. The Toronto Consensus Statements for the management of inflammatory bowel disease in pregnancy. Gastroenterology. 2016;150:734–57. https://doi.org/10.1053/j.gastro.2015.12.003.
24. Van Der Woude CJ, Ardizzone S, Bengtson MB, et al. ECCO guidelines/consensus paper the second European evidenced-based consensus on reproduction and pregnancy in inflammatory bowel disease. 2018:107–24. https://doi.org/10.1093/ecco-jcc/jju006.
25. Glantz A, Marschall H, Mattsson L. Intrahepatic cholestasis of pregnancy: relationships between bile acid levels and fetal complications rates. Hepatology. 2004;40:467–74.
26. Geenes V, Chappell L, Seed P, Steer P, Knight M, Williamson C. Association of severe intrahepatic cholestasis of pregnancy with adverse pregnancy outcomes: a prospective population-based case control study. Hepatology. 2014;59:1482–91.
27. Geenes V, Williamson C, Chappell L. Intrahepatic cholestasis of pregnancy. Obstet Gynaecol. 2016;18(4):273–81.
28. Ovadia C, Seed P, Sklavounos A, et al. Association of adverse perinatal outcomes of intrahepatic cholestasis of pregnancy with biochemical markers: results of aggregate and individual patient data meta-analyses. Lancet. 2019;393:899–909.
29. Royal College of Obstetricians and Gynaecologists. Green-top guideline no. 43: obstetric cholestasis. London: Royal College of Obstetricians and Gynaecologists; 2011.
30. British Medical Association, Royal Pharmaceutical Association. British national formulary. 74th ed. London: BMJ Group; Pharmaceutical Press; 2017.
31. Davidson J, Nelson-Piercy C, Kehoe S, Baker P. Renal disease in pregnancy. Cambridge: Cambridge University Press; 2008.
32. Palma-Reis I, Vais A, Nelson-Piercy C, Banerjee A. Renal disease and hypertension in pregnancy. Clin Med (Northfield IL). 2013;13(1):57–62.
33. Kapoor N, Makanjuola D, Shehata H. Management of women with chronic renal disease in pregnancy. Obstet Gynaecol. 2009;11:185–91.
34. Bramham K, Nelson-Piercy C, Pierce M, et al. Pregnancy in renal transplant recipients: a UK national cohort study. Clin J Am Soc Nephrol. 2013;8(2):290–8.
35. Kidney Disease: Improving Global Outcomes (KDIGO) Transplant Work Group. KDIGO clinical practice guideline for the care of kidney transplant recipients. Am J Transplant. 2009;9(Suppl 3):S1–155.
36. Cauldwell M, Nelson-Piercy C. Maternal and fetal complications of systemic lupus erythematosus. Obstet Gynaecol. 2012;14(3):167–74. https://doi.org/10.1111/j.1744-4667.2012.00113.x.
37. Steer PJ, James DK. High risk pregnancy. 4th ed. Amsterdam: Elsevier Health Sciences; 2011.
38. Flint J, Panchal S, Hurrell A, et al. Guidelines BSR and BHPR guideline on prescribing drugs in pregnancy and breastfeeding—part I: standard and biologic disease modifying anti-rheumatic drugs and corticosteroids. Rheumatology. 2016;55:1693–7. https://doi.org/10.1093/rheumatology/kev404.
39. Flint J, Panchal S, Hurrell A, et al. Guidelines BSR and BHPR guideline on prescribing drugs in pregnancy and breastfeeding—part II: analgesics and other drugs used in rheumatology practice. Rheumatology. 2016;55:1698–702. https://doi.org/10.1093/rheumatology/kev405.
40. Lateef A, Petri M. Managing lupus patients during pregnancy. Best Pract Res Clin Rheumatol. 2013;27(3):435–47.
41. Ince-Askan H, Dolhain RJEM. Pregnancy and rheumatoid arthritis. Best Pract Res Clin Rheumatol. 2015;29(4–5):580–96. https://doi.org/10.1016/j.berh.2015.07.001.

42. Myers B, Pavord S. Diagnosis and management of antiphospholipid syndrome in pregnancy. Obstet Gynaecol. 2011;13:15–21. https://doi.org/10.1576/toag.13.1.15.27636.
43. Soares RA, Castro M, Santiago M. Neonatal antiphospholipid syndrome. Lupus. 2006;15(5):301–3.
44. NICE. National Institute for Clinical Excellence (NICE). Diabetes in pregnancy: management from preconception to the postnatal period; 2015.
45. Lewis G, editor. The confidential enquiry into maternal and child health (CEMACH). Saving mothers lives: reviewing maternal deaths to make motherhood safer—2003–2005. In: The seventh report on confidential enquiries into maternal deaths in the United Kingdom. London: CEMACH.
46. Mathiesen E, Ringholm L, Damm P. Stillbirth in diabetic pregnancies. Best Pract Res Clin Obstet Gynaecol. 2011;25(1):105–11.
47. White S, Brackenridge A, Rajasingam D. Insulin pumps in pregnancy. Obstet Gynaecol. 2016;18(3):199–203.
48. De Groot L, Abalovich M, Alexander E, et al. Management of thyroid dysfunction during pregnancy and postpartum: an endocrine society clinical practice guideline. J Clin Endocrinol. Metab. 2012;97(8):2543–65.
49. Frise C, Williamson C. Endocrine disease in pregnancy. Clin Med (Northfield, IL). 2013;13(2):176–81.
50. Jeffreys A, Vanderpump M, Yasmin E. Thyroid dysfunction and reproductive health. Obstet Gynaecol. 2015;17:38–45.
51. Overton C, Davis C, West C, Davies M, Conway G. High risk pregnancies in hypopituitary women. Hum Reprod. 2002;17:1464–7.
52. Diabetes insipidus in pregnancy. Obstet Gynaecol. 2018;20:41–8.
53. Managing prolactinomas in pregnancy. Front Endocrinol. 2015;6:85.
54. Lindsay JR, Jonklaas J, Oldfield EH, Nieman LK. Cushing's syndrome during pregnancy: personal experience and review of the literature. J Clin Endocrinol Metab. 2016;90(5):3077–83. https://doi.org/10.1210/jc.2004-2361.
55. Care A, Pavord S, Knight M, Alfirevic Z. Severe primary autoimmune thrombocytopenia in pregnancy: a national cohort study. BJOG. 2018;125(5):604–12. https://doi.org/10.1111/1471-0528.14697.
56. Pavord S, Myers B, Robinson S, Allard S, Strong J, Oppenheimer C. UK guidelines on the management of iron deficiency in pregnancy. Br J Haematol. 2012;156:588–600. https://doi.org/10.1111/j.1365-2141.2011.09012.x.
57. Royal College of Obstetricians and Gynaecologists. Green-top guideline no. 61: management of sickle cell disease in pregnancy. London: Royal College of Obstetricians and Gynaecologists; 2011. https://doi.org/10.1016/j.apme.2012.07.002.
58. Howard L, Ryan E, Trevillion K, et al. Accuracy of Whooley questions and the Edinburgh Postnatal Depression Scale in identifying depression and other mental disorders in pregnancy. Br J Psychiatry. 2018;212(1):50–6.
59. McAllister-Williams R, Baldwin D. British Association for Psychopharmacology consensus guidance on the use of psychotropic medication preconception, in pregnancy and postpartum 2017. J Psychopharmacol. 2017;31(5):519–52.
60. UK Teratology Information Service. Use of lithium in pregnancy; 2015.
61. Thomas E, Peacock P, Bates S. Variation in the management of SSRI-exposed babies across England. BMJ Paediatr Open. 2017;1:e000060.
62. NICE. Antenatal and postnatal mental health. CG 192; 2015.
63. Vaughan Jones S, Ambros-Rudolph C, Nelson-Piercy C. Skin disease in pregnancy. Br Med J. 2014;348:g3489.
64. Oumeish O, Parish J. Impetigo herpetiformis. Clin Dermatol. 2006;24(2):101–4.
65. Maharajan A, Aye C, Ratnavel R, Burova E. Skin eruptions specific to pregnancy: an overview. Obstet Gynaecol. 2013;15:233–40.

66. Chi C, Wang S, Charles-Holmes R, et al. Pemphigoid gestationis: early onset and blister formation associated with adverse pregnancy outcomes. Br J Dermatol. 2009;160:1222–8.
67. Black M, Ambros-Rudolph C, Edwards L, Lynch P. Obstetric and gynaecologic dermatology. 3rd ed. London: Mosby Elsevier; 2008.
68. Moore SA, Dietl CA, Coleman DM. Extracorporeal life support during pregnancy. J Thorac Cardiovasc Surg. 2016;151(4):1154–60.
69. Agerstrand C, Abrams D, Biscotti M, et al. Extracorporeal membrane oxygenation for cardiopulmonary failure during pregnancy and postpartum. Ann Thorac Surg. 2016;102(3):774–9. https://doi.org/10.1016/j.athoracsur.2016.03.005.
70. Chu J, Hinshaw K, Paterson-Brown S, et al. Perimortem caesarean section—why, when and how. Obstet Gynaecol. 2018;20:151–8.
71. Royal College of Obstetricians and Gynaecologists. Green-top guideline no. 56: maternal collapse in pregnancy and the puerperium. London: Royal College of Obstetricians and Gynaecologist; 2011.

Chapter 3
Artificial Gestation

Dominic Wilkinson and Lydia Di Stefano

Introduction

Case

It is the year 2030. Eleanor presents in preterm labour following a normal pregnancy at 21 weeks of gestation. She is found to have cervical dilatation with bulging membranes, suggesting that delivery may be imminent. Eleanor and her partner are told that if she undergoes a vaginal delivery, even with the best obstetric and neonatal care the baby will die. However, a new technology has recently become available. It would involve having a Caesarean section to remove the baby before placing it in a liquid environment for at least 4 weeks, allowing its lungs and brain to mature sufficiently before a second 'birth'. Using this technique her baby will then have an outcome similar to those of infants born prematurely at 25 weeks of gestation. Most such infants survive, and the majority of survivors have no or only relatively minor long-term disability. On the down side, the process of Caesarean section at this gestation increases the chance of complications for Eleanor in future pregnancies (she is likely to need repeat Caesarean section, and has higher risks of bleeding or other serious complications such as placenta accreta or uterine rupture).

Should Eleanor consent to the procedure? What if she declines this intervention? This chapter will explore some of the ethical questions raised by a technique that we

---

D. Wilkinson (✉)
Oxford Uehiro Centre for Practical Ethics, Faculty of Philosophy, University of Oxford, Oxford, UK

John Radcliffe Hospital, Oxford, UK
e-mail: dominic.wilkinson@philosophy.ox.ac.uk

L. Di Stefano
Oxford Uehiro Centre for Practical Ethics, Faculty of Philosophy, University of Oxford, Oxford, UK

Monash University, Melbourne, VIC, Australia

© Springer Nature Switzerland AG 2020
E. M. Boyle, J. Cusack (eds.), *Emerging Topics and Controversies in Neonatology*, https://doi.org/10.1007/978-3-030-28829-7_3

will call 'ectogestation'. These questions overlap with ethical questions raised by other advances in neonatal care.

We will start by describing the current state of scientific research into ectogestation. We will then set out some of the ethical questions raised by this technology and its application to neonatology. We will focus in particular on the question of 'viability' and the implications of ectogestation for both neonatal and obstetric management.

Definition

Several different terms have been used to describe technologies that aim to mimic the uterine environment for a fetus or embryo. These are often not clearly defined, leading to some confusion in the literature (Table 3.1). We will use the term 'Ectogestation' in this chapter to refer to techniques that aim to extend gestation by transferring fetuses to an artificial uterine environment.

Animal Models of Ectogestation

The first documented production of artificial placenta (in this case, to determine the effect of flow direction on the placental transmission) was published in 1946 [1]. To be successful, ectogestation would require alternatives to the amniotic fluid environment (sterile fluid incubation) and the umbilical placental system (blood circulation and gas exchange not dependent on fetal lungs) [2]. Several circuits have been tested

Table 3.1 Terminology relating to the artificial womb

Term(s)	Meaning in this review
Artificial womb OR Artificial uterus	Technology that aims to mimic the physical environment of the fetus within the uterus. This may allow conception and fetal development to occur entirely independent of a woman, or allow a fetus to be transferred from a woman's womb to an artificial womb at a certain point during pregnancy to continue gestation
Artificial placenta	Technology that aims to artificially replace the extra-corporeal oxygen/ nutrient exchange function of the placenta. Sometimes used interchangeably with artificial womb/ uterus in the literature
Ectogenesis	Technology that would allow humans to be grown from embryos entirely in an artificial environment, without the need for a human womb at any stage
Ectogestation[a] OR Partial ectogenesis	Technology that allows a fetus to be transferred from a woman's womb to an artificial womb at a point some way through pregnancy to continue gestation. This could be applied to infants who would otherwise be born extremely prematurely (and may not survive, or may suffer significant complications)

[a]This is the term and technology that will be the focus of this chapter

Table 3.2 Published animal models of ectogestation since 2000

Group	Model	Survival	Mortality/morbidity
Pak 2002 [7]	Goat	Up to 34 h	Cardiovascular failure
Reoma 2009 [8]	Lamb	4 h	Four with hypoxaemia. Two cardiac arrest. Congestive heart failure, high cannula resistance
Arens 2011 [9]	Texel lamb	3 h	Increasing resistance of oxygenator leading to decreasing blood flow rate
Gray 2012 [10]	Lamb	24 h	Hypoxaemia, cardiac failure, sepsis
Miura 2012 [11]	Suffolk lamb	18.2 ± 3.2 h	Hypoxaemia, peripheral circulation failure
Gray 2013 [12]	Lamb	70 h	Hypoxaemia
Rochow 2014 [13]	Piglet	4 h	Hypotension and hypoxaemia with low flow rates
Schoberer 2014 [14]	Texel lamb	3.22 ± 1.89 h	Hypoxaemia, respiratory failure
Bryner 2015 [15]	Lamb	7 days	One with hypotension, two arrhythmia, two device failure
Miura 2015 [16]	Suffolk lamb	27.0 ± 15.5 h	Hypoxaemia, circuit clotting, circuit failure
Miura 2016 [17]	Suffolk lamb	60.4 ± 3.8 h	Hypoxaemia, peripheral. Circulation failure
Usuda 2017 [18]	Lamb	1 week	Euthanased after acute circuit failure in one lamb
Partridge 2017 [3]	Lamb	4 weeks	See text

Modified from Bird [5] and Metelo-Coimbra and Roncon-Albuquerque [6]
CA Carotid artery, *UV* Umbilical vein, *UA* Umbilical artery

on animal models, typically utilising Extracorporeal Membrane Oxygenation (ECMO) technology as the basis for the designs.

Some of the recent published attempts at ectogestation are summarised in Table 3.2. Although initial attempts had limited success (due to cardiovascular failure, hypoxaemia, sepsis etc.), these results have led to potentially more sustainable models, notably those by the paediatric surgery team at the Children's Hospital of Philadelphia [3, 4].

Current State of Science

In a landmark study [3], extremely premature lambs were delivered by Caesarean section at a level of lung maturity equivalent to 23 week gestation human infants. Blood vessels in the umbilical cord were connected rapidly to a low-resistance oxygenator circuit, which also provided artificial intravenous nutrition. The lambs were supported within a sealed fluid-filled bag (a "Biobag"), the fluid continuously exchanged to prevent infection. Eight of the lambs were sustained for between 20 and 28 days using this system, which researchers called the Extra-uterine

Environment for Neonatal Development (EXTEND). A summary of the main aspects of the EXTEND are included in Table 3.3 (Fig. 3.1).

Prior to the "Biobag" model, the researchers from the Children's Hospital of Philadelphia attempted less successful open and semi-closed incubator designs which resulted in sepsis or bacterial overgrowth in half of the ten lambs [3]. In comparison, none of the thirteen "Biobag" lambs developed such complications. However, the "Biobag" was not without complication: two of the lambs experienced oxygenator failure and did not survive to delivery/ventilation; four of the lambs

Table 3.3 Aspects of the EXTra-uterine environment for neonatal development (EXTEND), as described by Partridge et al. [3]

	Details of Philadelphia experiment	Effects
1. Continuous fluid exchange in a closed sterile environment	• The lambs were enclosed in a single use polythene bag constructed of a translucent, sonolucent and flexible film with multiple watertight ports • The bags were placed on mobile support platforms that provided temperature and pressure regulation	• The bag permitted monitoring, scanning and manipulation of the fetuses • Continued development of the lambs' lungs by preserving the fluid-filled environment of the womb, resulting in equivalent development to age-matched controls based on early neonatal pulmonary function • Reduced infection, and where low-level contamination did occur, this was eliminated by adjusting the fluid exchange rate and injecting antibiotics into the bag
2. Pumpless arteriovenous circuit connected to umbilical vessels	• Fetal lambs were transferred directly from the uterine environment to the circuit • The umbilical cord vessels were connected to a heparin-coated arteriovenous circuit where the blood flow was driven by the fetal heart • The circuit priming volumes were within the normal range of placental blood volumes, and the blood was passed through a low resistance oxygenator	• Preservation of fetal circulation • No systemic anticoagulation • No need for vasopressors • No evidence of progressive acidosis or circulatory failure
3. Medication and fluids	• Carbohydrates and amino acids with trace lipid were provided and titrated according to plasma levels of nutrients and waste products • The final two lambs also received an insulin infusion	• The lambs maintained stable metabolic parameters • Insulin infusion permitted higher caloric loads and led to an increase in fetal growth

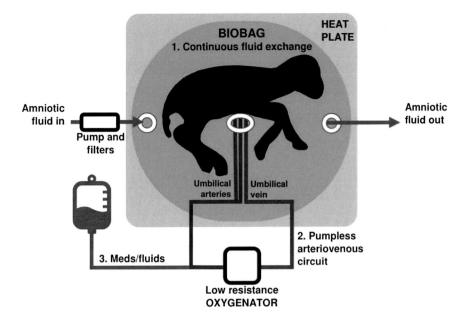

Fig. 3.1 The EXTra-uterine environment for neonatal development (EXTEND). Shown here with umbilical artery/umbilical vein cannulation. (Adapted from Partridge et al. [3])

were shown to have pulmonary inflammation; and one had pulmonary hypoplasia. Cardiac failure had been a common problem in previous ectogestation experiments, however the Philadelphia group only observed hydrops in very early gestational lambs and saw no instances in "developmentally relevant lambs" beyond 105 days gestation. The majority of the "Biobag" lambs were able to transition to normal post-natal life, with apparent normal neurological outcomes. However, the researchers acknowledged limitations in the assessment of lamb neurologic function.

In another paper, the Philadelphia research group evaluated three different arteriovenous cannulation strategies: carotid artery/jugular vein, carotid artery/umbilical vein and umbilical artery (×2)/umbilical vein [4]. Comparing circuit flow and pressure parameters across each cannulation strategy, the researchers found that umbilical vessel cannulation was the most successful, resulting in significantly superior flows and longer runs on the circuit. However, even in the umbilical catheterisation group, 3 died during cannulation, 1 had traumatic decannulation during the run, 1 had umbilical artery thrombosis, and 1 had iatrogenic air embolism.

The outcomes of these studies are promising; however clearly more research is needed before this technique can be applied to humans. Notably, developmentally-equivalent human fetuses are smaller than fetal lambs (0.5 kg rather than 1 kg), so questions remain as to whether this technology could be successfully applied to fetuses at the borderline of viability. Some of the limitations of the EXTEND technique are summarised in Table 3.4.

Table 3.4 Limitations of the extra-uterine environment for neonatal development (EXTEND)

Limitation	Details
Contents of the amniotic fluid	The researchers utilised a simple electrolyte solution in this study which was lacking trophic factors (for example epidermal growth factor, which has been shown to have an effect on immature intestinal cells [19]) and other beneficial components of normal amniotic fluid
Function of the placenta	The placenta has several functions, some of which have not been replicated with the Biobag e.g. provision of placental hormones, growth factors and maternal antibodies
Contact from caregivers and parents	Although the Biobag does allow for monitoring through ultrasound and other techniques, it does not facilitate physical examination or affectionate contact from parents
The need for Caesarean section	Caesarean sections at ~23 weeks of gestation currently involve major maternal risk[a]. It is unclear whether this system may be able to be used post vaginal delivery (for example, this would potentially stimulate transition to the post-natal circulation and reversal of those changes may be complicated)
Applicability in cases of chorioamnionitis	It is unclear whether it will be possible to clear infection in cases of preterm birth secondary to chorioamnionitis (an infection that is a common cause of premature labour [20])
Applicability of animal model to humans—size of lambs	Human fetuses at 23 weeks of gestation are much smaller than developmentally equivalent lambs. When attempts were made with human-size equivalent lambs (480–750 g) there were issues with excessive circuit flow, with development of hydrops and premature discontinuation (after 5–8 days) resulted [3]
Applicability of animal model to humans—intraventricular haemorrhage, uncertainty about developmental outcome	Lambs do not develop intraventricular haemorrhage, a common problem of prematurity in human infants [21]. Brain development in lambs also differs from humans

[a]At this gestation, the small uterus often requires a vertical incision rather than the transverse incision performed on women closer to term. This type of Caesarean increases maternal morbidity and has impacts on future pregnancies. One study showed the risk of uterine rupture after a periviable Caesarean was 4.5 times more likely than after a Caesarean at term [22]

Potential Applications of Ectogestation

In the future, ectogestation could have a range of clinical applications. The obvious direct extension of the animal model would be in infants who would otherwise be born extremely prematurely. Women in advanced preterm labour could choose to deliver their infant direct to ectogestational support—potentially extending gestation by a period of weeks, or maybe longer. The Philadelphia researchers claim that their "goal is not to extend the current limits of viability, but rather to offer the potential for improved outcomes for those infants who are already being routinely resuscitated and cared for in neonatal intensive care units." As noted above, it is not clear whether it would be technically possible to use the biobag model in human infants before 22/23 weeks of gestation. However, it seems possible that with time the model might be applied prior to this point.

Ectogestation could be used in fetuses who have had premature rupture of membranes at extremely preterm gestation, where it might extend gestation but also reduce the risk of chorioamnionitis, and provide an environment more conducive to lung development—preventing or reducing oligohydramnios-related pulmonary hypoplasia and pulmonary hypertension. Similarly, in fetuses with renal conditions leading to anhydramnios or oligohydramnios, the Biobag might facilitate more normal lung development and allow neonatal survival (with adjunctive renal replacement therapy, similar to the reported use of amnioinfusion in fetuses with renal agenesis [23, 24]). Ectogestation might be used for other severe life-threatening congenital abnormalities as an alternative to EXIT-to-ECMO (where infants are delivered onto an ECMO circuit immediately at delivery). The Philadelphia group have used a version of their ectogestation circuit to provide low resistance extracorporeal support to lambs with a model of congenital diaphragmatic hernia [25]. The same researchers have suggested that Biobags could be used to deliver infants with congenital malformations (e.g. spina bifida) and perform correctional surgeries while maintaining lung development [3]. This might allow greater innovations or flexibility in fetal surgery (for example repeated surgery) with less risks to the mother.

Other, even more speculative applications could include ectogestation in cases of placental insufficiency even when birth is not imminent, or the delivery of medical, stem cell or gene therapy directly to the fetus without maternal exposure.

Ethical Questions

The first ethical questions raised by ectogestation will relate to its evaluation in early phase and then more clinical trials.

Ectogestation: Research Ethics

Who Should Be Enrolled in Trials?

While the animal studies of ectogestation have focused on a model of extreme prematurity, this may not be the best place for first-in-human studies. The first problem is that an acceptable outcome is possible with existing forms of support for extremely preterm infants. For example, at 23 weeks of gestation, there is a 30% higher chance of survival if infants are treated actively, while 80% of survivors do not have severe neurodevelopmental disability [26]. While the outcome for a 23-week infant receiving ectogestation might be better than with standard care, the outcome may be significantly worse, raising the prospect of causing harm by enrolment in a trial. Infants of lower gestation (22 weeks or below) have lower survival chances with conventional care, but employing ectogestation may be more technically challenging (because of small physical size) and conflict with the stated goal of such therapy (i.e. not to extend 'viability').

Consent is crucial for clinical trials, particularly where the benefits of an intervention are unknown, and there may be significant risk. However, it could be ethically fraught to obtain consent for ectogestation from women facing extremely preterm delivery as there is sometimes little advance warning of delivery, and the risks to the mother (e.g. from classical caesarean section and an EXIT-procedure) may be significant. As with other fetal surgical interventions, such as surgery for spina bifida, ethics committees will need to decide what level of maternal risk is acceptable for possible fetal benefit [27].

As a consequence, the first human trials of ectogestation may be easier to justify in conditions like renal agenesis where fetal prognosis without intervention is extremely poor, there is potentially more time to obtain consent, and delivery could occur at a slightly later gestation, which would be technically easier and less risky for the mother. Alternatively, ectogestation might be used first in infants with such severe congenital abnormalities that they would otherwise be candidates for EXIT-to-ECMO procedures (e.g. very severe congenital diaphragmatic hernia/congenital heart disease), since such mothers would already be contemplating caesarean delivery and high risk extracorporeal support.

When Would Trials Be Ethical?

A second major challenge for trials of ectogestation will be the potential for loss of equipoise. When ECMO was first evaluated, there was intense ethical debate about whether it was ethical to randomise patients to standard treatment (without ECMO) [28]. If ectogestation is used for conditions with very high mortality (and appears to be successful), clinicians may lose equipoise rapidly. However, this could compromise the ability of researchers to evaluate the effectiveness of the new intervention. It may mean that other methods for evaluation are required (e.g. historical controls), that the evidence base for decisions about the use of the therapy is small, and that there remains uncertainty about the overall risks, costs and benefits of ectogestation.

Ectogestation: Clinical Ethics

If ectogestation appears to be effective in trials, its transition into clinical care is likely to be associated with similar ethical questions to other potentially life-saving interventions in newborn intensive care:

- Is this therapy in an infant's best interests (do the benefits outweigh the risks)?
- Does it represent a reasonable use of limited healthcare resources?

Both of these questions will be harder if the evidence base for evaluation is small, as may occur if trials are ceased early because of loss of equipoise. Questions relating to an infant's best interests are challenging since they require weighing up the harms of a potentially burdensome therapy (with potentially low chance of survival) against certain death without therapy [29]. If some or even all of the survivors have long-term morbidity or disability, the key ethical question is whether these are so bad that it would have been better for them to die [30]. If complications such as sepsis or intracranial haemorrhage, develop during the course of therapy, clinicians may feel that it would be better to withdraw treatment and allow the infant to die. However, as with other therapies in intensive care, that may lead to conflict in situations where parents strongly desire that treatment continue [31].

At this stage, it is unclear how much it might cost to support an infant using ectogestation. If ectogestation is a similar cost to existing technology, resource questions may be addressed similarly to current therapies in intensive care. In contrast, if ectogestation leads to prolonged support in intensive care for infants who would previously not have survived, that may require significant investment of resources in neonatal intensive care. There will then need to be careful ethical deliberation about whether this cost is justified. Should the cost threshold used for older patients be the same for therapies used to save fetuses [32]? Some may have the view that fetuses have full moral status, and that therefore equivalent levels of resources should be expended to save them. Others may hold that it would be better to spend limited resources on saving or improving the lives of older children or adults.

A more distinctive ethical question could be raised by the effect of ectogestation on viability. Will ectogestation change the threshold of viability of extremely preterm infants? If so, what implications will this have for medical decision-making?

The Concept of Viability

In both obstetrics and neonatal care, the concept of "viability" is often taken to have ethical implications. In neonatology, resuscitation is considered to be an option if infants are 'viable', while in many jurisdictions, termination of pregnancy is either prohibited or limited beyond a gestation where the fetus would be 'viable' [33]. However, it is not always clear what exactly is meant by viability: is it the point beyond which survival of newborns is possible, or likely? Does it depend on whether technology or techniques required to save infants are available? Is it just a question of survival, or do infants need to survive without a certain level of disability?

Viability and Neonatal Care

In neonatology, there is not a single threshold of viability. Instead, there are at least two different thresholds—a level of maturity beyond which prognosis is sufficiently high that resuscitation is mandatory (the Upper Threshold), and a level of maturity

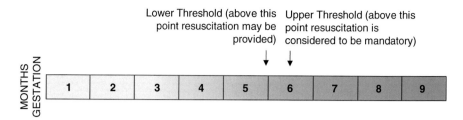

Fig. 3.2 Diagram illustrating thresholds for resuscitation

below which the prognosis is sufficiently poor that resuscitation is not an option (the Lower Threshold) (see Fig. 3.2). In between these two thresholds, resuscitation is seen to be optional (this is sometimes referred to as the 'grey zone').

As noted above, ectogestation may make it possible for neonatologists to save the lives of infants who are more immature than those currently able to survive. This would potentially shift the Lower Threshold for neonatal resuscitation and expand the grey zone. It would not, however, necessarily shift the Upper Threshold, even if the outcome following ectogestation were shown to be excellent.

That is because of the requirement (as currently appears to be the case) for infants to be delivered by Caesarean section. In most jurisdictions, women are not obliged to undergo Caesarean section, even if that would lead to the survival of a newborn—it would be regarded as an unacceptable breach of the woman's autonomy to perform a caesarean against her wishes [34]. Given that very early Caesarean section, before development of the lower uterine segment, and caesarean section/anaesthesia for EXIT procedures are associated with higher maternal risks [35, 36], it appears that ectogestation should be regarded as ethically optional. Ectogestation is therefore somewhat different from other advances in neonatal care, which might improve outcome for extremely preterm infants without requiring any additional interventions or risks for the mother.

Viability and Obstetric Care

Some people, and some jurisdictions, consider viability important for the question of when termination of pregnancy is permissible. This position has been defended using several arguments. For example, some people believe that viability confers *moral status*, and therefore post-viability abortions are the equivalent of infanticide. Others maintain that doctors should be *consistent* in the way that they treat fetuses and newborn infants of the same level of maturity: once a pregnancy is sufficiently advanced that doctors would resuscitate premature newborns, abortion should no longer be permitted.

It is worth noting that many on both sides of the abortion debate reject viability as important for the permissibility of abortion. Those with strongly pro-life views argue that an early embryo has full moral status and therefore would disallow termination of pregnancy even before the point of fetal viability; those who are strongly pro-choice often believe that the ethical significance of a woman's autonomy means that termination should be an option even beyond viability. On either of these views, technologies that alter the point of viability (such as ectogestation) should make no ethical difference to policy or law around abortion.

For those who believe that viability is ethically important for termination of pregnancy, the relevance of a technique like ectogestation will depend on why viability is important and how viability is defined. For example, if ethical *consistency* is the reason why viability is important, that may mean that the Upper Threshold, and not the Lower Threshold of neonatal resuscitation is where the viability line should be drawn. In other words, termination of pregnancy should be limited or prohibited beyond the point in pregnancy where resuscitation of a premature newborn would be ethically obligatory. Since (as noted above) ectogestation is likely to remain ethically optional, it should not affect policy around termination.

Conclusion

Medical advances in neonatal intensive care have often raised challenging ethical questions. Future developments, whether they are small and incremental, or more revolutionary (as with the potential technique of ectogestation) will require clinicians to consider carefully whether or when those treatments should be used.

We have outlined some of the ethical issues that are likely to be raised if and when ectogestation is attempted in human infants. Clinical trials will need to consider when it would be ethical to perform trials, but also when such trials should cease. In translation to clinical care, it will be important to consider whether ectogestation is in the best interests of an infant, and also whether it represents a reasonable use of limited medical resources. Treatment advances around the borderline of viability are likely to be particularly controversial since they intersect with and potentially affect debate around the ethically divisive question of abortion.

Acknowledgement Funding: DW was supported for this work by a grant from the Wellcome trust WT106587/Z/14/Z.

References

1. Noer R. A study of the effect of flow direction on the placental transmission, using artificial placentas. Anat Rec. 1946;96(4):383–9. https://doi.org/10.1002/ar.1090960405.
2. Partridge EA, Davey MG, Flake AW. Development of the artificial womb. Curr Stem Cell Rep. 2018;4(1):69–73. https://doi.org/10.1007/s40778-018-0120-1.
3. Partridge EA, Davey MG, Hornick MA, McGovern PE, Mejaddam AY, Vrecenak JD, et al. An extra-uterine system to physiologically support the extreme premature lamb. Nat Commun. 2017;8:15112. https://doi.org/10.1038/ncomms15112.

4. Hornick MA, Davey MG, Partridge EA, Mejaddam AY, McGovern PE, Olive AM, et al. Umbilical cannulation optimizes circuit flows in premature lambs supported by the EXTra-uterine Environment for Neonatal Development (EXTEND). J Physiol. 2018;596(9):1575–85. https://doi.org/10.1113/JP275367.

5. Bird SD. Artificial placenta: analysis of recent progress. Eur J Obstet Gynecol Reprod Biol. 2017;208:61–70. https://doi.org/10.1016/j.ejogrb.2016.11.005.

6. Metelo-Coimbra C, Roncon-Albuquerque R. Artificial placenta: recent advances and potential clinical applications. Pediatr Pulmonol. 2016;51(6):643–9. https://doi.org/10.1002/ppul.23401.

7. Pak SC, Song CH, So GY, Jang CH, Lee KH, Kim JY. Extrauterine incubation of fetal goats applying the extracorporeal membrane oxygenation via umbilical artery and vein. J Korean Med Sci. 2002;17(5):663–8. https://doi.org/10.3346/jkms.2002.17.5.663.

8. Reoma JL, Rojas A, Kim AC, Khouri JS, Boothman E, Brown K, et al. Development of an artificial placenta I: pumpless arterio-venous extracorporeal life support in a neonatal sheep model. J Pediatr Surg. 2009;44(1):53–9. https://doi.org/10.1016/j.jpedsurg.2008.10.009.

9. Arens J, Schoberer M, Lohr A, Orlikowsky T, Seehase M, Jellema RK, et al. NeonatOx: a pumpless extracorporeal lung support for premature neonates. Artif Organs. 2011;35(11):997–1001. https://doi.org/10.1111/j.1525-1594.2011.01324.x.

10. Gray BW, El-Sabbagh A, Rojas-Pena A, Kim AC, Gadepali S, Koch KL, et al. Development of an artificial placenta IV: 24 hour venovenous extracorporeal life support in premature lambs. ASAIO J. 2012;58(2):148–54. https://doi.org/10.1097/MAT.0b013e3182436817.

11. Miura Y, Matsuda T, Funakubo A, Watanabe S, Kitanishi R, Saito M, et al. Novel modification of an artificial placenta: pumpless arteriovenous extracorporeal life support in a premature lamb model. Pediatr Res. 2012;72(5):490–4. https://doi.org/10.1038/pr.2012.108.

12. Gray BW, El-Sabbagh A, Zakem SJ, Koch KL, Rojas-Pena A, Owens GE, et al. Development of an artificial placenta V: 70 h veno-venous extracorporeal life support after ventilatory failure in premature lambs. J Pediatr Surg. 2013;48(1):145–53. https://doi.org/10.1016/j.jpedsurg.2012.10.030.

13. Rochow N, Manan A, Wu WI, Fusch G, Monkman S, Leung J, et al. An integrated array of microfluidic oxygenators as a neonatal lung assist device: in vitro characterization and in vivo demonstration. Artif Organs. 2014;38(10):856–66. https://doi.org/10.1111/aor.12269.

14. Schoberer M, Arens J, Erben A, Ophelders D, Jellema RK, Kramer BW, et al. Miniaturization: the clue to clinical application of the artificial placenta. Artif Organs. 2014;38(3):208–14. https://doi.org/10.1111/aor.12146.

15. Bryner B, Gray B, Perkins E, Davis R, Hoffman H, Barks J, et al. An extracorporeal artificial placenta supports extremely premature lambs for 1 week. J Pediatr Surg. 2015;50(1):44–9. https://doi.org/10.1016/j.jpedsurg.2014.10.028.

16. Miura Y, Saito M, Usuda H, Woodward E, Rittenschober-Bohm J, Kannan PS, et al. Ex-vivo uterine environment (EVE) therapy induced limited fetal inflammation in a premature lamb model. PLoS One. 2015;10(10):e0140701. https://doi.org/10.1371/journal.pone.0140701.

17. Miura Y, Matsuda T, Usuda H, Watanabe S, Kitanishi R, Saito M, et al. A parallelized pumpless artificial placenta system significantly prolonged survival time in a preterm lamb model. Artif Organs. 2016;40(5):E61–8. https://doi.org/10.1111/aor.12656.

18. Usuda H, Watanabe S, Miura Y, Saito M, Musk GC, Rittenschober-Bohm J, et al. Successful maintenance of key physiological parameters in preterm lambs treated with Ex Vivo Uterine Environment (EVE) therapy for a period of one week. Am J Obstet Gynecol. 2017;217(4):457. e1–13. https://doi.org/10.1016/j.ajog.2017.05.046.

19. Hirai C, Ichiba H, Saito M, Shintaku H, Yamano T, Kusuda S. Trophic effect of multiple growth factors in amniotic fluid or human milk on cultured human fetal small intestinal cells. J Pediatr Gastroenterol Nutr. 2002;34(5):524–8.

20. Tita ATN, Andrews WW. Diagnosis and management of clinical chorioamnionitis. Clin Perinatol. 2010;37(2):339–54. https://doi.org/10.1016/j.clp.2010.02.003.

21. Roberts CT. Premature lambs grown in a bag. Nature. 2017;546:45. https://doi.org/10.1038/546045a.
22. Lannon SMR, Guthrie KA, Vanderhoeven JP, Gammill HS. Uterine rupture risk after periviable cesarean delivery. Obstet Gynecol. 2015;125(5):1095–100. https://doi.org/10.1097/AOG.0000000000000832.
23. Bienstock JL, Birsner ML, Coleman F, Hueppchen NA. Successful in utero intervention for bilateral renal agenesis. Obstet Gynecol. 2014;124(2 Pt 2 Suppl 1):413–5. https://doi.org/10.1097/AOG.0000000000000339.
24. Sugarman J, Anderson J, Baschat AA, Herrera Beutler J, Bienstock JL, Bunchman TE, et al. Ethical considerations concerning amnioinfusions for treating fetal bilateral renal agenesis. Obstet Gynecol. 2018;131(1):130–4. https://doi.org/10.1097/AOG.0000000000002416.
25. Partridge EA, Davey MG, Hornick M, Dysart KC, Olive A, Caskey R, et al. Pumpless arteriovenous extracorporeal membrane oxygenation: a novel mode of respiratory support in a lamb model of congenital diaphragmatic hernia. J Pediatr Surg. 2018;53(8):1453–60. https://doi.org/10.1016/j.jpedsurg.2018.02.061.
26. Rysavy MA, Li L, Bell EF, Das A, Hintz SR, Stoll BJ, et al. Between-hospital variation in treatment and outcomes in extremely preterm infants. N Engl J Med. 2015;372(19):1801–11. https://doi.org/10.1056/NEJMoa1410689.
27. Smajdor A. Ethical challenges in fetal surgery. J Med Ethics. 2011;37(2):88–91. https://doi.org/10.1136/jme.2010.039537.
28. Lantos JD, Frader J. Extracorporeal membrane oxygenation and the ethics of clinical research in pediatrics. N Engl J Med. 1990;323(6):409–13. https://doi.org/10.1056/NEJM199008093230610.
29. Wilkinson D. Death or disability? The Carmentis Machine and treatment decisions for critically ill children. Oxford: Oxford University Press; 2013.
30. Wilkinson D. Is it in the best interests of an intellectually disabled infant to die? J Med Ethics. 2006;32(8):454–9. https://doi.org/10.1136/jme.2005.013508.
31. Wilkinson D, Savulescu J. Ethics, conflict and medical treatment for children: from disagreement to dissensus. London: Elsevier; 2018.
32. Hayden D, Wilkinson D. Asymmetrical reasons, newborn infants, and resource allocation. Am J Bioeth. 2017;17(8):13–5. https://doi.org/10.1080/15265161.2017.1341000.
33. Han L, Rodriguez MI, Caughey AB. Blurred lines: disentangling the concept of fetal viability from abortion law. Womens Health Issues. 2018;28(4):287–8. https://doi.org/10.1016/j.whi.2018.02.006.
34. American College of O, Gynecologists' Committee on E. Committee opinion No. 664: refusal of medically recommended treatment during pregnancy. Obstet Gynecol. 2016;127(6):e175–82. https://doi.org/10.1097/AOG.0000000000001485.
35. Evans LC, Combs CA. Increased maternal morbidity after cesarean delivery before 28 weeks of gestation. Int J Gynaecol Obstet. 1993;40(3):227–33.
36. Subramanian R, Mishra P, Subramaniam R, Bansal S. Role of anesthesiologist in ex utero intrapartum treatment procedure: a case and review of anesthetic management. J Anaesthesiol Clin Pharmacol. 2018;34(2):148–54. https://doi.org/10.4103/joacp.JOACP_239_16.

Part II
The Term Infant: Evidence-Based Approach to Management

Chapter 4
Management of the Depressed Newborn; to Cool or Not to Cool

Divyen K. Shah

A Case Study

A 38 weeks gestation newborn is born unexpectedly depressed. The baby boy's heart rate at birth is between 80 and 100/min but he is not breathing spontaneously and the midwife is giving inflation breaths when the neonatal team arrive at 3 min of age. By the time the neonatal team assess him, his heart rate is >120 bpm. He is breathing regularly by 10 minutes of age. His arterial cord pH is 6.9, Base Excess −13 and lactate 8.

Before the team decide to start passive cooling on the delivery suite, a cursory neurologic examination is carried out. He does not open his eyes spontaneously, but does respond to painful stimuli. His pupils are 2 mm dilated, equal and probably reactive, but not convincingly so. On pulling to sit, he demonstrates marked head lag, and on ventral suspension there is marked central hypotonia. How should this baby be managed—should he be cooled?

The neonatal team decide not to start passive cooling on the delivery suite, opting to admit him to the neonatal intensive care unit (NICU) to repeat assessment and start amplitude-integrated EEG (aEEG) monitoring. The baby is 4 h old by the time monitoring with acceptable impedances and electrode signal is obtained allowing for an interpretable trace. The aEEG background shows a discontinuous normal voltage (lower margin <5 mcV and upper margin >10 mcV on the cross cerebral channel) with no evidence of electrical seizures. However, within half an hour of commencing the recording, the aEEG background improves to a continuous normal voltage (lower margin > 5mcV, upper margin >10 mcV) with an absence of sleep-wake cycling. Should mild therapeutic hypothermia be commenced?

D. K. Shah (✉)
Royal London Hospital, Barts and the London School of Medicine and Dentistry, London, UK
e-mail: d.shah@qmul.ac.uk

© Springer Nature Switzerland AG 2020
E. M. Boyle, J. Cusack (eds.), *Emerging Topics and Controversies in Neonatology*, https://doi.org/10.1007/978-3-030-28829-7_4

The neonatal team repeat the neurologic examination, the baby is now 5 h old. The baby is more active, the nurse looking after him has described him as slightly irritable. He has opened his eyes briefly, but cries when handled. He still has some head lag, but is felt to have more normal tone when leg recoil is checked. His pupils are now felt to be definitely reactive. In view of the improved neurologic condition with a normal aEEG background within 6 h of birth, the team decide not to start cooling but to continue aEEG monitoring. He is left nil-by-mouth and on maintenance fluids at 50 mL/kg/day.

At 18 h of age, as the nurse is about to check his observations, she calls the junior doctor as she has noticed some eye movements that she does not think are normal. The baby's heart rate coincidentally has increased above baseline and a clear seizure lasting about 10 min is identified on the aEEG monitor. There is a rise in the lower and upper aEEG margins with rhythmic spike and wave activity on the corresponding raw EEG trace showing evolution. Should cooling be commenced now?

Hypoxic-Ischaemic Encephalopathy

Described above, is a type of scenario that is not uncommon, illustrating the challenges that we, as clinicians, face in identifying which babies will most benefit from cooling. The first thing to say is that mild therapeutic hypothermia (cooling to a core temperature of 33–34 °C), when started within 6 h of birth and continued for 72 h, reduces death and disability in babies after HIE and improves neurologic outcomes [1].

Hypoxic-ischaemic encephalopathy (HIE) is a description, albeit a very useful description, of the pathophysiologic disturbance resulting from hypoxaemia and/or ischaemia to the fetus that may lead to brain injury and adverse neurodevelopmental outcome in newborn babies [2]. The fetal brain is thought to be relatively tolerant to hypoxaemia, the fetus being adapted to a relatively hypoxic intrauterine environment with the possibility of compensatory increases in cerebral blood flow to maintain oxygen delivery [3]. However the brain may become vulnerable if cerebral blood flow is reduced below a certain threshold (cerebral ischaemia).

HIE is sufficiently common, affecting approximately 1.5 in 1000 live births in western countries [4] (and more prevalent in developing nations) that we recognise the clinical pattern relatively easily. It is the commonest and arguably the most important neurologic condition affecting term newborns.

Our ideas about HIE and what we can do about it have changed over the last three decades. During many of our professional life times, it has gone from being (in many cases) a sad, rather hopeless condition for which all we were able to do was provide supportive treatment, in the knowledge that there were no active interventions available that would improve the outcome, to one with some optimism in the knowledge that interventions have the potential to make a difference to the outcome. Now that active intervention is available, it is possible that more careful evaluation, monitoring and active management to support all the systems of such babies may also be contributing to better outcomes for these babies.

Meta-analyses from systematic reviews of the randomised controlled trials of mild therapeutic hypothermia provide a number needed to treat (NNT) of 7 [1]. i.e. using the empirical criteria, such as those used by the UK TOBY (TOtal Body hYpothermia) study [5, 6], one baby will benefit for every seven we treat. So using these criteria, cooling does not seem to benefit every baby we treat. And conversely, although we have no evidence for this, it is possible that these cooling criteria may not capture all babies that may benefit from cooling.

Which Babies Will Most Benefit from Therapeutic Hypothermia?

To answer this question, we have to try and understand how cooling works. Although we don't know exactly how it works, a number of mechanisms have been demonstrated by which it may improve outcomes. These include reducing cellular metabolic demands, reduced accumulation of cytotoxins such as glutamate and oxygen free radicals, suppression of the post-ischaemic inflammatory reaction and inhibition of the intracellular pathways leading to programmed cell death (apoptosis) [7]. With their elegant fetal sheep model of ischaemia and cooling, Gunn and colleagues demonstrated that cooling was very beneficial when commenced 90 min after the ischemic insult, in terms of neuronal loss scores; it was still beneficial 5.5 h post insult but not beneficial if commenced 8.5 h post insult [7]. So what happens during this relatively early period immediately after hypoxic ischaemia?

Secondary Energy Failure

Biochemical neurotoxic cascades are set off involving increased activity of the excitatory neurotransmitter glutamate, leading to increased NMDA (N-methyl-D-aspartic acid) receptor activation, calcium flooding, mitochondrial failure and eventually neuronal cell death [8]. Mechanisms leading to brain injury postulated include inflammation involving cytokines and free radical activation to name but a few.

Ground breaking studies carried out by researchers at University College Hospital, London, among others examining the magnetic resonance spectra from the brain demonstrated that, after resuscitation post hypoxia-ischaemia, despite maintaining adequate cardio-respiratory support, there was a depletion in the high energy phosphates over the next 12 h or so and a rise in lactate despite maintaining adequate cardiorespiratory support [9, 10]. This has been termed as secondary energy failure and correlated with adverse outcomes [11]. We may postulate that an important aim of "brain sparing" treatments would be to try and prevent the onset of this secondary energy failure which seems to commence within hours after the insult. Hence a treatment such as cooling has to be commenced within a narrow time-critical window.

Why May Cooling Not Be Beneficial for All Babies Who Are Depressed After Birth?

Firstly it cannot be emphasised enough that not all babies who are depressed at birth have HIE. HIE is a pathophysiologic description, albeit a useful one [2]; the clinical features and pattern are recognisable by most experienced clinicians. It is, however, important to keep an open mind and to have a low threshold for considering other diagnoses such as inborn errors of metabolism, neuromuscular conditions and sepsis which may either co-exist or masquerade as HIE.

A baby with HIE is likely to be most encephalopathic soon after or within the first 12 h after birth. In most cases of HIE, the seizure burden peaks in the first 24 h and should reduce over the next few days and then seizures burn out [12]. If a baby has a relatively low grade encephalopathy that progressively worsens, alternative causes of encephalopathy must be considered e.g. non-ketotic hyperglycinemia. Similarly if the seizure burden does not abate or if seizures are extremely difficult to control, then other causes for seizures should also be considered. It is important to have a low threshold for considering other diagnoses and performing a basic metabolic screen as well as a lumbar puncture to exclude inborn errors of metabolism or early onset meningitis.

In a prospectively recruited cohort of 83 babies who underwent cooling in the Brain Injury Biomarkers in Newborn (BIBiN) Study, three children were later diagnosed to have neurometabolic disorders (Tharmapoopathy et al. 2019). Similarly it is not unusual for babies who have had required resuscitation at birth, to then be treated with therapeutic hypothermia because they have fulfilled the cooling criteria and have subsequently had features of persistent hypotonia leading eventually to a diagnosis of a neuromuscular condition.

Why May Some Babies with HIE Not Benefit from Cooling?

We have seen from the experimental data, that cooling is likely to be most beneficial if commenced one and a half hours after the insult in the fetal sheep model [7]. In the clinical scenario, how often do we know the timing of a hypoxic-ischaemic insult? In some cases there may be warning symptoms and signs of fetal distress such as decreased fetal movements or abnormalities of the cardiotocogram (CTG). In many cases, the baby is born unexpectedly depressed at birth with no prior warning, as in our case study. In a small proportion of cases there may be a documented sentinel event such as placental abruption, uterine rupture or cord prolapse. In the BIBiNS cohort of 80 babies with HIE, 19 (24%) had a sentinel event (Tharmapoopathy et al. 2019). Hence the timing of the hypoxic-ischaemic insult in the majority of cases with HIE is not known. If the insult has occurred several hours prior to delivery of the baby, we can postulate that cooling may not be as effective as if the insult had occurred shortly prior to birth.

Severity of Encephalopathy

Meta-analyses of the cooling trials show that moderately encephalopathic babies are much more likely to benefit from cooling treatment than severely enccphalo-pathic ones [13]. We can postulate that the most severely affected babies are less likely to benefit on the assumption that in these cases, the neurotoxic cascades that eventually lead to cell death have passed a point of "no return".

Pattern of Brain Injury

Given that the timing of the insult is likely to be important in how effective cooling treatment is likely to be, are there any other pointers apart from the clinical history that tell us about the nature of the insult? The pattern of brain injury on MRI may give us clues, although they will not assist us in selecting the baby for cooling. Classic studies of the primate model showed that the pattern of brain injury is related to severity and pattern of insult [14]. The signature pattern of brain injury noted on cerebral MRI is to the basal ganglia and thalami (BGT) and the posterior limb of the internal capsule (PLIC) [15]. This is thought to be because the BGT are regions of high metabolic demand and will be affected most by an acute severe ischaemic event. In case of subacute repeated insults, blood may be preferentially redistributed to regions of high metabolic demand thus sparing the BGT and the predominant pattern of abnormality noted on cerebral MRI is to the subcortical white matter in the watershed areas.

Although abnormality of the BGT and PLIC are the key findings noted on cerebral MRI after hypoxia-ischaemia in term babies most babies will have a combination of BGT, PLIC and SCWM (sub cortical white matter) abnormality reflecting the global nature of the insult.

What Objective Early Bedside Biomarkers of Brain Injury Are Available That May Allow Us to Select Babies for Cooling?

At present there is only one bedside tool in common use; the amplitude-integrated EEG (aEEG). The aEEG is a summary pattern obtained from devices such a "cerebral function monitor" or CFM, after the raw EEG signal is processed. The signal has been smoothed, attenuated, filtered and displayed on a semilog scale on the y-axis and compressed so that typically 6 cm of the x-axis represents an hour [16]. This technology was first described by Prior and Maynard at the London Hospital in the 1960s [16]. It arose from a need to monitor cerebral function in adults during intensive care or when patients were undergoing cardiac by-pass procedures, but it was not possible to monitor cerebral function easily. Using analog conventional EEG produced large amounts of data and trends were difficult to monitor.

The aEEG, allowed monitoring of trends of cerebral function relatively easily over a relatively long period of time. Hellstrom-Westas and colleagues were among early workers to explore the potential of the CFM in newborns [17]. In the pre-cooling era, studies showed that as early as 3 and 6 h after birth, the aEEG background pattern was predictive of later neurodevelopmental outcome [18]. This has assumed particular importance with the advent of therapeutic hypothermia for newborn babies; some of the cooling trials used the aEEG background to help stratify disease severity and select babies for treatment [5, 19].

When Should Cooling Be Commenced? Switching Off the Overhead Heater

Given that moderate hypothermia is most effective if started as soon after the insult as possible [7] it would seem logical to commence cooling treatment as early as possible. In some centres, the overhead heaters of resuscitaires are switched off during the resuscitation of a newborn. At present, there is not enough evidence to support this practice. One study has shown that the motor outcomes for survivors who had cooling commenced within the first 3 h after birth were better than those of survivors for whom cooling was commenced at between 3 and 6 h after birth [20, 21].

In our personal practice, we attempt to optimize cardiorespiratory stability before we start cooling. As part of active decision making, the baby's cooling criteria are evaluated and there is discussion with the attending consultant. On deciding to commence passive cooling, the baby's rectal temperature is measured before switching off the overhead heater.

Cooling Outside of Protocol, Cooling Longer, Deeper and Smaller

So what about commencing cooling after 6 h age? The experimental evidence suggests that there is an optimum time window for initiating cooling and in experimental models delayed onset of cooling outside of this window was not beneficial. Is there clinical evidence for commencing cooling outside of the 6 h window? Although not thought to be harmful, at present, the evidence for benefit is not clear either as shown by one large study [21].

Given that mild hypothermia—i.e. cooling babies down to a core temperature of 33–34 C for 72 h—improves outcome, would cooling babies to even lower temperatures or cooling for longer lead to even better outcomes? One trial cooling babies to lower temperatures down to 32 °C± cooling for 120 h (5 days) showed no additional benefit [22].

And what about cooling smaller babies e.g. preterm infants or extremely growth restricted babies? Data from the UK TOBY Cooling Register showed that once cooling practice was established, centres were cooling smaller babies with gestational age range down to 34 weeks and birth weight as low as 1530 g, perhaps a sign of "therapeutic creep" [23]. However at present there is no evidence for benefit of cooling in very small babies.

Cooling After Sudden Unexpected Postnatal Collapse

What about babies who undergo sudden unexpected postnatal collapse? This is a rare event and this group of babies is not well studied. Although a substantial proportion of these babies have an undiagnosed underlying pathology such as congenital anomalies, infection, metabolic diseases and pulmonary hypertension, the largest category of deaths is unexplained [24]. A large proportion of these babies have suffered hypoxia-ischaemia and also have encephalopathy. So in theory some of these babies may benefit from cooling, and Monnelly and Becher advise consideration for therapeutic hypothermia on a case by case basis after excluding pathologies such as sepsis that may be adversely affected by cooling [25]. They address this subject in greater detail in Chap. 11 of this book.

Therapeutic Hypothermia for Mild HIE

To select babies for cooling we use the empirical criteria used by the trials that showed benefit. There are probably babies who do not fulfil the criteria but may have benefited from cooling treatment. Where is the evidence for this? Studies show that some babies classified to have mild HIE, who do not get cooled, go on to have adverse neurodevelopmental outcomes [26, 27]. In fact there is so much concern about babies classified with mild HIE who go on to have adverse outcomes, that there are trials under way to cool babies who have mild HIE.

Given that mild therapeutic hypothermia is relatively safe in the way that it is used, why not cool all babies with mild HIE? Well, as safe as any treatment can be, there are potential side effects. Part of the success story of cooling, used as it is at the moment, was the solid foundation of experimental studies that preceded the clinical human trials. At present we do not have the same amount of experimental work to support the hypothesis that cooling may benefit babies with mild HIE.

Assuming that, of all the babies with truly mild HIE, the vast majority would go on to have a "normal" outcome with conservative management, a relatively small proportion of babies with mild HIE will benefit from cooling. Hence the numbers needed to treat may be rather large. As such, there is an argument that we may potentially be subjecting a large number of babies who may not benefit, to an unnecessary treatment, and hence exposing them to potential harm. This is aside from the huge resource implications that cooling so many additional babies would entail. A phase 3 trial of cooling for mild HIE would not only require a large sample size to show effect, but substantial resources to carry out neurodevelopmental follow-up (the gold standard outcome measure) for babies who may not be followed up routinely in all clinical practice. Recent neuroprotection studies have resorted to using less well utilised surrogate outcome measures such as MRS (magnetic resonance spectroscopy) [28].

In the opinion of the author, there are two theoretical explanations for why some babies with mild HIE go on to have adverse neurodevelopmental outcomes: (1) (with the devil's advocate hat on) it is possible that some of these babies may have been misclassified and did not truly have mild HIE and (2) (much more likely) at the present the selection criteria we use do not capture all the babies who may benefit from cooling, hence the urgent need for additional biomarkers at the bedside for more objective selection of babies for cooling.

Novel Biomarkers for Selecting Babies for Cooling?

At present there are no tissue (i.e. blood or other body fluid) biomarkers in clinical practice for selecting babies for cooling; tests that say "yes, cool", or "no, don't cool' because this baby will not benefit. Although a number of biomarkers have been tested over the last few decades and show promise, as yet none have made it to clinical translation. These include markers of inflammation (specifically cytokines), markers of neuronal injury and repair, as well as the more novel discovery markers [29].

There are multiple reasons for this lack of translation to the clinic; the single most important being that we have not as yet identified a single biomarker that specifically identifies the group of babies who will most benefit from cooling. Although our focus with therapeutic hypothermia is on the central nervous system, perinatal hypoxia-ischaemia affects multiple organ systems. Similar processes of inflammation, injury and repair may occur in other organ systems as they do in the brain.

The ideal biomarker is sensitive and specific with an acceptably low false positive and false negative rate. It should be relatively cheap, easy to obtain and also have a fast turnaround time. There are some biomarkers being tested that show promise; e.g. the neurofilament light protein [30] and microRNAs [31, 32]. Ultimately a whole panel comprising tissue and non-tissue biomarkers may be required for better selection of babies that benefit from cooling.

Back to the Case Study

Our baby in the case study above fulfilled the cooling criteria soon after birth in that his cord pH was less than 7.0 and he had a moderate degree of encephalopathy, in that he was not very responsive to begin with (altered state of consciousness), he had abnormal tone (hypotonia) and he had pupillary abnormality (sluggishly reactive pupils). At 4 h of age, his neurology had improved and, although the aEEG background was moderately abnormal to begin with, it normalised within the 6 h window. However, at 18 h of age, he had suffered a clinical-electrical seizure, hence suggesting a moderate encephalopathy and one that would benefit from therapeutic hpothermia.

With hindsight (and someone did say that hindsight is a wonderful thing!), he should have been cooled from his first evaluation for cooling in the delivery suite despite his apparent improvement within the 6 h window.

Conclusions

So having said that HIE is a label, albeit a useful label as we recognise the clinical pattern, and may cover various underlying aetiologies with an unclear time of insult in most cases, a "sledge-hammer" treatment such as cooling seems to work and has been shown to improve outcomes. Our ideas of injury and repair in the newborn brain have changed substantially over the last few decades. The success of mild therapeutic hypothermia has changed the field of neonatal neurology to one of optimism and an exciting field for cutting edge research.

The translation of therapeutic hypothermia from experimental models to the neonatal unit is one of the most important success stories in neonatology, representing careful and thorough experimental work prior to clinical trials. The coordination, collaboration and cooperation between researchers and clinicians around the world ensured uniformity between the various cooling trials. This has allowed for meaningful interpretation and conclusions when put together in meta-analyses, even when the results from individual trials may have been more nuanced. Future research in the field of neuroprotection will benefit from following this example.

We, as clinicians on the "coal face", may all be able to contribute to optimising outcomes by fine tuning our existing management and clinical practice. This includes improving neurologic examination of the newborn by regular teaching and practice sessions, optimising MR imaging services for newborns and developing and maintaining neurodevelopmental follow-up services with the wider multidisciplinary team.

Note Due to the very broad nature of the topic, only key selected references have been cited. Also the terms "cooling" and therapeutic hypothermia have been used interchangeably.

References

1. Jacobs SE, Berg M, Hunt R, et al. Cooling for newborns with hypoxic ischaemic encephalopathy. Cochrane Database Syst Rev. 2013;(1):CD003311. https://doi.org/10.1002/14651858. CD003311.pub3. [published Online First: 2013/01/31].

2. Volpe JJ. Neonatal encephalopathy: an inadequate term for hypoxic-ischemic encephalopathy. Ann Neurol. 2012;72(2):156–66. https://doi.org/10.1002/ana.23647.
3. Giussani DA. The fetal brain sparing response to hypoxia: physiological mechanisms. J Physiol. 2016;594(5):1215–30. https://doi.org/10.1113/JP271099. [published Online First: 2016/01/06].
4. Kurinczuk JJ, White-Koning M, Badawi N. Epidemiology of neonatal encephalopathy and hypoxic-ischaemic encephalopathy. Early Hum Dev. 2010;86(6):329–38. https://doi.org/10.1016/j.earlhumdev.2010.05.010. [published Online First: 2010/06/16].
5. Azzopardi DV, Strohm B, Edwards AD, et al. Moderate hypothermia to treat perinatal asphyxial encephalopathy. N Engl J Med. 2009;361(14):1349–58. https://doi.org/10.1056/NEJMoa0900854. [published Online First: 2009/10/03].
6. Azzopardi D. UK TOBY cooling register clinician's handbook. Version 4; 2010.
7. Gunn AJ, Thoresen M. Hypothermic neuroprotection. NeuroRx. 2006;3(2):154–69. https://doi.org/10.1016/j.nurx.2006.01.007.
8. Northington FJ, Chavez-Valdez R, Martin LJ. Neuronal cell death in neonatal hypoxia-ischemia. Ann Neurol. 2011;69(5):743–58. https://doi.org/10.1002/ana.22419.
9. Groenendaal F, Veenhoven RH, van der Grond J, et al. Cerebral lactate and N-acetyl-aspartate/choline ratios in asphyxiated full-term neonates demonstrated in vivo using proton magnetic resonance spectroscopy. Pediatr Res. 1994;35(2):148–51. https://doi.org/10.1203/00006450-199402000-00004.
10. Penrice J, Cady EB, Lorek A, et al. Proton magnetic resonance spectroscopy of the brain in normal preterm and term infants, and early changes after perinatal hypoxia-ischemia. Pediatr Res. 1996;40(1):6–14. https://doi.org/10.1203/00006450-199607000-00002.
11. Azzopardi D, Wyatt JS, Cady EB, et al. Prognosis of newborn infants with hypoxic-ischemic brain injury assessed by phosphorus magnetic resonance spectroscopy. Pediatr Res. 1989;25(5):445–51. https://doi.org/10.1203/00006450-198905000-00004.
12. Shah DK, Wusthoff CJ, Clarke P, et al. Electrographic seizures are associated with brain injury in newborns undergoing therapeutic hypothermia. Arch Dis Child Fetal Neonatal Ed. 2014;99(3):F219–24. https://doi.org/10.1136/archdischild-2013-305206. [published Online First: 2014/01/17].
13. Edwards AD, Brocklehurst P, Gunn AJ, et al. Neurological outcomes at 18 months of age after moderate hypothermia for perinatal hypoxic ischaemic encephalopathy: synthesis and meta-analysis of trial data. BMJ. 2010;340:c363. https://doi.org/10.1136/bmj.c363. [published Online First: 2010/02/11].
14. Myers RE. Four patterns of perinatal brain damage and their conditions of occurrence in primates. Adv Neurol. 1975;10:223–34.
15. Okereafor A, Allsop J, Counsell SJ, et al. Patterns of brain injury in neonates exposed to perinatal sentinel events. Pediatrics. 2008;121(5):906–14. https://doi.org/10.1542/peds.2007-0770.
16. Maynard D, Prior PF, Scott DF. Device for continuous monitoring of cerebral activity in resuscitated patients. Br Med J. 1969;4(5682):545–6. [published Online First: 1969/11/29].
17. Hellström-Westas L, Rosén I, Svenningsen NW. Predictive value of early continuous amplitude integrated EEG recordings on outcome after severe birth asphyxia in full term infants. Arch Dis Child Fetal Neonatal Ed. 1995;72(1):F34–8.
18. Toet MC, Hellstrom-Westas L, Groenendaal F, et al. Amplitude integrated EEG 3 and 6 hours after birth in full term neonates with hypoxic-ischaemic encephalopathy. Arch Dis Child Fetal Neonatal Ed. 1999;81(1):F19–23. [published Online First: 1999/06/22].
19. Gluckman PD, Wyatt JS, Azzopardi D, et al. Selective head cooling with mild systemic hypothermia after neonatal encephalopathy: multicentre randomised trial. Lancet. 2005;365(9460):663–70 . S014067360517946X [pii] [published Online First: 2005/02/22]. https://doi.org/10.1016/S0140-6736(05)17946-X.
20. Thoresen M, Tooley J, Liu X, et al. Time is brain: starting therapeutic hypothermia within three hours after birth improves motor outcome in asphyxiated newborns. Neonatology. 2013;104(3):228–33. https://doi.org/10.1159/000353948. [published Online First: 2013/09/14].

21. Laptook AR, Shankaran S, Tyson JE, et al. Effect of therapeutic hypothermia initiated after 6 hours of age on death or disability among newborns with hypoxic-ischemic encephalopathy: a randomized clinical trial. JAMA. 2017;318(16):1550–60. https://doi.org/10.1001/jama.2017.14972. [published Online First: 2017/10/27].

22. Shankaran S, Laptook AR, Pappas A, et al. Effect of depth and duration of cooling on death or disability at age 18 months among neonates with hypoxic-ischemic encephalopathy: a randomized clinical trial. JAMA. 2017;318(1):57–67. https://doi.org/10.1001/jama.2017.7218.

23. Azzopardi D, Strohm B, Linsell L, et al. Implementation and conduct of therapeutic hypothermia for perinatal asphyxial encephalopathy in the UK--analysis of national data. PLoS One. 2012;7(6):e38504. https://doi.org/10.1371/journal.pone.0038504. [published Online First: 2012/06/22].

24. Becher JC, Bhushan SS, Lyon AJ. Unexpected collapse in apparently healthy newborns—a prospective national study of a missing cohort of neonatal deaths and near-death events. Arch Dis Child Fetal Neonatal Ed. 2012;97(1):F30–4. https://doi.org/10.1136/adc.2010.208736. [published Online First: 2011/06/28].

25. Monnelly V, Becher JC. Sudden unexpected postnatal collapse. Early Hum Dev. 2018;126:28–31. https://doi.org/10.1016/j.earlhumdev.2018.09.001. [published Online First: 2018/09/25].

26. Murray DM, O'Connor CM, Ryan CA, et al. Early EEG grade and outcome at 5 years after mild neonatal hypoxic ischemic encephalopathy. Pediatrics. 2016;138(4):e20160659. https://doi.org/10.1542/peds.2016-0659. [published Online First: 2016/09/20].

27. Chalak LF, Nguyen KA, Prempunpong C, et al. Prospective research in infants with mild encephalopathy identified in the first six hours of life: neurodevelopmental outcomes at 18–22 months. Pediatr Res. 2018;84(6):861–8. https://doi.org/10.1038/s41390-018-0174-x. [published Online First: 2018/09/13].

28. Azzopardi D, Robertson NJ, Bainbridge A, et al. Moderate hypothermia within 6 h of birth plus inhaled xenon versus moderate hypothermia alone after birth asphyxia (TOBY-Xe): a proof-of-concept, open-label, randomised controlled trial. Lancet Neurol. 2016;15(2):145–53. https://doi.org/10.1016/s1474-4422(15)00347-6. [published Online First: 2015/12/29].

29. Chalak LF, Sánchez PJ, Adams-Huet B, et al. Biomarkers for severity of neonatal hypoxic-ischemic encephalopathy and outcomes in newborns receiving hypothermia therapy. J Pediatr. 2014;164(3):468–74.e1. https://doi.org/10.1016/j.jpeds.2013.10.067. [published Online First: 2013/12/12].

30. Shah DK, Ponnusamy V, Evanson J, et al. Raised plasma neurofilament light protein levels are associated with abnormal MRI outcomes in newborns undergoing therapeutic hypothermia. Front Neurol. 2018;9:86. https://doi.org/10.3389/fneur.2018.00086. [published Online First: 2018/03/21].

31. Looney AM, Walsh BH, Moloney G, et al. Downregulation of umbilical cord blood levels of miR-374a in neonatal hypoxic ischemic encephalopathy. J Pediatr. 2015;167(2):269–73.e2. https://doi.org/10.1016/j.jpeds.2015.04.060. [published Online First: 2015/05/24].

32. Ponnusamy V, Kapellou O, Yip E, et al. A study of microRNAs from dried blood spots in newborns after perinatal asphyxia: a simple and feasible biosampling method. Pediatr Res. 2016;79(5):799–805. https://doi.org/10.1038/pr.2015.276. [published Online First: 2016/01/01].

Chapter 5
Neonatal Hypotonia

Robin Miralles and Deepa Panjwani

The term hypotonia describes a decrease in muscle tone, a diminished resistance to passive movements or stretch [1]. The decrease in tone can be accompanied by an increased range of movement around joints as well as a decrease in muscle power or weakness. The infant with hypotonia (or 'floppy infant') will frequently be identified by an abnormal posture as well as a reduction in spontaneous movements. The limbs are often less flexed and abducted, leading to what is often described as a 'frog-leg' posture (Fig. 5.1). Confirmation of hypotonia may also come in the form of head lag, a positive scarf sign or increased popliteal angle. Examination may reveal the absence of antigravity movements or reduced reflexes.

Features in the History

The maternal history and pregnancy history can provide important clues as to the diagnosis. A lack of fetal movements (in the absence of fetal compromise) or polyhydramnios (which can suggest reduced fetal swallowing) indicate that an underlying condition is likely to be found. A family history can be helpful in many cases [2]. A description of a mother who has difficulties releasing a grip (e.g. door handle or handshake) or cataracts at an expectedly young age would strongly point to a diagnosis of myotonic dystrophy. Parental consanguinity would increase the chance of any of the autosomal recessive conditions, such as spinal muscular atrophy (SMA).

R. Miralles (✉) · D. Panjwani
University Hospitals of Leicester NHS Trust, Leicester, UK
e-mail: robin.miralles@uhl-tr.nhs.uk; deepa.panjwani@uhl-tr.nhs.uk

© Springer Nature Switzerland AG 2020
E. M. Boyle, J. Cusack (eds.), *Emerging Topics and Controversies in Neonatology*, https://doi.org/10.1007/978-3-030-28829-7_5

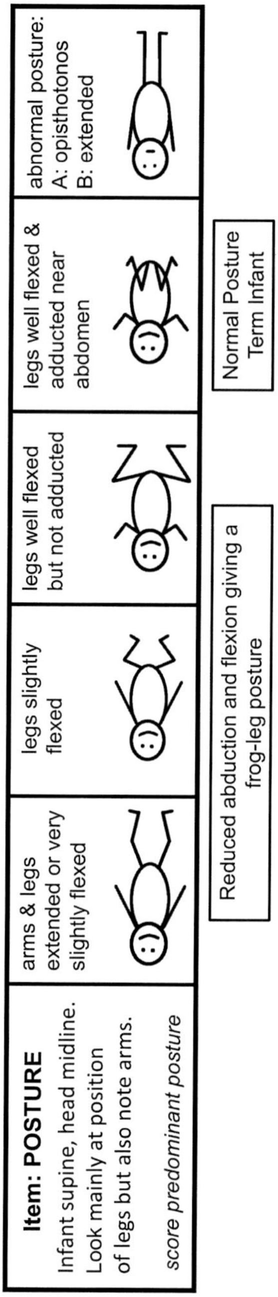

Fig. 5.1 Guide to the assessment of posture, one of the items on the Hammersmith Neonatal Neurological Examination proforma (adapted from [7, 8])

The Anatomical Perspective: Central and Peripheral Hypotonia

Neonatal hypotonia can result from systemic illnesses such as sepsis or hypoxic-ischaemic encephalopathy, and these illnesses should first be excluded. Given that hypothyroidism is a treatable illness, thyroid function also needs to be assessed. Less commonly, because of the contribution of connective tissues to muscle tone, low tone may be a presenting feature of conditions such as Ehlers-Danlos or Marfan syndrome which can be considered as well.

Any problem affecting the motor pathway may lead to presentation with hypotonia. The causes can then be divided into central causes (correlating with upper motor neuron—brain, spinal cord, excluding the motor neuron) and peripheral causes (lower motor neuron, including motor neuron, axon, neuromuscular junction and muscle) [3–5]. Central hypotonia may be due to chromosome abnormalities, cerebral malformations and some metabolic conditions. Peripheral neuromuscular disorders are listed in table by anatomical location (Table 5.1).

A useful starting point in considering the likely diagnoses and relevant investigations is to assess, from the history and examination, whether an infant is more likely to have a central cause, or a peripheral cause for the hypotonia.

Table 5.1 'Peripheral' neuromuscular causes of hypotonia, listed by anatomical location

Anatomical location	
Anterior horn cell	Type 0/1 spinal muscular atrophy
	Non 5q spinal muscular atrophy
	Traumatic myelopathy
Peripheral nerve	Congenital demyelinating neuropathy
	Hypomyelinating neuropathy
	Axonal neuropathy
	Acquired inflammatory demyelinating neuropathy
Neuromuscular junction	Transient acquired myasthenia gravis
	Congenital myasthenia
	Magnesium toxicity
	Aminoglycoside toxicity
	Infantile botulism
Muscle	Congenital myotonic dystrophy
	Congenital muscular dystrophies
	Congenital myopathies
	Metabolic and mitochondrial myopathies

Clinical Examination

The clinical evaluation should include both a general physical examination and a neurological examination. A more general examination may reveal dysmorphic features in infants with chromosome abnormalities. Some features can be specific to particular conditions, such as the facial appearance in in Prader-Willi syndrome (bitemporal narrowing and thin upper lip) [6]. Dysmorphic features point towards a central cause of hypotonia, but it should be noted that other conditions with a combination of central and peripheral features can also present with dysmorphic features.

Neurological Examination

A structured neurological exam, such as the Hammersmith Neonatal Neurological Examination, can be useful in documenting the degree of hypotonia [7–9]. Instructions are on the proforma, and include overall posture (Fig. 5.1), head lag (with shoulders supported), limb tone, traction response and recoil. Improvements or deteriorations can be determined by serial examinations. In addition, there can be a comparison with gestational age norms. Increasing flexor tone becomes apparent earlier in the lower limbs by 32 weeks and in the upper limbs by 36 weeks [7].

Further to tone and posture, it is important to assess the strength of limb movements. The observation of anti-gravity limb movements suggests that reasonable strength is present. In such cases, a central cause of hypotonia is more likely. Lack of movements against gravity, or hypotonia with weakness, are suggestive of a peripheral cause. Deep tendon reflexes will generally be reduced or absent with peripheral causes of hypotonia. The typical clinical findings in central and peripheral causes are listed in Table 5.2 [5, 10]. Further to this, Table 5.3 outlines some of the clinical features of neuromuscular disease by anatomical site. The flowchart in Fig. 5.2 indicates the way in which clinical assessment can be used to guide the various investigations [11].

While there are some conditions that can fit nicely into central-peripheral classification, such as SMA (appearing alert but with peripheral hypotonia) it is important to appreciate that this distinction is not always clear-cut. There can be an overlap in

Table 5.2 Clinical clues to central or peripheral causes of neonatal hypotonia

	Central	Peripheral
General examination	Dysmorphic features	Muscle atrophy
	Microcephaly	Joint contractures
	Decreased alertness	Tongue fasciculations (SMA)
	Seizures	
Strength	Some preserved strength	Hypotonic and weak
Antigravity movements	Present	Absent
Tendon reflexes	Normal or brisk, clonus	Hypo/areflexia

Table 5.3 Clinical features of neuromuscular disease by anatomical site

Site	Facial involvement	Oculomotor	Deep tendon reflexes	Pattern of weakness
Central	Normal		Normal or brisk	Relatively preserved strength
Anterior horn cell	Normal but can occur	–		Prominent limb weakness
Peripheral nerve	Normal	–	Decreased	Prominent: distal > proximal
Neuromuscular junction	Prominent—ptosis	Yes	Normal	Prominent limb weakness
Muscle—muscular dystrophy	Not usually	Not usually	Decreased	Proximal > distal
Muscle—myopathy	Myopathic facies[a]	Unusual—can be seen in myotubular myopathy	Decreased	Proximal > distal

[a]Also seen in myotonic dystrophy

clinical findings [10, 12]. For instance, on our unit we have observed neuropathies with antigravity movements even though a neuropathy is a peripheral cause of hypotonia. Cervical spine injury will initially appear as hypotonia with weakness even though it is central cause anatomically [5]. A recommendation that Prader-Willi syndrome with central hypotonia should be excluded before undertaking a muscle biopsy has been put forward because of the overlap in clinical presentations. In addition, there can be disorders that have both central and peripheral features, such as congenital myotonic dystrophy, metabolic conditions, peroxisomal disorders, and mitochondrial myopathies.

Investigations

Genetic Investigations

The introduction of chromosome microarrays (array-based comparative genomic hybridisation: aCGH) in the place of traditional G-banded chromosome karyotype analysis has allowed the identification of more anomalies because of the superior resolution of detection (10–50 kb compared to 5 Mb for karyotype analysis) [13, 14]. However, because the microarray method assesses copy number variants it cannot detect balanced chromosome rearrangements. A karyotype with fluorescent in situ hybridisation is still the recommended investigation for whole chromosome aneuploidy (e.g. trisomies 21, 18, 13). Further tools available include targeted mutation testing, single gene sequencing and multigene panel testing based on next-generation sequencing [13]. Whole exome sequencing can be performed in cases where the genetic cause is elusive and other tests have been negative [14]. This is discussed further in Chap. 33. Methylation studies are needed for the diagnosis of

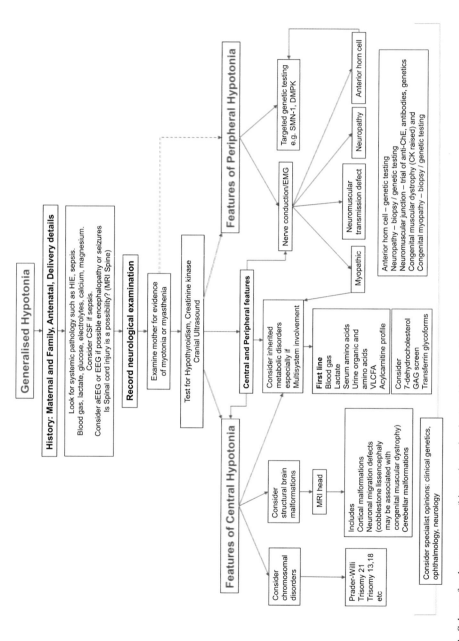

Fig. 5.2 Scheme for the assessment (history/examination) and investigation of neonatal hypotonia

Prader-Willi syndrome where imprinting may be the issue without a deletion being present. With the increasing number of techniques available, guidance from the clinical genetics team is essential beyond first-line testing.

Cranial Imaging

A cranial MRI may be performed to look for structural abnormalities (e.g. cortical dysplasias/neuronal migration defects) particularly if a central cause of hypotonia is suspected. For most babies with a peripheral neuromuscular condition the MRI will be normal. However, brain abnormalities can be associated with specific conditions, such as the group of muscular dystrophies with CNS abnormalities (the dystroglycanopathies) [15, 16]. Cranial ultrasonography may also be able to demonstrate various structural abnormalities and identify acute pathology such as intraventricular haemorrhage. The availability of cranial ultrasound on neonatal units means that preliminary information will often be obtained before an MRI scan is performed.

Nerve Conduction Studies/Electromyography

Nerve conduction studies (NCS) and electromyography (EMG) can prove useful in localising a cause of hypotonia, particularly in peripheral hypotonia. NCS is thought to be reliable after 32 weeks gestation [17, 18]. In disorders with central hypotonia, the results are likely to be normal. With the loss of anterior horn cells in spinal muscular atrophy, muscle fasciculations (group of fibres) and fibrillation potentials (single fibres) may be seen at rest. A reduced nerve conduction velocity will be observed in some neuropathies. A myopathic pattern can also be identified in muscle disorders, although it is also recognised that EMG can be normal. When congenital myotonic dystrophy is suspected, the study will be more usefully performed in the mother as maternal inheritance is the general rule and myotonia is not present in the newborn. An abnormal response to repetitive nerve stimulation would point towards an issue at the neuromuscular junction (Fig. 5.2 and Table 5.4).

Creatinine Kinase and Other Blood Investigations

A very raised level of creatinine kinase (5–10 times normal) is suggestive of a muscular dystrophy, while in other conditions, such as myopathies and SMA, creatinine kinase (CK) can be mildly elevated (Table 5.4) [18, 19]. CK can be raised in the first week after vaginal delivery which can make interpretation of an early measurement more difficult [20]. Levels can also be elevated after performing an EMG. In addition to CK (also referred to as creatinine phosphokinase), we check routine biochemistry:

Table 5.4 Overview of creatinine kinase (CK), EMG and muscle biopsy results by location of deficit

Site	CK	EMG	Muscle biopsy
Central	Normal	Normal	Normal
Anterior horn cell	Normal or mild rise	Fasciculation/fibrillations at rest	Denervation pattern
Peripheral nerve	Normal	Fibrillation at rest/no fasciculations	Denervation pattern
Neuromuscular junction	Normal	Decremental (incremental in botulism)	Normal
Muscle—muscular dystrophies	Raised or very raised	Myopathic[a]	Dystrophic changes
Muscle—congenital myopathies	Normal	Myopathic or can be normal	Characteristic types

[a]Slowed nerve conduction velocity in merosin-deficient (LAMA-2 related) CMD

serum electrolytes, liver function tests, calcium and magnesium. We test for congenital hypothyroidism and would screen for metabolic conditions in many cases, particularly if there is multi-system involvement or a suggestive biochemical derangement.

Muscle and Nerve Biopsy

A muscle biopsy may be performed if the clinical picture or EMG points to a muscle disorder. Muscle biopsy with immunohistochemistry is used to distinguish between causes of muscular weakness and forms part of the investigation of myopathies, with characteristic histological appearances, and muscular dystrophies. Results can point to which genetic tests would be most appropriate. Muscle tissue may also be required for respiratory chain testing. Nerve biopsy may be needed if NCS indicates a neuropathy.

Lumbar Puncture

A lumbar puncture may be performed to look for CNS infection. Protein may be raised in the absence of a white cell response in inflammatory demyelinating neuropathy.

Specific Conditions

Spinal Muscular Atrophy

Spinal muscular atrophy (SMA) is a condition characterised by hypotonia and weakness due to degeneration of the anterior horn cells in the spinal cord and motor nuclei of the lower brainstem. SMA is also the leading single gene cause of death in infancy [21]. It is now well-established that this degeneration is usually due to a lack of the survival motor neuron (SMN) protein caused by mutations in the SMN-1 gene. The SMN protein is known to have an important role in mRNA splicing [21, 22] and other cellular pathways [23].

As a condition affecting motor neurons, there is no impact on cognitive ability. It is unusual to find disturbance of eye movements or weakness of the facial muscles in SMA, so facial expression and feeding can be normal at diagnosis. Therefore, infants with SMA present as an alert infant with significant limb weakness and respiratory difficulties. Muscle fasciculation, and in particular tongue fasciculation (spontaneous contraction of a group of muscle fibres—a denervation phenomenon), strongly suggest the diagnosis of SMA. Further findings are in keeping with peripheral hypotonia with a lack of antigravity movements and reduced or no deep tendon reflexes [21, 24]. EMG is consistent with denervation, but with fasciculations and fibrillations at rest.

Classification of SMA

Earlier onset of SMA correlates with severity of the disease [24, 25] (Table 5.5). Type 1 SMA (Werdnig-Hoffman disease) presents in the first 6 months. Such infants do not acquire the ability to sit and respiratory deterioration is the main (primary) cause of death. This is a life-limiting illness with death by the age of 3 years. Where the onset of symptoms has started before delivery, with antenatal features such as reduced fetal movements, polyhydramnios and contractures, this can be termed type 0 SMA with a life expectancy of less than 6 months [25].

Genetics of Spinal Muscular Atrophy

The vast majority of SMA occurs due to deletions of the survival motor gene, SMN-1 with autosomal recessive inheritance. The SMN-1 gene is located on the long arm of chromosome 5 (5q13) and contains nine exons. Ninety-five percent of

Table 5.5 Classification of SMA by age of onset and severity, including SMN-2 copy numbers

SMA type		Age of onset	Motor milestones	Life expectancy	SMN-2 copy numbers
0	Very severe SMA	Prenatal	Reduced fetal movements	<6 months	1 copy
1	Werdnig-Hoffman disease	<6 months	Sitting not achieved	<3 years	1–2 copies in 80%
2	Intermediate	6–18 months	Sits but not stand	10–40 years	3 copies in 80%
3	Krugelberg-Welander disease	>18 months	Stands/walks as adult (assisted)	Adult	3–4 copies in 96%
4	Late onset, adult	2nd/3rd decade[a]	Walks unaided	Adult	4–8 copies

[a]Not clearly defined

patients will have homozygous deletions of SMN-1 exon 7 (together with exon 8 in most cases). Two to five percent will be compound heterozygotes with an exon 7 deletion on one allele, and an intragenic point mutation in the other allele. The incidence of SMA has been reported to be around 1 in 6000 to 1 in 10,000, which is in keeping with the estimated gene frequency of 1 in 40 to 1 in 50.

The 5q13 region also contains an almost identical copy gene SMN-2 (centromeric copy). However, one of base changes which distinguishes SMN-2 from SMN-1 leads to alternative splicing of the transcription product (pre-RNA) causing the omission of exon 7 from mRNA. This in turn means that around 90% of the protein produced from SMN-2 genes is truncated and non-functioning, while around 10% is full-length (FL-SMN) and functioning (Fig. 5.3). Therefore normally, most functional SMN protein comes from the SMN-1 gene, with a small proportion coming from SMN-2 [22, 26].

The number of SMN-2 genes on each chromosome can vary, with up to four copies [27, 28]. There is some correlation between the severity of the disease and the number of SMN-2 copies with more copies being associated with less severe disease (Table 5.5). It appears that to some extent, the SMN-2 gene can act as a backup gene and is responsible for significant part of the variation in severity of SMA [27, 28]. Other factors may also have an impact.

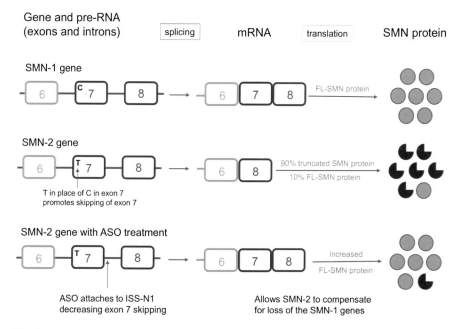

Fig. 5.3 Top section: transcription, splicing and translation from the normal SMN-1 gene leading to full-length SMN protein (FL-SMN). Middle section: SMN-2 gene with skipping of exon 7 and the production of mainly truncated SMN protein. Bottom section: treatment with the antisense oligonucleotide (ASO), Nusinersen, which binds to the ISS-N1 site, allowing increased production of full-length SMN protein

Specific Treatment for SMA

One of the most significant developments in the treatment of SMA is the development of a specific, disease-modifying treatment to increase the levels of SMN protein by increasing the amount of intact full-length SMN protein produced by the SMN-2 genes. Nusinersen is an antisense oligonucleotide (ASO) which binds to a site downstream of exon 7 (ISS-N1). This modifies splicing in a way that promotes inclusion of exon 7 allowing production of an increased amount of FL-SMN protein [22, 26] (Fig. 5.3).

Effectiveness has been demonstrated in a recent trial [29] and intrathecal Nusinersen has been approved by NICE (National Institute of Clinical Excellence, UK) for treatment of SMA type 1 (but excluding type 0, most likely due to the established severity of disease and lack of evidence of benefit [30]). As treatment is intrathecal and repeated doses are required, the logistics of administration need careful consideration. In the U.S., Nusinersen has also been approved for treatment but the ethics of costly treatments have been highlighted [31, 32].

Other treatments are also in the process of being investigated. This includes gene therapy with intravenous administration of a viral capsid vector to deliver DNA that codes for the SMN protein [33].

Non-5q SMA

A small number of conditions (collectively 'non-5q SMA') also present as SMA but do not involve the SMN-1 gene [24]. The best known is probably spinal muscular atrophy with respiratory distress type 1 (SMARD1). Early diaphragmatic involvement means that an affected infant usually presents first with respiratory distress rather than hypotonia, although a weak cry and distal weakness may be noted. Other conditions include SMA with pontocerebellar hypoplasia, and X-linked infantile SMA with arthrogryposis [24].

Congenital Myotonic Dystrophy

Myotonic dystrophy is the commonest of muscular dystrophies. It is also a multisystem disease with cardiac effects, gastrointestinal effects and intellectual impairment. The earlier the onset of the condition, the more severe the disease. In keeping with this, the severest form of type 1 myotonic dystrophy (DM1) is the congenital form. The incidence is estimated to be 1 in 8000 to 1 in 10,000.

Characteristic features of congenital myotonic dystrophy in the newborn include hypotonia with facial weakness, poor swallow (bulbar weakness) and respiratory insufficiency (Table 5.6). The respiratory difficulties can be severe and lead to ventilator-dependence in around 80% [34]. The facial appearance is often described

Table 5.6 Main features associated with congenital myotonic dystrophy adapted from [34]

Clinical features	
Consistent 90–100%	Hypotonia
	Facial diplegia
	Feeding difficulties
	Cognitive disability—100%
Very frequent 80–90%	Respiratory distress
	Hyporeflexia
	Arthrogryposis (especially distal)
	Polyhydramnios
Frequent (50–80%)	Reduced fetal movements
	Elevated right hemidiaphragm
	Oedema

as 'myopathic' with tenting (inverted V-shape) of the upper lip due to facial diplegia. Gastro-oesophageal reflux can be problematic when trying to feed. Diaphragmatic weakness has been reported. Polyhydramnios, presumed to be due to impaired fetal swallowing, is often noted in the pregnancy history. Reduced fetal movements and talipes are consistent with an antenatal onset of the disease [34]. The CK is usually normal. Treatment includes respiratory support, physiotherapy, tube feeding and treatment for reflux.

Myotonic dystrophy is an autosomal dominant condition which also displays the phenomenon of *anticipation*, where the severity of the condition worsens in each successive generation [35, 36]. In the case of congenital myotonic dystrophy, inheritance is from the mother who generally has some features of the condition but then passes a more severe form on to the infant. In many mothers, the diagnosis of myotonic dystrophy may not have been recognised prior to pregnancy. Myotonic dystrophy can also account for symptoms in a grandparent who may have had more subtle symptoms. As congenital myotonic dystrophy is one of the more frequent diagnoses in the hypotonic infant it is worth looking for features of the condition in the mother.

Myotonic Dystrophy: Clinical Features in the Mother

Physical findings in the mother result from progressive muscle weakness and myotonia (impaired muscle relaxation). Muscle weakness tends to affect the eyelids, leading to ptosis with facial and jaw muscles giving a relatively expressionless face. The facial contour can be long and thin and be affected by muscle wasting. Indistinct speech may be a feature. Suspicious findings would include a history of cataracts at an early age. Myotonia, a cardinal feature of myotonic dystrophy, commonly manifests as difficulties relaxing a grip when shaking hands or grasping a door handle [35]. Because myotonia is not a feature of myotonic dystrophy until early childhood, neurophysiological testing is usually performed on the mother rather than the baby. The finding of a myotonic discharges on EMG (waxing and waning in frequency) can be useful in confirming the diagnosis [37].

Outcome of Congenital Myotonic Dystrophy

Neonatal mortality has varied between studies, but it is estimated to be around 15–20%, rising to 40% in more severely affected patients [34]. Outcomes are worse for those infants who require prolonged ventilation [38, 39]. While motor abilities can improve beyond the neonatal period, the tendency is to worsen again with the later onset of myotonia. Looking at survivors in the longer-term through childhood, virtually all had some intellectual disability, with moderate to severe impairment in 30%. Weakness, fine motor difficulties and facial diplegia continued to be observed in all children. Twenty per cent were using a wheelchair for longer distances. Gastrointestinal complications included faecal incontinence in 70% and urinary incontinence in around 40% [40].

Genetics of Congenital Myotonic Dystrophy

Congenital myotonic dystrophy is a form of Myotonic dystrophy type 1 (DM1) and is inherited in an autosomal dominant fashion with the gene affected on the long arm of chromosome 19 (19q13.3). It is estimated that congenital myotonic dystrophy will be seen in around 15–25% of affected mothers. The disease results from the expansion of 'unstable' CTG repeats in an untranslated region of DMPK (myotonic dystrophy protein kinase) gene. Disease severity roughly correlates with the size of the expansion. The number of repeats ranges from 5 to 36 in normal individuals to over a thousand in most cases of congenital myotonic dystrophy. (Table 5.7).

The number of CTG repeats is liable to increase during cell division in a DMPK allele with more than 37 repeats. The phenomenon of anticipation mentioned above results from an increase in the number of CTG repeats from one generation to the next. *Somatic mosaicism* has also been reported, with higher numbers of CTG

Table 5.7 Number of CTG repeats by clinical phenotype of myotonic dystrophy

Phenotype	CTG repeats
Normal	5–37
Premutation	38–49
Mild/late onset	50–100
Classic adult onset	50–1000
Childhood onset	Usually 800 or more
Congenital	Usually 1000 or more

Higher numbers of repeats are associated with an increased severity of disease repeats found in different tissues, such as brain, skeletal muscle and heart, as compared to blood taken from the same individual.

The main mechanism by which triplet repeat expansions lead to disease appears to be RNA toxicity. The CTG repeats allow production of CUG RNA expansions which then disrupt processing and splicing of other genes. Altered splicing of a chloride channel RNA transcript causes myotonia, while the effect on insulin receptor transcripts leads to insulin resistance. The mechanism of RNA toxicity is supported by the fact that a milder form of myotonic dystrophy (type 2—DM2) is caused by quadruple CCTG repeats but from an unrelated gene (ZNF9).

Prader-Willi Syndrome

A combination of central hypotonia, poor feeding and specific appearance may suggest a diagnosis of Prader-Willi syndrome (PWS) [3, 41]. Typically reported findings include bitemporal narrowing, thin upper lip, almond shaped palpebral fissures and thin nasal bridge [6]. However, these characteristics are not always present at birth and may only become apparent with age. Genital hypoplasia is feature in both males and females (small penis with hypoplastic scrotum, or small clitoris/labia minora). Unilateral or bilateral cryptorchidism is present in an estimated 80–90% of male infants. There can be hypopigmentation compared to their family. Even though PWS is associated with overeating and obesity from early childhood, the neonatal presentation frequently includes a need for nasogastric feeding support which gradually improves. Tendon reflexes may be diminished. In a recent review of perinatal complications, infants with PWS were more likely to be born preterm, and reduced fetal movements were reported in around 70%. All infants were hypotonic at birth [42]. In the longer term, the development of hyperphagia occurs from a year of age. Mild to moderate learning difficulties are seen with motor and coordination difficulties and delay in speech development [6, 41]. In one study, the UK estimate of PWS prevalence was 1 in 45,000 in one study but with higher prevalence reported in other countries [43]. However, in one study around 10% of infants referred for hypotonia (with normal conventional karyotype) were found to have PWS [44].

Genetics of Prader-Willi Syndrome

The genetic cause of Prader-Willi syndrome is the loss of expression of *paternally* inherited genes that lie on 4-6 kb region on the long arm of chromosome 15 (15q11.2–13) [41, 45]. Patterns of imprinting (methylation) mean that some genes in this region are only expressed when inherited from the father (PWS region), while others are only expressed when maternally derived (AS, Angelman Syndrome region) (Fig. 5.4).

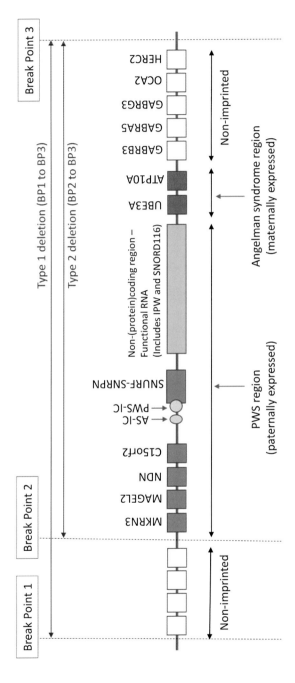

Fig. 5.4 Simplified map of the 15q region showing paternally expressed genes (PWS region) and maternally expressed regions. *PWS-IC* Prader-Willi imprinting centre, *AS-IC* Angelman syndrome imprinting centre

Large deletions occur most commonly at the breakpoints illustrated (type 1 and type 2 deletions) and it is such deletions in the paternally inherited chromosome that form the commonest mechanism of PWS (around 65–75%). In 20–30% of individuals the mechanism is uniparental disomy (UPD), where both chromosomes have been inherited from the mother. As a result, there is again loss of expression of the paternally inherited genes of the PWS region. UPD is associated with increased maternal age. For both UPD and deletions, the recurrence risk is less than 1% [45].

The imprinting centre (PWS-IC in Fig. 5.4) is an area controlling the imprinting of surrounding genes. A defect in the imprinting centre is responsible for around 1–2% of PWS. The majority results from an imprinting centre with a maternal methylation pattern, but there can also be a microdeletion of this area. The latter is only found in a very small proportion of those with PWS (<0.5%), but if a microdeletion is the cause then the recurrence risk is high (50%) [45].

Methylation studies for PWS will diagnose most cases, but without necessarily identifying the mechanism. A CGH array can detect copy number changes and so UPD can be distinguished from a large deletion.

Neuromuscular Disorders by Anatomical Site

Peripheral Nerve: Neuropathies

In the neonatal period, neuropathies can also present as generalised hypotonia, and can resemble SMA. Distal muscle weakness would be expected to be more prominent than proximal weakness. Nerve conduction studies may localise the cause of the hypotonia to the peripheral nerve. A nerve biopsy would then be considered along with specific genetic testing. NCS can also be of help in distinguishing between types of neuropathy where the problem is the myelin sheath and those where it is the axon itself that has been affected.

In axonal neuropathy, a reduction in the number of motor neuron axons will lead to a reduction in the size of the compound muscle action potential (CMAP) and sensory nerve amplitudes (sensory nerve action potential: SNAP). There may be a mild slowing in the velocity. With loss of myelin the main finding is a significant reduction in nerve conduction velocities, and an increase in distal latency [46].

Under the umbrella of the hereditary motor and sensory neuropathies (HMSN or Charcot-Marie-Tooth diseases) there are two congenital myelinopathies. The first is the severe congenital demyelinating neuropathy, Dejerine-Sottas disease (hypotonia with absent reflexes, arthrogryposis, poor feeding and respiratory insufficiency). Nerve biopsy shows a reduction in myelinated fibres, thin myelin sheaths and 'onion bulb' layers around axons, representing repeated cycles of demyelination and remyelination [47]. In the second, congenital hypomyelinating neuropathy, there is complete absence of a myelin sheath and no onion bulb formation [48].

Axonal neuropathies with onset in infancy are less common, but as indicated above, can be distinguished by the main finding of a reduction in CMAP but with relatively less reduction in conduction velocity. These neuropathies are said to be more commonly associated with CNS or other features [49].

Riley-Day syndrome is a form of hereditary sensory and autonomic neuropathy which may present with neonatal hypotonia. This is rare outside the Ashkenazi Jewish population but has specific features such as absent corneal reflex and lack of normal response to intradermal histamine (i.e. a deficiency in the autonomic response). Nerve biopsy shows a severe reduction in unmyelinated nerve fibres with much less impact on myelinated fibres [50].

Acquired inflammatory demyelinating neuropathies are very rare in the neonatal period but have been described. There is an acute form (acute inflammatory demyelinating polyneuropathy, ADIP or Guillain-Barré) and chronic form. NCS may show patchy, asymmetrical reductions in nerve conduction velocity and temporal dispersion [51]. These conditions are associated with raised CSF protein in the absence of a white cell response. The importance of this diagnosis is the potential for recovery.

The Neuromuscular Junction

Disorders of the neuromuscular junction are generally characterised by variable weakness and fatiguability including ptosis. The EMG may indicate such a diagnosis with a decremental response on repetitive nerve stimulation [46], which is the neurophysiological correlate of fatiguability.

A transient disturbance in neuromuscular transmission can be due to antibodies (usually anti-acetylcholine receptor and rarely anti-MuSK) that have been transplacentally acquired from a mother who has myasthenia gravis [52, 53]. This is estimated to occur in 10–20% of mothers with myasthenia gravis, but in some cases, disease in the mother may not have been identified. The inherited congenital myasthenic syndromes (CMS), in contrast, are caused by genetic defects disrupting the pathway of signal transmission across the neuromuscular junction. These defects can be classified as pre-synaptic, synaptic and post-synaptic (receptor deficiency and end-plate development) as shown in Table 5.8 [54, 55].

The adult acetylcholine receptor (AChR) consists of five subunits (2 alpha, beta, delta, epsilon) forming a central ion channel pore (Fig. 5.5). Receptor defects can be further subdivided into primary deficiency, slow-channel syndrome (prolonged opening of the receptor channel) or fast-channel syndrome (relatively brief channel opening). Some deficiencies relate to interference with the clustering of ACh receptors, a crucial part of the development of the motor end-plate. While the acetylcholinesterase inhibitor, pyridostigmine, is of benefit in some cases of CMS, for those who have acetylcholinesterase deficiency or prolonged opening of the receptor channel (both causing a depolarising block), this treatment would not be helpful [54]. Other treatments include beta-2 agonists and fluoxetine.

Table 5.8 Classification of congenital myasthenic syndromes: biochemical deficiencies and associated functions that can impact on neuromuscular transmission

Location	Function affected	Deficiency
Pre-synaptic	Presynaptic development	Myo9 deficiency
	Manufacture of acetylcholine	CHAT deficiency
	Synaptic vesicle exocytosis	SNAP25, synaptogen-2
Synaptic	Component of acetylcholine	ColQ gene (ACh tail/anchor)
	Synaptic extracellular matrix	Beta-2 laminin deficiency
Post-synaptic		
Acetylcholine receptor	Primary receptor deficiency	Most commonly mutation of epsilon subunit (CHRE)
	Slow channel syndrome (prolonged channel opening)	Most commonly mutation of alpha subunit (CHRA)
	Fast channel syndrome (abnormally brief channel opening)	Most commonly mutation of epsilon subunit (CHRE)
End-plate development	ACh receptor clustering pathway	Agrin (signalling molecule)
		MuSk (Muscle specific kinase)
		DOK-7
		LRP4
	Stabilisation of ACh receptor clusters	Rapsyn

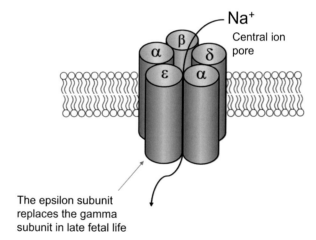

Fig. 5.5 Diagram of the acetylcholine receptor, made up of five subunits with a central ion pore (adapted from [55])

The epsilon subunit replaces the gamma subunit in late fetal life

CMS in infancy and childhood is rare. The UK the prevalence was 9.2 per million children [53], with the most common mutations being in CHRE ('Choline Receptor E' gene coding for the epsilon subunit of AChR), RAPSN and DOK7. Neonatal presentation has been reported [56] but in most cases CMS has only become apparent outside the neonatal period.

The fetal form of the ACh receptor up to 33 weeks gestation contains a gamma subunit instead of the epsilon subunit. It is interesting to note that some cases of Escobar syndrome (multiple pterygium syndrome, a form of arthrogryposis), are due to mutations affecting the gamma subunit (CHRG gene mutation). While an infant with mutation may be born with webbing and contractures due to impairment of the neuromuscular junction in fetal life, evidence of myasthenia will be lacking because the fetal ACh receptors will have been replaced by the adult ACh receptors by the time the baby is born.

True autoimmune myasthenia gravis is not seen in the neonate, with the earliest reported presentation at 6 months [50, 53]. Infantile botulism (toxin-mediated) is a further cause of hypotonia due to transmission at the neuromuscular junction but with an incremental response on EMG. The toxin binds to the pre-synaptic surface, preventing the release of ACh. In addition to hypotonia and weakness the disease is characterised by poor feeding, constipation, and in at least two thirds, a need for ventilatory support. There is usually an abnormal pupillary reaction with an impaired reaction to light [50]. The condition has been associated with honey ingestion but appears to be rare in the UK [57, 58] despite being reported more frequently elsewhere [50].

Magnesium has been reported to cause hypotonia following administration to mothers in high doses for pre-eclampsia (with unusually high levels in the infant >4.5 mmol/L) [50]. There is impairment of release of ACh at the neuromuscular junction. Aminoglycoside antibiotics such as gentamicin can also interfere with neuromuscular transmission. Clinically this has only been observed in situations where large doses have been administered [50] but it may be worth noting where the effect of a neuromuscular agent is greater or more prolonged than expected.

Muscle Disorders: Muscular dystrophies and Myopathies

Muscle disorders can be classified by histological appearance on muscle biopsy, although more recently classifications have also combined protein deficiencies and loss of biochemical function in addition to the gene affected.

Congenital Muscular Dystrophies

The dystrophic appearance on biopsy characteristic of the muscular dystrophies consists of fibrosis, muscle fibre degeneration and replacement of muscle tissue with adipose tissue. The most common form of muscular dystrophy is myotonic dystrophy, but this has a distinct clinical presentation and is discussed above. Creatinine kinase is usually moderately or markedly elevated. The incidence of congenital muscular dystrophies in Northern England was found to be 0.75 per 100,000 [59]. Traditionally, congenital muscular dystrophies (CMDs) have been divided into those without structural CNS abnormalities ('classic' muscular dystrophies) and those with CNS abnormalities [5, 60].

The muscular dystrophy group with structural CNS abnormalities include conditions such as Walker-Warburg syndrome (WWS), muscle-eye brain disease (MEB) and Fukuyama muscular dystrophy. Walker-Warburg syndrome represents the severest form of this group with a combination of cobblestone lissencephaly, thin cortical mantle with ex-vacuo hydrocephalus, cerebellar malformations and eye abnormalities [15]. Life expectancy is less than a year. MEB is similar but with a milder phenotype (Table 5.9). Geographical clusters can be seen in the CMD with CNS abnormalities group. Fukuyama Congenital Muscular Dystrophy, while the commonest CMD in Japan, is rare elsewhere. MEB disease is commonest in Finland with a low incidence in other countries [5].

The classic CMDs i.e. those without overt structural brain abnormalities, were previously classified into merosin-deficient or merosin-positive (by merosin staining on histology). The merosin-deficient conditions were associated a worse prognosis with the clinical picture of a weak hypotonic infant with absent reflexes, who does not achieve standing or walking, but with otherwise preserved cognitive development. There could be a relatively high CK level with white matter abnormalities on MRI in addition to the muscular findings. The likelihood of ambulation in the merosin-positive group was higher.

CMDs are now also classified according to the protein deficiency or loss of function [61] (Table 5.9), but there is a relationship with the previous classification [62]. The CMDs previously classified as being associated with structural brain abnormalities, such as WWS, have been found to be due to deficiencies in the glycosylation of alpha-dystroglycan and so are termed alpha-dystroglycanopathies (Fig. 5.6). Merosin is an extracellular matrix protein, laminin-2. The laminin alpha-2 protein chain, coded for by the LAMA2 gene, is a critical component of laminin-2 (Fig. 5.6), so that any deficiency due to LAMA2 mutations leads to a lack of laminin-2. Following on from this, 'LAMA2-associated CMD' or 'CMD with alpha-2 chain deficiency' are alternative terms for the previously described merosin-deficient congenital muscular dystrophy MDC1A or *primary* merosin deficiency (Table 5.9). Collagen-6, like laminin-2, is also a protein located in the extracellular matrix. The fact that extracellular matrix protein deficiency can lead to early onset CMDs underlines the dependence of skeletal muscle on the extracellular matrix for function. (Fig. 5.6).

Congenital Myopathies

Congenital myopathies were originally described as muscle conditions presenting at birth without dystrophic appearances on histology [63]. Myopathies are still classified by their distinctive histological appearances [64]. The commonest types are nemaline myopathy, central core disease, centronuclear myopathy (including X-linked myotubular myopathy) and congenital fibre-type disproportion (CFTD) [65], shown in Table 5.10.

Although most myopathies may have a stable or slowly progressive course, myopathy with onset in the neonatal period will usually present with significant respiratory involvement and marked facial weakness. Facial weakness is suggestive

Table 5.9 Classification of the main congenital muscular dystrophies (CMD) presenting in the neonatal period (current and previous classification included)

Classification by protein/biochemical defect	Disease phenotype	Traditional classification by merosin and structural CNS anomalies
Extracellular matrix protein: Laminin alpha-2 chain (LAMA2) component of laminin-2	**Primary merosin deficiency (MCD1A)** Hypotonia at birth or early infancy. Most do not achieve independent ambulation and can have white matter changes on MRI	**Merosin deficient**
Extracellular matrix protein: Collagen 6 (COL6A1, COL6A2, COL6A3)	**Ullrich CMD** Hypotonia, proximal contractures, hip dislocation, distal hyperlaxity Respiratory insufficiency, first to second decade **Bethlem CMD**—milder phenotype—mild weakness, hypermobility	**Merosin positive**
Endoplasmic reticulum protein (SEPN1 gene)	**CMD with Spinal Rigidity** (SEPN1 gene)	**Merosin positive**
Defective glycosylation of alpha-dystroglycan (Alpha dystroglycanopathies) Commonest genes affected: POMT1, POMT2, FKTN, FKRP, LARGE1, POMGNT1 and ISPD	**Walker-Warburg Syndrome** Severest phenotype of the alpha-dystroglycanopathies Cobblestone malformation, thin cortical mantle, hydrocephalus, encephalocoele, midline brain structure hypoplasia, severe eye involvement, life span <1 year	**CMD with structural CNS anomalies**
	Muscle–Eye–Brain disease Pachygyria and polymicrogyria Ocular involvement, severe myopia, retinal hypoplasia Most achieve sitting, standing, walking. Life expectancy 6–16 years	
	Fukuyama Congenital CMD Microcephaly, polymicrogyria, pachygyria, cerebellar involvement seizures. Death usually by 10 years. Mostly do not achieve walking	

Other congenital muscular dystrophies include those related to nuclear envelope/mitochondrial membrane proteins and integrins

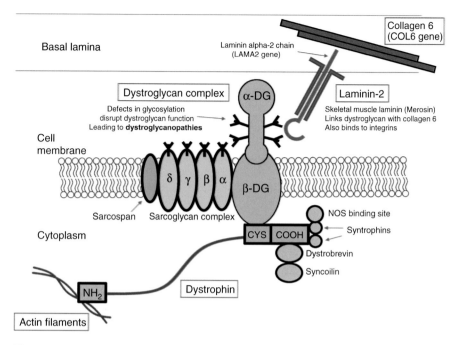

Fig. 5.6 Diagrammatic representation of the binding relationships between the dystroglycan subunits (alpha and beta DG), laminin-2 (merosin), collagen 6, dystrophin and actin filaments

of a myopathy, but with congenital myotonic dystrophy in the differential diagnosis. Oculomotor muscle involvement tends to be restricted to centronuclear / myotubular myopathy [5, 64, 65]. Cardiac involvement is unusual. In contrast to the muscular dystrophies, the creatinine kinase is usually normal or only mildly elevated. EMG may be normal or myopathic with normal repetitive nerve stimulation.

Of the myopathies with early onset, myotubular myopathy may have a prenatal onset with death during infancy. Associated features can include a dysmorphic appearance (dolichocephaly and elongated face) in addition to hypotonia and respiratory insufficiency [3, 66]. Nemaline myopathy *congenital* subtypes include 'typical', intermediate, and severe. The severe form can present before birth (fetal akinesia) or during the neonatal period leading to death in the first month [5]. A severe perinatal-neonatal form of core myopathy (RYR1 gene-related) has also been reported [67].

Progress in genetic diagnosis has revealed that the congenital myopathies are a genetically heterogeneous. Different gene mutations may lead to the same histological appearance, while mutations in the same gene can lead to different histopathological appearances. For instance, 90% of central core disease (associated with malignant hyperthermia) is caused by mutation in the skeletal muscle ryanodine receptor gene (RYR1). For nemaline myopathy, the commonest genes involved are ACTA-1 (alpha actin) and NEB (also known as NEM2). However, both ACTA1 and RYR1 gene mutations can also be seen in CFTD. It seems likely, therefore, that the histological appearances represent the end-product of a variety of pathological processes. Some genes are more specific such as X-linked MTM1 causing a centronuclear myopathy.

Table 5.10 Classification of congenital myopathies by histological appearance

Myopathy type	Histological appearance		Associated subtypes
Normal myocyte		Nucleus to the side	
Nemaline myopathy 'rods'		Nemaline rods Purple staining rods at the periphery of most fibres (trichrome stain)	Nemaline myopathy—rods Rods and cores Cap myopathy Zebra body myopathy
Core myopathies 'cores'		Lack of oxidative staining centrally (the 'core') in central core myopathy	Central core myopathy Multiminicore
Centronuclear myopathies		Centrally-placed nuclei	Centronuclear myopathy (AD) Myotubular myopathy (X-linked)
Congenital fibre-type disproportion (CFTD)		Small size type 1 fibres	

Other types include—myosin storage myopathy

There is a cross-over with congenital muscular dystrophies. Mutations in SEPN1 (CMD with spinal rigidity) can be seen in CFTD and core myopathy (multi-mini-core). RYR1 gene mutations can also present with congenital muscular dystrophy. With the increasing use of genetic panels, it has been suggested that the classification of myopathies and identification of potential treatment may become more focused on the underlying genetic defect.

Metabolic and Mitochondrial Disorders Presenting with Neonatal Hypotonia

Various metabolic disorders and mitochondrial dysfunction can present with hypotonia in the neonatal period [68]. An encephalopathy associated with hypotonia (central and peripheral features) or multi-system involvement should prompt investigations for inborn errors of metabolism. The presence of a metabolic or mito-chondrial disorder may be supported by lactic acidosis, persistent hypoglycaemia or raised ammonia. First-line metabolic investigations should include blood gas and lactate, serum amino acids, urine amino and organic acids, acylcarnitine profile and very long chain fatty acids.

Mitochondrial myopathies involve abnormalities of mitochondrial structure and function that interfere with the process of releasing energy from substrates. A mitochondrial disorder may be suggested by an elevated lactate that fails to resolve. It is cytochrome oxidase deficiency (COX or complex IV of the respira-tory chain) which is the most likely to present in the neonatal period although deficiencies of other complexes are possible [5, 15]. The presentation is with severe generalised weakness which may be accompanied by lactic acidosis, respi-ratory and feeding difficulties, hepatomegaly and cardiomyopathy. The life expec-tancy is only a few months ('fatal infantile myopathy'). However, COX deficiency can also be seen in a severe neonatal myopathy which then starts to resolve after the first few months, with significant recovery by 3 years ('benign infantile myop-athy'). This condition which has also been described as a 'reversible infantile respiratory chain deficiency' appears to be a problem of mitochondrial DNA translation. Reported genetic defects include maternally inherited mitochondrial mutations coding for transfer rRNA (tRNA), or a nuclear *gene,* TRMU, encoding a mitochondrial tRNA-modifying enzyme [69]. Immunohistochemistry and genetic studies are needed to assist in distinguishing the benign condition from the fatal form [34, 69].

Pompe's disease, an autosomal recessive lysosomal storage disorder may need to be considered where there is a combination of heart enlargement and hypotonia after the first few weeks of life. Deficiency of the enzyme acid alpha-glucosidase (GAA—'acid maltase') leads to an abnormal accumulation of gly-cogen within cells. Features may include hepatomegaly and macroglossia in addition to hypotonia and cardiomyopathy. Presentation is usually in the first few months of life rather than the newborn period, but neonatal onset has been reported [70]. Other metabolic disorders that need to be considered include fatty acid oxidation defects.

The Zellweger spectrum disorders are genetically heterogeneous peroxisome biogenesis disorders characterized by disruption of peroxisome formation [71]. They are autosomal recessive conditions caused by mutations in one of 13 PEX genes [71]. The severest form, Zellweger disease, presents in the neonatal period with marked hypotonia and weakness combined with facial dysmorphism [71, 72]. Features include an enlarged fontanelle, high forehead, epicanthic folds, and redun-dant neck skin folds. Investigations may reveal renal cysts and calcific stippling of epiphyses, impaired liver function, hearing loss and seizures. Investigations include very long chain fatty acids which accumulate as a result of the peroxisome defi-ciency. Other metabolites that accumulate include phytanic, pristanic and pipecolic acid. Diagnosis can be confirmed with genetic testing.

Case Illustration 1

A 41-week infant was born by vaginal delivery to non-consanguineous parents following an uncomplicated pregnancy (no report of polyhydramnios). The paediatric team was asked to review the baby at 2 hours because of floppiness. There was no respiratory distress.

Examination revealed very low tone in all four limbs, with absent reflexes and no spontaneous antigravity movements. Nasogastric feeding was commenced, but by day 5 breastfeeding had been established. Tongue fasciculations were observed. SMN-1 gene testing was performed, but with an estimated 2 weeks required for results. Creatinine kinase was at 608 units/l. Cranial ultrasound was normal. A nerve conduction study/EMG revealed a loss of motor axons with profuse spontaneous (at rest) activity in left biceps and right tibialis anterior (consistent with SMA). Subsequently genetic testing revealed homozygous loss of the SMN-1 gene.

In this case the clinical features were very suggestive of SMA. The combination of hypotonia, hyporeflexia, absence of spontaneous anti-gravity movements pointed to a lower motor neuron neuromuscular disorder. The facial appearance was normal, with breastfeeding established by day 5—an alert infant with profound hypotonia and with tongue fasciculations. The EMG was highly suggestive and 5q spinal muscular atrophy was confirmed with genetic testing. The creatinine kinase level was initially raised, and this shows how CK can be elevated following vaginal delivery. It had fallen to normal levels by the second week.

Case Illustration 2

A 33-week infant was born by elective caesarean section to a 27-year-old mother. Intubation and ventilator support from birth was required. Transfer to the local tertiary neonatal unit was undertaken. There had been a history of polyhydramnios and the pregnancy had been complicated by a maternal pulmonary embolus at 30 weeks gestation. The mother's medical history also included cataract removal in her twenties. It was noted that the baby had low limb tone and paucity of facial movements. Creatinine kinase was normal. Despite low ventilatory requirements, a trial of extubation on day 3 was unsuccessful. Once the mother was well enough to visit, she was noted to have a relatively expressionless face with muscle wasting. She acknowledged that she did have difficulties with releasing her grip with door handles. Further to this, she also recalled that her mother had an unusual gait, but without any formal medical diagnosis being made. Arrangements were made for an EMG in the mother and this demonstrated the myotonic signature of myotonic dystrophy. Genetic testing for myotonic dystrophy demonstrated >1000 CTG repeats in the DMPK gene, confirming a diagnosis of congenital myotonic dystrophy in the infant.

The initial differential diagnosis of a baby requiring respiratory support at birth was wide. The finding of polyhydramnios with hypotonia in the infant suggested that a neuromuscular condition was a possibility. The biggest clue to the diagnosis here was the history and examination of the mother. Given the lack of myotonia in infancy, it was more appropriate to perform the EMG in the mother. Normal testing in the mother would have made the diagnosis of myotonic dystrophy very unlikely.

Case Illustration 3

A 34-week infant was the first baby born by caesarean section to consanguineous parents of middle eastern descent. Delivery by caesarean section was performed because of IUGR and dilated loops of bowel. Resuscitation at birth consisted of ventilation breaths only. Once spontaneous respirations were established it was observed that she remained profoundly floppy. There was a transient requirement for CPAP and then nasal prong oxygen.

A number of features were noted—a large forehead, epicanthic folds and redundant neck skin folds. The anterior fontanelle was large. In addition to the hypotonia she appeared quiet with reduced facial movements. There were few spontaneous movements and no antigravity limb movements. Feeding was by nasogastric tube and there was no suck reflex.

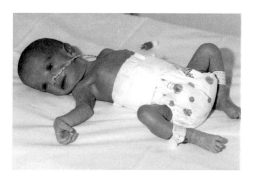

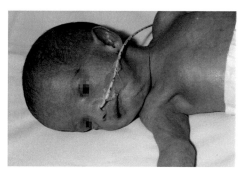

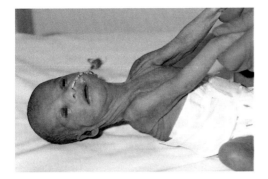

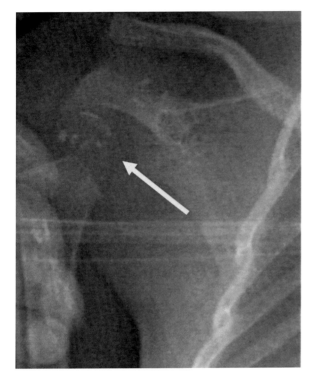

A cranial ultrasound revealed colpocephaly with a thinned corpus callosum. Cortical cysts were found on renal tract ultrasound. Calcific stippling of the humeral epiphysis was seen (above). The newborn hearing screen was failed. Creatinine kinase and NCS/EMG were both normal. Onset of apnoeas was noted on day 30. These episodes were confirmed as seizures on aEEG and were treated with levetiracetam. Further investigations included analysis of very long chain fatty acids (VLCFA). The result was consistent with a severe peroxisomal disorder, such as Zellweger's disease.

This infant had profound hypotonia with dysmorphic features and large fontanelle. There was additional CNS involvement and renal cysts. The NCS/EMG did not point to a specific anatomical location. The history of consanguinity would have increased the chance of this infant having an autosomal recessive condition. She was found to be homozygous for a mutation in the PEX5 gene, confirming the diagnosis of Zellweger disease, the severe end of Zellweger spectrum disorders. As an autosomal recessive disorder, there would be a 1 in 4 chance of a further child with Zellweger's disease.

Neonatal hypotonia is a common clinical presentation but with a wide differential diagnosis that includes systemic illness, central nervous system pathology and peripheral neuromuscular diseases. There are key components to elicit from both the history and examination which can then lead to the appropriate investigations. Understanding the range of possible underlying causes can help in the recognition and treatment of the main conditions associated with reduced tone in the newborn infant.

References

1. Sparks SE. Neonatal hypotonia. Clin Perinatol. 2015;42(2):71, ix.
2. Birdi K, Prasad AN, Prasad C, Chodirker B, Chudley AE. The floppy infant: retrospective analysis of clinical experience (1990-2000) in a tertiary care facility. J Child Neurol. 2005;20(10):803–8.
3. Hartley L, Ranjan R. Evaluation of the floppy infant. Paediatr Child Health. 2015;25(11):498–504.
4. Leyenaar J, Camfield P, Camfield C. A schematic approach to hypotonia in infancy. Paediatr Child Health. 2005;10(7):397–400.
5. Chan K-K, Darras BT. Neonatal hypotonia. In: Perlman JM, editor. Neurology. 2nd ed. Philadelphia: Elsevier; 2008. p. 172–94.
6. Wattendorf DJ, Muenke M. Prader-Willi syndrome. Am Fam Physician. 2005;72(5):827–30.
7. Dubowitz LM, Dubowitz V, Mercuri E. The neurological assessment of the preterm and full-term newborn infant. 2nd ed. London: Mac Keith Press; 1999.
8. Dubowitz L, Ricciw D, Mercuri E. The Dubowitz neurological examination of the full-term newborn. Ment Retard Dev Disabil Res Rev. 2005;11(1):52–60.
9. Wusthoff CJ. How to use: the neonatal neurological examination. Arch Dis Child Educ Pract Ed. 2013;98(4):148–53.
10. Harris SR. Congenital hypotonia: clinical and developmental assessment. Dev Med Child Neurol. 2008;50(12):889–92.
11. Yazowitz E, Delfiner L, Moshé SL. Neonatal hypotonia. NeoReviews. 2018;19(8):e455.
12. Richer LP, Shevell MI, Miller SP. Diagnostic profile of neonatal hypotonia: an 11-year study. Pediatr Neurol. 2001;25(1):32–7.
13. Ankala A, Hegde MR. Gamut of genetic testing for neonatal care. Clin Perinatol. 2015;42(2):26, vii.
14. Lalani SR. Current genetic testing tools in neonatal medicine. Pediatr Neonatol. 2017;58(2):111–21.

15. Mercuri E, Muntoni F. The neonate with a neuromuscular disorder. In: Rutherford MA, editor. MRI of the neonatal brain. London: W.B. Saunders; 2002.
16. Barkovich AJ, Guerrini R, Kuzniecky RI, Jackson GD, Dobyns WB. A developmental and genetic classification for malformations of cortical development: update 2012. Brain. 2012;135(Pt 5):1348–69.
17. Kang PB. Pediatric nerve conduction studies and EMG. In: Blum AS, Rutkove SB, editors. The clinical neurophysiology primer. Totowa: Humana Press; 2007. p. 369–89.
18. Ahmed MI, Iqbal M, Hussain N. A structured approach to the assessment of a floppy neonate. J Pediatr Neurosci. 2016;11(1):2–6.
19. Natarajan N, Ionita C. Neonatal neuromuscular disorders. In: Gleason CA, Juul SE, editors. Avery's diseases of the newborn. 10th ed. New York: Elsevier Health Sciences; 2017. p. 952–60.
20. Amato M, Nagel R, Huppi P. Creatine-kinase MM in the perinatal period. Klin Padiatr. 1991;203(5):389–94.
21. Darras BT, Kang PB. Clinical trials in spinal muscular atrophy. Curr Opin Pediatr. 2007;19(6):675–9.
22. Wan L, Dreyfuss G. Splicing-correcting therapy for SMA. Cell. 2017;170(1):5.
23. Singh RN, Howell MD, Ottesen EW, Singh NN. Diverse role of survival motor neuron protein. Biochim Biophys Acta Gene Regul Mech. 2017;1860(3):299–315.
24. D'Amico A, Mercuri E, Tiziano FD, Bertini E. Spinal muscular atrophy. Orphanet J Rare Dis. 2011;6:71.
25. Al Dakhoul S. Very severe spinal muscular atrophy (type 0). Avicenna J Med. 2017;7(1):32–3.
26. Singh NN, Howell MD, Androphy EJ, Singh RN. How the discovery of ISS-N1 led to the first medical therapy for spinal muscular atrophy. Gene Ther. 2017;24(9):520–6.
27. Feldkotter M, Schwarzer V, Wirth R, Wienker TF, Wirth B. Quantitative analyses of SMN1 and SMN2 based on real-time lightCycler PCR: fast and highly reliable carrier testing and prediction of severity of spinal muscular atrophy. Am J Hum Genet. 2002;70(2):358–68.
28. Butchbach ME. Copy number variations in the survival motor neuron genes: implications for spinal muscular atrophy and other neurodegenerative diseases. Front Mol Biosci. 2016;3:7.
29. Finkel RS, Mercuri E, Darras BT, Connolly AM, Kuntz NL, Kirschner J, et al. Nusinersen versus sham control in infantile-onset spinal muscular atrophy. N Engl J Med. 2017;377(18):1723–32.
30. Gidaro T, Servais L. Nusinersen treatment of spinal muscular atrophy: current knowledge and existing gaps. Dev Med Child Neurol. 2019;61(1):19–24.
31. Neil EE, Bisaccia EK. Nusinersen: a novel antisense oligonucleotide for the treatment of spinal muscular atrophy. J Pediatr Pharmacol Ther. 2019;24(3):194–203.
32. Burgart AM, Magnus D, Tabor HK, Paquette ED, Frader J, Glover JJ, et al. Ethical challenges confronted when providing Nusinersen treatment for spinal muscular atrophy. JAMA Pediatr. 2018;172(2):188–92.
33. Mendell JR, Al-Zaidy S, Shell R, Arnold WD, Rodino-Klapac LR, Prior TW, et al. Single-dose gene-replacement therapy for spinal muscular atrophy. N Engl J Med. 2017;377(18):1713–22.
34. Darras BT, Volpe JJ. Muscle involvement and restricted disorders. In: Volpe JJ, editor. Volpe's neurology of the newborn. 6th ed. Philadelphia: Elsevier; 2018. p. 922–70.
35. Turner C, Hilton-Jones D. The myotonic dystrophies: diagnosis and management. J Neurol Neurosurg Psychiatry. 2010;81(4):358–67.
36. Ho G, Cardamone M, Farrar M. Congenital and childhood myotonic dystrophy: current aspects of disease and future directions. World J Clin Pediatr. 2015;4(4):66–80.
37. Mills KR. The basics of electromyography. J Neurol Neurosurg Psychiatry. 2005;76(Suppl 2):5.
38. Rutherford MA, Heckmatt JZ, Dubowitz V. Congenital myotonic dystrophy: respiratory function at birth determines survival. Arch Dis Child. 1989;64(2):191–5.
39. Campbell C, Sherlock R, Jacob P, Blayney M. Congenital myotonic dystrophy: assisted ventilation duration and outcome. Pediatrics. 2004;113(4):811–6.
40. Ho G, Carey KA, Cardamone M, Farrar MA. Myotonic dystrophy type 1: clinical manifestations in children and adolescents. Arch Dis Child. 2019;104(1):48–52.

41. Cassidy SB, Driscoll DJ. Prader-Willi syndrome. Eur J Hum Genet. 2009;17(1):3–13.
42. Singh P, Mahmoud R, Gold J, Tamura RN, Miller JL, Butler MG, et al. Perinatal complications associated with Prader-Willi syndrome (PWS)—comparison to the general population and among the different genetic subtypes. Pediatrics. 2018;142(1 MeetingAbstract):230A.
43. Whittington JE, Holland AJ, Webb T, Butler J, Clarke D, Boer H. Population prevalence and estimated birth incidence and mortality rate for people with Prader-Willi syndrome in one UK Health Region. J Med Genet. 2001;38(11):792–8.
44. Tuysuz B, Kartal N, Erener-Ercan T, Guclu-Geyik F, Vural M, Perk Y, et al. Prevalence of Prader-Willi syndrome among infants with hypotonia. J Pediatr. 2014;164(5):1064–7.
45. Smith A, Hung D. The dilemma of diagnostic testing for Prader-Willi syndrome. Transl Pediatr. 2017;6(1):46–56.
46. Mallik A, Weir AI. Nerve conduction studies: essentials and pitfalls in practice. J Neurol Neurosurg Psychiatry. 2005;76(Suppl 2):31.
47. Ouvrier RA, McLeod JG, Conchin TE. The hypertrophic forms of hereditary motor and sensory neuropathy. A study of hypertrophic Charcot-Marie-Tooth disease (HMSN type I) and Dejerine-Sottas disease (HMSN type III) in childhood. Brain. 1987;110(Pt 1):121–48.
48. Wilmshurst JM, Pollard JD, Nicholson G, Antony J, Ouvrier R. Peripheral neuropathies of infancy. Dev Med Child Neurol. 2003;45(6):408–14.
49. Yiu EM, Ryan MM. Genetic axonal neuropathies and neuronopathies of pre-natal and infantile onset. J Peripher Nerv Syst. 2012;17(3):285–300.
50. Darras BT, Volpe JJ. Levels above lower motor neurone to neuromuscular junction. In: Volpe J, editor. Volpe's neurology of the newborn. 6th ed. Philadelphia: Elsevier. p. 887–921.
51. Choi HW, Kuntz NL. Peripheral nerve disorders in the neonate. NeoReviews. 2016;17(12):e728.
52. Jovandaric MZ, Despotovic DJ, Jesic MM, Jesic MD. Neonatal outcome in pregnancies with autoimmune myasthenia gravis. Fetal Pediatr Pathol. 2016;35(3):167–72.
53. Parr JR, Andrew MJ, Finnis M, Beeson D, Vincent A, Jayawant S. How common is childhood myasthenia? The UK incidence and prevalence of autoimmune and congenital myasthenia. Arch Dis Child. 2014;99(6):539–42.
54. Engel AG, Shen XM, Selcen D, Sine SM. Congenital myasthenic syndromes: pathogenesis, diagnosis, and treatment. Lancet Neurol. 2015;14(4):420–34.
55. Rodriguez Cruz PM, Palace J, Beeson D. The neuromuscular junction and wide heterogeneity of congenital myasthenic syndromes. Int J Mol Sci. 2018;19(6). https://doi.org/10.3390/ijms19061677.
56. Khan A, Hussain N, Gosalakkal JA. Bulbar dysfunction: an early presentation of congenital myasthenic syndrome in three infants. J Pediatr Neurosci. 2011;6(2):124–6.
57. Smith JK, Burns S, Cunningham S, Freeman J, McLellan A, McWilliam K. The hazards of honey: infantile botulism. BMJ Case Rep. 2010;2010. https://doi.org/10.1136/bcr.05.2010.3038.
58. Abdulla CO, Ayubi A, Zulfiquer F, Santhanam G, Ahmed MA, Deeb J. Infant botulism following honey ingestion. BMJ Case Rep. 2012;2012. https://doi.org/10.1136/bcr.11.2011.5153.
59. Norwood FL, Harling C, Chinnery PF, Eagle M, Bushby K, Straub V. Prevalence of genetic muscle disease in northern England: in-depth analysis of a muscle clinic population. Brain. 2009;132(Pt 11):3175–86.
60. Falsaperla R, Pratico AD, Ruggieri M, Parano E, Rizzo R, Corsello G, et al. Congenital muscular dystrophy: from muscle to brain. Ital J Pediatr. 2016;42(1):9.
61. Bonnemann CG, Wang CH, Quijano-Roy S, Deconinck N, Bertini E, Ferreiro A, et al. Diagnostic approach to the congenital muscular dystrophies. Neuromuscul Disord. 2014;24(4):289–311.
62. Fu XN, Xiong H. Genetic and clinical advances of congenital muscular dystrophy. Chin Med J. 2017;130(21):2624–31.
63. North KN. Clinical approach to the diagnosis of congenital myopathies. Semin Pediatr Neurol. 2011;18(4):216–20.
64. North KN, Wang CH, Clarke N, Jungbluth H, Vainzof M, Dowling JJ, et al. Approach to the diagnosis of congenital myopathies. Neuromuscul Disord. 2014;24(2):97–116.

65. Cassandrini D, Trovato R, Rubegni A, Lenzi S, Fiorillo C, Baldacci J, et al. Congenital myopathies: clinical phenotypes and new diagnostic tools. Ital J Pediatr. 2017;43(1):z.
66. Frazer L, Florence A, Warner D. Why the long face? A case of neonatal hypotonia. Pediatrics. 2018;142(1 Meeting Astract).
67. Bharucha-Gocbcl DX, Santi M, Medne L, Zukosky K, Dastgir J, Shieh PB, et al. Severe congenital RYR1-associated myopathy: the expanding clinicopathologic and genetic spectrum. Neurology. 2013;80(17):1584–9.
68. Prasad AN, Prasad C. The floppy infant: contribution of genetic and metabolic disorders. Brain Dev. 2003;25(7):457–76.
69. Uusimaa J, Jungbluth H, Fratter C, Crisponi G, Feng L, Zeviani M, et al. Reversible infantile respiratory chain deficiency is a unique, genetically heterogenous mitochondrial disease. J Med Genet. 2011;48(10):660–8.
70. Martinez M, Romero MG, Guereta LG, Cabrera M, Regojo RM, Albajara L, et al. Infantile-onset Pompe disease with neonatal debut: a case report and literature review. Medicine (Baltimore). 2017;96(51):e9186.
71. Klouwer FC, Berendse K, Ferdinandusse S, Wanders RJ, Engelen M, Poll-The BT. Zellweger spectrum disorders: clinical overview and management approach. Orphanet J Rare Dis. 2015;10:9.
72. Rais Dana J, Tunnessen WW. Picture of the month. Zellweger (cerebro-hepato-renal) syndrome. Arch Pediatr Adolesc Med. 1999;153(10):1105–6.

Chapter 6
Critical Congenital Heart Disease

Katie Linter and Thomas Mukasa

Introduction

Concepts in diagnosis and management of critical, ductus dependent, congenital heart disease that are life threatening to the fetus and the neonate continue to be both challenging and exciting since the first neonatal surgeries over 40 years ago [1]. The team ethos of exceeding expectations has led to individual survival stories, previously, thought to be inconceivable to become a reality. For example, a baby born with the heart outside the body, despite a miserable prognosis and expectation of death ex-utero, can survive through the innovation and determination of multiple professionals [2, 3]. There are now cohorts of adults who are employed and have their own families, who just 30 years ago would not have been expected to live beyond the first few days of life.

This chapter focuses on the types of duct-dependent critical congenital heart disease for which survival beyond the neonatal period is close to zero without intervention. For most lesions in which a biventricular circulation is achievable, prognosis is good but despite excellent surgical technique most of these infants will need multiple procedures during their life. An example would be Tetralogy of Fallot when the arterial duct is the only source of pulmonary blood flow. The risks of surgery and subsequent re-intervention become higher when there is an anomaly within the heart, for example a ventricular septal defect (VSD) seen together with aortic arch interruption or obstruction [4, 5].

K. Linter (✉) • T. Mukasa
East Midlands Congenital Heart Centre, University Hospitals of Leicester NHS Trust, Leicester, UK
e-mail: katie.linter@uhl-tr.nhs.uk; thomas.mukasa@uhl-tr.nhs.uk

© Springer Nature Switzerland AG 2020
E. M. Boyle, J. Cusack (eds.), *Emerging Topics and Controversies in Neonatology*, https://doi.org/10.1007/978-3-030-28829-7_6

The spectrum for single ventricle anomalies is wide. There are relatively established surgical pathways for single ventricle palliation and the short and midterm outcomes are reasonable. Longer term outcomes continue to be guarded, but there are now many adults who were born with these conditions living full and productive lives. Malevolent combinations of atrial isomerism, ventricular hypoplasia right or left, with pulmonary venous obstruction or complete heart block carry a far bleaker, mid and longer term prognosis.

Surgical risk is increasingly determined by, and made significantly higher by, the unmodifiable risk factors of prematurity, low birth weight or an underlying medical condition such as a chromosomal/syndromic diagnosis. As postoperative survival improves, our focus looks to reaching the maximum physical and neurodevelopmental, potential of each individual affected by congenital heart disease [6, 7].

What is crystal clear is that information about the underlying morphology of the anomaly, the nuances of the diagnosis and the specific characteristics of the individual fetus or patient is critical. Advances in the understanding of cardiac gene expression and morphogenesis, and how this is linked with brain morphogenesis will be discussed here. Technological advances in both surgery and catheter intervention continue to evolve and debate about the proposed interventional plan heightens with more international, single and multicentre, published data. The challenges of established best surgical practice are reviewed using the two ventricle example of Pulmonary Atresia, VSD and a ductus dependent pulmonary circulation and the single ventricle example of Hypoplastic Left Heart Syndrome (HLHS).

For the congenital cardiac community there is a duty to collect and publish outcome data with regard to management strategy and survival. Alongside the success in improving survival comes the importance of the assessment and monitoring of neurodevelopmental outcome and overall quality of life.

Genetics

The majority of congenital heart anomalies occur sporadically and currently recognised risk factors or identified gene variants do not always provide an answer to the question of how these occurred. When a recognised chromosomal anomaly or gene change can be identified, more definitive information about prognosis can be given to the individual and their family. The combination of and interaction between environment, chromosomal and single gene anomalies is very complex. Reflecting this is the increasing identification of multiple combinations of genes, gene-modifiers and the interaction of these with environmental factors [8–10]. Despite this complexity, there is tremendous potential for developing a personalised approach to the care of a patient with congenital cardiac disease and tailored counselling for their relatives.

Teratogens

Many population based databases for the collection of data for congenital anomalies or birth defect surveillance exist. Analysis of data, between 2003 and 2012, from the European Surveillance of Congenital Anomalies (EUROCAT) observed a statistically significant increasing trend for severe congenital heart disease as a whole and, individually for single ventricle, Tetralogy of Fallot and Atrioventricular Septal defects.

Datasets are from live births, fetal deaths and terminations of pregnancy, excluding chromosomal anomalies, reported in 25 population based registries across Europe [11, 12]. Embryonic exposure to maternal illness such as congenital infection, diabetes, obesity, exposure to maternal smoking or alcohol abuse and assisted reproduction techniques are considered to be the main risk factors associated with congenital heart disease. The increased prevalence of diabetes, high maternal body mass index and assisted reproductive techniques in the same population in the same period may explain some of this.

Chromosomal Microarray and DNA Analysis

Variations in DNA, for example, clinically significant micro-duplications, rearrangements or microdeletions (copy note variations) can now be identified using chromosomal microarray analysis. This has become the standard for pre and postnatal genetic diagnosis when a cardiac anomaly has been identified. As this technique evolved, areas in a genomic region could be recognised as having an association with risk for a congenital heart defect (Tables 6.1 and 6.2). In a study designed to determine whether pathogenic copy note variants among infants with a single ventricle anomaly were associated with a worse neurocognitive outcome, greater than 70% of children had a copy note variation (CNV) associated with genomic, pathogenic disorders but no dysmorphic or extra-cardiac anomaly.

Potentially, in the future, consideration could be given to incorporating copy note variant status in the design of clinical trials [13]. Possession of a specific CNV could put an infant at more risk of an extreme inflammatory response related to cardiopulmonary bypass for example.

Finding a specific, identified single gene variant within a genomic region may help to inform an individual or their family of the predicted outcome for their disease and potential for other family members to be affected and screened. In the research setting microarray data has shed light on the complex morphogenesis of cardiac development [14, 15]. There are intricate signalling pathways directing the transformation of cardiac progenitor cells, cardiomyocyte differentiation, migration and cell death. Mutation in genes can be identified and with appropriate analysis, a mutation could be linked with altered expression of the genes, which have a central role in the aspects of such pathways.

Table 6.1 Typical cardiac anomalies associated with a syndromic diagnosis identifiable using chromosomal microarray

Syndromic		
Copy number variation		
22q11.2 deletion	DiGeorge	Left and right outflow tract
7q11.23 deletion	Williams	Supra aortic stenosis
XO	Turners	Coarctation of aorta
8p23.1 duplication		Atrioventricular septal defect Single ventricle
1q21.1 deletion		Aortic arch anomalies
Single gene anomaly		
PTPN11, RAS	Noonan	Pulmonary stenosis Hypertrophic cardiomyopathy
JAG1, NOTCH2	Alagille	Peripheral pulmonary stenosis
TBX5	Holt-oram	Atrial septal defect Ventricular septal defect
DHCR7	Smith-lemli-opitz	Atrioventricular septal defect Patent arterial duct Ventricular septal defect
TAZ	Barth	Cardiomyopathy

Table 6.2 Typical cardiac anomalies associated with a single gene anomaly identifiable using chromosomal microarray

Non-syndromic		
Familial	NOTCH1	Bicuspid aortic valve Aortopathy
	GATA4	Atrioventricular septal defect
	FBN1	Aortopathy
Mitochondial	ACAD9	Cardiomyopathy

Genome Sequencing

The technologies that allow massive parallel sequencing (MPS) are newer and allow multiple fragments of genome sequences at nucleic acid level to be screened at once. This DNA sequencing technology, either as exome sequencing or whole-genome sequencing, has immensely increased power to identify sources of genetic variation. This is further explored in Chapter 33.

Genomic sequencing has confirmed that assumed "pathogenic" variants are present at higher rates among patients with observed congenital heart disease, neurodevelopmental disorders and other extracardiac anomalies. This type of sequencing has also shown that additional variation within genes provides some explanation of why reduced penetrance and variable expressivity are seen within the same family. Targeted exome sequence analysis by identifying "de novo" mutations in a gene highly expressed in both heart and brain together demonstrate a definite link existing between heart anomalies and neurodevelopmental function quite separate to postnatal factors detrimental to the developing brain.

In the United Kingdom and Republic of Ireland, there are two recent studies, the results of which are expected to be particularly important for individuals with congenital heart disease [16, 17]. The Deciphering Developmental Disorders (DDD) study uses microarray and sequencing techniques to potentially identify new genetic diagnoses in children with a developmental disorder in whom a diagnosis using conventional testing has not yet been identified. The 100,000 Genome Project sequences the whole genome—every nucleic acid, for every participant in the project. Each individual has a known rare disease. The genome is then compared to a reference genome and compared to a specialist gene panel when appropriate.

The aim of linking rare conditions with the same or similar mutation potentially allows improved patient specific care, better knowledge of the anticipated outcome and better risk counselling in future pregnancies. With insight from this information it may be possible to modify the disease, target medical therapies at patients that will specifically benefit from them, for example, which patients with a single ventricle are likely to benefit from transplantation and when.

Modification of Short Term Outcome

Prenatal Diagnosis

When a prenatal diagnosis is made, an improvement in postoperative survival seems intuitive, but there is no convincing evidence that a prenatal diagnosis influences postoperative survival. Consistently a prenatal diagnosis has not been shown to confer a post-surgical advantage in immediate or 1 year survival [17] or in the longer term neurodevelopmental outcome.

There are multi-factorial considerations, both innate and modifiable, to take into account when assessing outcomes. Attempts to successfully tease out potential benefits are thwarted by findings coming from retrospective population based studies in which there is an inevitable temporal effect on the interpretation of results. Outcome data from specialist tertiary centres affiliated with a surgical congenital heart centre are not easy to compare to the wider population, which includes postnatal deliveries in a non-specialist centre at a distant location requiring neonatal transfer. Transposition of the great arteries is the only specific cardiac diagnosis in which a prenatal diagnosis has been shown to provide some benefit. Balloon atrial septostomy can occur promptly before decompensation as the atrial septum becomes restrictive.

Whilst it is difficult to prove better longer term postoperative survival when there has been an antenatal diagnosis, it is hard to ignore potential benefits. A prenatal diagnosis allows optimisation of the pre-operative status from birth, informed counselling and decisions to be made around the timing and location of delivery [18].

A genetic diagnosis can be made through amniocentesis and this can help to recognise and plan for other co-morbidities. The more stable pre-operative course facilitated by this, whilst not affecting post-surgical survival, may impact on brain maturation, avoidance of end-organ insult and long term neurodevelopment.

A multidisciplinary team, including the fetal maternal medicine team, neonatology, interventional cardiology and surgery, can be prepared and primed for immediate postnatal intervention. In the case, for example, of an expected delivery of a fetus having Hypoplastic Left Heart Syndrome (HLHS) with a thickened restrictive or intact atrial septum, it may be necessary for the infant to be delivered by caesarean section with immediate postnatal intervention to decompress the left atrium and availability of mechanical support. It is possible to identify this antenatally and, when there is a high level of anticipation that an infant will be critically unstable immediately after delivery, the parents can be counselled of the likely futility of active treatment. In this situation, the emotional needs of the expectant parents and family may be better served by avoiding the devastating impact of such an extreme diagnosis and even the possible guilt they may feel when their baby has presented, out of hospital, critically ill. There is opportunity to digest objective information, and to discuss any association with potential neurodevelopmental delay, [19] establish contacts in a positive, supportive way via social networks and the wider family can be prepared and hopefully primed to support the parents. It also allows parents the time to consider the future and some conclude that continuing with the pregnancy is not an option when taking many personal factors into account.

There are also financial implications for healthcare providers associated with a prenatal diagnosis. The costs of a collapsed infant requiring emergency resuscitation, neonatal transfer to a surgical centre and a period of intensive care resulting in a time delay on reaching surgery are significant.

Targets for Antenatal and Fetal Intervention

Decreasing the Likelihood of Premature and Early Term Delivery

Intervention targeted at decreasing the likelihood of premature delivery, when a severe congenital heart defect is diagnosed in utero, is a conceivable antenatal option that could positively impact on the neonatal outcome.

Database analyses of large cohort populations of very/extremely preterm babies have shown a strong correlation between gestation at birth and an increased birth prevalence of severe defects when compared to the same size group of term neonates (7.4/1000 vs. 1.5/1000) [20, 21]. In the same study, when evaluating groups by gestational age, unsurprisingly there was a markedly higher mortality in babies born between 25–26 and 31–32 weeks of gestation.

The advantages of delivering at term and the benefits of a vaginal delivery are also internationally recognised and advocated. Studies of early term babies (37–38 weeks of gestation) demonstrated statistically higher in-hospital mortality and higher risks of one or more major post-operative complications when compared to group of infants born at 39 weeks and above, even when data were adjusted according to risk. There may also be a longer term benefit beyond perioperative mortality and morbidity when considering neurodevelopment. At term, brain maturation in neonates with HLHS or TGA is shown to be delayed by approximately 1 month compared with a normative sample [22]. The neurodevelopmental profile of this group of children exposed to cardiopulmonary bypass is similar to that of premature infants. Each group shares a vulnerability to hypoxia-ischaemia that is consistent with brain immaturity at the time of the insult. Delivering a further 2–3 weeks earlier potentially may predispose a more immature brain still, further to hypoxia prior to, during and after the operation.

Fetal Aortic Valvuloplasty

Fetal aortic valvuloplasty, undertaken usually at about 24 weeks of gestation, is an intervention to optimise left ventricular size in cases of critical aortic valve disease, in order to establish a biventricular circulation, postnatally, is at least in theory, irresistible. The reality is less inviting and results are mixed [23, 24]. For a successful outcome, biventricular repair should be obtainable. This may be completed initially or as staged surgery. If, after delivery, the left ventricular size remains borderline and unlikely to support an adequate cardiac output, the first surgery would be to reconstruct the aortic arch and place a shunt to secure pulmonary blood flow (for example, the Norwood operation). The next surgery, usually performed within a few months of life would be a subsequent conversion to a biventricular circulation.

Aortic valvuloplasty in fetal life is only the first step of a dedicated strategy with expectation of repeat transcatheter and surgical intervention with the goal of reaching a biventricular circulation. Acknowledgement has to be given to the risks to the mother and to the fetus. Due to small numbers, longer term outcome is not known. With ongoing improvements in surgical outcomes after the Norwood operation some would consider surgery after delivery to be a less risky and better option at least in the short to midterm.

In-Utero Stabilisation

Procedural and registry outcome data from the Fetal Cardiac Intervention Registry show that, in selected cases, when a prenatal diagnosis of the potentially lethal combination of hypoplastic left heart with intact atrial septum is made in utero, techniques to perforate the atrial septum and place an inter-atrial stent in-utero are technically feasible [25]. When the procedure is undertaken earlier in gestation, when the fetal heart is large enough to accommodate the needle, sheaths and stents that are required, the intention is to reverse or attenuate the pulmonary vascular changes that lead to a very high mortality in the infant after birth and postoperatively.

In later gestation, creating a non-restrictive foramen ovale at delivery may reduce the need for caesarean section and immediate, high risk, intervention. However, the procedure itself carries a high risk of fetal demise.

Maternal Hyperoxygenation Therapy

There is long standing research into the haemodynamics of placental, fetal and cere-brovascular blood flow from studies of intrauterine growth restriction and placental dysfunction. Giving high levels of oxygen to mothers antenatally can increase blood oxygen level of the fetus.

In congenital heart disease with small left sided structures this concept is impor-tant for two reasons. In fetal life, when the left ventricle is small and diastolic filling is restricted, there is preferential flow through the arterial duct with less flow to the developing lungs and pulmonary venous/preload to the left ventricle. With inade-quate flow through the left side of heart, delivery of oxygen to the developing brain is retrograde from the arterial duct, which may compromise cerebral oxygenation and brain maturation. Increasing the blood oxygen level of the fetus should produce an increase in pulmonary blood flow and thus increased venous return to the left side of the heart. Giving supplemental oxygen to the mother, and thereby optimising left ventricular growth and brain maturation, with a level of neuroprotection, in utero by manipulating fetal blood flow is very appealing [26, 27].

There have been a multitude of pilot and feasibility studies but the amount of oxygen, the length of therapy, the optimal gestation of therapy and potential risk to mother remain as yet undetermined.

Decision Making Around Surgical Approach

Neonatal cardiac surgery is high risk and this risk for each infant will vary consider-ably according to gestational age, weight and risk factors. This group of patients could have either a chromosomal or syndromic diagnosis as well as pre-procedural co-morbidities such as prematurity, necrotising enterocolitis, septicaemia, mechani-cal support, shock, acidosis, pulmonary hypertension and impaired heart function. Collecting mortality data is an integral part of quality assurance for centres under-taking surgical procedures, and differing systems have been used to take into account these risks according to procedure and case. Interpretation of data can be fraught due to wide range of case mix and case complexity.

Gestational Age and Birth Weight

With the advances in myocardial preservation, cannulation techniques and postoperative intensive care, most cardiac surgery for a duct dependent cardiac anomaly in a neonate is feasible at term and at a weight as low as 2.5 kg with acceptably low mortality and morbidity. There are increasing numbers of reports to show that, despite birth weights less than 2.5 kg, although associated with higher mortality, and longer hospital stay, the short term and midterm outcomes are reasonable. Poorer outcomes may not be intrinsically related to surgery at low birth weight but more to do with a lower gestational age as the major independent risk factor [28, 29].

Regardless of chronological age or weight, as the pulmonary arterial pressures decrease. Inevitably, a duct dependent circulation becomes progressively more unbalanced and risk of serious complication of death of infant increases. If tissue oxygen demand is not met, hypoxia with anaerobic metabolism ensues and, uncorrected, this will culminate in multiple organ failure and death [30, 31]. The increased risk of operating on a low birthweight or premature baby in a stable, well balanced status may be considered preferable to deferring surgery to reach a larger weight or more maturity. Earlier surgery may avoid the complications of acute destabilisation, necrotising enterocolitis, brain injury and sepsis in a premature or low birth weight neonate with increased pulmonary blood flow and borderline cardiac output.

Individualised decisions are made taking all these factors together with the details of the underlying heart defect and feasibility of different interventions into account.

Surgical Strategy

The surgical approach to congenital heart disease will be discussed for two conditions; Tetralogy of Fallot with pulmonary atresia (TOF/PA) and Hypoplastic Left Heart Syndrome.

In TOF/PA the combination of a ventricular septal defect (VSD) and duct dependent pulmonary blood flow, manifests as a diverse spectrum. Differing approaches, including staged palliative surgeries, percutaneous intervention or early neonatal surgical repair, have been published as case reviews, cohort studies and large, multicentre trials [31–34].

The goal of treatment is to provide a secure source of pulmonary blood flow that will promote growth of the pulmonary arteries, whilst avoiding distortion. Too little pulmonary blood flow will result in reduced oxygen saturations, and too much can compromise systemic output. When considering the merits of each approach the number of repeat interventions in the future must also be taken into account. The approach that is chosen will depend on the precise anatomy, the pre-operative status including the presence of low birth weight or chromosomal anomaly and the philosophy of the surgeon or surgical centre.

Seventy five years ago, in order to improve profound cyanosis, the first cases of an anastomosis between the end of the subclavian artery and the side of the pulmonary artery by Drs Thomas, Taussig and Blalock at the John Hopkins Hospital, Baltimore, US were reported [35]. Now a 3–3.5 mm tube of Gore-Tex between the subclavian artery and pulmonary artery is favoured. Inevitably, somatic growth of the infant together with complications of acute or chronic obstruction of the shunt by thrombus or neointimal proliferation will compromise the function of the shunt.

With the introduction of, and advances in cardiopulmonary bypass techniques for the neonate, a different approach was possible. Continuity between the right ventricle and the pulmonary artery became feasible via a conduit or a direct anastomosis. Optimism around better oxygen saturations and a more stable postoperative period prevailed, but evidence of better mid and long term results in terms of pulmonary arterial growth is difficult. Disadvantages include repeat intervention to address proximal or juxtaductal stenosis prior to final stage surgery, shunt inflow blockage or RVOT aneurysm with potential need for repeat surgery before final repair is possible.

Driving the development of percutaneous interventions is the logical benefit of avoiding cardiopulmonary bypass, and consequent neurological insult in the small or preterm baby. Percutaneous procedures, which use radiofrequency to perforate an atretic pulmonary valve, are feasible in selected cases as is placement of a stent within the arterial duct.

Neonatal surgical repair has the advantage of establishing normal oxygen supply to a rapidly maturing brain and potentially better development of the pulmonary arterial tree. Closure of the VSD and establishing secure forward flow from the right ventricle to the pulmonary arteries can be performed on cardiopulmonary bypass in a neonate or young infant and this is also reported as having good outcomes. The VSD is closed and right ventricle to pulmonary artery continuity can be as a RV to PA conduit, a transannular patch or a valve-sparing procedure. Preserving the pulmonary valve tackles the problem of a transannular patch in a small baby and longer term complications of chronic pulmonary regurgitation.

To shorten length of time on cardiopulmonary bypass, with careful consideration, a newer, hybrid approach with closure of VSD and intraoperative balloon dilatation of the pulmonary annulus could be considered. Reported mortality rates from neonatal surgery are low but there is a significantly higher need for reintervention, soon after surgery, particularly if the size of the pulmonary valve annulus is inadequate, when a right ventricle to pulmonary artery conduit becomes necessary. New technologies evolving with time and experience, in the absence of randomised controlled trials, is likely to continue to sustain differing approaches.

Hypoplastic Left Heart Syndrome and Variants: Staged Palliation for a Single Ventricle Circulation

A full review of the management of Hypoplastic Left Heart Syndrome (HLHS) and variants with poorly developed left sided heart structures is beyond the scope of this chapter. There are many excellent reviews detailing different management options for HLHS which comprises 1.5–4% of congenital heart disease from antenatal diagnosis to adulthood [36–40] Heart transplantation is also reviewed, as first surgery for a neonate with HLHS and for the group of single ventricle patients in whom such staged palliation eventually fails. Survivors of the early surgical era are now in their forties.

Surgery in the neonatal period is the first stage of establishing a single ventricle circulation either with left or right ventricle morphology with the final aim of separating the pulmonary and systemic circulations, and normalising oxygen saturations. The Norwood Operation, first attempted in 1979 [41, 42] has evolved as a surgical technique to establish an unobstructed systemic circulation by reconstructing the aorta with incorporation of the main pulmonary artery and patching of a small hypoplastic aortic arch. The atrial septum is removed, permitting unobstructed pulmonary venous return, and a source of controlled pulmonary blood flow is established either with a BT shunt or a right ventricle to pulmonary artery shunt.

Coronary compromise during diastole is a feared complication of the continuous flow through a BT shunt. The alternative is pulmonary blood flow secured with a shunt from the right ventricle to the pulmonary artery protecting myocardial perfusion but with the disadvantage of a ventriculotomy in the systemic right ventricle. Evidence of benefit of one type of shunt versus the other has not been shown, despite studies comparing the two [43].

Initial mortality after the Norwood Procedure has improved significantly. Analysis of National UK data collected between 2014 and 2017 demonstrated an average 30 day survival for the Norwood Procedure of 90% [44]. As the immediate postoperative mortality decreases, there still remains a high risk of morbidity affecting multiple systems—respiratory, neurological and nutrition and associated long length of hospital stay. Beyond, the first 30 days, there is still significant attrition with only 60–70% of infants requiring surgical palliation and following a single ventricle pathway, surviving to adulthood.

After the Norwood operation, the second stage of surgery will be performed between 4 and 5 months of age. This is a bidirectional Glenn procedure to take down the arterial shunt and anastomose the superior caval vein to the pulmonary arteries providing a more secure source of blood supply to the lungs.

The hybrid procedure was developed and utilised to avoid cardiopulmonary bypass in the immediate neonatal period [45–47] The hypoplastic aorta is bypassed by stenting of the arterial duct providing systemic supply and bilateral pulmonary artery bands are surgically applied to control pulmonary blood flow thus balancing the systemic and pulmonary circulations. The second stage of surgery takes place between 4 and 5 months of age. It is subsequently more complex but in a more physically and neurologically mature infant. The aortic arch is reconstructed using a modified Norwood technique, the pulmonary artery bands are removed and an anastomosis between the superior vena cava and the pulmonary arteries is constructed. For some surgical centres, the hybrid procedure will be the surgical approach of choice with good reported outcomes [48, 49]. Other centres will use the hybrid procedure only when the Norwood operation is considered too high risk.

The third surgery following either a surgical Norwood and Glenn procedure or a hybrid surgical approach will be, between 3 and 5 years, to anastomose the inferior caval vein to the pulmonary arteries usually via an extracardiac conduit—the Fontan operation. Heart failure is inevitable, mostly during adulthood, and heart transplantation or palliative care are the only options when heart failure becomes end-stage.

Outcome Data

Mortality

The Common International Paediatric and Congenital Cardiac Disease Code (IPCCD) arose following the establishment of International Congenital Heart Surgery Nomenclature and Database Project of the Society of Thoracic Surgeons (STS) and the European Paediatric Cardiac Code (EPCC) of the Association for European Paediatric Cardiology (AEPC). Both International and European databases were created with goal of collecting data to assess surgical outcome [50].

Risk Adjustment in Congenital Heart Surgery (RACHS-1) categories and Aristotle Basic Complexity (ABC) scores are used to compare the quality of care received by children undergoing heart surgery [51, 52]. These systems can be used to measure expected mortality rates and calculate standardised mortality rates for an institution over time or between institutions in a more meaningful way than mortality rates alone. They are a retrospective review of hospital discharge data, with a consensus of medical experts assigning individual procedures a risk category between 1 and 6. The highest risk cases include cases such as the Norwood procedure for Hypoplastic Left Heart Syndrome. The simplest method of risk adjustment was based on procedure alone but the more complex multivariate method incorporated four additional clinical factors: age stratified as 30 days or less, 31 days to 1 year, and 1 year or older; prematurity and presence of a major non-cardiac structural anomaly in addition to the cardiac defect (for example a tracheoesophageal fistula, cleft lip, and/or palate); and presence of combinations of cardiac surgical procedures. Many studies in centres internationally have validated the relationship between these risk stratification scales and mortality and hospital length of stay.

A disadvantage of these earlier methods was that the assignment of risk was led by expert-based opinion and not by objective data. This led to the establishment of a new system with a range of categories for classifying congenital heart surgery procedures based on their potential for in-hospital mortality. These categories are intended to serve as a stratification variable that can be used to adjust for case mix for the analysis of outcomes.

In the United Kingdom, the National Congenital Heart Disease Audit (NCHDA) has required compulsory submission of data from all centres since 2000. NCHDA is part of a National Clinical Audit and Patient Outcomes Programme (NCAPOP) and is clinically led by the British Congenital Cardiac Association and the Society for Cardiothoracic Surgery in Great Britain and Ireland. Mortality data is generated primarily for cardiac centres for their own quality assurance, and is ongoing to flag changes in performance rapidly and with the data that is collected designed to be time relevant.

Survival

The survival data for each procedure is demonstrated as a funnel plot over a 3 year period. NICOR reports from data collected between 2013 and 2016 in the UK and RoI show survival 30 days after paediatric cardiac surgery for children aged <16 years with congenital heart disease currently close to 98%. None the less, the neonatal population is more vulnerable with considerably higher mortality.

The desire to compare surgical results within a cardiac unit or hospital performance nationally as a marker of performance and for local quality assurance is natural for patients and clinicians. To interpret data in context though survival rates needs to take into account case mix. An unprecedented collaboration of cardiologists, intensivists, surgeons, mathematicians, and statisticians worked to create a Partial Risk Adjustment in Surgery (PRAiS) formula which was first developed in 2011 [53–55]. This model not only takes into account diagnosis and procedural risk but also incorporates risk factors such as congenital and acquired co-morbidities, whether the procedure is performed on or off cardiopulmonary bypass, when surgery for a single ventricle cardiac diagnosis occurs, and the severity of illness in the time preceding surgery.

Conclusions

Through historical trend and published experiences, strategies have become well established for almost every type of congenital heart disease. Pioneering work by all members of this multifaceted team including geneticists, neurobiologists, fetal medicine specialists, clinicians, nurses and surgeons, is continuously opening up new lines of research and technology. The effect of congenital heart disease to the patient is personal and far reaching, both socially and economically. Fundamental to improving care delivery are the skills to share knowledge and inevitable uncertainty with colleagues, our patients and their families.

References

1. Edmunds L, Fishman N, Gregory G, Heymann M, Hoffman J, Robinson S, Roe B, Rudolph A, Stanger P. Cardiac surgery in infants less than six weeks of age. Circulation. 1972;XLVI:250–6.
2. https://www.leicesterhospitalscharity.org.uk/baby-vanellope-hope. Accessed 21 June 2019.
3. Türkyilmaz G, Avcı S, Sıvrıkoz T, Erturk E, Altunoglu U, Turkyilmazlmaz SE, Kalelioglu IH, Has R, Yuksel A. Prenatal diagnosis and management of ectopia cordis: varied presentation spectrum. Fetal Pediatr Pathol. 2019;38(2):127–37.
4. McCrindle B, Tchervenkov C, Konstantinov I, Williams W, Neirotti R, Jacobs M, Blackstone E, Congenital Heart Surgeons Society. Risk factors associated with mortality and interventions in 472 neonates with interrupted aortic arch: a Congenital Heart Surgeons Society study. J Thorac Cardiovasc Surg. 2005;129(2):343–50.

5. Murphy MO, Bellsham-Revell H, Morgan GJ, Krasemann T, Rosenthal E, Qureshi SA, Salih C, Austin CB, Anderson DR. Hybrid procedure for neonates with hypoplastic left heart syndrome at high-risk for Norwood: midterm outcomes. Ann Thorac Surg. 2015;100(6):2286–92.
6. Pizarro C, Davies RR, Woodford E, Radtke WA. Improving early outcomes following hybrid procedure for patients with single ventricle and systemic outflow obstruction: defining risk factors. Eur J Cardiothorac Surg. 2014;47(6):995–1001.
7. Gaynor JW, Stopp C, Wypij D, Andropoulos DB, Atallah J, Atz AM, Beca J, Donofrio MT, Duncan K, Ghanayem NS, Goldberg CS. International Cardiac Collaborative on Neurodevelopment (ICCON) Investigators. Neurodevelopmental outcomes after cardiac surgery in infancy. Pediatrics. 2015;135(5):816–25.
8. Gaynor JW, Stopp C, Wypij D, Andropoulos DB, Atallah J, Atz AM, Beca J, Donofrio MT, Duncan K, Ghanayem NS, Goldberg CS. Neurodevelopmental outcomes after cardiac surgery in infancy. Pediatrics. 2015;135(5):816.
9. Hacıhamdioğlu B, Hacıhamdioğlu D, Delil K. 22q11 deletion syndrome: current perspective. Appl Clin Genet. 2015;8:123.
10. Russell MW, Chung WK, Kaltman JR, Miller TA. Advances in the understanding of the genetic determinants of congenital heart disease and their impact on clinical outcomes. J Am Heart Assoc. 2018;7(6):e006906.
11. Blue GM, Kirk EP, Giannoulatou E, Sholler GF, Dunwoodie SL, Harvey RP, Winlaw DS. Advances in the genetics of congenital heart disease: a clinician's guide. J Am Coll Cardiol. 2017;69(7):859–70.
12. Morris JK, Springett AL, Greenlees R, Loane M, Addor MC, Arriola L, Barisic I, Bergman JE, Csaky-Szunyogh M, Dias C, Draper ES. Trends in congenital anomalies in Europe from 1980 to 2012. PLoS One. 2018;13(4):e0194986.
13. Lynch TA, Abel DE. Teratogens and congenital heart disease. J Diagn Med Sonogr. 2015;31(5):301–5.
14. Carey AS, Liang L, Edwards J, Brandt T, Mei H, Sharp AJ, Hsu DT, Newburger JW, Ohye RG, Chung WK, Russell MW. Effect of copy number variants on outcomes for infants with single ventricle heart defects. Circ Cardiovasc Genet. 2013;6(5):444–51.
15. Homsy J, Zaidi S, Shen Y, Ware JS, Samocha KE, Karczewski KJ, DePalma SR, McKean D, Wakimoto H, Gorham J, Jin SC. De novo mutations in congenital heart disease with neurodevelopmental and other congenital anomalies. Science. 2015;350(6265):1262–6.
16. Luna-Zurita L, Stirnimann CU, Glatt S, Kaynak BL, Thomas S, Baudin F, Samee MAH, He D, Small EM, Mileikovsky M, Nagy A. Complex interdependence regulates heterotypic transcription factor distribution and coordinates cardiogenesis. Cell. 2016;164(5):999–1014.
17. Wright CF, McRae JF, Clayton S, Gallone G, Aitken S, FitzGerald TW, Jones P, Prigmore E, Rajan D, Lord J, Sifrim A. Making new genetic diagnoses with old data: iterative reanalysis and reporting from genome-wide data in 1,133 families with developmental disorders. Genet Med. 2018;20(10):1216.
18. Landis BJ, Levey A, Levasseur SM, Glickstein JS, Kleinman CS, Simpson LL, Williams IA. Prenatal diagnosis of congenital heart disease and birth outcomes. Pediatr Cardiol. 2013;34(3):597–605.
19. Carvalho JS. Antenatal diagnosis of critical congenital heart disease. Optimal place of delivery is where appropriate care can be delivered. Arch Dis Child. 2016;101(6):505–7.
20. Paladini D, Alfirevic Z, Carvalho JS, Khalil A, Malinger G, Martinez JM, Rychik J, Ville Y, Gardiner H, ISUOG Clinical Standards Committee. ISUOG consensus statement on current understanding of the association of neurodevelopmental delay and congenital heart disease: impact on prenatal counseling. Ultrasound Obstet Gynecol. 2017;49(2):287–8.
21. Chu PY, Li JS, Kosinski AS, Hornik CP, Hill KD. Congenital heart disease in premature infants 25-32 weeks' gestational age. J Pediatr. 2017;181:37–41.
22. Cheng HH, Almodovar MC, Laussen PC, Wypij D, Polito A, Brown DW, Emani SM, Pigula FA, Allan CK, Costello JM. Outcomes and risk factors for mortality in premature neonates with critical congenital heart disease. Pediatr Cardiol. 2011;32(8):1139–46.

23. Licht DJ, Shera DM, Clancy RR, Wernovsky G, Montenegro LM, Nicolson SC, Zimmerman RA, Spray TL, Gaynor JW, Vossough A. Brain maturation is delayed in infants with complex congenital heart defects. J Thorac Cardiovasc Surg. 2009;137(3):529–37.
24. Barry OM, Friedman KG, Bergersen L, Emani S, Moeyersoms A, Tworetzky W, Marshall AC, Lock JE. Clinical and hemodynamic results after conversion from single to biventricular circulation after fetal aortic stenosis intervention. Am J Cardiol. 2018;122(3):511–6.
25. Donofrio MT, Moon-Grady AJ, Hornberger LK, Copel JA, Sklansky MS, Abuhamad A, Cuneo BF, Huhta JC, Jonas RA, Krishnan A, Lacey S. Diagnosis and treatment of fetal cardiac disease: a scientific statement from the American Heart Association. Circulation. 2014;129(21):2183–242.
26. Jantzen DW, Moon-Grady AJ, Morris SA, Armstrong AK, Berg C, Dangel J, Fifer CG, Frommelt M, Gembruch U, Herberg U, Jaeggi E. Hypoplastic left heart syndrome with intact or restrictive atrial septum: a report from the International Fetal Cardiac Intervention Registry. Circulation. 2017;136(14):1346–9.
27. Schidlow DN, Tworetzky W, Wilkins-Haug LE. Percutaneous fetal cardiac interventions for structural heart disease. Am J Perinatol. 2014;31(07):629–36.
28. Co-Vu J, Lopez-Colon D, Vyas HV, Weiner N, DeGroff C. Maternal hyperoxygenation: a potential therapy for congenital heart disease in the fetuses? A systematic review of the current literature. Echocardiography. 2017;34(12):1822–33.
29. Costello JM, Pasquali SK, Jacobs JP, He X, Hill KD, Cooper DS, Backer CL, Jacobs ML. Gestational age at birth and outcomes after neonatal cardiac surgery: an analysis of the Society of Thoracic Surgeons Congenital Heart Surgery Database. Circulation. 2014;129(24):2511–7.
30. Kalfa D, Krishnamurthy G, Duchon J, Najjar M, Levasseur S, Chai P, Chen J, Quaegebeur J, Bacha E. Outcomes of cardiac surgery in patients weighing<2.5 kg: affect of patient-dependent and-independent variables. J Thorac Cardiovasc Surg. 2014;148(6):2499–506.
31. Marwali E, Heineking B, Haas N. Pre and postoperative management of pediatric patients with congenital heart diseases. Paediatric and neonatal surgery. Edited by Joanne Baerg; Published by InTech open, DOI 10.5772/63041 Published 2017.
32. Schiller O, Sinha P, Zurakowski D, Jonas RA. Reconstruction of right ventricular outflow tract in neonates and infants using valved cryopreserved femoral vein homografts. J Thorac Cardiovasc Surg. 2014;147(3):874–9.
33. Van Puyvelde J, Meyns B, Rega F. Pulmonary atresia and a ventricular septal defect: about size and strategy. Eur J Cardiothorac Surg. 2016;49(5):1419–20.
34. Gerelli S, van Steenberghe M, Murtuza B, Bojan M, Harding ED, Bonnet D, Vouhé PR, Raisky O. Neonatal right ventricle to pulmonary connection as a palliative procedure for pulmonary atresia with ventricular septal defect or severe tetralogy of Fallot. Eur J Cardiothorac Surg. 2013;45(2):278–88.
35. Bentham JR, Zava NK, Harrison WJ, Shauq A, Kalantre A, Derrick G, Chen RH, Dhillon R, Taliotis D, Kang SL, Crossland D. Duct stenting versus modified Blalock-Taussig shunt in neonates with duct-dependent pulmonary blood flow: associations with clinical outcomes in a multicenter national study. Circulation. 2018;137(6):581–8.
36. Thomas VT. Partners of the heart: Vivien Thomas and his work with Alfred Blalock: an autobiography. Philadelphia: University of Pennsylvania Press; 1998.
37. Ohye RG, Schranz D, D'udekem Y. Current therapy for hypoplastic left heart syndrome and related single ventricle lesions. Circulation. 2016;134(17):1265–79.
38. Yabrodi M, Mastropietro CW. Hypoplastic left heart syndrome: from comfort care to long-term survival. Pediatr Res. 2017;81(1–2):142.
39. Kenny LA, DeRita F, Nassar M, Dark J, Coats L, Hasan A. Transplantation in the single ventricle population. Ann Cardiothorac Surg. 2018;7(1):152.
40. Wilson WM, Valente AM, Hickey EJ, Clift P, Burchill L, Emmanuel Y, Gibson P, Greutmann M, Grewal J, Grigg LE, Gurvitz M. Outcomes of patients with hypoplastic left heart syndrome reaching adulthood after Fontan palliation: multicenter study. Circulation. 2018;137(9):978–81.

41. Norwood WI, Lang P, Casteneda AR, Campbell DN. Experience with operations for hypoplastic left heart syndrome. J Thorac Cardiovasc Surg. 1981;82(4):511–9.
42. Kishimoto H, Kawahira Y, Kawata H, Miura T, Iwai S, Mori T. The modified Norwood palliation on a beating heart. J Thorac Cardiovasc Surg. 1999;118(6):1130–2.
43. Reemtsen BL, Pike NA, Starnes VA. Stage I palliation for hypoplastic left heart syndrome: Norwood versus Sano modification. Curr Opin Cardiol. 2007;22(2):60–5.
44. https://www.nicor.org.uk/wp-content/uploads/2018/11/National-Congenital-Heart-Disease-Audit-Summary-Report-2014-17.pdf. Accessed 21 June 2019.
45. Rehman SM, Ravaglioli A, Singappuli K, Roman K, Gnanapragasam J, Samarasinghe D, Viola N. Hybrid strategies for high-risk non-hypoplastic left heart syndrome patients. J Card Surg. 2018;33(7):399–401.
46. Coe JY, Olley PM. A novel method to maintain ductus arteriosus patency. J Am Coll Cardiol. 1991;18(3):837–41.
47. Gibbs JL, Wren C, Watterson KG, Hunter S, Hamilton JR. Stenting of the arterial duct combined with banding of the pulmonary arteries and atrial septectomy or septostomy: a new approach to palliation for the hypoplastic left heart syndrome. Heart. 1993;69(6):551–5.
48. Cao JY, Lee SY, Phan K, Ayer J, Celermajer DS, Winlaw DS. Early outcomes of hypoplastic left heart syndrome infants: meta-analysis of studies comparing the hybrid and Norwood procedures. World J Pediatr Congen Heart Surg. 2018;9(2):224–33.
49. Yerebakan C, Valeske K, Elmontaser H, Yörüker U, Mueller M, Thul J, Mann V, Latus H, Villanueva A, Hofmann K, Schranz D. Hybrid therapy for hypoplastic left heart syndrome: myth, alternative, or standard? J Thorac Cardiovasc Surg. 2016;151(4):1112–23.
50. Franklin RC, Jacobs JP, Krogmann ON, Béland MJ, Aiello VD, Colan SD, Elliott MJ, Gaynor JW, Kurosawa H, Maruszewski B, Stellin G. Nomenclature for congenital and paediatric cardiac disease: historical perspectives and The International Pediatric and Congenital Cardiac Code. Cardiol Young. 2008;18(S2):70–80.
51. Jenkins KJ, Gauvreau K. Center-specific differences in mortality: preliminary analyses using the Risk Adjustment in Congenital Heart Surgery (RACHS-1) method. J Thorac Cardiovasc Surg. 2002;124(1):97–104.
52. Lloyd DF, Cutler L, Tibby SM, Vimalesvaran S, Qureshi SA, Rosenthal E, Anderson D, Austin C, Bellsham-Revell H, Krasemann T. Analysis of preoperative condition and interstage mortality in Norwood and hybrid procedures for hypoplastic left heart syndrome using the Aristotle scoring system. Heart. 2014;100(10):775–80.
53. Rogers L, Pagel C, Sullivan ID, Mustafa M, Tsang V, Utley M, Bull C, Franklin RC, Brown KL. Interventional treatments and risk factors in patients born with hypoplastic left heart syndrome in England and Wales from 2000 to 2015. Heart. 2018;104(18):1500–7.
54. Pagel C, Rogers L, Brown K, Ambler G, Anderson D, Barron D, Blackshaw E, Crowe S, English K, Franklin R, Jesper E. Improving risk adjustment in the PRAiS (Partial Risk Adjustment in Surgery) model for mortality after paediatric cardiac surgery and improving public understanding of its use in monitoring outcomes. Health Serv Delivery Res. 2017;5(23):1–164.
55. https://www.ucl.ac.uk/clinical-operational-research-unit/AnalysisTools/PRAiS. Accessed 21 June 2019.

Chapter 7
Evidence Based Approach to the Management of Persistent Pulmonary Hypertension of the Newborn (PPHN)

Venkatesh Kairamkonda and Sumit Mittal

Introduction

Although there is better understanding of the pathophysiology, the optimal approach to the management of persistent pulmonary hypertension of the newborn (PPHN) remains controversial. The mainstay of therapy is treatment of the underlying condition along with optimising oxygen delivery, mechanical ventilation and inhaled nitric oxide (iNO). However, mortality remains unchanged despite the reduced need for extracorporeal membrane oxygenation (ECMO). There is a lack of iNO and ECMO facilities particularly in resource limited settings, prompting the need to develop new treatments. There are several promising therapeutic modalities including systemic and inhaled vasodilators, phosphodiesterase inhibitors, prostaglandin analogues and endothelin receptor antagonists. Newer modalities of treatment are increasingly being used in resistant cases albeit without evidence from randomised trials.

This chapter will explore the diagnosis of PPHN and review the current evidence for newer treatments, particularly for babies who are unresponsive to inhaled nitric oxide, or do not have access to this treatment.

What Is on the Horizon in this Area?

Newer therapies such as systemic and inhaled vasodilators such as sildenafil, prostaglandin E1 (Alprostadil), prostacyclin, milrinone and endothelin antagonists are being investigated in the light of advances in the understanding of the

V. Kairamkonda · S. Mittal (✉)
University Hospitals of Leicester NHS Trust, Leicester, UK
e-mail: venkatesh.kairamkonda@uhl-tr.nhs.uk; sumit.mittal@uhl-tr.nhs.uk

© Springer Nature Switzerland AG 2020   119
E. M. Boyle, J. Cusack (eds.), *Emerging Topics and Controversies in Neonatology*, https://doi.org/10.1007/978-3-030-28829-7_7

pathophysiology of PPHN. Several novel treatment modalities have also been proposed including antioxidants, L-citrulline, soluble guanylate cyclase (sGC) activators, Rho-kinase inhibitors and peroxisome proliferator-activated receptor-γ (PPAR-γ) agonists. Many of these pharmacologic agents are not approved for use in PPHN and current understanding is based on case reports and small trials. There is a need for large multicentre randomised controlled trials with long term follow-up to evaluate these agents in PPHN.

Case Study

A 40 + 2 week gestation, male infant weighing 3580 g was born by spontaneous vaginal delivery with APGAR scores of 9, 9, and 10 at 1, 5 and 10 min of life respectively. There were no antenatal concerns. He had one attempt at breast feeding and passed urine. He failed routine pulse oximetry screening at 4 h of age and was admitted to the neonatal unit for monitoring, oxygen therapy and antibiotics administration. Based on the history, what factors influence making the differential diagnosis for this infant?

Etiology and Risk Factors

Pulmonary hypertension in neonates represents a heterogeneous group of diagnoses associated with a 10–20% mortality rate [1]. Causes of pulmonary hypertension in neonates include congenital heart disease (CHD), congenital diaphragmatic hernia (CDH) and sepsis. PPHN is a specific type of pulmonary hypertension in neonates [2]. The aetiology of PPHN is listed in Table 7.1.

PPHN occurs when the high pulmonary vascular resistance, characteristic of fetal circulation fails to decrease at birth, resulting in right-to-left shunting of blood through fetal-channels, diminished pulmonary blood flow, and profound hypoxaemia. It can be secondary (90% of cases) to a variety of disorders causing hypoxic respiratory failure including meconium aspiration syndrome (MAS), congenital

Table 7.1 Etiology of PPHN

1.	Idiopathic Or "Black Lung"	
2. Secondary PPHN	Meconium aspiration syndrome
	Pneumonia and infection (mainly Group B streptococcus)
	Congenital diaphragmatic hernia
	Respiratory distress syndrome
	Transient tachypnoea of the newborn
	Hypoxic ischaemic encephalopathy
3. Severe and intractable PPHN	Alveolar capillary dysplasia
	RDS due to mutations in surfactant protein B (SP-B) gene
	ATP binding cassette protein member A3 (ABCA3) deficiency
	Genetic variants in corticotropin-releasing hormone (cRh) receptor 1 (CRHR1) and cRh-binding protein (CRHBP)

Table 7.2 Risk factors for hypoxic respiratory failure in term or near-term neonates

Antenatal	Postnatal
Meconium stained amniotic fluid	Male gender and African or Asian race
Perinatal acidosis and asphyxia	Late preterm and large for gestational age and birth by Caesarean section
Maternal fever, prolonged rupture of membranes, or Group B streptococcal carrier status	Perinatal exposure to nicotine, SSRIs, NSAIDs
Chorioamnionitis and/or funisitis	Polycythemia
Preconception maternal obesity	Hypothermia
Maternal diabetes and asthma	Hypocalcemia

infection, CDH and chronic lung disease of prematurity (CLDP). PPHN is also seen in infants with moderate to severe hypoxic ischaemic encephalopathy (HIE) and is associated with lung disease, sepsis, systemic hypotension, and increased mortality. Idiopathic or "black lung" PPHN (10% of cases) is mainly due to abnormal muscularisation of pulmonary arterioles in the absence of any parenchymal disease or lung hypoplasia [3, 4].

Rare causes of severe and intractable PPHN are alveolar capillary dysplasia [5], respiratory distress syndrome (RDS) due to mutations in surfactant protein B (SP-B) gene [6], ATP binding cassette protein member A3 (ABCA3) deficiency [7] and variants in corticotropin-releasing hormone (cRh) receptor 1 (CRHR1) and cRh-binding protein (CRHBP) [8].

Risk factors [9, 10] associated with PPHN have been described and are listed in Table 7.2.

There was a theoretical concern of aggravating PPHN following the introduction of therapeutic hypothermia in the management of HIE. However, studies have not shown any association between cooling and PPHN despite observing some pulmonary dysfunction [11, 12].

Pathophysiology

The pathophysiology of PPHN (Fig. 7.1) involves the interplay of endothelium derived vasodilators, prostacyclin (PGI2) and nitric oxide (NO), on pulmonary arterial smooth muscle cells. Nitric oxide is a free radical and can avidly combine with superoxide anions to form a toxic vasoconstrictor, peroxynitrite. Endothelin (ET-1) is a powerful vasoconstrictor and exerts its action via ET-A receptors on the smooth muscle cell. ET-B is the other endothelin receptor on the endothelial cell and causes vasodilation by nitric oxide release. The main enzymes responsible are cyclooxygenase (COX), endothelial nitric oxide synthase (eNOS), soluble guanylate cyclase (sGC), phosphodiesterase 5 (PDE5), phosphodiesterase 3A (PDE3A), prostacyclin synthase (PGIS), cyclic adenosine monophosphate (cCMP), cyclic guanosine monophosphate (cGMP) and adenylate cyclase (AC).

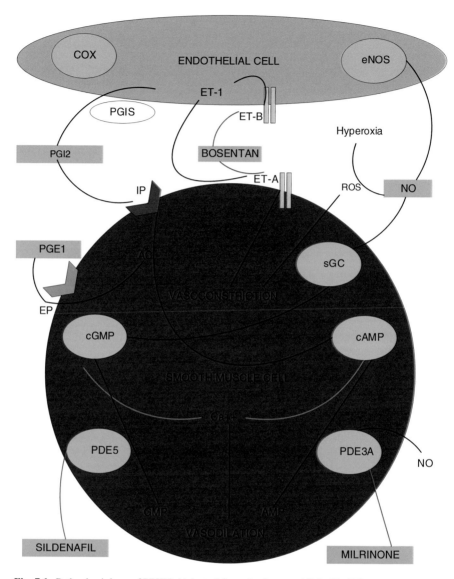

Fig. 7.1 Pathophysiology of PPHN. (Adapted from the figure published in [3])

Current therapies are mainly directed towards influencing eNOS, PDE3A and PDE5. Milrinone inhibits PDE3A and increases cAMP levels in pulmonary arterial smooth muscle cells and cardiac myocytes resulting in pulmonary (and systemic) vasodilation and inotropy. Sildenafil inhibits PDE5 and increases cGMP levels in pulmonary arterial smooth muscle cells. Bosentan is a non-specific inhibitor of endothelin receptors. Prostacyclin and PGE1 (aerosolised alprostadil) cause vasodilation by increasing cAMP by action on prostacyclin receptors (IP) and prostacyclin E receptors (EP) respectively and AC.

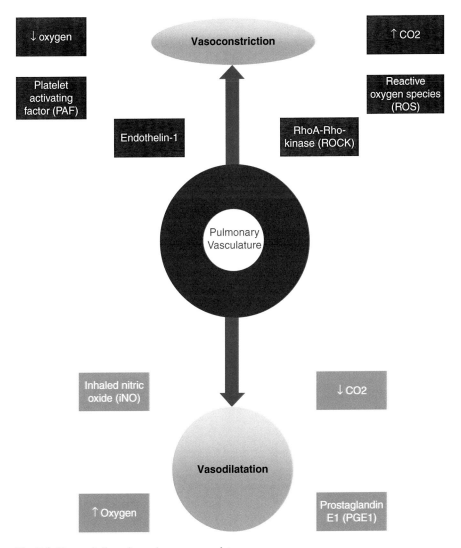

Fig. 7.2 Factors influencing pulmonary vasculature

Figure 7.2 details the various factors influencing pulmonary vasculature to cause vasoconstriction and vasodilatation.

Case Study

Continuous positive airway pressure (CPAP) was commenced due to an increase in the infant's work of breathing, respiratory acidosis and hypoxia requiring 50% oxygen. Pre-ductal and post-ductal saturations intermittently showed more than 10% difference during the placement of umbilical venous and arterial lines placement.

What clinical signs and symptoms will help in differentiating between PPHN and cyanotic heart disease?

Approach to a Diagnosis

Pulse oximetry screening is a safe and feasible test that is increasingly being employed in the UK in term and near-term infants before discharging home. Newborn pulse oximetry screening identifies critical congenital heart disease (CCHD) in addition to respiratory disease and sepsis [13].

Figure 7.3 shows an approach to the clinical work up of a baby with risk factors for suspected PPHN. PPHN should be suspected clinically in term and near-term infants with risk factors who have failed pulse oximetry screening with or without signs of perinatal distress. Idiopathic or "black lung" PPHN can present without clinical signs of perinatal distress. Physical examination may show the presence of a loud, single second heart sound or harsh systolic murmur due to tricuspid regurgitation.

In an infant with hypoxemia (arterial PaO_2 less than 2.6 kPa in 100% FiO_2), pre-post ductal saturation difference of 10% or higher (preductal saturations being higher) and PaO_2 difference of ≥ 2.6 kPa is indicative of right-to-left shunting at the ductal level and is highly suggestive of PPHN [3]. This diagnosis can only be made in the absence of duct dependent systemic flow lesions such as interrupted aortic arch, coarctation of the aorta, critical aortic stenosis, hypoplastic left heart syndrome or other anatomic pulmonary vascular disease (total anomalous pulmonary venous drainage and pulmonary venous stenosis). It is important to remember that the absence of a difference in pre and post ductal oxygenation in a hypoxemic infant only indicates that there is no right-to-left ductal shunting and does not exclude PPHN.

A hyperoxia test, a quick bedside test, can be performed to help make the diagnosis of PPHN. This consists of obtaining an arterial blood gas (ABG) after exposing the infant to 100% oxygen for 5–10 min. PPHN or a cyanotic heart disease are suspected if the ABG shows a PaO_2 of less than 13.3 kPa (100 mmHg). Secondary PPHN commonly presents with labile hypoxemia. Cyanotic congenital heart conditions may present with fixed hypoxemia and be clinically indistinguishable from PPHN [14]. Currently, echocardiography remains the gold standard diagnostic tool in PPHN.

Cotside echocardiography by an appropriately skilled neonatologist is an invaluable tool in diagnosis, management and progression of PPHN (Table 7.3, Figs. 7.3 and 7.4). Right-to-left or bidirectional shunting of blood at the foramen ovale and/or the ductus arteriosus is seen in 73–100% [15–19], as well as high pulmonary arterial and right ventricular systolic pressure estimated by Doppler velocity measurement of the tricuspid regurgitation jet.

Among the various methods used to measure the pulmonary pressure, the pressure drop across the PDA is a reliable method followed by the measurement of TR (tricuspid regurgitation) jet velocity. However, TR jet velocity has limitation in the presence of right ventricular dysfunction which may be a feature of severe PPHN. In the absence of a TR jet, systolic ventricular septal flattening which indicates whether the right ventricular pressures are more than half or less than half of left ventricular systolic pressure may be useful to the diagnosis of PPHN. Normally the septum bows into the right ventricle (O-shaped Left ventricle) and with increasing right

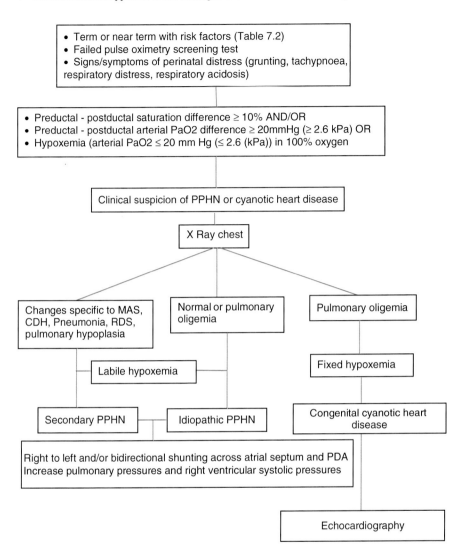

Fig. 7.3 PPHN diagnosis and management flow chart

ventricular pressure, the interventricular septum will flatten (D-shaped LV) and eventually curves into the left ventricle (crescent-shaped LV) [20]. It is best analysed at the end of systole in the parasternal short axis view above the level of the papillary muscles [21].

The direction of the shunt at atrial and ductal level also provides clues to aid management (Figs. 7.3 and 7.4). Left-to-right shunting at the foramen ovale and ductus arteriosus with marked hypoxemia suggests predominant intrapulmonary shunting, and interventions should focus on optimizing lung recruitment (increasing positive end expiratory pressure and mean airway pressure and/or administering

Table 7.3 A guide to transthoracic echocardiography for the neonatologist in the management of PPHN

Confirm cardiac anatomy to rule out congenital heart conditions
Confirm atrial level and ductal shunting (right-to-left or bidirectional)
Estimate and confirm increased systolic pulmonary arterial pressure (SPAP) for grading, choice of treatment, and monitor response, and weaning of therapy
• Bernoulli equation to pulmonary regurgitation peak velocity = SPAP ∞ RVSP (in mmHg) = 4 × (VmaxTR)2 + RAP (right atrial pressure = 3–5 mmHg)
• Bernoulli equation to transductal right-to-left blood flow peak velocity = SPAP (in mmHg) = 4 × (VmaxDA)2 + SSAP (systolic systemic arterial pressure)
• Left ventricular configuration = O-shaped (<50% of estimated RVP), D-shaped (50–100% of RVP), and Crescent shaped (≥100% of LVP)
Estimate ventricular function for choice of inotrope and monitor response and weaning of inotrope

surfactant). The presence of right-to-left shunting at the foramen ovale and/or the ductus arteriosus is suggestive of extra-pulmonary shunting, which may respond to pulmonary vasodilator therapy.

A pure right-to-left shunt at the atrial level suggests total anomalous pulmonary venous connection until proven otherwise. Similarly, right-to-left shunting at the ductal level and left-to-right shunting at the atrial level suggest PPHN with left ventricular dysfunction due to pulmonary venous hypertension as seen in CDH, asphyxia or sepsis. It is important to note that ductal dependent systemic circulation syndromes listed previously may be associated with a similar shunt pattern. Vasodilator therapy with milrinone may be considered in this setting. Echocardiographic findings of impaired ejection fraction and stroke volume carry a poor prognosis [22]. An ECG is not usually helpful for the diagnosis.

Imaging studies can be valuable to make the diagnosis of PPHN: chest X-ray can show oligemic lung fields in idiopathic PPHN and may also be helpful in diagnosing lung disease.

A blood work-up may be helpful to identify the etiological factors responsible for PPHN. A complete blood count may show abnormal white blood cell counts and polycythaemia. Blood glucose and calcium level are helpful to rule out metabolic causes. Recently, B-type natriuretic peptide (BNP) was proposed as a biomarker in PPHN, especially to assess efficacy of treatment and to predict rebound PPHN [23, 24]. Reynolds et al. in a prospective cohort study showed that BNP measuring ≥550 pg/mL is predictive of PPHN with a sensitivity of 85% and a specificity of 100% [23]. However, its value in the practical management of PPHN is presently unclear.

Case Study
At 12 h of age he was intubated, put on conventional ventilation, sedated and paralysed due to worsening respiratory acidosis, hypoxemia and hypotension. What are the early interventions and supportive management to prevent hypoxia spiral?

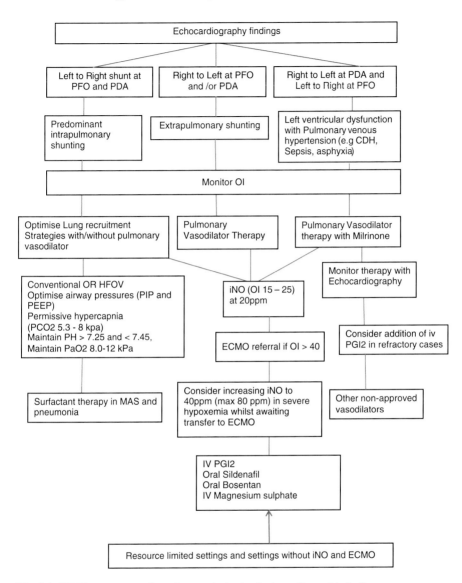

Fig. 7.4 PPHN management flow chart on the basis of echocardiographic findings

Delivery Room Resuscitation

Neonates with PPHN are often cyanotic and significant resuscitative efforts may be required in the delivery room. Standardised resuscitation should be carried out and should focus on optimal lung recruitment and ventilation. Oxygen is a potent pulmonary vasodilator and should be given promptly to maintain pre-ductal saturations in the recommended range.

Supportive Measures

Supportive measures following diagnosis of PPHN are vital in successful management efforts. It is important to maintain normothermia and correct hypoglycaemia, hypocalcaemia, acidosis and polycythaemia. Parenteral nutrition should be administered preferably through a central line.

Monitoring and prompt correction of trend changes in pre- and post-ductal saturation differences are important. Due to underlying shunts, any stimulus can result in a precipitous drop in oxygen saturations. It is common practice to minimise stimulation by preventing vaso-vagal manoeuvres, covering the infant's eyes and ears and maintaining a low-noise environment. Judicious use of sedation and analgesia with narcotic analgesics such as morphine and fentanyl or benzodiazepines such as midazolam is appropriate. Therapeutic muscle relaxation should be avoided if possible as it has been associated with hypotension, oedema, hearing impairment [25], ventilation perfusion mismatch and increased mortality [26].

Systemic blood pressure should be maintained at normal values for the infant's gestational age. If there is hypotension and/or poor perfusion indicating hypovolemia, volume replacement in the form of one or two fluid boluses should be administered. If hypotension persists despite volume replacement, inotropic agents such as dopamine, dobutamine, and epinephrine are indicated. These agents are not selective to the systemic circulation and may be associated with pulmonary vasoconstriction and elevation of pulmonary vascular resistance (PVR) at high doses. Norepinephrine has been shown to be efficacious in improving lung function in PPHN by decreasing PVR:SVR ratio and improving cardiac function [27, 28].

Surfactant administration reduces the severity of pulmonary morbidity, air leaks and length of hospital stay in infants with MAS and pneumonia [29]. In a multicentre randomised controlled study comparing surfactant to placebo in babies with meconium aspiration, surfactant use significantly decreased the need for ECMO [29, 30]. In another study, surfactant lung lavage showed an improvement in oxygenation, a decrease in mean airway pressure (MAP), and alveolar-arterial gradients, however it did not improve the duration of mechanical ventilation, the use of inhaled NO, length of hospitalisation, or overall complications [31].

Hyperventilation and alkali infusions to maintain an alkaline pH were strategies previously in use but are now considered outdated. There were concerns of impaired cerebral perfusion and sensorineural deafness when deliberate respiratory alkalosis was used [32, 33]. Similar or better outcomes with less chronic lung disease were observed in infants with PPHN maintaining 6–8 kPa PCO_2 [34, 35]. Alkali infusion was associated with increased use of ECMO and need for oxygen at 28 days [26]. Most centres aim to avoid acidosis as animal studies demonstrated exaggerated hypoxic pulmonary vasoconstriction with pH < 7.25 [36].

Mechanical Ventilation

The management of PPHN aims to restore postnatal cardiopulmonary adaptation by the provision of adequate tissue oxygenation without inflicting an iatrogenic pulmonary injury. There is no difference between various mechanical ventilatory modes and outcome. HFOV may be attempted to minimize lung injury. Meta-analysis has failed to show a clear benefit of HFOV (elective or as a rescue mode) over conventional ventilation in term or preterm infants with PPHN [22, 29, 37]. However, HFOV may be beneficial [38] when high mean airway pressure on conventional ventilation impedes venous return. The severity of disease and treatment response can be monitored by calculating oxygen index OI = [mean airway pressure $\times$ FiO$_2$ $\div$ PaO$_2$] $\times$ 100. OI > 20 indicates severe hypoxemic respiratory failure and OI > 40 is an indication for ECMO referral.

There has been a strong association between hypocarbia (partial pressures of carbon dioxide (PaCO$_2$) levels <3.3–4.0 kPa) and an increased incidence of cystic periventricular leukomalacia and cerebral palsy in preterm and near term infants [29]. Therefore, mechanical ventilation should be targeting PaCO$_2$ levels of 5.3–8 kPa and a PaO$_2$ of 8–12 kPa. During ventilation and respiratory support, special care should be taken to avoid hyperoxia; since this has been shown, in multiple animal models, to cause significant lung injury and increase in peroxynitrite, a potent vasoconstrictor, in the presence of NO [39].

Case Study

During the further clinical course the baby received >40 mL/kg of normal saline boluses and was commenced on dopamine, dobutamine and adrenaline infusions. Chest X-ray was indicative of congenital pneumonia. Echocardiography showed a structurally normal heart with supra-systemic pulmonary pressures and right to left ductal shunt. His respiratory failure and hypoxemia continued to worsen, requiring change from conventional ventilation to high frequency oscillatory ventilation (HFOV). At that time, his oxygen index was 26, so he was started on inhaled nitric oxide.

Are there any safety concerns with iNO and what do clinicians need to be aware of?

Specific Management

Interventions are targeted to improve pulmonary and systemic circulation to achieve balance or reversal of right-to-left shunt and thereby improve oxygenation and preserve end organ functions.

Inhaled Nitric Oxide

Inhaled nitric oxide can be started in term or late preterm infants when the OI is between 15–25 or when the PaO$_2$, while receiving 100% FiO$_2$, is <14 kPa. The starting dose of iNO is 20 parts per million (ppm) and improvement in oxygenation is usually seen within 30–60 min [40–42]. The response to iNO is defined as an improvement in PaO$_2$ or reduction in FiO$_2$ [43]. Early response is generally associated with good long-term outcome and reflects the reversibility of lung pathology. Several randomised controlled trials have demonstrated the effectiveness of iNO as a selective pulmonary vasodilator without significant side effects [44]. In a randomised controlled trial, combined iNO and HFOV therapy were found to be more effective in rescue treatment of severe PPHN compared to HFOV or iNO alone [38]. iNO has been shown to reduce the need for ECMO by 40% without reduction in mortality [44]. Up to 40% of neonates with severe PPHN fail to respond to iNO therapy [3, 41]. Furthermore, meta-analysis of randomised controlled trials failed to show the beneficial effects of iNO in patients with pulmonary hypertension secondary to CDH [44]. The common reasons for failure to respond to iNO include poor lung inflation, myocardial dysfunction, systemic hypotension, severe pulmonary vascular structural disease, undiagnosed anatomical cardiovascular lesions and alveolar capillary dysplasia [44, 45].

An early randomised controlled study [41] demonstrated 20 ppm iNO to be most effective although 6% responded only after increasing to 80 ppm. In patients who do not respond to 20 ppm of iNO, a brief exposure to higher doses (40–80 ppm) can be attempted; however rigorous monitoring of the concentration of methaemoglobin (MetHb) should be undertaken. Methaemoglobinemia is a recognised complication of iNO in patients with methaemoglobin reductase deficiency and overdose of iNO. MetHb levels should be recorded 1 and 6 h after starting iNO and thereafter twice a day. Levels of MetHb below 2.5% of haemoglobin (normal range 1–3%) is considered safe [46]. In a trial, 80 ppm of iNO was associated with methaemoglobinemia at a concentration of 7% and higher, 35% of the time [47]. Methaemoglobinemia is fatal if not detected early in hypoxia due to its refractoriness to oxygen therapy. Urgent treatment with methylene blue is indicated when metHb levels reach above 20%. Figure 7.5 outlines the approach to management of methaemoglobinemia.

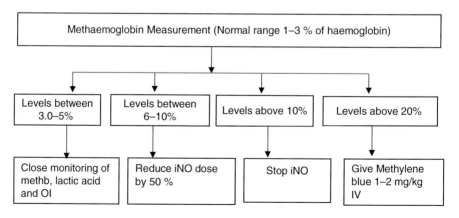

Fig. 7.5 Management of methaemoglobinemia during iNO therapy

The half-life of iNO is 5 seconds. Babies can clinically deteriorate and develop rebound pulmonary hypertension if iNO is discontinued suddenly [48]. Therefore, weaning from iNO should be done gradually especially once the baby has achieved stability.

Case Study

His respiratory failure and hypoxaemia continued to worsen. He was on maximum infusions of dopamine, dobutamine and epinephrine for his hypotension. Blood cultures were redrawn, and antibiotic changed to vancomycin and cefotaxime. There was mention of newer/alternative therapies in management of PPHN. In what circumstances would you turn to those and how aggressive would your approach be?

Alternative and Newer Therapies

In resource limited settings and in babies unresponsive to iNO, alternative therapies such as Sildenafil or Milrinone, MgSO$_4$, Prostacyclin and Bosentan are increasingly gaining popularity. The use of these medications is currently "off label" and their definitive role in PPHN treatment is yet to be established.

Sildenafil

Sildenafil (Viagra®, Revatio®, Pfizer) is a PDE5 inhibitor that is approved in oral form for the treatment of pulmonary arterial hypertension in children (European Union) and oral/intravenous preparation in adults (global). A systematic review has demonstrated a significant reduction in mortality rate and improvement in oxygenation index 6–8 h following the oral sildenafil dose up to 2 mg/kg [1, 2]. In developed countries there has been limited experience in the use of oral sildenafil for acute PPHN, as nitric oxide is readily available. There is a paucity of publications on IV sildenafil use and only one multinational study involving 36 patients showed that its use is associated with improved oxygenation [49]. Case reports of "off label" use of sildenafil in conjunction with iNO indicate that sildenafil could enhance the efficacy of iNO and reduce the time on iNO therapy. Recommended dosing regimen for IV sildenafil: loading dose of 0.4 mg/kg delivered over 3 h, followed by a maintenance infusion at 1.6 mg/kg/day over 24 h. Alternative intermittent IV dose: 0.4 mg/kg over 1–2 h infusion [50]. The effects of addition of IV Sildenafil to standard iNO therapy in neonates with hypoxic respiratory failure is currently subject to an ongoing multicentre, randomised, placebo controlled, double blind, two-armed, parallel group study. Long term follow-up of developmental progress at 12 and 24 months after completion is also included in this study.

Milrinone

Milrinone has been recommended in severe PPHN with suboptimal response to iNO and evidence of myocardial dysfunction [51, 52] due to its inotropic, lusotropic (myocardial relaxation) and vasodilation action. Dosage regimen varies from 0.25 µg/kg/min to maximum 0.75 µg/kg/min by continuous infusion [50]. A loading dose preceding continuous infusion should not be used in sick neonates as it may induce hypotension. Although Milrinone is commonly used and has been found to be effective post cardiac surgery and low cardiac output states, evidence for its efficacy and safety in infants with PPHN is yet to be established [52]. Intravenous milrinone infusion in severe PPHN (iNO non-responders) leads to an early improvement in OI, reduction in tachycardia, improved response to iNO, better systemic blood pressure, improved LV and RV outputs, reduction in right-to-left shunt across PDA, improved urine output, better blood pH values, reduction in blood lactate levels and an overall reduction in inotropic use [52, 53]. Milrinone seems to have a beneficial effect in the management of PPHN secondary to CDH by increasing left ventricular haemodynamic however this effect needs to be confirmed by properly conducted studies.

Prostacyclin

Prostacyclin I2 (PGI2) and prostaglandin E1 (PGE1) are two classes of prostaglandin (PG) that have therapeutic applications in PPHN. The role of intravenous PGI2 therapy is well established in adults with pulmonary hypertension. PGI2 analog, Epoprostenol, is available in IV formulation which has been used as aerosolised inhaled form. Intravenous PGI2 is a non-selective pulmonary vasodilator; it can lead to systemic hypotension, so it is generally avoided in neonatal population. In infants with iNO refractory PPHN, IV epoprostenol decreased OI within 4 h of treatment with a significant response persisting for 24 h [54].

Prostacyclin analog, Iloprost (intravenous, inhaled), is a selective pulmonary vasodilator and has been used endotracheally and in the inhaled form. It has been shown to be a useful adjunct to iNO therapy due to its additive effects in cases refractory to iNO therapy alone [55]. However further evaluation and research is needed before it can become an approved treatment for PPHN.

There are anecdotal reports of benefit from the use of IV infusion of Prostin to relieve right ventricular (RV) dysfunction, associated with CDH and PPHN.

Bosentan

Bosentan is an oral non-selective dual endothelin-1 receptor antagonist; Sitaxentan and ambrisentan are selective ET_A receptor inhibitors. They improve symptoms and exercise capacity in adult patients with pulmonary hypertension [56]. Randomised controlled studies and systematic reviews in adults have shown improvement in outcomes of patients with pulmonary hypertension [57]. Nakwan et al. have reported the benefits of bosentan in neonates with PPHN [58]. A recent randomised controlled trial has shown its efficacy over placebo in a setting where iNO was not available [59].

Magnesium Sulphate

Magnesium decreases influx of extracellular calcium ions in vascular smooth muscle cells (therefore low Ca++) and hence causes relaxation of blood vessels. However, being a non-selective vasodilator, it can cause systemic hypotension. A Cochrane review [60] did not show any evidence from randomised controlled trials (RCT) for its use. One RCT [61] involving magnesium sulphate and nitric oxide followed by cross over if there was no response in either arm was terminated early due to excessive mortality in the overall study group, especially in the nitric oxide arm [60, 61]. The current recommendation would be to maintain normal magnesium levels. It may be helpful to keep the level closer to 1 mmol/L in infants with PPHN.

Vasopressin

There is experimental evidence to show that low-dose arginine vasopressin leads to selective vasodilatation in pulmonary, cerebral, renal and coronary vasculature bed under hypoxic conditions by its action on V1 receptors stimulation of which induces the release of endothelial-derived NO.

A published case series [62] has shown that very low dose vasopressin is an effective adjunctive therapy in neonates with a diagnosis of PPHN where there is refractory systemic hypotension and hypoxemia despite conventional treatments. In this case series, vasopressin use was associated with improvement in systemic blood pressure, reduction in OI, steady reduction in iNO use and enabled weaning of other inotropes. Recommended dose used was 0.02–0.1 unit/kg/min in UK case series [63].

If an infant responds to vasopressin, one should reduce the dose of adrenaline and dopamine infusions to avoid excessive tachycardia and intense peripheral vasoconstriction.

Concomitant use of milrinone and vasopressin has been shown to stabilise sick infants who have not responded to nitric oxide and are awaiting transfer for ECMO [62].

Case Study
His OI worsened despite escalation of intensive care and he required ECMO treatment for 3 days followed by 5 days of HFOV. Chest CT scan was normal. His investigations, including immunology and investigation for surfactant deficiencies syndromes were normal. He was extubated soon after return to the neonatal unit to

humidified high flow oxygen at 8 L for a few days and subsequently nasal cannula oxygen prior to discharge home.

Extracorporeal Membrane Oxygenation

ECMO has significantly improved survival of neonates with severe but reversible lung disease without increased risk of severe disability [63, 64]. It is the ultimate rescue therapy for infants with PPHN with an oxygenation index persistently above 40 despite treatment with NO and optimal ventilator management. Neonatal mobile ECMO is also available in some centres to rescue neonates with PPHN who are not stable enough to transfer due to severe cardio-respiratory embarrassment. To be suitable candidates for ECMO, infants should be more than 2 kg in weight, and should have no contraindication to heparinisation such as severe IVH or non-survivable congenital anomalies. Overall, the survival of neonates with PPHN after ECMO therapy is 80% and veno-arterial ECMO is most often used for ease of access [65]. There are a few predictors of good outcome in infants with PPHN requiring ECMO. Higher birth weight, higher 5-min Apgar score, absence of CDH, and postnatal diagnosis of CDH are associated with an improvement in survival [65]. The most common complications of ECMO therapy are cardiovascular, followed by mechanical (clots in the circuit) and renal problems. Neurodevelopmental disability can be as common as 15–20% among ECMO survivors. The rate of complications increases as the number of days on ECMO increases [65].

Long Term Outcome

Neurodevelopmental disabilities ranging from 14–46% has been reported following PPHN—which includes sensorineural hearing loss, cerebral palsy and delay in either cognitive or motor performance [66]. Feeding problems and short-term respiratory morbidities can also be seen in 24% of PPHN survivors [66]. The long-term outcome of infants with PPHN may depend on their underlying conditions and the therapeutic interventions they have received at birth. Interestingly, there were no differences in medical, neurodevelopmental, and social/emotional/behavioural outcomes at school age, between children with PPHN who were treated with iNO, with or without ECMO, and infants who were treated without exposure to iNO [66]. Similarly, neurodevelopmental, behavioural, or medical abnormalities at 18–24 months were similar in infants who were treated for PPHN with or without iNO [67]. In another long-term follow up study, it was found that infants, who were treated for PPHN at birth, had a higher prevalence of sensorineural hearing loss, chronic health problems, need for bronchodilator therapy, and remedial education at the age of 5–10 years in comparison to their controls [68]. Long-term medical and neurodevelopmental follow up of infants with PPHN is warranted.

Novel Therapies Under Investigation

There is a need for additional therapies for PPHN that may supplement the use of iNO or ECMO, reduce time on the ventilator and duration of stay. Several newer therapies for PPHN are under investigation in animal studies. These include antioxidant recombinant human superoxide dismutase (SOD) [69], Apocynin (NADPH oxidase inhibitor) [70], antenatal betamethasone [71], sGC activators [72], L-citrulline [73], Rho-kinase inhibitors (Fasudil and Y27632) [74] and peroxisome proliferator-activated receptor-γ (PPARγ) [75]. There is a need to prove their safety and clinical efficacy in humans.

Conclusions

PPHN is a neonatal emergency that requires early diagnosis and treatment to prevent severe hypoxia and various short-term and long-term morbidities. The mainstay of therapy is the treatment of the underlying condition, oxygen supplementation, mechanical ventilation, and iNO. Several promising therapeutic modalities are being employed in resistant PPHN such as PDE inhibitors, PG analogues, ET receptor antagonists, and ECMO. However, the optimal approach to the management of PPHN remains controversial. Future high quality randomised controlled studies of current and newer therapeutic modalities are needed to develop evidence-based guidelines for the management of PPHN. After discharge from the NICU, infants with PPHN warrant long-term follow up due to the risk of neurodevelopmental disabilities and chronic health conditions.

Key Points
- PPHN should be suspected when severe hypoxemic respiratory failure is out of proportion to the degree of lung disease.
- Pre-postductal saturation and PaO_2 differential of more than 10% and more than or equal to 2.6 kPa respectively is indicative of right-to-left ductal shunting and highly suggestive of PPHN.
- Therapy includes treatment of underlying causes, maintenance of adequate systemic blood pressure, optimised ventilator support for lung recruitment and alveolar ventilation, and pharmacotherapy to increase pulmonary vasodilation and decrease pulmonary vascular resistance.
- Inhaled nitric oxide improves oxygenation in 60–70% of PPHN patients and significantly reduces the need for ECMO.
- Despite the availability of iNO and ECMO in specialised centres, hypoxic respiratory failure and PPHN remain life threatening conditions.
- About 14–46% of the survivors develop long term impairments such as hearing deficits, chronic lung disease, cerebral palsy and other neurodevelopmental disabilities.

References

1. Perez KM, Laughon M. Sildenafil in term and premature infants: a systematic review. Clin Ther. 2015;37(11):2598–2607.e1.
2. Kelly LE, Ohlsson A, Shah PS. Sildenafil for pulmonary hypertension in neonates. Cochrane Database Syst Rev. 2017;8:CD005494.
3. Nair J, Lakshminrusimha S. Update on PPHN: mechanisms and treatment. Semin Perinatol. 2014;38(2):78–91.
4. Wild LM, Nickerson PA, Morin FC. Ligating the ductus arteriosus before birth remodels the pulmonary vasculature of the lamb. Pediatr Res. 1989;25(3):251–7.
5. Szafranski P, Gambin T, Dharmadhikari AV, Akdemir KC, Jhangiani SN, Schuette J, et al. Pathogenetics of alveolar capillary dysplasia with misalignment of pulmonary veins. Hum Genet. 2016;135(5):569–86.
6. Hamvas A, Cole FS, Nogee LM. Genetic disorders of surfactant proteins. Neonatology. 2007;91(4):311–7.
7. Shulenin S, Nogee LM, Annilo T, Wert SE, Whitsett JA, Dean M. ABCA3 gene mutations in newborns with fatal surfactant deficiency. N Engl J Med. 2004;350(13):1296–303.
8. Byers HM, Dagle JM, Klein JM, Ryckman KK, McDonald EL, Murray JC, et al. Variations in CRHR1 are associated with persistent pulmonary hypertension of the newborn. Pediatr Res. 2012;71(2):162–7.
9. Van Marter LJ, Hernandez-Diaz S, Werler MM, Louik C, Mitchell AA. Nonsteroidal antiin-flammatory drugs in late pregnancy and persistent pulmonary hypertension of the newborn. Pediatrics. 2013;131(1):79–87.
10. Winovitch KC, Padilla L, Ghamsary M, Lagrew DC, Wing DA. Persistent pulmonary hyper-tension of the newborn following elective cesarean delivery at term. J Matern Neonatal Med. 2011;24(11):1398–402.
11. Thoresen M. Hypothermia after perinatal asphyxia: Selection for treatment and cooling proto-col. J Pediatr. 2011;158(Suppl 2):e45–9.
12. Eicher DJ, Wagner CL, Katikaneni LP, Hulsey TC, Bass WT, Kaufman DA, et al. Moderate hypothermia in neonatal encephalopathy: efficacy outcomes. Pediatr Neurol. 2005;32:11–7.
13. Ewer AK, Middleton LJ, Furmston AT, Bhoyar A, Daniels JP, Thangaratinam S, et al. Pulse oximetry screening for congenital heart defects in newborn infants (PulseOx): a test accuracy study. Lancet. 2011;378(9793):785–94.
14. Lakshminrusimha S, Wynn RJ, Youssfi M, Pabalan MJ, Bommaraju M, Kirmani K, et al. Use of CT angiography in the diagnosis of total anomalous venous return. J Perinatol. 2009;29(6):458–61.
15. Berenz A, Vergales JE, Swanson JR, Sinkin RA. Evidence of early pulmonary hyperten-sion is associated with increased mortality in very low birth weight infants. Am J Perinatol. 2017;34(8):801–7.
16. Puthiyachirakkal M, Mhanna MJ. Pathophysiology, management, and outcome of persistent pulmonary hypertension of the newborn: a clinical review. Front Pediatr. 2013;1:23.
17. Skinner JR, Hunter S, Hey EN. Haemodynamic features at presentation in persistent pul-monary hypertension of the newborn and outcome. Arch Dis Child Fetal Neonatal Ed. 2008;74(1):F26–32.
18. Fraisse A, Geva T, Gaudart J, Wessel DL. Doppler echocardiographic predictors of outcome in newborns with persistent pulmonary hypertension. Cardiol Young. 2004;14(3):277–83.
19. Aggarwal S, Natarajan G. Echocardiographic correlates of persistent pulmonary hypertension of the newborn. Early Hum Dev. 2015;91(4):285–9.
20. Bendapudi P, Rao GG, Greenough A. Diagnosis and management of persistent pulmonary hypertension of the newborn. Paediatr Respir Rev. 2015;16(3):157–61.
21. King ME, Braun H, Goldblatt A, Liberthson R, Weyman AE. Interventricular septal configu-ration as a predictor of right ventricular systolic hypertension in children: a cross-sectional echocardiographic study. Circulation. 1983;68(1):68–75.

22. Dhillon R. The management of neonatal pulmonary hypertension. Arch Dis Child Fetal Neonatal Ed. 2012;97(3):F223–8.
23. Reynolds EW. Brain-type natriuretic peptide in the diagnosis and management of persistent pulmonary hypertension of the newborn: in reply. Pediatrics. 2005;114(5):1297–304.
24. Vijlbrief DC, Benders MJ, Kemperman H, van Bel F, de Vries WB. B-type natriuretic peptide and rebound during treatment for persistent pulmonary hypertension. J Pediatr. 2012;160(1):111–5.e1.
25. Cheung PY, Tyebkhan JM, Peliowski A, Ainsworth W, Robertson CMT. Prolonged use of pancuronium bromide and sensorineural hearing loss in childhood survivors of congenital diaphragmatic hernia. J Pediatr. 1999;135(2 Pt 1):233–9.
26. Walsh-Sukys MC, Tyson JE, Wright LL, Bauer CR, Korones SB, Stevenson DK, et al. Persistent pulmonary hypertension of the newborn in the era before nitric oxide: practice variation and outcomes. Pediatrics. 2000;105(1 Pt 1):14–20.
27. Agrawal. Persistent pulmonary hypertension of the newborn: recent advances in the management. Int J Clin Pediatr. 2013;89(3):226–42.
28. Tourneux P, Rakza T, Bouissou A, Krim G, Storme L. Pulmonary circulatory effects of norepinephrine in newborn infants with persistent pulmonary hypertension. J Pediatr. 2008;153(3):345–9.
29. Ostrea EM, Villanueva-Uy ET, Natarajan G, Uy HG. Persistent pulmonary hypertension of the newborn: pathogenesis, etiology, and management. Pediatr Drugs. 2006;8(3):179–88.
30. Lotze A, Mitchell BR, Bulas DI, Zola EM, Shalwitz RA, Gunkel JH, et al. Multicenter study of surfactant (beractant) use in the treatment of term infants with severe respiratory failure. J Pediatr. 1998;132(1):40–7.
31. Gadzinowski J, Kowalska K, Vidyasagar D. Treatment of MAS with PPHN using combined therapy: SLL, bolus surfactant and iNO. J Perinatol. 2008;28(Suppl 3):S56–66.
32. Bifano EM, Pfannenstiel A. Duration of hyperventilation and outcome in infants with persistent pulmonary hypertension. Pediatrics. 1988;81(5):657–61.
33. Hendricks-Munoz KD, Walton J. Hearing loss in infants with persistent fetal circulation. Pediatrics. 1988;81(5):650–6.
34. Dworetz A, Moya F, Sabo B, et al. Survival of infants with persistent pulmonary hypertension without extracorporeal membrane oxygenation. Pediatrics. 1989;84(1):1–6.
35. Wung JT, James LS, Kilchevsky E, James E. Management of infants with severe respiratory failure and persistence of the fetal circulation, without hyperventilation. Pediatrics. 1985;76(4):488–94.
36. Rudolph AM, Yuan S. Response of the pulmonary vasculature to hypoxia and H+ ion concentration changes. J Clin Invest. 1966;45(3):399–411.
37. Konduri GG, Kim UO. Advances in the diagnosis and management of persistent pulmonary hypertension of the newborn. Pediatr Clin North Am. 2009;56(3):579–600.
38. Kinsella JP, Abman SH. Clinical approach to inhaled nitric oxide therapy in the newborn with hypoxemia. J Pediatr. 2000;136(6):717–26.
39. Gao Y, Ray J. Regulation of the pulmonary circulation in the fetus and newborn. Circulation. 2010;90(4):1291–335.
40. Barrington K, Finer N. Inhaled nitric oxide for respiratory failure in preterm infants. Cochrane Database Syst Rev. 2007;(12):CD000509.
41. The Neonatal Inhaled Nitric Oxide Study Group. Inhaled nitric oxide in full-term and nearly full-term infants with hypoxic respiratory failure. N Engl J Med. 1997;336(9):597–604.
42. Konduri GG, Solimano A, Sokol GM, Singer J, Ehrenkranz RA, Singhal N, et al. A randomized trial of early versus standard inhaled nitric oxide therapy in term and near-term newborn infants with hypoxic respiratory failure. Pediatrics. 2004;113(3 Pt 1):559–64.
43. Shivananda S, Ahliwahlia L, Kluckow M, Luc J, Jankov R, McNamara P. Variation in the management of persistent pulmonary hypertension of the newborn: a survey of physicians in Canada, Australia, and New Zealand. Am J Perinatol. 2012;29(7):519–26.
44. Soll RF. Inhaled nitric oxide in the neonate. J Perinatol. 2009;29(Suppl 2):S63–7.

45. Kinsella JP. Clinical trials of inhaled nitric oxide therapy in the newborn. Pediatr Rev. 2018;20(11):e110–3.
46. Peliowski A, Jefferies AL, Lacaze-Masmonteil T, Sorokan ST, Stanwick R, Whyte HEA, et al. Inhaled nitric oxide use in newborns. Paediatr Child Health. 2012;17(2):95–7.
47. Davidson D, Barefield ES, Kattwinkel J, Dudell G, Damask M, Straube R, et al. Inhaled nitric oxide for the early treatment of persistent pulmonary hypertension of the term newborn: a randomized, double-masked, placebo-controlled, dose-response, multicenter study. The I-NO/PPHN Study Group. Pediatrics. 1998;101(3 Pt 1):325–34.
48. Davidson D, Barefield ES, Kattwinkel J, Dudell G, Damask M, Straube R, et al. Safety of withdrawing inhaled nitric oxide therapy in persistent pulmonary hypertension of the newborn. Pediatrics. 1999;104(2 Pt 1):231–6.
49. Steinhorn RH, Kinsella JP, Pierce C, Butrous G, Dilleen M, Oakes M, et al. Intravenous sildenafil in the treatment of neonates with persistent pulmonary hypertension. J Pediatr. 2009;155(6):841–847.e1.
50. Lakshminrusimha S, Mathew B, Leach CL. Pharmacologic strategies in neonatal pulmonary hypertension other than nitric oxide. Semin Perinatol. 2016;40(3):160–73.
51. Lakshminrusimha S, Steinhorn RH. Inodilators in nitric oxide resistant persistent pulmonary hypertension of the newborn. Pediatr Crit Care Med. 2013;14(1):107–9.
52. Bassler D, Kreutzer K, McNamara P, Kirpalani H. Milrinone for persistent pulmonary hypertension of the newborn. Cochrane Database Syst Rev. 2010;(11):CD007802.
53. McNamara PJ, Laique F, Muang-In S, Whyte HE. Milrinone improves oxygenation in neonates with severe persistent pulmonary hypertension of the newborn. J Crit Care. 2006;21(2):217–22.
54. Ahmad KA, Banales J, Henderson CL, Ramos SE, Brandt KM, Powers GC. Intravenous epoprostenol improves oxygenation index in patients with persistent pulmonary hypertension of the newborn refractory to nitric oxide. J Perinatol. 2018;38(9):1212–9.
55. Golzand E, Bar-Oz B, Arad I. Intravenous prostacyclin in the treatment of persistent pulmonary hypertension of the newborn refractory to inhaled nitric oxide. Isr Med Assoc J. 2005;7(6):408–9.
56. Gabbay E, Fraser J, McNeil K. Review of bosentan in the management of pulmonary arterial hypertension. Vasc Health Risk Manag. 2007;3(6):887–900.
57. Rao S, Bartle D, Patole S. Current and future therapeutic options for persistent pulmonary hypertension in the newborn. Expert Rev Cardiovasc Ther. 2010;8(6):845–62.
58. Nakwan N, Choksuchat D, Saksawad R, Thammachote P, Nakwan N. Successful treatment of persistent pulmonary hypertension of the newborn with bosentan. Acta Paediatr Int J Paediatr. 2009;98(10):1683–5.
59. Mohamed WA, Ismail M. A randomized, double-blind, placebo-controlled, prospective study of bosentan for the treatment of persistent pulmonary hypertension of the newborn. J Perinatol. 2012;32(8):608–13.
60. Ho JJ, Rasa G. Magnesium sulfate for persistent pulmonary hypertension of the newborn. Cochrane Database Syst Rev. 2007;(3):CD005588.
61. Boo NY, Rohana J, Yong SC, Bilkis AZ, Yong-Junina F. Inhaled nitric oxide and intravenous magnesium sulphate for the treatment of persistent pulmonary hypertension of the newborn. Singapore Med J. 2010;51(2):144–50.
62. Mohamed A, Nasef N, Shah V, McNamara PJ. Vasopressin as a rescue therapy for refractory pulmonary hypertension in neonates: case series. Pediatr Crit Care Med. 2014;15(2):148–54.
63. Bennett CC, Johnson A, Field DJ, Elbourne D. UK collaborative randomised trial of neonatal extracorporeal membrane oxygenation: follow-up to age 4 years. Lancet. 2001;357(9262):1094–6.
64. Mugford M, Elbourne D, Field D. Extracorporeal membrane oxygenation for severe respiratory failure in newborn infants. Cochrane Database Syst Rev. 2008;(3):CD001340.
65. Lazar DA, Cass DL, Olutoye OO, Welty SE, Fernandes CJ, Rycus PT, et al. The use of ECMO for persistent pulmonary hypertension of the newborn: a decade of experience. J Surg Res. 2012;177(2):263–7.

66. Rosenberg AA, Lee NR, Vaver KN, Werner D, Fashaw L, Hale K, Waas N, et al. School-age outcomes of newborns treated for persistent pulmonary hypertension. J Perinatol. 2010;30(2):127–34.
67. Finer N. Inhaled nitric oxide in term and near-term infants: neurodevelopmental follow-up of The Neonatal Inhaled Nitric Oxide Study Group (NINOS). J Pediatr. 2000;136(5):611–7.
68. Eriksen V, Nielsen LH, Klokker M, Greisen G. Follow-up of 5- to 11-year-old children treated for persistent pulmonary hypertension of the newborn. Acta Paediatr. 2009;98(2):304–9.
69. Lakshminrusimha S, Russell JA, Wedgwood S, Gugino SF, Kazzaz JA, Davis JM, et al. Superoxide dismutase improves oxygenation and reduces oxidation in neonatal pulmonary hypertension. Am J Respir Crit Care Med. 2006;174(12):1370–7.
70. Wedgwood S, Lakshminrusimha S, Farrow KN, Czech L, Gugino SF, Soares F, et al. Apocynin improves oxygenation and increases eNOS in persistent pulmonary hypertension of the newborn. Am J Physiol Cell Mol Physiol. 2011;302(6):L616–26.
71. Chandrasekar I, Eis A, Konduri GG. Betamethasone attenuates oxidant stress in endothelial cells from fetal lambs with persistent pulmonary hypertension. Pediatr Res. 2008;63(1):67–72.
72. Deruelle P, Balasubramaniam V, Kunig AM, Seedorf GJ, Markham NE, Abman SH. BAY 41-2272, a direct activator of soluble guanylate cyclase, reduces right ventricular hypertrophy and prevents pulmonary vascular remodeling during chronic hypoxia in neonatal rats. Biol Neonate. 2006;90(2):135–44.
73. Fike CD, Dikalova A, Kaplowitz MR, Cunningham G, Summar M, Aschner JL. Rescue treatment with L-citrulline inhibits hypoxia-induced pulmonary hypertension in newborn pigs. Am J Respir Cell Mol Biol. 2015;53(2):255–64.
74. Parker TA, Roe G, Grover TR, Abman SH. Rho kinase activation maintains high pulmonary vascular resistance in the ovine fetal lung. Am J Physiol Cell Mol Physiol. 2006;291(5):L976–82.
75. Wolf D, Tseng N, Seedorf G, Roe G, Abman SH, Gien J. Endothelin-1 decreases endothelial PPARγ signaling and impairs angiogenesis after chronic intrauterine pulmonary hypertension. Am J Physiol Cell Mol Physiol. 2013;306(4):L361–71.

Chapter 8
Neonatal Surgical Conditions: Congenital Diaphragmatic Hernia and Short Bowel Syndrome

Yew-Wei Tan, Andrew Currie, and Bala Eradi

Congenital Diaphragmatic Hernia

The prevalence of Congenital Diaphragmatic Hernia (CDH) is about 3.5 in every 10,000 pregnancies [1]. The overall survival of babies diagnosed prenatally to have this condition is only about 55% once intrauterine fetal demise and termination of pregnancy are taken into account [1]. Although survival of infants born alive with this condition has improved over the years, it is still only 60–80% in high-volume centres [2, 3]. Contrast this with a condition such as oesophageal atresia, where survival now approaches 100% for infants born alive with an isolated anomaly [4]. In addition, there is significant morbidity associated with the condition, especially in the more severely affected infants with huge implications in terms of health-care costs [3].

Antenatal Imaging and Prognosis

There is a wide spectrum of severity of disease in babies affected by CDH. Therefore, when the condition is diagnosed prenatally, it is desirable to be able to predict the severity of disease with as much accuracy as possible in order to counsel the expectant parents as well as for important decisions regarding management and resource allocation [5].

Y.-W. Tan
Paediatric Surgery, Evelina Childrens Hospital, London, UK

A. Currie
Neonatology, Leicester Royal Infirmary, Leicester, UK
e-mail: Andrew.e.currie@uhl-tr.nhs.uk

B. Eradi (✉)
Paediatric Surgery, Leicester Royal Infirmary, Leicester, UK
e-mail: bala.eradi@uhl-tr.nhs.uk

© Springer Nature Switzerland AG 2020
E. M. Boyle, J. Cusack (eds.), *Emerging Topics and Controversies in Neonatology*, https://doi.org/10.1007/978-3-030-28829-7_8

The initial diagnosis is invariably by ultrasound examination (US) and the first described prognostic factor on antenatal ultrasound was the Lung to Head Ratio (LHR). LHR is an estimate of lung volume normalised for head circumference. LHR of less than one is a strong predictor of mortality [6]. There is however, differential growth of the lung and head in the fetus and therefore, the observed to expected LHR (o/e LHR) has been introduced to eliminate the effect of gestational age [7]. For left-sided CDH, there are virtually no survivors when o/e LHR is below 15% but survival is greater than 75% when o/e LHR is greater than 45% [7].

Fetal magnetic resonance imaging (MRI) measurements of lung volume have the advantage of being less affected by maternal body habitus and fetal position. Total fetal lung volume (TFLV) is the sum total volume of both lungs as measured by MRI. The observed to expected TFLV (o/e TFLV) is TFLV that is corrected for gestation as well as for fetal body volume, and percentage thresholds similar to o/e LHR are found to correlate closely with mortality [8]. Prognostic accuracy of o/e LHR is similar to MRI based TFLV when the tracing method is used for US estimation of lung volume [5, 9].

The presence of the liver within the chest has traditionally been considered an independent poor prognostic factor [10]. Though there is now uncertainty whether this is truly independent, recent studies have found that prognostic accuracy may be increased by combining the percentage of liver herniation with o/e LHR [11, 12]. Prenatally diagnosed right sided defects are associated with greater mortality. However, a recent study demonstrated that it is the size of the defect that determines mortality risk, as well as the potential for prenatal diagnosis and that similar size defects were associated with similar mortality irrespective of side or time of diagnosis [13].

Genetic Testing

Numerous genetic defects and syndromes are associated with CDH [14]. The genetic aetiology of CDH is highly heterogeneous and aneuploidies, cytogenetic rearrangements, copy number variants (CNVs) and single-gene mutations have been identified as being associated with isolated CDH [15]. However, these are not clinically useful at the present time as the resulting phenotype is unpredictable [14, 15]. Future large scale genetic studies may reveal more genes as well as factors affecting penetrance.

Antenatal Intervention

The primary cause of mortality and morbidity in CDH is the associated developmental lung abnormality. It seems reasonable, therefore, to attempt to interrupt the development of the lung abnormality by antenatal intervention. Initial attempts to repair the CDH prenatally were disappointing as returning the liver to the abdomen tended to obstruct umbilical venous blood flow [9].

Fetoscopic endoluminal tracheal occlusion (FETO) has been postulated as a method to make the lungs grow based on observations made in fetuses affected by congenital high airway obstruction. Currently this is the only prenatal intervention that is available and is offered by selected centres within the ambit of the TOTAL research trials (www.totaltrial.eu) which includes leading centres in Europe, North America and Australia. In these trials, the intervention is offered to fetuses stratified as having severe or moderate lung hypoplasia based on O/E LHR as well as liver position. Tracheal occlusion is done by using an intra-tracheal balloon that is placed by fetoscopy, ideally between 26 and 28 weeks of gestation and then removed at 34 weeks [16]. While the outcome of the TOTAL research trial is awaited, some FETO centres have reported improvements in mortality and morbidity [9].

A few workers have looked at use of antenatal pharmaceutical agents. Sildanefil (phosphodiesterase 5 inhibitor) [17], Bosentan (Endothelin-1 receptor antagonist) [18], Simvastatin (lipid lowering agent) [19] and Imatinib (platelet derived growth factor antagonist) [20] have all been shown to reduce pulmonary vascular changes in animal CDH models. Of these, maternal Sildenafil administration is closest to clinical application [16].

There is ongoing research into stem cell therapy to treat neonatal respiratory disorders such as bronchopulmonary dysplasia (BPD) and pulmonary hypertension (PH). Some stem cells have shown promise in preclinical studies and have already led to phase 1 clinical trials in infants at risk of developing BPD [21]. Similar developments are envisaged in antenatal interventions for CDH [22].

Neonatal Interventions

Ventilatory Strategy

Historically, mechanical ventilation strategies for newborn infants with CDH involved high respiratory rates and airway pressures in view of experimental evidence that pulmonary vascular resistance worsened with hypoxia and acidosis. This strategy resulted in pulmonary barotrauma and its deleterious effects soon became apparent. After the initial study reporting the benefit of restricting airway pressure, numerous other studies confirmed improved outcomes by using lung-protecting ventilation strategies [23]. Consensus guidelines from Europe [24] and from North America [25, 26] now recommend that conventional mechanical ventilation be used as the initial ventilatory strategy. The target $PaCO_2$ should be between 6.9 and 9.3 kPa (50–70 mmHg), pre-ductal oxygen saturation should be 80–95% and post ductal saturations above 70%. Pressure controlled ventilator settings should be adjusted so that peak inspiratory pressure (PIP) does not exceed 25 cm H_2O and positive end expiratory pressure (PEEP) of 3–5 cm H_2O is maintained. High frequency oscillatory ventilation should be considered for 'rescue' therapy if PIP of greater than 25–28 cm becomes necessary to maintain oxygenation [24–26].

Helium is an inert gas with lower density than air. It therefore flows through airways with less turbulence, lowering the driving pressure required to deliver it.

Heliox (oxygen and helium mixture) has been used in neonatal respiratory distress syndrome under research conditions and the available evidence suggests that it improves gas exchange and reduces the duration of mechanical ventilation. Similarly, use of Heliox in CDH has been reported to allow reduction of ventilator settings and oxygen exposure though further impact on outcomes is unknown [27]. This may be a useful addition for future ventilator strategies but further studies are needed.

Management of Pulmonary Hypertension

Congenital diaphragmatic hernia is associated with characteristic abnormalities of pulmonary vasculature such as a hypoplastic pulmonary vascular bed with fewer branches and increased muscular tissue that extends more distally than is normal. The adventitia of the pulmonary vasculature is also abnormally thickened. In addition to these anatomical, "irreversible" changes, the pulmonary vasculature reacts abnormally to physiological and pharmacological stimuli. These changes result in a higher than normal pulmonary artery pressure, the severity of which is an important determinant of outcome in infants affected by CDH [28, 29].

Direct measurement of the pulmonary artery pressure is not feasible in neonates with CDH, and there is no agreed definition for CDH associated pulmonary hypertension (PH). Echocardiography is therefore used to estimate the level of PH. The tricuspid regurgitant jet, bowing of the inter-ventricular septum and degree of shunt across the ductus arteriosus provide a useful estimate of the right ventricular systolic pressure (RVSP) in relation to the systemic blood pressure (SBP) and thus the severity of pulmonary hypertension. Survival is high (98.6%) when the ratio of RVSP to SBP is less than 0.5 and thus this is considered normal. Mortality approaches 100% when the RSVP/SBP ratio is >1.0 (i.e. RSVP is suprasystemic) at 3 weeks of age [30].

PH related to CDH is challenging to manage as the pulmonary vascular response to various pharmacological agents is altered in CDH, often resulting in a variable and inconsistent response.

Inhaled nitric oxide (iNO) is the most frequently used pharmacological agent to reduce pulmonary pressure. There is evidence that iNO does not reduce mortality or ECMO utilisation in neonates with CDH [24–26, 31]. Despite this the use of iNO is increasing. Consensus guidelines and other publications support the use of iNO for severe CDH associated PH once it is established that left ventricular function is preserved and that adequate lung recruitment has occurred, but recommend that it be discontinued if clinical improvement is not observed within a short, defined time frame [24–26].

Sildenafil is a phosphodiesterase-5 inhibitor and is gaining popularity in the management of CDH associated PH. Case series have demonstrated improvements in oxygenation and echocardiographic parameters [32]. Whether this would translate into improved outcomes is not clear. However, consensus guidelines suggest that Sildenafil may be used when PH is refractory to iNO or during weaning from iNO [24–26].

Milrinone (phosphodiesterase 3 inhibitor) has been shown in a small study of CDH patients to improve oxygenation and right ventricle function. A recent pilot survey has revealed more widespread use in patients with CDH and a more rigorous trial is proposed [33].

Bosentan (endothelin 1 receptor antagonist) has been shown in a trial to have benefit in infants with persistent pulmonary hypertension (PPHN) and has been used to treat CDH PH [34]. Other agents that have been used in the context of PPHN are prostaglandin E1 and prostacyclins (epoprostinol and treprostanil). Their use in CDH may be limited by the left ventricular dysfunction often encountered in severe CDH associated PH [34].

Role of Extracorporeal Membrane Oxygenation

CDH is the most common indication for neonatal Extracorporeal Membrane Oxygenation (ECMO) according to the ELSO (Extracorporeal Life Support Organisation) registry. Yet it is associated with the worst outcomes of all indications for ECMO with 50% survival [35], a number that has been static despite advances in technique, though the risk characteristics of infants treated with ECMO have also worsened with time [36, 37]. Its use varies widely, with 30–50% of CDH infants being treated by ECMO in large centres in the United States and Europe [38] whilst ECMO utilisation was only 7.1% in Canada [39] and 4% in Britain [40]. Reported survival rates are similar, which raises the question about either the comparability of patients [38] or indeed the utility of ECMO [24]. European consensus guidelines now suggest that ECMO be offered to CDH infants who fail conventional management [24]. By contrast, Canadian guidelines recommend that the parents also be counselled about lack of survival advantage based on current evidence [25].

The question also remains of how long support should be offered for if improvement is not seen, with some arguing against arbitrary time limits [38] and others suggesting that palliative care be offered after 2 weeks on ECMO [25] without sign of recovery.

The timing of repair of CDH is another matter of contention. Repair off ECMO is associated with best outcomes [41] but, in some infants discontinuation of ECMO may not be possible, and mortality is assured if repair is not done at all [38]. There seems to be a survival advantage when CDH repair is performed early on ECMO (before 72 h) compared to late [42]. It would appear therefore, that repair is best done either early on ECMO or after decannulation, but the evidence to support one approach over the other is weak [43].

Minimally Invasive Surgery (MIS)

Minimally invasive techniques are being used with increasing frequency for the repair of CDH. Intraoperative hypercarbia and acidosis is common and can be severe on occasion [44]. The long-term effects of this are not known.

The CDH Study group multicentre experience of MIS is that it was associated with higher recurrence rates during their initial experience compared to other studies [45, 46]. Recent series [47] and the latter part of the CDH study group experience [45] have shown equivalent recurrence rates to open repair and possibly reflect growing experience and expertise with MIS. However, there is a selection bias and MIS patients tend to be low-risk in terms of defect size and comorbidity [45, 48]. The advantages of MIS are a shorter hospital stay, reduced postoperative pain as well as lower risk of post-operative intestinal obstruction due to adhesions [45–48]. MIS may therefore have a role in experienced hands and in selected patients with appropriate counselling regarding risks; especially that of recurrence.

Short Bowel Syndrome

Definition of Short Bowel Syndrome and Intestinal Failure

Intestinal failure (IF) is defined as inability of an infant to achieve enteral autonomy(i.e. enteral nutrition alone is not enough to sustain growth and development) and therefore parenteral nutrition (PN) is required for more than 42 days (Canadian Association of Paediatric Surgeons definition) [49] or more than 60 days (Pediatric Intestinal Failure Consortium—PIFCON, USA, definition) [50].

Short bowel syndrome (SBS) is the most common cause of intestinal failure (IF) in infancy [51]. IF due to SBS is associated with significant loss or non-availability of absorptive surface area, whereas non-SBS IF is due to lack of satisfactory absorption [52]. This section focuses on IF due to intestinal loss.

Though consensus is lacking, one definition of SBS is residual small bowel length of less than 25% of that expected [53]. There is a subgroup of SBS known as ultra-SBS (USBS) whereby the length of small intestine is less than 10% of expected length [54].

Reference lengths for comparison have been attained from post-mortem measurements. Based on the patient's gestational age, the expected mean small intestine lengths are, approximately: 70 cm at 24–26 weeks, 120 cm at 33–35 weeks and 160 cm at 39–40 weeks of gestation. At 6 months and 1 year of age, intestinal length is approximately 240 and 280 cm respectively [55].

Aetiology of SBS in early life, in decreasing order of frequency include: necrotising enterocolitis (NEC), gastroschisis, jejunoileal atresia, volvulus, complex meconium ileus, and Hirschsprung's disease [49, 50].

Management of Short Bowel Syndrome

When major bowel compromise is encountered at initial laparotomy, and there is a real risk of USBS, the first decision is to determine whether the patient should continue to receive active treatment or palliative care. This is a decision best made jointly by neonatologists, gastroenterologists and paediatric surgeons, while considering the impact of co-morbidities and taking into account the parents' wishes [54]. A second-look laparotomy preceded by laparostomy or closure with a transparent silo may be indicated when there is considerable bowel of dubious viability and in order to gain time to ascertain the decision of the parents and the multidisciplinary team regarding continuation of care with USBS [56].

It was suggested in the 1950s that an infant could not part with more than 38 cm of small intestine and survive [57]. The management of SBS and IF has evolved tremendously since then, especially with the introduction of parenteral nutrition in the 1960s [58].

A protocolised, multidisciplinary approach to SBS and IF called intestinal rehabilitation program (IRP) has been credited with improved overall outcomes [58–61]. Referral to an IRP should be triggered once SBS and IF are identified based on definitions [49, 50, 53, 54]. The main aim of intestinal rehabilitation programs is to support the patient on PN and prevent complications while awaiting intestinal adaption and enteral autonomy. Medical and surgical adjuncts are used to help with this process.

Malabsorption and Dysmotility

It is well recognised that ileum is able to compensate for jejunal loss, but the opposite is not as well tolerated, as jejunum is not able to absorb bile salts and vitamin B12 [62, 63]. This is also because patients with a jejunostomy suffer from rapid transit, lack of digestion from pancreatobiliary secretions and lack of contact with enterocytes. Significant loss of ileum results in attenuation of the 'ileal brake' controlled by signaling from glucagon-like peptide (GLP-1 and GLP-2), neurotensin, and peptide tyrosine tyrosine (PYY) which results in loose stools [64, 65].

Loss of the ileocaecal valve may also result in colonic bacterial colonisation in the small bowel, causing inflammatory changes and villous atrophy and worsening malabsorption [65].

GLP-2 analogue (Teduglutide) helps with intestinal mucosal growth and repair, and reducing gastric secretion, and has been shown to improve fluid and nutritional absorption in short bowel syndrome. A multicentre randomised controlled trial in adults demonstrated advantage of teduglutide over placebo in terms of PN volume [66]. Post-hoc analysis also showed that such improvement is greatest in patients with a jejunostomy or ileostomy [67]. This was backed up by a phase 3 trial on paediatric patients on PN beyond infancy, demonstrating improvement in PN dependence [68]. Teduglutide is licensed for use in the United Kingdom [69] and is the subject of evaluation by the National Institute for Health and Care Excellence (NICE) [70].

Glutamine, which in animal models has been shown to promote enterocyte growth, integrity, and immunity, has not been demonstrated to be effective in helping to achieve enteral autonomy, either given enterally [71] or parenterally [72, 73].

SBS-IF patients often have intestinal dysmotility, including bowel inflammation and damage, distension resulting in mechanical failure of peristalsis, smooth muscle hypertrophy and hyperplasia (e.g. gastroschisis), interstitial cell of Cajal failure of differentiation (e.g. gastroschisis), and myenteric nerve aganglionosis (e.g. bowel atresia).

Prokinetic agents are often used to treat dysmotility, but are associated with unacceptable side effects and poor effectiveness [74].

Antimotility agents such as codeine and loperamide are effective in reducing stool volume and electrolyte losses but do not improve nutrient absorption [74].

Intestinal Failure Associated Liver Dysfunction (IFALD)

Cholestasis related to IF can be due to a combination of sepsis, lack of enteral feeds, hepatic immaturity, and total parenteral nutrition toxicity [75]. Systematic reviews [76, 77] have shown that:

- The risk factors for PN associated cholestasis (PNAC) are prematurity, low birth weight, NEC, long PN duration and sepsis.
- Fish-oil based lipid emulsions are safe and effective in reversing PNAC
- Enteral trophic feeding significantly reduces the incidence and severity of PNAC, though this may not always be practical. Discontinuation of PN for short periods of time (cycling) also prevents progression of liver dysfunction in mild to moderate PNAC.
- Bile acid (e.g. Ursodeoxycholic acid) supplementation for the prevention of IFALD or indeed its reversal is only supported by weak evidence. Its absorption is questionable when the terminal ileum is not available.
- Newer bile salts such as chenodeoxycholic acid and obeticholic acid have shown promise in early studies on animal models and in adults.
- Anti TNFalpha antibodies (Inflixamab) has been tested and found to be beneficial in murine models of IFALD.
- Exogenous GLP-2 has been shown to improve IFALD in a neonatal piglet model.
- Interruption of signaling pathways that activate Kupffer cells has been shown to reduce liver injury in certain mice models.

Central Venous Catheter Care

There is overwhelming evidence to support prevention of central line associated bloodstream infection (CLABSI) in reducing morbidity and mortality. Incidence of CLABSI in children on PN ranges from 1.3 to 10.2 per 1000 catheter-days [78]. SBS and age <1 year are risk factors. CLABSI reduction strategies, apart from meticulous aseptic technique, include: use of single lumen central line, avoidance of femoral veins and use of ethanol lock [59]. Ethanol lock however, is supported only by weak evidence and is associated with other issues such as catheter degradation and thrombosis. The consequences of failure in preventing CLABSI leads to poorer development, worsening IFALD, venous thrombosis and repeated procedure for line change, hospital admission (35% of admissions), and mortality (11% of all mortality) [78, 79].

Surgical Management

The indications for surgery in the management of SBS are: (1) to improve absorptive surface area; (2) to overcome dysmotility and stasis associated with grossly dilated segments of bowel; and (3) to slow down intestinal transit [80].

Improve Absorptive Surface Area

In the presence of an enterostomy, mucous fistula refeeding may enable early recruitment of the distal remaining intestine and has been claimed to have benefit in reducing PN duration and consequently cholestasis [81]. This practice however, is associated with risk of intestinal perforation, and is nursing intensive. It may be prudent to radiologically confirm distal patency prior to starting recycling of feed into the mucous fistula. Used carefully, it may serve as a means to improve distal intestinal function and growth. Early closure of the stoma would also enable recruitment of distal bowel for absorption.

Overcome Dysmotility and Stasis

This can simply be achieved with bowel tapering to excise the ante-mesenteric side of the dilated intestine, thus reducing calibre and improving the efficacy of peristalsis. With time, autologous intestinal lengthening procedures have supplanted bowel tapering. The term 'lengthening' is potentially misleading, as no increase in absorptive surface is achieved. Instead, reduction in intestinal caliber and improvement of peristalsis are the outcomes. The main contraindication for performing these procedures is end-stage liver failure. The most commonly performed is the Bianchi procedure or longitudinal intestinal lengthening (LILT) and serial transverse enteroplasty (STEP) achieving an average 'lengthening' of about 70% [82]. LILT, described in 1980, works on the principle of halving the dilated segment of bowel longitudinally, with each half being supplied by the preserved branching mesenteric vessels, followed by anastomosis of the two segments [83]. The STEP procedure was introduced in 2003, and involves applying a stapler across more than half the diameter of a dilated segment of bowel alternately in opposite directions, to create z-shape segments which are less dilated and longer in configuration [84].

Slow Down Intestinal Transit

This is now rarely performed due to potential stasis and consequently sepsis, but includes antiperistaltic segments, colonic interposition and intestinal valve creation [80].

Long Term Outcome

Survival

Most centres report about 90% survival over several years follow-up, but this varies from 75% to 97% due to time-period and baseline population [30]. An earlier multicentre series from 14 North American centres with intestinal rehabilitation programs reported outcome of 272 infants (2000–2006) with a median follow-up of 2 years. They found that enteral autonomy was achieved in 47%, survival in 73%, and intestinal transplant in 74% [50]. However more recent large series from Boston (n = 313) and Paris (n = 217) showed better results with transplant-free survival of 89–91%, and overall survival 94–97% at 5-year follow-up [78, 85].

   Two commonest causes of death were IF associated liver disease and central line associated infection. The ability to wean off PN greatly improved survival by eliminating these two factors [86].

Intestinal Transplant

There are three types of intestinal transplants: isolated intestinal, intestinal with liver, and multivisceral transplant. According to American data from Organ Procurement and Transplant Network derived from 2009 to 2011, 1-year and 5-year graft survival for paediatric (below 18 years) intestinal transplant, with or without liver, were 72% and 54%. Complications which developed following transplant included acute rejection (65.7%), and post-transplant lymphoproliferative disorder (9.2%) [87].

Adaptation and Enteral Autonomy (Growth, Development)

Achieving enteral autonomy is the central goal of intestinal rehabilitation. The ability to achieve enteral autonomy has been defined as successful PN discontinuation for more than 3 months [88], which has been reported to be between 42% and 86% [89–91]. PIFCON has identified three key independent factors associated with achieving enteral autonomy over a median follow-up of 33 months: NEC (Odds Ratio—OR—2.42), intact ileo-caecal valve (OR 2.8), and residual length of small bowel of more than 40 cm [89]. Interestingly, Wilmore et al. described that a cut-off of 40 cm of residual small bowel carried 100% mortality in the 1970s [92], but contemporary evidence suggests that a threshold value of 40 cm of small intestine is regarded as the best predictor of achieving enteral autonomy. Nevertheless, less residual small bowel than this is no reason to abandon intestinal rehabilitation. This is supported by another study showing children with SBS (less than 100 cm but more than 50 cm) have 88% chance of enteral autonomy by 1 year, and 96% by 2 years; whereas those with less than 50 cm residual bowel have 23% chance of enteral autonomy by 1 year, 38% by 2 years and 71% by 4.75 years [93].

Conclusion

There is no doubt that considerable ground has been gained in the outcomes of patients with CDH and SBS. Progress has been slow and painstaking however, and many promising interventions have had to be reconsidered in the light of emerging evidence. The ingenuity and industry of clinical and laboratory researchers provides abundant reason for optimism as existing interventions are refined further and nascent therapies are evaluated in a clinical setting.

References

1. Burgos CM, Frenckner B. Addressing the hidden mortality in CDH: a population based study. J Pediatr Surg. 2017;52:522–5.
2. Soek KG, Greenough A, van Rosmalen J, Capolupo I, Schaible T, Ali K, et al. Congenital diaphragmatic hernia: 10-year evaluation of survival, extracorporeal membrane oxygenation, and foetoscopic endotracheal occlusion in four high volume centres. Neonatology. 2018;113:63–8.
3. Lally KP. Congenital diaphragmatic hernia—the past 25 (or so) years. J Pediatr Surg. 2016;51:695–8.

4. Yamoto M, Nomura A, Fukumoto K, Takahashi T, Nakaya K, Sekioka A, et al. New prognostic classification and management in infants with oesophageal atresia. Pediatr Surg Int. 2018;11. https://doi.org/10.1007/s00383-018-4322-5.

5. Oluyomi-Obi T, Kuret V, Puligandla P, Lodha A, Lee-Robertson H, Lee K, et al. Antenatal predictors of outcome in prenatally diagnosed congenital diaphragmatic hernia(CDH). J Pediatr Surg. 2017;52:881–8.

6. Metkus AP, Filly RA, Stringer MD, Harrison MR, Adzick NS. Sonographic predictors of survival in fetal diaphragmatic hernia. J Pediatr Surg. 1996;31:148–51.

7. Deprest JA, Flemmer AW, Gratacos E, Nicolaides K. Antenatal prediction of lung volume and in-utero treatment by fatal endoscopic tracheal occlusion in severe isolated congenital diaphragmatic hernia. Semin Fetal Neonatal Med. 2009;14:8–13.

8. Cannie M, Jani J, Meersschaert J, Allegeart K, Done E, Marchal G, et al. Prenatal prediction of survival using observed to expected total fatal lung volume determined by magnetic resonance imaging based on either gestational age or foetal body volume. Ultrasound Obstet Gynecol. 2008;32:633–9.

9. Oluyomi-Obi T, Meighem TV, Ryan G. Fetal imaging and therapy for CDH—current status. Semin Pediatr Surg. 2017;26:140–6.

10. Mullassery D, Ba'ath ME, Jesudason EC, Losty PD. Value of liver herniation in prediction of outcome in fatal congenital diaphragmatic hernia: a systematic review and meta-analysis. Ultrasound Obstet Gynecol. 2010;35:609–14.

11. Jani J, Nicolaides KH, Keller RL, Benachi A, Peralta CFA, Favre R, et al. Observed to expected lung area to head circumference ratio in the prediction of survival in foetuses with isolated diaphragmatic hernia. Ultrasound Obstet Gynecol. 2007;30:67–71.

12. Ruano R, Lazar DA, Cass DL, Zamora IJ, Lee TC, Cassady CI, et al. Fetal lung volume and quantification of liver herniation by magnetic resonance imaging in isolated congenital diaphragmatic hernia. Ultrasound Obstet Gynecol. 2014;43:662–9.

13. Burgos CM, Frenckner B, Luco M, Harting MT, Lally PA, Lally KP. Prenatally versus postnatally diagnosed congenital diaphragmatic hernia—side, stage and outcome. J Pediatr Surg. 2018. https://doi.org/10.1016/j.jpedsurg.2018.04.008.

14. Deprest J, Brady P, Nicolaides K, Benachi A, Berg C, Vermeesch J, et al. Prenatal management of the foetus with isolated congenital diaphragmatic hernia in the era of the TOTAL trial. Semin Fetal Neonatal Med. 2014;19:338–48.

15. Kardon G, Ackerman KG, McCulley DJ, Shen Y, Wynn J, Shang L, et al. Congenital diaphragmatic hernias: from genes to mechanisms to therapies. Dis Model Mech. 2017;10:955–70.

16. Russo FM, Coppi PD, Allegaert K, Toelen J, van der Veerken L, Attilakos G. Current and future management of isolated congenital diaphragmatic hernia. Semin Fetal Neonatal Med. 2017;22:383–90.

17. Russo FM, Toelen J, Eastwood MP, Jiminez J, Miyague AH, Vande Velde G, et al. Transplacental sildenafil rescues lung abnormalities in a rabbit model of diaphragmatic hernia. Thorax. 2016;71:517–25.

18. Lemus-Varela Mde L, Soliz A, Gomez-Meda BC, Zamora-Perez AL, Ornelas-Aguirre JM, Melnikov V, et al. Antenatal use of bosentan and/or sildenafil attenuates pulmonary features in rats with congenital diaphragmatic hernia. World J Pediatr. 2014;10:354–9.

19. Makanga M, Maruyama H, Dewachter C, Mendes Da Costa A, Hupkens E, de Medina G, et al. Prevention of pulmonary hypoplasia and pulmonary vascular remodelling by antenatal simvastatin treatment in nitrofen-induced congenital diaphragmatic hernia. Am J Physiol Lung Cell Mol Physiol. 2015;308:L672–82.

20. Chang YT, Ringman Uggla A, Osterholm C, Tran PK, Eklof AC, et al. Antenatal imatinib treatment reduces pulmonary vascular remodeling in a rat model of congenital diaphragmatic hernia. Am J Physiol Lung Cell Mol Physiol. 2012;302:L1159–66.

21. Thebaud B. Stem cell-based therapies in neonatology: a new hope. Arch Dis Child Fetal Neonatal Ed. 2018. https://doi.org/10.1136/archdischild-2017-314451.

22. Coppi PD, Deprest J. Regenerative medicine solutions in congenital diaphragmatic hernia. Semin Pediatr Surg. 2017;26:171–7.
23. Boloker J, Bateman DA, Wung JT, Stolar CJH. Congenital diaphragmatic hernia in 120 infants treated consecutively with permissive hypercapnia/spontaneous respiration/elective repair. J Pediatr Surg. 2002;37:357–66.
24. Snoek K, Reiss IKM, Greenough A, Capolupo I, Urlesberger B, Wessel L, et al. CDH EURO consortium. Standardized postnatal management of infants with congenital diaphragmatic hernia in Europe: the CDH EURO Consortium Consensus—2015 update. Neonatology. 2016;110:66–74.
25. The Canadian Congenital Diaphragmatic Hernia Collaborative. Diagnosis and management of congenital diaphragmatic hernia: a clinical practice guideline. CMAJ. 2018;190:E103–12.
26. Puligandla PS, Grabowski J, Austin M, Hedrick H, Renaud E, Arnold M, et al. Management of congenital diaphragmatic hernia: a systematic review from the APSA outcomes and evidence based practice committee. J Pediatr Surg. 2015;50:1958–70.
27. Wise AC, Boutin MA, Knodel EM, Proudfoot JA, Lane BP, Evans ML, et al. Heliox adjunct therapy for neonates with congenital diaphragmatic hernia. Respir Care. 2018;63:1147–53.
28. Mous DS, Kool HM, Wijnen R, Tibboel D, Rottier RJ. Pulmonary vascular development in congenital diaphragmatic hernia. Eur Respir Rev. 2018;27:170104. https://doi.org/10.1183/16000617.0104-2017.
29. Thebaud B, Pierro M. Understanding and treating pulmonary hypertension in congenital diaphragmatic hernia. Semin Fetal Neonatal Med. 2014;19:357–63.
30. Harting MT. Congenital diaphragmatic hernia-associated pulmonary hypertension. Semin Pediatr Surg. 2017;26:147–53.
31. Neonatal Inhaled Nitric Oxide Study Group. Inhaled nitric oxide and hypoxic respiratory failure in infants with congenital diaphragmatic hernia. Paediatrics. 1997;99:838–45.
32. Kipfmuller F, Schroeder L, Berg C, Heindel K, Bartmann P, Mueller A. Continuous intravenous sildenafil as an early treatment in neonates with congenital diaphragmatic hernia. Paediatric Pulmonology. 2018;53:452–60.
33. Lakshminrusimha S, Kezler M, Kirpalani H, Meurs KV, Chess P, Ambalavanan N, et al. Milrinone in congenital diaphragmatic hernia—a randomised pilot trial: study protocol, review of literature and survey of current practices. Matern Health Neonatol Perinatol. 2017;3:27. https://doi.org/10.1186/s40748-017-0066-9.
34. Lakshminrusimha S, Mathew B, Leach CL. Pharmacological strategies in neonatal pulmonary hypertension other than nitric oxide. Semin Perinatol. 2016;40:160–73.
35. Barbaro RP, Paden ML, Guner YS, Raman L, Ryerson LM, Alexander P, et al. Pediatric extracorporeal life support organisation registry international report 2016. ASAIO J. 2017;63:456–63.
36. Turek JW, Nellis JR, Sherwood BG, Kotagal M, Mesher AL, Thiagarajan RR, et al. Shifting risks and conflicting outcomes—ECMO for neonates with congenital diaphragmatic hernia in the modern era. J Pediatr. 2017;190:163–8.
37. Guner YS, Delaplain PT, Zhang L, Nardo MD, Brogan T, Chen Y, et al. Trends in mortality and risk characteristics of congenital diaphragmatic hernia treated with extracorporeal membrane oxygenation. ASAIO J. 2018;65(5):509–15. https://doi.org/10.1097/MAT.0000000000000834.
38. Kays DW. ECMO in CDH: is there a role? Semin Pediatr Surg. 2017;26:166–70.
39. Beaumier CK, Beres AL, Puligandla PS, Skarsgård ED, The Canadian Pediatric Surgery Network. Clinical characteristics and outcomes of patients with right congenital diaphragmatic hernia: a population based study. J Pediatr Surg. 2015;50:731–3.
40. Long AM, Bunch KJ, Knight M, Kurinczuk JJ, Losty PD, on behalf of BAPS-CASS. Early population-based outcomes of infants born with congenital diaphragmatic hernia. Arch Dis Child Fetal Neonatal Ed. 2018;103(6):F517–22. https://doi.org/10.1136/archdischild-2017-313933.
41. Partridge EA, Peranteau WH, Rintoul NE, Herkert LM, Flake AW, Adzick S. Timing of repair of congenital diaphragmatic hernia in patients supported by extracorporeal membrane oxygenation (ECMO). J Pediatr Surg. 2015;50:260–2.

42. Fallon SC, Cass DL, Olutoye OO, Zamora IJ, Lazar DZ. Larimer EL et al Repair of congenital diaphragmatic hernia on extracorporeal membrane oxygenation (ECMO): does early repair improve survival? J Pediatr Surg. 2013;48:1172–6.
43. Desai AA, Ostlie DJ, Juang D. Optimal timing of congenital diaphragmatic hernia repair in infants on extracorporeal membrane oxygenation. Semin Pediatr Surg. 2015;24:17–9.
44. Bishay M, Giacomello M, Retrosi G, Thyoka M, Garriboli M, Brierley J, et al. Hypercapnia and acidosis during open and thoracoscopic repair of congenital diaphragmatic hernia and oesophageal atresia: results of a pilot randomised controlled trial. Ann Surg. 2013;258:895–900.
45. Putnam LR, Tsao K, Lally KP, Blakely ML, Jancelewicz T, Lally PA, et al. Minimal invasive vs open congenital diaphragmatic hernia repair: is there a superior approach. Am Coll Surg. 2017;224:928–32.
46. Vijfhuize S, Deden AC, Costerus SA, Sloots CE, Wijnen RM. Minimal access surgery for repair of congenital diaphragmatic hernia: is it advantageous? -An open review. Eur J Pediatr Surg. 2012;22:364–73.
47. Tyson AF, Sola R Jr, Arnold MR, Cosper GH, Schulman AM. Thoracoscopic vs open congenital diaphragmatic hernia repair: single tertiary centre review. J Laparoendosc Adv Surg Tech A. 2017;27:1209–16.
48. Criss CN, Coughlin MA, Matusko N, Gadepalli SK. Outcomes of thoracoscopic repair of small to moderate congenital diaphragmatic hernias. J Pediatr Surg. 2018;53:635–9.
49. Diamond IR, de Silva N, Pencharz PB, Kim JH, Wales PW, Group for the improvement of intestinal function and treatment (GIFT). Neonatal short bowel syndrome outcomes after the establishment of the first Canadian multidisciplinary intestinal rehabilitation program: preliminary experience. J Pediatr Surg. 2007;42:806–11.
50. Khan FA, Squires Robert H, Litman HJ, Balint J, Carter BA, Fisher JG, et al. Pediatric Intestinal Failure Consortium. Predictors of enteral autonomy in children with intestinal failure: a multicentre cohort study. J Pediatr. 2015;167:29–34.
51. Goulet O, Ruemmele F. Causes and management of intestinal failure in children. Gastroenterology. 2006;130:S16–28.
52. Wessel JJ, Kocoshis SA. Nutritional management of infants with short bowel syndrome. Semin Perinatol. 2007;31:104–11.
53. Hess RA, Welch KB, Brown PI, Teitelbaum DH. Survival outcomes of pediatric intestinal failure patients: analysis of factors contributing to improved survival over the past two decades. J Surg Res. 2011;170:27–31.
54. Batra A, Keys SC, Johnson MJ, Wheeler RA, Beattie RM. Epidemiology, management and outcome of ultrashort bowel syndrome in infancy. Arch Dis Child Fetal Neonatal Ed. 2017;102:1–6.
55. Struijs MC, Diamond IR, de Silva N, Wales PW. Establishing norms for intestinal length in children. J Pediatr Surg. 2009;44:933–8.
56. Tan YW, Merchant J, Sharma V, Davies B, Singh S, Stewart R, More B. Extensive necrotising enterocolitis: objective evaluation of the role of second-look laparotomy in bowel salvage and survival. World J Surg. 2015;39:3016–22.
57. Brown JJM. Small intestine obstruction in the newly born. Ann R Coll Surg Engl. 1957;20(5):280–97. Lecture delivered at the Royal College of Surgeons of England on 5th October 1956. https://europepmc.org/articles/pmc2413473/pdf/annrcse00325-0016.pdf.
58. Colomb V, Dabbas-Tyan M, Taupin P, Talbotec C, Revillon Y, Jan D, et al. Long-term outcome of children receiving home parenteral nutrition: a 20-year single-center experience in 302 patients. J Pediatr Gastroenterol Nutr. 2007;44:347–53.
59. Stanger JD, Oliveira C, Blackmore C, Avitur Y, Wales PW. The impact of multidisciplinary intestinal rehabilitation programs on the outcome of pediatric patients with intestinal failure: a systematic review and meta-analysis. J Pediatr Surg. 2013;48:983–92.
60. Modi BP, Langer M, Ching YA, Valim C, Waterford SD, Iglesias J, et al. Improved survival in a multidisciplinary short bowel syndrome program. J Pediatr Surg. 2008;43:20–4.
61. Merritt RJ, Cohran V, Raphael BP, Sentongo T, Volpert D, Warner BW, et al. on behalf of the Nutrition Committee of the North American Society for Pediatric Gastroenterology,

Hepatology and Nutrition. Intestinal Rehabilitation Programs in the Management of Pediatric Intestinal Failure and Short Bowel Syndrome. J Pediatr Gastroenterol Nutr. 2017;65:588–96.

62. Appleton GVN, Bristol JB, Williamson RCN. Proximal enterectomy provides a stronger systemic stimulus to intestinal adaptation than distal enterectomy. Gut. 1987;28(Suppl):165–8.

63. Chaves M, Smith MW, Williamson RCN. Increased activity of digestive enzymes in ileal enterocyte adaptation to small bowel resection. Gut. 1987;28:981–7.

64. Jeppesen PB, Hartmann B, Thulesen J, Hansen BS, Holst JJ, Poulsen SS, Mortensen PB. Elevated plasma glucagon-like peptide 1 and 2 concentrations in ileum resected short bowel patients with a preserved colon. Gut. 2000;47(3):370–6.

65. Carlson SJ, Chang MI, Nandivada P, Cowan E, Puder M. Neonatal intestinal physiology and failure. Semin Pediatr Surg. 2013;22:190–4.

66. Jeppesen PB, Gilroy R, Pertkiewicz M, Allard JP, Messing B, O'Keefe SJ. Randomised placebo-controlled trial of teduglutide in reducing parenteral nutrition and/or intravenous fluid requirements in patients with short bowel syndrome. Gut. 2011;60:902–14.

67. Jeppesen PB, Gabe SM, Seidner DL, Lee HM, Olivier C. Factors associated with response to teduglutide in patients with short-bowel syndrome and intestinal failure. Gastroenterology. 2018;154:874–85.

68. Carter BA, Cohran VC, Cole CR, Corkins MR, Dimmitt RA, Duggan C, et al. Outcomes from a 12-week, open-label, multicenter clinical trial of teduglutide in pediatric short bowel syndrome. J Pediatr. 2017;181:102–11.

69. https://bnf.nice.org.uk/treatment-summary/short-bowel-syndrome.html.

70. https://www.nice.org.uk/guidance/indevelopment/gid-ta10048.

71. Duggan C, Stark AR, Auestad N, Collier S, Fulhan J, Gura K, et al. Glutamine supplementation in infants with gastrointestinal disease: a randomized, placebo-controlled pilot trial. Nutrition. 2004;20:752–6.

72. Ong EG, Eaton S, Wade AM, Horn V, Losty PD, Curry JI, et al. SIGN Trial Group. Randomized clinical trial of glutamine-supplemented versus standard parenteral nutrition in infants with surgical gastrointestinal disease. Br J Surg. 2012;99:929–38.

73. Albers MJ, Steyerberg EW, Hazebroek FW, Mourik M, Borsboom GJ, Rietveld T, et al. Glutamine supplementation of parenteral nutrition does not improve intestinal permeability, nitrogen balance, or outcome in newborns and infants undergoing digestive-tract surgery: results from a double-blind, randomized, controlled trial. Ann Surg. 2005;241:599–606.

74. Dicken BJ, Sergi C, Rescorla FJ, Breckler F, Sigalet D. Medical management of motility disorders in patients with intestinal failure: a focus on necrotizing enterocolitis, gastroschisis, and intestinal atresia. J Pediatr Surg. 2011;46:1618–30.

75. Carter BA, Shulman RJ. Mechanisms of disease: update on the molecular etiology and fundamentals of parenteral nutrition associated cholestasis. Nat Clin Pract Gastroenterol Hepatol. 2007;4:277–87.

76. Rangel SJ, Calkins CM, Cowles RA, Barnhart DC, Huang EY, Abdullah F, et al. 2011 American Pediatric Surgical Association Outcomes and Clinical Trials Committee. Parenteral nutrition-associated cholestasis: an American Pediatric Surgical Association Outcomes and Clinical Trials Committee systematic review. J Pediatr Surg. 2012;47:225–40.

77. Orso G, Mandato C, Veropalumbo C, Cecchi N, Garzi A, Vajro P. Pediatric parenteral nutrition-associated liver disease and cholestasis: novel advances in pathomechanisms-based prevention and treatment. Dig Liver Dis. 2016;48:215–22.

78. Fullerton BS, Hong CR, Jaksic T. Long term outcomes of pediatric intestinal failure. Semin Pediatr Surg. 2017;26:328–35.

79. Beath SV, Davies P, Papadopoulou A, Khan AR, Bulck RG, Corkery JJ, et al. Parenteral nutrition-related cholestasis in postsurgical neonates: multivariate analysis of risk factors. J Pediatr Surg. 1996;31(4):604–6.

80. Hollwarth ME. Chapter 25. Short bowel syndrome. In: Puri P, Hollwarth M, editors. Springer surgery atlas series—pediatric surgery. New York: Springer; 2004.

81. Lau EC, Fung AC, Wong KK, Tam PK. Beneficial effects of mucous fistula refeeding in necrotizing enterocolitis neonates with enterostomies. J Pediatr Surg. 2016;51:1914–6.
82. Frongia G, Kessler M, Weih S, Nickkholgh A, Mehrabi A, Holland-Cunz S. Comparison of LILT and STEP procedures in children with short bowel syndrome—a systematic review of the literature. J Pediatr Surg. 2013;48:1794–805.
83. Bianchi A. Intestinal loop lengthening—a technique for increasing small intestinal length. J Pediatr Surg. 1980;15:145.
84. Kim HB, Lee PW, Garza J, Duggan C, Fauza D, Jaksic T. Serial transverse enteroplasty for short bowel syndrome: a case report. J Pediatr Surg. 2003;38:881.
85. Abi Nader E, Lambe C, Talbotec C, Pigneur B, Lacaille F, Garnier-Lengline H, et al. Outcome of home parenteral nutrition in 251 children over a 14-y period: report of a single center. Am J Clin Nutr. 2016;103:1327–36.
86. Oliveira C, de Silva NT, Stanojevic S, Avitzur Y, Bayoumi AM, Ungar WJ, et al. Change of outcomes in pediatric intestinal failure: use of time-series analysis to assess the evolution of an intestinal rehabilitation program. J Am Coll Surg. 2016;222:1180–8.
87. Smith JM, Weaver T, Skeans MA, Horslen SP, Harper AM, Snyder JJ, et al. OPTN/SRTR 2016 annual data report: intestine. Am J Transplant. 2018;18(Suppl 1):254–90.
88. Khan FA, Squires Robert H, Litman HJ, et al. For Pediatric Intestinal Failure Consortium. Predictors of enteral autonomy in children with intestinal failure: a multicentre cohort study. J Pediatr. 2015;167:29–34.
89. Goulet O, Revillon Y, Jan D, De Potter S, Maurage C, Lortat-Jacob S, et al. Neonatal short bowel syndrome. J Pediatr. 1991;119:18–23.
90. Guarino A, DeMarco G, Italian National Network for Pediatric Intestinal Failure. Natural history of intestinal failure, investigated through a national network-based approach. J Pediatr Gastroenterol Nutr. 2003;37:136–41.
91. Nucci A, Burns R, Armah T, Lowery K, Yaworski J, Strohm S, et al. Inter-disciplinary management of pediatric intestinal failure: a 10-year review of rehabilitation and transplantation. J Gastrointest Surg. 2008;12:429–36.
92. Wilmore D. Factors correlating with a successful outcome following extensive intestinal resection in newborn infants. J Pediatr. 1972;80:88–95.
93. Fallon EM, Mitchell PD, Nehra D, et al. Neonates with short bowel syndrome: an optimistic future for parenteral nutrition independence. JAMA Surg. 2014;149:663–70.

Chapter 9
Managing the Difficult Airway in a Neonate

James Blythe and Jonathan Cusack

Introduction

Intubation is one of the fundamental clinical skills needed on the neonatal unit. A straightforward 'routine' intubation is a commonplace occurrence and usually goes well. However, a complicated intubation due to a 'difficult airway' can be encountered anywhere, at any time, and even the most experienced clinician can struggle in this situation.

This chapter seeks to help readers with an introduction to the difficult airway, outlining what is meant by this term, and how it might be anticipated, along with details of adjuncts that can be used and a proposed approach to the management in such a scenario. It should be noted that the vast majority of intubations are uncomplicated, resulting in successful placement of a tracheal tube. However, on the rare occasion in which a difficult airway presents itself, the skills described in this chapter could make a significant difference to the outcome.

This chapter builds on the previous sections in this book, with an assumed basic understanding of the techniques involved in routine intubation.

Definition of a 'Difficult Airway'

Figure 9.1 shows a diagram of the oropharynx, showing the important structures that are visualised during intubation.

J. Blythe · J. Cusack (✉)
Leicester Neonatal Service, University Hospitals of Leicester NHS Trust, Leicester Royal Infirmary, Leicester, UK
e-mail: jamesblythe@nhs.net; jonathan.cusack@uhl-tr.nhs.uk

© Springer Nature Switzerland AG 2020
E. M. Boyle, J. Cusack (eds.), *Emerging Topics and Controversies in Neonatology*, https://doi.org/10.1007/978-3-030-28829-7_9

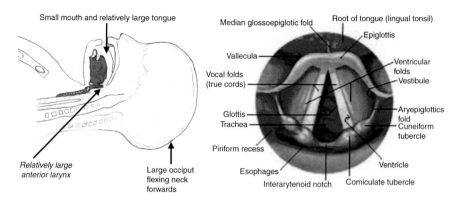

Fig. 9.1 Annotated diagram of the neonatal oropharynx

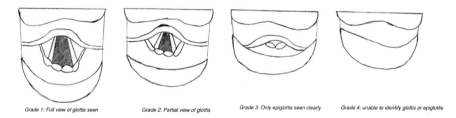

Grade 1: Full view of glottis seen   Grade 2: Partial view of glottis   Grade 3: Only epiglottis seen clearly   Grade 4: unable to identify glottis or epiglottis

Fig. 9.2 The Cormack Lehane grading system

Adult medicine has long recognised that intubations differ in their level of difficulty from one patient to the next. Some clinicians will be familiar with the Cormack-Lehane system (Fig. 9.2), that allows an intubation to be given a level or 'grade' of difficulty. This system was developed in 1984 as a tool to assess an airway, allowing identification of potential difficulties in tracheal intubation, based on the view obtained of the supraglottic region when performing direct laryngoscopy [1]. Further studies have suggested modifications or augmentations to the Cormack-Lehane system, to allow estimations of likely success and time taken to perform intubation [2, 3]. This grading system is based on data from adult patients.

It is worth highlighting that the difficulties encountered in neonatal intubations can be different to that of adult patients, with obesity in the adult population being the most obvious. Conversely, neonatal intubation can be more challenging due to anatomy of oropharyngeal structures. The glottis is smaller (and can be very small in the extremely preterm neonate) and more anterior. It can be physically more challenging to insert equipment into the mouth and obtain a good view of the airway. Neonatal patients have a larger tongue relative to the size of their mouth, which can present challenges in gaining an adequate view of the glottis, and a larger occiput which can complicate head positioning [4, 5]. The epiglottis is 'floppier' and a different shape to that in an adult. This makes it more likely to obscure the view of the vocal cords. There is often decreased muscle tone leading to potential partial or complete occlusion of the airway by the tongue [5]. Added to these things can be a variety of structural congenital anomalies that can further complicate intubation.

In summary, a 'difficult airway' in a neonate is difficult to define, and should perhaps instead be limited to the clinician's interpretation of how the procedure unfolded at that time. Experienced clinicians will recognise cases whereby an intubation has been entirely 'routine' on one occasion, and 'difficult' in another situation with the same patient, even with the same clinician performing the task.

The grading system above has some value in neonatal intubation, if only as a method of documenting any issues which may be of use to the next clinician undertaking intubation in the infant, but is far from being the only tool needed to assess and define the neonatal airway.

Many infants do not require immediate intubation and there is an increasing emphasis on non-invasive ventilation in neonatal intensive care. This should be the first thought if intubation is expected to be challenging, especially for the less experienced clinician, who should ask themselves 'is intubation essential?'. If clinical stability can be maintained with simple manoeuvres such as head position and mask technique, or the use of adjuncts such as an oropharyngeal or nasopharyngeal airway, it might be that intubation can be deferred pending the arrival of senior support.

Anticipation of a Difficult Airway

There are some instances where a difficult airway can be predicted antenatally, which allows for advanced planning and the assembly of a team with appropriate expertise at delivery. An example of this would be a case of upper airway atresia that has been identified antenatally. There is increasing evidence that this can be managed as an 'EXIT' procedure (ex-utero intra-partum treatment). The airway can be instrumented and if necessary an emergency tracheostomy can be performed when the infant's head, neck and chest have been partly delivered by Caesarean section. The baby remains attached to the placenta so that oxygenation is maintained during the procedure [6].

Unfortunately, however, a difficult airway at delivery is often unanticipated, and neonatal teams should plan for this in advance and have processes and procedures in place to manage an unexpected emergency.

The list below gives examples of patients with conditions that may lead to difficulty with intubation that may be predicted antenatally. This list not exhaustive:

- Achondroplasia (mid-facial hypoplasia, limited neck mobility [7])
- Beckwith Wiedemann (macroglossia [8])
- Cleft palate
- Craniofacial conditions e.g. Aperts, Crouzons (with associated maxillary hypoplasia [9])
- Cystic hygroma or other neck masses (often referred to as CHAOS (Congenital High Airway Obstruction Syndrome [10])

- Down syndrome (mid-face hypoplasia, macroglossia [11])
- Goldenhar syndrome (unilateral anomalies, higher incidence of airway anomalies [12])
- Pierre-Robin sequence (glossoptosis, micrognathia, cleft palate [13])
- Treacher Collins syndrome (mandibulo–facial dysostosis, cleft palate [14])

Other features that can result in a difficult intubation, but which are harder to anticipate include:

- Subglottic stenosis
- Laryngeal atresia
- Laryngeal web
- Glottic oedema post previous intubation/multiple previous attempts
- Vascular malformations that may compress the airway e.g. vascular ring
- Venous/lymphatic malformation

Clearly, if a potential airway issue can be identified in advance, plans can be put in place to allow for this. Early recognition in the delivery room can allow a clinician to call for help in a timely fashion rather than mid-procedure. Having the ability and foresight to identify a potentially difficult intubation, and allowing for this by seeking help and adjusting management could save lives. An example of this would be a 'semi-elective' intubation—for example, a patient with an increasing oxygen requirement needing exogenous surfactant administration in the early neonatal period. Rather than a junior member of the team working alone overnight administering pre-medications only to find themselves in a 'can't intubate, can't ventilate' scenario, early identification of a potential airway issue might lead to a discussion with senior colleagues, a request for assistance from another network centre, discussion with the anaesthetic and ENT teams, and subsequent intubation by senior staff in the operating theatre—a far safer method, with the slight detriment of a delay in surfactant therapy being far outweighed by the potential risks of being unable to ventilate.

Early identification of a potential airway issue allows a clinician to share the burden of intubation with colleagues of different specialties, drawing on their field of expertise and is safer than an inexperienced or out-of-practice clinician attempting a difficult intubation single-handedly.

Any clinician can encounter difficulties during an intubation where there does not appear to be a contributing pre-existing condition. The causes of this can be wide-ranging, from any of the neonatal specific difficulties detailed in the section above, to simply a clinician being unable to perform the task on a given day—human factors can play a large part in this, and are discussed later in this chapter. Being able to identify, where possible, a potentially difficult airway in advance of intubation is a valuable skill. However, an understanding of the equipment and techniques used in the approach to the difficult airway discussed below are important skills for all clinicians.

Equipment to Manage a Difficult Airway

Bougies

A bougie, or tracheal tube introducer, is a device that allows insertion of a tracheal tube in a fashion not dissimilar to the Seldinger technique used in vascular access (Fig. 9.3).

The bougie is inserted, usually by direct laryngoscopy, through the vocal cords and advanced a short distance before an endo-tracheal tube (ETT) is advanced over the bougie and through the cords. The bougie is then removed. The use of a bougie to aid tracheal intubation was first described by Macintosh in 1949 [15]. Originally a urethral dilation catheter was used (the word bougie is also used in medicine to describe both urethral and oesophageal dilators) in the fashion described above. The bougie was modified in the early 1970s by Venn [16], with an angulated tip that is designed to allow the bougie to point towards the cords once introduced into the oral cavity.

The bougie has been recognised as a useful tool in the management of a difficult airway in the adult population for a long time [17]. The use of a bougie is generally considered to increase the likelihood of intubation in cases of a difficult airway, with a recent randomised controlled trial in adult patients reporting a 96% success rate at first attempt with a bougie versus 82% with endo-tracheal tube with stylet alone [18].

Bougies allow the user to access the trachea even if partially or totally occluded by the epiglottis, by gently inserting just below a visualised epiglottis, even if the cords are not seen—the angulated tip helps with this, and can be augmented by the user further angling the bougie as necessary. The bougie should not be advanced more than 2 cm below the cords/beyond the epiglottis due to the risk of trauma. Whilst maintaining direct vision a tracheal tube can then be placed over the end of the bougie, usually by an assistant, and the tube advanced along the bougie to the level of the cords. The view may well have improved once the trachea has been accessed by the bougie. There can be some resistance felt at the level of the aryte-noids, where the beveled tip of the tracheal tube might catch, in which case the tube can be gently rotated 90° and then further advanced [19]. Once the tracheal tube appears to be in position the bougie is removed and confirmatory checks are performed to ensure correct tracheal tube placement.

Bougies are generally available in three sizes—neonatal, paediatric and adult. Neonatal bougies are designed to be used with tracheal tubes of sizes 2.0–3.5 mm; a larger sized bougie is used in paediatric practice. Complications of bougies are uncommon, but are recognised. Older products were used on multiple occasions, with complications including problems such as fractured tips and dispersal of

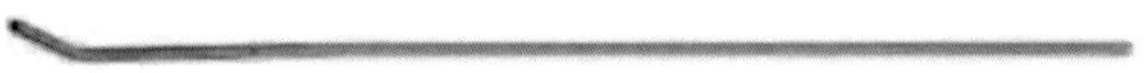

Fig. 9.3 A neonatal bougie

Fig. 9.4 Image of the glottic region obtained using an Airtraq® device

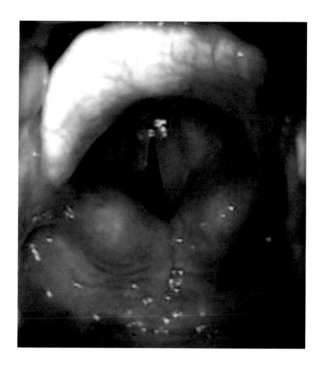

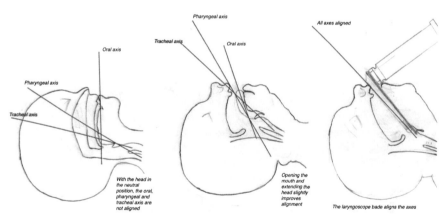

Fig. 9.5 Illustration depicting the alignment of the oropharyngeal-laryngeal axis

fragments into the airway—the authors believe all products available currently for the neonatal population are now single use. Traumatic complications are recognised, with pneumothorax [20], tracheal trauma [21], pharyngeal perforation [22], significant bleeding [23] and oesophageal trauma all potential issues. However, with care in use detailed above the likelihood of these is reduced and should not prevent a clinician using a bougie during a difficult intubation (Figs. 9.4 and 9.5).

Familiarity with equipment and technique is important and regular training using task trainers and simulators is recommended.

Indirect Laryngoscopy

Video laryngoscopy is a form of indirect laryngoscopy. Of historical interest, the oropharynx and glottis were first visualised indirectly using mirrors, as early as the mid-nineteenth century by Manuel Garcia [24]. The method since the late nineteenth century has been that of direct laryngoscopy using initially a crude, then later a formal, laryngoscope, with Alfred Kirstein an early pioneer [25]. In an apparent return to primitive methods, indirect laryngoscopy is once again becoming more popular, albeit with more modern equipment. With the relatively recent emergence of video laryngoscopy around the turn of the century [26], the user visualises the area of interest via a camera attached to a form of laryngoscope that can remove the need for direct visualisation. Thus, it is not always necessary to align the oral-pharyngeal-laryngeal axes [27] to allow a direct line of sight of the glottis, one of the main advantages of video laryngoscopy when faced with a difficult intubation.

Patients with a difficult airway due to limited mouth opening or neck movement are often easier to intubate using video guided intubation, as are patients with markedly anterior cords or those with a cleft palate. Video laryngoscopy is generally accepted to offer improved visualisation of the glottis [28]—though this does not necessarily translate into improved intubation rates, as discussed below. Other potential advantages [27] are that team members are concurrently able to visualise proceedings, enabling them to make suggestions and give advice based on what they can see, and also manipulate any cricoid pressure more effectively, though it should be noted these benefits are not evidenced at present. Video laryngoscopes have a role in teaching and can be useful in complex intubation in an operating theatre setting.

Video Laryngoscopes for Neonatal Use

It is generally accepted that 'straight' versus 'curved' blades in video laryngoscopy have different attributes and uses. A 'traditional' neonatal straight blade (usually a Miller or Wisconsin blade equivalent) requires the usual alignment of the airway, but using a camera provides a wide angled magnified view that can aid intubation. This can also be useful in teaching intubation. Those with a curved anatomical blade can allow the user to gain an indirect 'view' of the vocal cords and glottic region (via the camera) without having to align the cords with the blade. This can be particularly useful in patients with abnormal anatomy and congenital airway anomalies.

In practice, there are several companies providing neonatal video laryngoscopy equipment in the UK, some of which are illustrated below, offering a range of products. Blade sizes 00, 0 and 1 are available. The camera at the tip of the laryngoscope attaches to a screen which displays a real time colour image of the structures visualised. The screen is either separate to the laryngoscope, on a stand-alone monitor, or attached to the end of the laryngoscope handle (Figs. 9.6 and 9.7).

Fig. 9.6 Storz Cmac®
videolaryngoscope

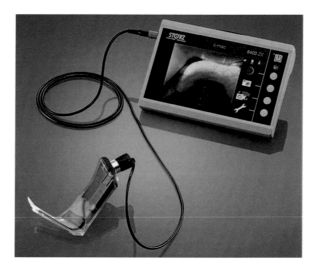

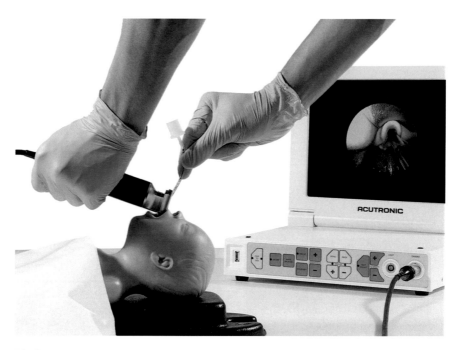

Fig. 9.7 Acutronic infant view system

Video laryngoscopy has demonstrated quicker and more effective visualisation of the oropharynx and glottis [29], including in patients with difficult airways. This has not yet equated, in trials, to an improved rate of successful intubation by experienced clinicians, though may be of more use to inexperienced or 'non-expert' users [29] both in success rates and length of time of intubation attempt. There is limited data to suggest video-laryngoscopy offers improved successful intubation rates at the first attempt, but this requires further study [30].

Airtraq®

The Airtraq device has a similar shape to a curved laryngoscope blade but instead of a camera positioned on the blade of the laryngoscope, a series of 'lenses, prisms and mirrors' [31] works to allow the user a view of the oropharynx from a viewing area at the proximal end of the laryngoscope handle—one might liken the method to a traditional periscope. The 'infant' model available is suitable for use on endotracheal tubes of size 2.5–3.5 (Fig. 9.8).

A lens heating system is present to prevent fogging and recent advances in the company now mean camera technology is also available. Small-number studies have suggested Airtraq outperforms other indirect visualisation methods of intubation with regards to time to intubation in the paediatric population [32], though not in actual rates of successful intubation. Other advantages are that Airtraq is generally more portable and cost effective than camera-reliant methods with separate monitors, though this may be less problematic now that other companies have developed screens incorporated into the laryngoscope itself.

In summary, indirect video laryngoscopy is a relatively new method of visualising the oropharynx and glottis. The various methods and products discussed above have all been shown to improve visualisation and thus could improve the likelihood of intubation, with new studies beginning to evidence this further. Each system has its own benefits, potential drawbacks and costs. Local teams should review what equipment is available in their unit and give some thought to establishing a 'difficult airway box.' Larger units and/or those providing full neonatal intensive care should

Fig. 9.8   Neonatal Airtraq® device

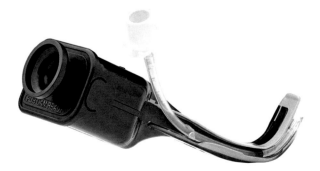

consider incorporating video laryngoscopy into their repertoire of intubation equipment as it will likely become standard practice in coming years.

Supra Glottic Airways

Supraglottic airway devices, also referred to as laryngeal mask airways (LMAs) were first developed in the 1980s, initially for use in relatively short elective surgical procedures as an alternative to tracheal intubation [32]. Laryngeal mask ventilation is classed as non-invasive, as the device is positioned in the supraglottic region, with a distal oval mask shaped specifically to sit in the hypopharynx, snugly over the glottis. Many devices have an inflatable cuff, which works to further create a seal between the device and the glottis. This allows positive pressure ventilation to be delivered to the trachea with minimal or no gastric distension when properly sited [33]. More recently, its use has been recognised both in resuscitation situations where users are untrained in tracheal intubation and in patients with difficult airways in whom intubation is difficult, with inclusion in several national and international difficult airway guidelines worldwide [34, 35]. Supraglottic airway devices are increasingly used in adult resuscitation.

These devices are available in a variety of sizes, with size 1 (manufactured as appropriate for use in infants with birthweight of 2.5–5 kg) used in neonatology, though some studies and case studies report the successful use of size 1 LMAs in infants with a birthweight as low as 800 g [36, 37] (Fig. 9.9).

The insertion technique for a cuffed supraglottic airway device is as follows: [38]

Fig. 9.9 Igel® supraglottic airway device in position (used with permission)

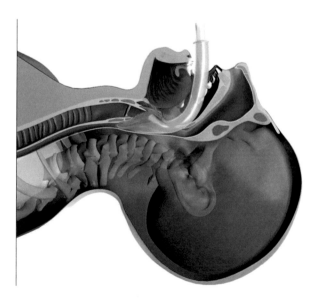

- Fully deflate the cuff, and lubricate the posterior aspect of mask at distal end of LMA;
- Grasp the LMA between thumb and forefinger at the junction of oval mask and airway shaft, as if holding a pen;
- Press the lubricated (posterior) aspect of the mask against the hard palate, and advance in one movement gently pressing against the hard then soft palate until it cannot be advanced further;
- Inflate the cuff, observing a slight rise or lift in the LMA, which serves as confirmation of correct position;
- Further confirmation can be gained by positive pressure ventilation, during which chest rise can be seen and air entry heard on auscultation.

Complications of insertion including sticking at the base of the tongue, 'down-folding' of the epiglottis causing (partial) occlusion of the airway, or simply sitting too high in the oropharynx leading to suboptimal ventilation [38, 39].

Publications suggest insertion of LMA has high success rates in a timely fashion. A study of medical students placing LMAs in the simulation setting after a 15 min training package showed an average insertion time of 5 s [40], whilst a study of 2–10 year olds having elective surgery produced rates of successful placement as high as 94% versus a tracheal intubation success rate of 53% [41].

Clearly, a marked advantage of the LMA versus tracheal intubation is the relative ease of insertion, especially in the patient with a difficult airway. Many of the previously listed congenital anomalies can be managed with a supraglottic airway device—for example cranio-facial deformities and Pierre-Robin sequence [42, 43]. Equally, the use of an LMA can help in intubating a patient with difficult to view, anterior cords.

Other potential uses for the LMA include using them to aid tracheal intubation [44], with a tracheal tube passed down the airway shaft of a correctly positioned LMA, through the mask then vocal cords down into the trachea. This is particularly useful in larger patients. Another important use, perhaps specific to neonatology more than other specialties, is the use of an LMA as a temporary, non-definitive airway in complex patients requiring transfer to a specialist centre by a transport team [45].

It is generally accepted that an LMA is not appropriate for long term ventilation, with isolated case reports of use for up to 6 days [46]. Potential complications include gastric distension and vomiting, though some studies have shown that this is not the case when the device is correctly positioned. It has been shown that, above a peak inspiratory pressure of around 25 cm H_2O, mask leak occurs, with a presumed inability to provide intra-thoracic pressures higher than this [47]. Localised trauma is rarely reported and has not been reported to have long term complications.

iGel© Supraglottic Airway Device

Newer supraglottic airway devices include the Igel® supraglottic airway device. This uses the same concept but instead of an inflatable cuff has a gel surrounding the mask, which is designed to fit over the glottis in a fashion similar to the inflatable

Fig. 9.10 Neonatal IGel®

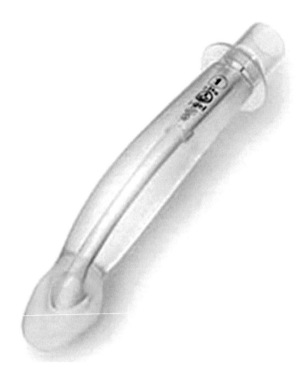

cuff in traditional models. Once inserted, the gel softens slightly due to the patient's body heat and then 'moulds' itself to the shape of the glottis, aiming to achieve a better seal than the traditional LMA. There are a range of paediatric size iGel devices available, with size 1 for use in neonatology, manufactured as suitable for weights between 2 and 5 kg (Fig. 9.10).

There is little evidence in neonates at present regarding the efficacy of the Igel compared to a cuffed LMA [48], but early adult studies have found quicker insertion times and fewer adverse effects (mainly 'sore throat'); however, use of higher pressures suggestive of improved seal have yet to be demonstrated (49).

In summary, a Supraglottic airway device is a well-recognised tool in the management of the neonatal airway, in particular those patients with a difficult airway in whom tracheal intubation is challenging. It is quick and easy to insert and can be life-saving in 'can't intubate, can't ventilate' situations and/or in patients who need transferring for escalation of care. We feel that these devices are often underused, despite being listed in several respected national and international guidelines. They are relatively cheap, especially in comparison to some products using video technology. As with indirect laryngoscopic methods, it is suggested that clinicians familiarise themselves with the device, either in elective cases or in the simulation environment, and consider the introduction of LMAs to their ward equipment for use in emergency situations.

Digital Intubation

An historical but now infrequently used technique, digital (or 'finger') intubation was likely the first used method of tracheal intubation, with Vesalius describing the insertion of a tracheal tube via this method in 1543 [49]. The first documented neonatal digital tracheal intubation was by Blundell in 1838 [50]. Further instances were reported in 1941 and 1968 [51]. A randomised controlled trial of neonatal intubation from 2006 [52] compared digital intubation with intubation using laryngoscope: success rates were 90.5% for the digital method and only 50% for laryngoscopic; in addition, it took an average of 8.2 s to intubate digitally and 13.1 s to intubate with a laryngoscope. While the numbers involved were small, they support at least the possibility that this method is effective and may be of real use in the patient with a difficult airway.

There are a number of slight variations in methods suggested in the literature for the clinician undertaking neonatal digital intubation, but all follow a common theme—the 'non-dominant' hand is directed along the tongue until the index finger reaches the epiglottis, at which point the ETT is advanced via the dominant hand, with the non-dominant index finger used as a guide to direct the ETT towards the glottic region then down through the cords [53]. This is a rarely used technique, and, understandably, one which might be considered primitive or inferior to other methods. However, in a 'can't intubate, can't ventilate' situation when a clinical team has exhausted all other possibilities the literature suggests it may be worthwhile attempting this.

Nasal Intubation

Whilst not a new or 'advanced' technique, nasal intubation is worth mentioning in this chapter. This technique involves passing the tracheal tube through the nostril, after application of lubricant, and with gentle pressure advancing the tracheal tube up along the superior aspect of the hard palate before curling round and dropping into view at the back of the oropharynx. Once the tip of the tracheal tube is visualised, it can be advanced through the vocal cords with Magill's forceps. Complications include local trauma, and ischaemia of the nares which can be avoided by ensuring the tracheal tube is not causing blanching at the entry site, and injury to the turbinates, piriform sinus or rarely penetrative brain injury [54, 55]. The likelihood of this is minimised with the use of lubricant, never using a stylet or introducer, gentle pressure only, and arranging the tube on insertion so as the bevel is facing superior encouraging the natural progression of the tube along the intended route.

A Cochrane review comparing nasal intubations with oral intubations did not find any difference in success rates or complications [56]. However, some clinicians feel the natural path that a tracheal tube follows with nasal intubation 'directs' the tip of the tracheal tube towards the supraglottic region and vocal cords, providing an angle that assists in successful intubation. Many readers will be familiar with stylets, or introducers, which are commonly used both to make a tracheal tube more 'sturdy', and to allow the clinician to angle the tip of the tube so it is directed towards the vocal cords when undertaking intubation. The pathway an endo-tracheal tube naturally takes with nasal intubation achieves this without the need for an introducer, but the 'sturdy' aspect of using a stylet is lost. Furthermore, it is not unreasonable to consider that the increased manoeuvrability of a tracheal tube afforded by the use of Magill's forceps within the oral cavity might assist in patients who are difficult to intubate, particularly those with anterior cords. Anecdotally nursing staff report nasal tubes are easier to care for, allowing improved mouth care and improved security of the tube itself.

Additional Airway Adjuncts

Babies with difficulty maintaining an airway can often be managed using oropharyngeal or nasopharyngeal airways.

Intubation view can be improved by altering the head position and using a roll under the neck to provide a slight neck extension.

When planning emergency equipment, it useful to consider different lengths and shapes of laryngoscopic blades. A wider 'Macintosh' or Seward® blade can be useful if the tongue is difficult to control in a larger infant.

Difficult Airway Kit

With the above in mind, it seems reasonable to consider the development of a difficult airway 'kit', or 'box', or 'trolley'—the choice is determined by what would work best for an individual neonatal unit.

We recommend that appropriate contents would include the following:

- Laryngoscope blades of various shapes and sizes—including wider curved blades
- ETT tubes of a various sizes and/or manufacturers
- Oropharyngeal airways
- Stylet
- Bougie(s)
- Supraglottic Airway Devices/iGel
- Video-laryngoscope/'Airtraq'
- Magills Forceps
- Difficult airway algorithm
- Usual equipment—ETT fixation devices, Colour change capnography, NGT/syringe, towel for neck-roll

There is much debate about what to do in the event of a critical airway situation: should a neonatologist attempt surgical access?

The chance of survival following an attempt at emergency tracheostomy in non-surgical hands is very low and we would not recommend this. It is possible to insert a wide bore cannula through the cricothyroid membrane, but no evidence to show that this is safe or effective in the neonatal population. This should only be considered when all other options have been exhausted and should ideally be performed by an ENT surgeon.

Human Factors

Human factors are increasingly recognised as the cause of medical errors in emergency situations. The Clinical Human Factors Group was established following an unexpectedly difficult intubation in theatre, the case of Elaine Bromiley [57] that perhaps suits the underlying message of this chapter more than any other in this book.

In summary, a clinical team involved with performing a routine surgical procedure found themselves unable to intubate or ventilate the patient which, sadly, led to an irretrievable situation whereby the patient died. Subsequent analysis of the event demonstrated significant contributors to the episode included human factors—the physical and mental characteristics of team members that can impact on patient care and outcome, along with organisational factors within a system.

One can foresee, far too easily, that in the case of a neonate who has a difficult airway, these factors can come into play and influence a scenario that is already fraught with tension, where clear communication and a high level of effective teamwork is paramount.

The Clinical Human Factors Group classifies these factors into organisational and individual areas, both of which are discussed in more detail below:

Organisational Factors

- Systems
  Hospitals are complex, often involving many teams in different locations. A neonatal difficult intubation scenario could take place in one of several areas with members from different teams. It is important to plan how these will work together, considering:
  - Equipment: correct equipment available, working, checked, accessible, in a location known to team members, different kits for different areas or one mobile kit?

 – Bed/Room Design: can the patient/airway be easily accessed, and can a call
    for help be easily made?
 – Signage: can emergency teams find the location quickly?
 – Guidelines/Algorithms: are these easily and quickly accessible?

• Workforce
  Any intubation can be challenging, as alluded to at the beginning of this chapter.
  Consideration should be given to the workforce available in an intubation emergency, in terms of neonatal unit staff, level of seniority and experience, and other
  specialties—this will vary depending on location and local setup but might
  include anaesthetists, intensivists and ENT team members. Again, planning
  before an event allows pathways to be developed which help guide teams in
  emergency situations.

• Training
  A difficult intubation is a relatively rare occurrence. This makes it all the more
  important to practise skills regularly, allowing all team members to develop competencies and feel more comfortable in a genuine emergency.
  Training can be delivered using a variety of different methods. There are internationally recognised and approved certified life support courses in neonatology,
  which have an emphasis on airway management. Simulation training is becoming an increasingly used method of education in healthcare, and many units now
  have on site simulation training programmes. Simulation scenarios are invaluable, not only for clinical skills training, but also for educating team members
  about human factors and even identifying potential systems human factor issues
  with 'in situ' simulations undertaken in the ward environment. Alongside these,
  task trainers allow trainees to practice specific skills which are not used regularly
  in the clinical setting.
  As touched upon throughout this chapter, many items of equipment discussed
  above will not be in use on a day-to-day basis and therefore regular refreshers
  using simulation or task trainers are vital for the user to be confident in their use
  during an emergency situation.

Individual Factors

Team Working

In a difficult neonatal intubation, working as a team becomes all the more complex
due to the high pressure nature of the situation. This can be further complicated by
team members attending who are not routinely involved in neonatal care, for example anaesthetists or ENT surgeons. The familiarity and good team working neonatal
staff have developed with their colleagues, often over years of working together,
does not exist with 'new' staff members who attend only in an emergency—a time
when team working needs to be at its most effective.

The team needs to have a dedicated leader to provide a central point of communication and an overview of the situation. As well as strong leadership, the concept of good followership is of equal importance.

Clearly, communication plays a huge part in the ability of a team to work together effectively. Team leaders are encouraged to practice **'closed-loop' communication**: team members are addressed by name, given a task, repeat this task back to the team leader and then report back once this task is complete, giving feedback and/or suggestions as appropriate. Using this method, comments such as 'can someone get ENT' become far more focused and likely to be completed. **Checklists** are coming into regular practice more commonly, with 'command and response' style interactions between professionals. Their use in everyday practice can only improve team performance in an emergency situation.

Team members should be aware of common issues which can lead to error:

- **Confirmation bias**
  This is the concept of arriving at an (incorrect) diagnosis prematurely, then subconsciously misinterpreting developing clinical information in such a way that it appears to support the diagnosis made. An example might be an oesophageal intubation, where there is no colour change on a CO_2 detector, explained away by the team as secondary to an infant being extremely premature. In these situations, it is vital a team can work together to generate ideas and work together without fear of criticism for making suggestions.

- **Situational Awareness**
  The team leader should maintain a global overview of a developing scenario, allowing themselves to manage an unfolding emergency effectively, utilizing team members as necessary. Ideally, this would mean that the leader would not become involved in tasks that will distract them from the overview they seek to maintain. This can be difficult in a difficult intubation scenario, in which the natural team leader is often the clinician most experienced in intubation. It is worthwhile considering formally delegating the role of team leader to an experienced colleague in this eventuality.

- **Overload and 'thinking aloud'**
  A difficult intubation can only ever be stressful and difficult for the team, and in particular the team leader. It is easy for the team leader to be overloaded with information and lose track of the progression of a scenario. This can be overcome by thinking aloud, detailing to the team the current clinical status of the patient, the working diagnosis and intended management plan moving forward. This allows the team to maintain an understanding of the situation, and feel comfortable in making suggestions contributing to the ongoing plan, or indeed, disagreeing with the team leader if necessary.

- **Task Fixation**
  Touching on some of the themes discussed above in situational awareness, it can be all too easy to focus in on a task such as cannulation and in the meantime have missed the fact that a patient is hypoxic and bradycardic. Team leaders should try as much as possible to delegate such tasks allowing them to maintain an overview

- **Distraction and Interruption**

  These should be minimised as much as possible to allow the team to communicate and work together effectively. Neonatal units and delivery rooms are busy places. Discussions unrelated to the developing scenario should take place away from the patient and team, alarms should be silenced once acknowledged and actioned if needed, and on-call bleeps or mobile phones should not be in the possession of active team members.

- **Fatigue, hunger and stress**

  The effect of fatigue on motor skills is well recognised. Many readers will be aware from their own clinical work their performance is dulled when hungry, and will improve after a meal break. A clinician involved in a difficult intubation scenario requires full focus on the task in hand, and should ideally not be worrying about other stressors in their life, be it personal or work related. Some advance thought into these areas can enhance personal performance significantly, both with clarity of thought when managing a crisis, and delivering clinical skills such as a difficult intubation.

  After any complex patient scenario, whatever the outcome, debriefs should be encouraged to allow group reflection and learning. 'Hot' debriefs, immediately after the event, can be a good method of discussing good practice points so these can be noted and taken forward, which can sometimes be forgotten if debriefing several days or weeks after the event.

  The significance of human factors are increasingly being recognised in clinical medicine. When dealing with a difficult neonatal intubation, it is easy to see how the themes discussed above could directly impact on team performance and patient outcome. Giving thought to these both in advance of, and during, such an intubation is important for all clinicians.

Suggested Approach to the Patient with a Difficult Airway

The British Association of Perinatal Medicine has recently formed a 'working group' to produce a national framework to help guide practice. This framework for practice in the UK is expected to publish in early 2020.

Conclusions

This chapter has discussed the definition of the difficult airway, and reviewed the conditions that might be detected antenatally or postnatally that may predict a potentially difficult intubation.

We have reviewed available equipment and made suggestions about what to include in a difficult airway kit.

It is important that teams recognise the effect of human factors in managing an acutely difficult situation and that teams remember the basic airway techniques taught on life support courses. Often applying a face mask correctly and minimising leak can provide effective ventilation without needing a tracheal tube.

We have summarised the new BAPM framework guidance and suggest that local teams use this to create their own local guidelines for management of a baby who is difficult to intubate.

References

1. Cormack RS, Lehane J. Difficult tracheal intubation in obstetrics. Anaesthesia. 1984;39:1105–11.
2. Cook TM. A new practical classification of laryngoscopy. Anaesthesia. 2000;55:274–9.
3. Mallampati SR, Gatt SP, Gugino LD, et al. A clinical sign to predict difficult tracheal intubation: a prospective study. Can Anaesth Soc J. 1985;32:429–34.
4. Harless J, Ramaiah R, Bhananker S. Pediatric airway management. Int J Crit Illn Inj Sci. 2014;4(1):65–70.
5. Adewale L. Anatomy and assessment of the pediatric airway. Paediatr Anaesth. 2009;19(Suppl 1):1–8.
6. Abraham RJ, Sau A, Maxwell D. A review of the EXIT (Ex utero Intrapartum Treatment) procedure. J Obstet Gynaecol. 2010;30(1):1–5.
7. Karnalkar A, Deshpande A. Anesthesia management of patient with achondroplasia for abdominal hysterectomy. Int J Sci Rep. 2015;1(6):264–6.
8. Tsukamoto M, Hitosugi T, Yokoyama T. Perioperative airway management of a patient with Beckwith-Wiedemann syndrome. J Dent Anesth Pain Med. 2016;16(4):313–6.
9. Kumar A, Goel N, Sinha C, Singh A. Anesthetic implications in a child with Crouzon syndrome. Anesth Essays Res. 2017;11(1):246–7.
10. Gurulingappa, Awati MN, Asif Aleem M. Cystic hygroma: a difficult airway and its anaesthetic implications. Indian J Anaesth. 2011;55(6):624–6.
11. Kanamori G, Witter M, Brown J, Williams-Smith L. Otolaryngologic manifestations of Down syndrome. Otolaryngol Clin North Am. 2000;33:1285–92.
12. Khan WA, Salim B, Khan AA, Chughtai S. Anaesthetic management in a child with Goldenhar syndrome. J Coll Physicians Surg Pak. 2017;27(3):S6–7.
13. Li W-Y, et al. Airway management in Pierre Robin sequence: the Vancouver classification. Plast Surg (Oakv). 2017;25(1):14–20.
14. Goel L, Bennur S, Jambhale S. Treacher-Collins syndrome–a challenge for anaesthesiologists. Indian J Anaesth. 2009;53(4):496–500.
15. Macintosh RR. An aid to Oral intubation. Br Med J. 1949;1(4591):28.
16. Venn PH. The gum elastic bougie. Anaesthesia. 1993;48:274–5.
17. Bokhari A, Benham SW, Popat MT. Management of unanticipated difficult intubation: a survey of current practice in the Oxford region. Eur J Anaesthesiol. 2004;21:123–7.
18. Driver BE, et al. Effect of use of a Bougie vs endotracheal tube and stylet on first-attempt intubation success among patients with difficult airways undergoing emergency intubation: a randomised controlled trial. JAMA. 2018;319(21):2179–89.
19. de Andrade Reis L, et al. Bougie. Rev Bras Anestesiol. 2009;59(5):618–23.
20. Rajagopal R, Jayaseelan V, George M. A case of pneumothorax following bougie-guided intubation in a patient undergoing excision of an intraventricular space occupying lesion. J Anaesthesiol Crit Care. 2017;4(2):117–9.

21. Özcan ATD, Balci CA, Aksoy SM, Ugur G, Kanbak O, Müderrris T. Upper airway injury caused by gum elastic bougie. Int J Case Rep Images. 2017;8(7):439–43.
22. Kadry M, Popat M. Pharyngeal wall perforation—an unusual complication of blind intubation with gum elastic bougie. Anaesthesia. 1999;54:404–5.
23. Prabhu A, et al. Bougie trauma: it is still possible. Anaesthesia. 2003;58(8):811–3.
24. Jahn A, Blitzer A. A short history of laryngoscopy. Logoped Phoniatr Vocol. 1996;21(3–4):181–5.
25. Burkle CM, et al. A historical perspective on use of the laryngoscope as a tool in anesthesiology. Anesthesiology. 2004;100:1003–6.
26. Pieters BM, et al. Pioneers of laryngoscopy: indirect, direct and video laryngoscopy. Anaesth Intensive Care. 2015;43 Suppl:4–11.
27. Chemsian RV, et al. Videolaryngoscopy. Int J Crit Illn Inj Sci. 2014;4(1):35–41.
28. Paolini JB, et al. Review article: video-laryngoscopy: another tool for difficult intubation or a new paradigm in airway management? Can J Anaesth. 2013;60:184–91.
29. Griesdale DEG, et al. Glidescope video-laryngoscopy versus direct laryngoscopy for endotracheal intubation: a systematic review and meta-analysis. Can J Anaesth. 2012;59(1):41–52.
30. De Jong A, et al. Video laryngoscopy versus direct laryngoscopy for orotracheal intubation in the intensive care unit: a systematic review and meta-analysis. Intensive Care Med. 2014;40(5):629–39.
31. Soerensen MK, et al. Airtraq outperforms VL and CMAC for pediatric intubations. BMC Anesthesiol. 2012;12:7.
32. Brain AI. The development of the laryngeal mask—a brief history of the invention, early clinical studies and experimental work from which the laryngeal mask evolved. Eur J Anaesthesiol Suppl. 1991;4:5–17.
33. Maltby RJ, Beriault MT, Watson NC, et al. Gastric distension and ventilation during laparoscopic cholecystectomy: LMA-classic vs. tracheal intubation. Can J Anesth. 2000;47:622–6.
34. American Society of Anesthesiologists Task Force on Management of the Difficult Airway. Practice guidelines for management of the difficult airway. Anesthesiology. 1993;78:597–602.
35. ILCOR, Wyllie J, Bruinenberg J, Roehr CC, Rüdiger M, Trevisanuto D, Urlesberger B. European Resuscitation Council Guidelines for Resuscitation 2015. Section 7. Resuscitation and support of transition of babies at birth. Resuscitation. 2015;95:249–63.
36. Gandini D, Brimacombe JR. Neonatal resuscitation with the laryngeal mask airway in normal and low birth weight infants. Anesth Analg. 1999;89(3):642.
37. Brimacombe J. Airway rescue and drug delivery in an 800 g neonate with the laryngeal mask airway. Paediatr Anaesth. 1999;9:178.
38. Trevisanuto D, Micaglio M, Ferrarese P, et al. The laryngeal mask airway: potential applications in neonates. Arch Dis Child Fetal Neonatal Ed. 2004;89:F485–9.
39. Schmiesing CA, Brock-Utne JG. An airway management device: the laryngeal mask airway: a review. J Intensive Care Med. 1998;13:32–43.
40. Gandini D, Brimacombe J. Manikin training for neonatal resuscitation with the laryngeal mask airway. Pediatr Anaesth. 2004;14:493–4.
41. Jamil SN, Alam M, Usmani H, Khan MM. A study of the use of laryngeal mask airway (LMA) in children and its comparison with endotracheal intubation. Indian J Anaesth. 2009;53(2):174–8.
42. Markakis DA, Sayson SC, Schreiner MS. Insertion of the laryngeal mask airway in awake infants with the Robin sequence. Anesth Analg. 1992;75:822–4.
43. Ellis DS, Potluri PK, O'Flaherty JE, et al. Difficult airway management in the neonate: a simple method of intubating through a laryngeal mask airway. Paediatr Anaesth. 1999;9:460–2.
44. Sung A, Kalstein A, Radhakrishnan P, Yarmush J, Raoof S. Laryngeal mask airway: use and clinical applications. J Bronchol Interv Pulmonol. 2007;14(3):181–8.
45. Fraser J, Hill C, McDonald D, Jones C, Petros A. The use of the laryngeal mask airway for inter-hospital transport of infants with type 3 laryngotracheo-oesophageal clefts. Intensive Care Med. 1999;25:714–6.

46. Bucx MJ, Grolman W, Kruisinga FH, Lindeboom JA, Van Kempen AA. The prolonged use of the laryngeal mask airway in a neonate with airway obstruction and Treacher Collins syndrome. Paediatr Anaesth. 2003;13:530–3.
47. Brimacombe J, Brain AI, Berry A. The laryngeal mask airway: review and practical guide. Philadelphia: WB Saunders; 1997.
48. de Montblanc J, Ruscio L, Mazoit JX, Benhamou D. A systematic review and meta-analysis of the i-gel vs laryngeal mask airway in adults. Anaesthesia. 2014;69:1151–62.
49. Vesalius A. De humani corporis fabrica. 1543.
50. Dunn PM. Dr. James Blundell (1790–1878) and neonatal resuscitation. Arch Dis Child. 1988;64:494.
51. Hancock PJ, et al. Finger intubation of the trachea in newborns. Paediatrics. 1992;89(2):325–7.
52. Moura JH, et al. Neonatal laryngoscope intubation and the digital method: a randomised controlled trial. J Pediatr. 2006;148(6):840–1.
53. Christodoulou C, et al. Blind digital intubation. In: Hag-berg C, editor. Benumof's airway management: principles and practice. 2nd ed. Philadelphia: Mosby Elsevier; 2007. p. 393–9.
54. Black AE, Hatch DJ, Nauth-Misir N. Complications of nasotracheal intubation in neonates, infants and children: a review of 4 years experience in a children's hospital. Br J Anaesth. 1990;65:461–7.
55. de Vries MJ, et al. Traumatic perforation of the lamina cribrosa during nasal intubation of a preterm infant. Pediatrics. 2014;133(3):e762–5.
56. Spence K, Barr P. Nasal versus oral intubation for mechanical ventilation of newborn infants. Cochrane Database Syst Rev. 2000;(2):CD000948.
57. Bromiley M. The husband's story: from tragedy to learning and action. BMJ Qual Saf. 2015;24(7):425–7.

Chapter 10
Sudden Unexpected Postnatal Collapse

Vix Monnelly and Julie-Clare Becher

Abbreviations

ALTE   Acute life threatening event
MRI   Magnetic resonance imaging
SIDS   Sudden infant death syndrome
SUDI   Sudden unexpected death in infancy
SUEND   Sudden unexpected early neonatal death
SUPC   Sudden unexpected collapse

The Challenges of Definition

Sudden unexpected postnatal collapse (SUPC), is a rare, but well described entity with potentially catastrophic consequences including death or severe disability. In 2011, a UK expert group defined SUPC as 'a term or near-term infant who is well at birth, assigned to routine postnatal care and who collapses unexpectedly within the first 7 days of life, requiring resuscitation with intermittent positive pressure ventilation and who either dies, requires ongoing intensive care or develops an encephalopathy' [1]. This definition of SUPC, which has been endorsed by the British Association of Perinatal Medicine (BAPM) is increasingly used internationally.

The majority of cases of SUPC occur within the first 24 h of life: 36% within the first 2 h of birth, 29% between 2 and 24 h after birth, while 24% occur between 24 and 72 h after birth and 9% between day 4–7 of life [2]. There are around 2000 cases described in the medical literature describing a widely variable incidence of SUPC, with estimates ranging from 1.92 per 100,000 live births [3] to 38 per 100,000 [4] and as high as 133 per 100,000 [5] (Table 10.1).

V. Monnelly · J.-C. Becher (✉)
Department of Neonatology, Simpson Centre for Reproductive Health, Royal Infirmary of Edinburgh, Edinburgh, Scotland
e-mail: vix.monnelly@nhslothian.scot.nhs.uk; vmonnelly@doctors.org; julie-clare.becher@nhslothian.scot.nhs.uk

© Springer Nature Switzerland AG 2020
E. M. Boyle, J. Cusack (eds.), *Emerging Topics and Controversies in Neonatology*, https://doi.org/10.1007/978-3-030-28829-7_10

Table 10.1 Population-based studies describing the incidence and outcome of SUPC (case series excluded)

	Study	Age at collapse	Gestation (weeks)	Incidence per 100,000 live births	No of cases reported	% SUPC infants dying before discharge	% SUPC survivors with adverse neurodevelopmental outcome
Studies reporting deaths and survivors							
UK and Ireland [6]	National	≤12 h	37+	5	45	27%	24% at 1 year
Germany [7]	National	≤24 h	37+	2.6	17	41%	Not reported
Australia [8]	National	≤7 days	37+	5.6	48	56%	Not reported
France [9]	Regional	≤2 h	36+	4.8	3	33%	50%
Taiwan [10]	Regional	≤7 days	37+	19	13	41%	Not reported
France [11]	Regional	≤7 days	37+	3.8	18	39%	Not reported
Studies reporting deaths only							
USA [3]	National	<7 days	35+	1.92	1558	100%	NA
Sweden [12]	Regional	≤4 days	38+	12	16	100%	NA
England [13]	Regional	≤7 days	34+	3.5	30	100%	NA

This variation is largely due to differences in the definition of SUPC including age of infant, variation in the severity of the collapse, and in inclusion and exclusion criteria; some studies include only deaths, some include collapse within the first 12–24 h of life [6, 7] and others up to 7 days postpartum [2]. Studies which include 'mild' collapse, where the infant requires stimulation without intermittent positive pressure and subsequent intensive care support [5] have a much higher incidence than those using a stricter definition of collapse where advanced resuscitation is required. Moreover, some studies exclude infants with a subsequently identified aetiology, which underestimates the true incidence of SUPC. It is likely that the true incidence of all SUPC is more common than that quoted in the literature, which reflects only the most critical events [7] and infants with rapid and favourable outcomes may be omitted from reports or surveys.

As SUPC is rare in any one centre, reports from single centres may not be as robust as larger population data due to recall bias. Other factors which may impact the interpretation of the incidence of SUPC is the increasing professional awareness of SUPC as a clinical entity, including the availability of therapeutic hypothermia (TH) as a potential treatment for asphyxia. In a single centre in Italy the reported incidence of SUPC has risen from 5.3 per 100,000 cases to 15.5 per 100,000 live births [14] in a centre offering TH to such infants. There are also diagnostic coding challenges for those dying from hypoxic-ischaemic complications some time after collapse, and the cause of death may be rationally coded as hypoxic ischaemic encephalopathy, further hindering identification of cases of SUPC.

The use of alternative diagnostic terminology such as acute life-threatening event (ALTE), sudden unexplained death in infancy (SUDI) and sudden infant death syndrome (SIDS) fail to capture the unique differences between extreme events in the newborn period and those later in infancy. Further complicating matters is that SUPC is not yet an official category in the *International Classification of Diseases* (ICD). It is therefore vital that we adopt an international standardised definition of SUPC to acknowledge such crucial differences between populations and enable robust estimates of incidence.

The Relationship Between SUPC and SUDI

There is no single aetiology of SUPC with a wide number of underlying conditions described in the literature which lead to a final common pathway (Table 10.2). This process is almost certainly complex. The triple risk theory for sudden unexplained death in infancy (SUDI) was first described in the 1990s [15] and has since been widely endorsed. It focuses on the multifactorial mechanisms, which culminate in SUDI when certain risk factors coincide [16]. It is likely that a similar multifactorial mechanism exists for SUPC, although this is unproven:

Table 10.2 List of conditions and relevant investigations for SUPC during life

Condition	Investigation
Infection E.g. systemic and meningitis, bacterial and viral	Maternal and placental samples for bacteriology and virology Infant samples (blood culture, CSF, urine, endotracheal, surface swabs) for bacteriology and virology
Cardiac E.g. cyanotic conditions, left outflow tract obstruction, arrhythmias, cardiomyopathies	ECG, CXR, echocardiogram, genetic blood tests
Respiratory E.g. pneumonia, haemorrhage, pulmonary hypertension, diaphragmatic hernia	CXR, echocardiogram
Haematological E.g. anaemia	FBC/CBC, maternal Kleihauer test, viral studies
Endocrine E.g. hypoglycaemia, hyperinsulinism, congenital adrenal hypoplasia	Blood glucose, electrolytes, full metabolic screen (including lactate, ammonia, beta-hydroxybutyrate, AA, insulin, FFA, acylcarnitines, urate), cortisol, renal ultrasound
Metabolic E.g. fatty acid oxidation defects, urea cycle defects, organic acid defects	Full metabolic screen as above, VLCFA, genetic blood tests, blood spot, CSF (lactate, AA, glycine), Urine (OA, AA), skeletal survey, muscle biopsy, skin biopsy
Neurological E.g. any cause of seizure, apnoea, antenatal brain injury	EEG or aEEG/CFM, cranial ultrasound scan, MRI brain, maternal and infant toxicology, genetic blood tests
Neuromuscular E.g. congenital myasthenia, myopathies	Cranial ultrasound, MRI brain, skeletal survey, genetic blood tests, muscle biopsy, ophthalmoscopy

Table modified from the BAPM Investigation of an infant with sudden unexpected postnatal collapse, 2011, Appendix 4 [1]

AA amino acids, *aEEG* amplitude integrated electroencephalogram, *CBC* complete blood count, *CFM* cerebral function monitor, *CSF* cerebrospinal fluid, *CXR* chest radiograph, *ECG* electrocardiogram, *EEG* electroencephalogram, *FBC* full blood count, *FFA* free fatty acids, *MRI* magnetic resonance imaging, *VLCFA* very long chain fatty acids

Triple risk theory [15] when applied to SUPC:

- *Intrinsic vulnerability*: e.g. underlying anomaly, metabolic disorder or antenatal hypoxic-ischaemic insult
- *Extrinsic risk factor*: e.g. potentially asphyxiating position, maternal factors impairing awareness
- *Developmental vulnerability*: newborn status of the infant: time of postnatal adaptation, inability to self-correct airway obstruction, high pulmonary resistance.

Although many believe that SUPC and SUDI are heterogeneous and represent two completely different clinical entities, in reality there is probably an overlap in a subgroup of infants. SUDI refers to the sudden death of an infant younger than one year, which remains unexplained after formal examination, and is the leading cause of death in the post-neonatal period [17]. Both SUDI and SUPC are sudden, unexpected and are associated with some overlapping risk factors.

However, several fundamental differences between SUPC and SUDI exist; the most pivotal being that not all infants with SUPC die. Approximately 50% of infants will survive after SUPC, most likely due to prompt recognition of collapse while in hospital and immediate access to newborn life support.

Of the 50% who die, over half of these have an underlying cause identified at post mortem examination compared to around a third of SUDI cases. The most frequently identified causes of death after SUPC include congenital anomalies, pulmonary hypertension, congenital infection and metabolic disorders [18]. As such there is guidance in some countries recommending that, similar to the approach following SUDI, a detailed review of the death and its circumstances should be undertaken after a SUPC [19], that age-specific investigations are performed (Table 10.2) and that a Coronial post mortem examination should be obligatory [1]. Even with a high post mortem diagnostic yield, the largest category of deaths after SUPC is unexplained, accounting for 40–56% of cases. In such cases, co-sleeping remains an important association [18, 20] implying that there may be modifiable factors in the pathogenesis of SUPC, as is observed in SUDI.

Extrinsic Risk Factors for SUPC

There are several well described risk factors for SUPC (Table 10.3). Those most commonly reported relate to potentially asphyxiating position of the infant [6, 11, 21–24, 27] and other risk factors which have been hypothesised to affect the mother's awareness of her baby's wellbeing either through relative inexperience, distraction or fatigue [2, 9, 21, 23, 27–29, 33, 34]. Maternal mobile phone use has also been implicated in several case reports of SUPC [4, 26]. The distracting influence of a mobile phone has been reported to impair driving performance [35] and is hypothesised to contribute to a failure or delay in recognising deterioration in the infant.

Table 10.3 Risk factors described in SUPC

Baby factors	Maternal factors	Situational factors
Underlying pathology [18] Bias towards time of birth [2] Position: – Prone [6, 11, 21–23] – Skin to skin [24] – Cobedding [25] – Breastfeeding [6, 26]	Inexperience: Primigravida [21, 23, 27–29] Maternal habitus [26] Reduced awareness: – Distracted: mobile phone use [4, 26], pain, procedures [29] – Drowsiness: fatigue [25, 30, 31], sedation [8] – Position: supine [32], unable to see baby [6]	Lack of surveillance by staff [6, 8]: – Parents alone [9, 33, 34] – Staff preoccupied with tasks Dim lighting [25]

This association may become more apparent with time, as mobile phones are increasingly ubiquitous in modern day life.

Because the developmental vulnerability of the newborn cannot be modified, and intrinsic risk factors are usually difficult to identify before birth, it is important that extrinsic risk factors are understood such that they can be addressed in any postnatal safety bundle aiming to reduce the risk of SUPC [30].

Controversies in SUPC

Skin to Skin Care (SSC) in the Post-partum Period

SSC is the practice of placing infants directly onto the chest of their mothers, usually in a prone position, typically with the infant naked to maximise the surface area in contact between the mother-infant dyad.

The World Health Organisation (WHO) and UNICEF as part of the Baby-Friendly Hospital Initiative (World Health Organisation, Baby Friendly Hospital Initiative [36]) has called upon all maternity facilities globally to implement the "Ten steps to successful breastfeeding" (World Health Organisation [37]) with step four referring to SSC. It states that "skin to skin contact should be immediate and uninterrupted and mothers should be supported to initiate breast feeding as soon as possible after birth, offering help if need". This was endorsed by the American Academy of Pediatrics (AAP [38]) in 2009 and subsequently this practice has been widely adopted worldwide [31, 39].

The most current evidence for SSC in the immediate newborn period is summarised in a Cochrane review of 46 trials including 3850 women and their term or near term infants [40]. This concludes that SSC promotes breast feeding, and that it may result in 'a trend to more stable physiological parameters and higher blood glucose levels in term infants', *without apparent adverse short or long-term consequences*. However, the systematic review was limited by the methodological quality of included trials with the majority including less than 100 women hence this conclusion should be interpreted with caution.

There is a consistent and concerning observation that SUPC most commonly occurs in the context of SSC, either with the infant breast feeding or in the prone position [2, 4, 11, 24, 29, 41, 42]. Observational data from Spain indicated a rise in SUPC following the introduction of routine SSC, with cases increasing from 6 per 100,000 to 74 per 100,000 live births [23]. This association has been further highlighted in France [41].

It has been acknowledged for decades that the prone position is associated with an increased risk of sudden unexplained death in infancy (OR 4.47, 95% confidence interval 1.3–13.43) [43] although it remains unclear why the prone position is dangerous for infants [44]. Proposed mechanisms include airway obstruction leading to suffocation, perhaps by flattening on the nose leading to posterior displacement of the tongue and airway obstruction [45] and that the presence of maternal arm or hand may render an infant unable to extend its neck to relieve obstruction. An excess of petechial haemorrhages and congested lungs in SUPC infants who die implies an asphyxial mode of death [20].

Irrespective of proposed mechanism of harm, the prone position is not recommended at any time for infants due to the significantly increased risk of sudden death [46, 47], yet it has become standard practice to overlook this advice immediately after birth. Indeed, on a global scale newborn infants undergoing the precarious transition to extra-uterine life are being placed prone on their mother's chest to facilitate SSC and early breast feeding. Nevertheless, in the UK, in recognition of the emerging risk of SUPC, UNICEF-UK now recommends that during SSC 'midwives check on the infant's condition frequently during the first two to three hours after birth, with particular emphasis on ensuring that the infant's position is safe and the nose and mouth are not occluded' [48]. Furthermore, it has been proposed that SSC can be more safely undertaken if the mother adopts a semi-recumbent position of 45° avoiding a fully prone position of the baby, but this remains unproven [32]. It is important to acknowledge that the risks associated with prone positioning do not disappear during SSC and are potentially exaggerated in the presence of other risk factors.

The fact that most SUPC occurs in proximity to birth at a time when SSC is strongly advocated may simply reflect the time that infants are most vulnerable; they are undergoing a complex sequence of physiological transition processes and may be less tolerant of hypoxia induced by airway obstruction during this time [7]. Although many infants are found collapsed at the breast, it is unlikely that breast feeding *per se* is directly implicated as thousands of infants are successfully breast fed shortly after birth without adverse effect. Indeed, breast feeding is protective for later sudden unexpected death. There is however a theory that newborn infants exhibit increased vagal tone during breastfeeding, which may be a contributing factor to cardiorespiratory collapse [33], and exclusive breast feeding is a risk factor for early death in infants with fatty acid oxidation defects and other rare metabolic conditions [49].

There is an urgent need to promote 'safe' SSC [31] with an emphasis on safety to ensure that the benefits gained from skin to skin care are not counteracted by acute collapse.

Therapeutic Hypothermia After SUPC

Therapeutic hypothermia (TH) is an effective and safe intervention in term infants with moderate to severe intrapartum hypoxic ischaemic encephalopathy, but the evidence for its benefit after SUPC is scarce. No clinical trial has assessed the role of TH in the context of encephalopathy resulting from SUPC, and such a trial would be difficult to undertake in view of the rare nature of SUPC and the subsequent small numbers of eligible infants.

There is uncertainty about whether to offer TH after SUPC, as such infants were excluded from the original cooling trials. However, there are emerging case reports of infants undergoing TH in this context [4, 50–52]. Whilst these data report 'success', the outcomes reported are variable and long-term data is lacking. Moreover, the potential limitations and even harm that may arise should be acknowledged.

Underlying infection is a recognised cause of SUPC [18] and the evidence regarding the interaction between infection and therapeutic hypothermia is deficient [53], at best suggesting that infection may abolish neuroprotective effects of TH [54] or indeed may increase mortality [55, 56].

The perils of extrapolating the benefit of TH has been illustrated in preliminary trials in low and middle income areas where there is evidence of increased mortality rather than the benefit observed in the developed world [57, 58]. Other aetiologies in which TH might potentially result in harm include intracranial haemorrhage, cardiac anomalies or dysrhythmias, pulmonary hypertension and some metabolic conditions.

Nevertheless around three quarters of infants where a cause for SUPC is not identified develop a typical post-asphyxial encephalopathy [6]. There is therefore a theoretical plausibility for benefit from TH in such context and so it should be carefully considered on an individual case basis. Importantly, TH should only be instigated after exclusion of conditions which may be adversely affected by TH and after discussion of the potential benefits and risks with parents. A clinical trial to assess benefit would be challenging to perform given the small numbers of infants with SUPC and the wide variation in underlying causes. It is vital that information from other sources is reported and collated, including both short and long-term outcomes.

Medico-Legal Aspects of SUPC

As awareness of SUPC and associated modifiable factors grows within the general population, there are increasing numbers of SUPC following which litigation is pursued [59]. Table 10.4 lists some emerging themes relating to breach of duty.

Table 10.4 Potential breaches of duty in SUPC

Failure to ensure transition is adequately established after birth
Failure to recognise preceding risk factors for deterioration e.g. prolonged rupture of membranes, small for gestational age
Failure to conduct appropriate assessments of baby after birth e.g. Apgar scores, observations
Failure to act on abnormal observations
Failure to give appropriate parental advice e.g. skin to skin, co-sleeping, co-bedding
Lack of, or failure to follow hospital policies e.g. skin to skin, co-sleeping, co-bedding
Failure to ensure safety and/or appropriate surveillance of baby during skin to skin care

The clinical histories of two cases where medical negligence claims have been successfully pursued are reproduced with parental permission:

Case 1

A baby was born at 39 weeks of gestation to a primigravida who had had an uneventful pregnancy. There had been prolonged rupture of membranes for 72 h before vaginal delivery. The birthweight was 4510 g and Apgar scores were 9 at 1 min and 10 at 5 min. There was parental concern about persistent abnormal respiratory noises in the minutes after birth but no further clinical assessment was recorded as having been undertaken.

Collapse of the infant was identified in the first hour of life whilst being held by the father. The heart rate was 40/min, there was apnoea, and the baby was white and floppy. Resuscitation commenced including ventilation and chest compressions and the heart rate rose to over 100/min at 9 min following collapse.

A blood gas was taken 17 min after collapse and showed pH of 6.56, PCO_2 23 kPa and base excess −21 mmol/L.

There was clinical, radiological, haematological and biochemical evidence of congenital pneumonia and sepsis without meningitis. The baby received TH for severe hypoxic ischaemic encephalopathy and there was hypoxic-ischaemic multi-organ involvement.

An early MRI and subsequent severe neurological impairment were consistent with an acute severe near total asphyxial event.

Case 2

A primigravida with an uneventful pregnancy had a vaginal delivery at 41 weeks. The birthweight was 3830 g and Apgar scores were 9 at 1 min and 10 at 5 min. The baby was placed immediately on the mother's chest for skin to skin and repositioned to breast feed at an hour of age at a 45° angle. The mother was moved into a supine lithotomy position for suturing of perineal tear and the baby remained on the breast. The suturing procedure was complicated by equipment failures during which the father and a second healthcare worker were required to assist.

One hour after breast feeding commenced and during ongoing repair, the baby was found in a state of collapse on the mother's chest: the heart rate was 80–100/min, and the baby was apneic, grey and hypotonic. Mask and endotracheal ventilation was delivered, and the circulation recovered within 10 min of collapse.

A blood gas taken 36 min after collapse showed a venous pH of 6.9, PCO_2 5.1 kPa, base excess −25.5 mmol/L, glucose 5.1 mmol/L and lactate 14 mmol/L.

No underlying condition was diagnosed, and accidental airway obstruction was presumed. The baby received TH for severe hypoxic ischaemic encephalopathy and there was no evidence of other organ involvement.

An early MRI and subsequent severe neurological impairment were consistent with an acute severe near total asphyxial event.

The first case demonstrates that, where an underlying condition ultimately results in collapse, there is usually a prodromal period during which early recognition and intervention may prevent profound cardiorespiratory arrest [29]. Notably, the consequences of the hypoxic-ischaemic collapse may be more injurious than that of the underlying pathology. Careful consideration of risk factors, for example for sepsis and hypoglycaemia, can help to guide surveillance in the first postnatal hours and avoid deterioration.

The second case demonstrates the need for additional surveillance of infant well-being by another individual when the baby's airway and colour cannot be visualised by the mother during SSC or breastfeeding. In this case both the prone position of the baby in the context of supine position of the mother, and distraction of the mother by the procedure mandated that another person be responsible for safeguarding her baby's wellbeing while she could not. Of note in neither case did therapeutic hypothermia appear to confer significant benefit.

Improving Safety in the Early Postpartum Period

The growing understanding of the potentially avoidable factors in SUPC within the perinatal community has prompted discussion about how best to maintain the safety of all infants after birth.

As a proportion of infants with SUPC prove to have an underlying condition [6], stratified risk assessment at birth for sepsis and hypoglycaemia should be implemented for all infants at birth [60]. It is rare for an underlying condition to be fatal in itself and many SUPC infants die or suffer consequences as a result of severe hypoxia-ischaemia, indicating that a window of opportunity exists in which deteriorating infants could be identified and treated earlier, potentially avoiding catastrophic asphyxia.

The deteriorating infant is more likely to be noticed when healthcare workers are present [6], although SUPC does occur when parents are not alone. It is therefore reasonable to conclude that increased frequency of observation during SSC and early breast feeding attempts during the first two hours postpartum might reduce the risk of SUPC or adverse events. This targeted approach of increased unobtrusive surveillance at high risk times and in high risk cases has been suggested by several authors as a pragmatic way to improve safety which in turn may result in a reduction in SUPC [2, 4, 6, 24, 31] and is now recommended by the New Zealand Ministry of Health [61], the Italian Paediatrics Society [19] and UNICEF UK [48]. This approach of increased surveillance may also prevent newborn falls, which occur more frequently during co-sleeping [62]. The risks associated with practices such as co-sleeping should be discussed with parents soon after birth and prone position should be actively discouraged during hospital stay and after discharge.

Continuous pulse oximetry monitoring has been suggested as a potential intervention to promote safety. On a practical level this would be challenging to perform, and may not improve safety of the infant [31]. Evolving wireless technology is a less intrusive alternative and may have a role in the future, although benefit from such an intervention should be investigated prior to instigation.

Infant assessment tools have been developed to try to identify adverse event precursors whilst promoting safe mother infant bonding. Examples include the RAPPT tool, devised in the US, which scores infants under the domains of respiratory effort, activity, perfusion, position and tone [30]; and a postnatal surveillance protocol in an Italian centre with similar aims [39]. In developing both tools, the authors report identification of infants who had signs of hypoxia. Such tools have the benefit of identifying early signs of illness whilst improving awareness of risk factors for SUPC but as assessment is intermittent may not identify a rapid deterioration.

The parallels between SUPC and SUDI have previously been discussed. Perhaps the most significant similarity is the potential to reduce SUPC through a successful high-profile awareness campaign, comparable to the 'back to sleep' campaign of the 1990s. Written information for parents to enhance their awareness of signs of 'general wellbeing' may be useful and might empower them to be aware of the importance of positioning and the infant airway [39]. A study utilising more contemporary methods of communication such as text [63], email and video demonstrated improved parental compliance with safe sleep practices. Although there is a risk that such an approach may induce additional anxiety in parents at an already stressful time, the benefits are likely to outweigh the risk for the vast majority of parents [39, 47]. Increased education for staff is also a key component of any risk reduction strategy. Owing to its rarity, clinical staff may have no experience of SUPC, nor appreciate the risk factors.

Undoubtedly, a major challenge will be proving the efficacy of any intervention or surveillance programme aimed at reducing SUPC, as its individual occurrence in individual centres is rare. Irrespective of these challenges, the perinatal community should strive for a collaborative effort of maternity, neonatal and obstetric teams to mitigate avoidable harm in all newborn infants.

Conclusion

SUPC is a rare but potentially fatal event, with devastating consequences for survivors. Most importantly, it is potentially avoidable. Increased vigilance and parental empowerment may help to reduce SUPC and prevent thousands of avoidable deaths and disability worldwide. A pragmatic approach to improving the safety of infants after birth should be developed whilst support of beneficial practices such as breast feeding and SSC continues.

References

1. British Association of Perinatal Medicine. Guidelines for the investigation of newborn infants who suffer a sudden and unexpected postnatal collapse in the first week of life. Recommendations from a professional group on sudden unexpected postnatal collapse. 2011.
2. Herlenius E, Kuhn P. Sudden unexpected postnatal collapse of newborn infants: a review of cases, definitions, risks, and preventive measures. Transl Stroke Res. 2013;4(2):236–47.
3. Bass JL, Gartley T, Lyczkowski DA, Kleinman R. Trends in the incidence of sudden unexpected infant death in the newborn: 1995-2014. J Pediatr. 2018;196:104–8.

4. Pejovic NJ, Herlenius E. Unexpected collapse of healthy newborn infants: risk factors, supervision and hypothermia treatment. Acta Paediatr. 2013;102(7):680–8.
5. Grylack LJ, Williams AD. Apparent life-threatening events in presumed healthy neonates during the first three days of life. Pediatrics. 1996;97(3):349–51.
6. Becher J-C, Bhushan SS, Lyon AJ. Unexpected collapse in apparently healthy newborns–a prospective national study of a missing cohort of neonatal deaths and near-death events. Arch Dis Child Fetal Neonatal Ed. 2012;97(1):F30–F4.
7. Poets A, Steinfeldt R, Poets CF. Sudden deaths and severe apparent life-threatening events in term infants within 24 hours of birth. Pediatrics. 2011;127(4):e869–73.
8. Lutz TL, Elliott EJ, Jeffery HE. Sudden unexplained early neonatal death or collapse: a national surveillance study. Pediatr Res. 2016;80(4):493–8.
9. Dageville C, Pignol J, De Smet S. Very early neonatal apparent life-threatening events and sudden unexpected deaths: Incidence and risk factors. Acta Paediatr. 2008;97(7):866–9.
10. Tsao PC, Chang FY, Chen SJ, Soong WJ, Jeng MJ, Lee YS, et al. Sudden and unexpected and near death during the early neonatal period: a multicenter study. J Chin Med Assoc. 2012;75(2):65–9.
11. Branger B, Savagner C, Roze JC, Winer N. [Eleven cases of early neonatal sudden death ou near death of full term and healthy neonates in maternity wards]. J Gynecol Obstet Biol Reprod (Paris). 2007;36(7):671–9.
12. Polberger S, Svenningsen NW. Early neonatal sudden infant death and near death of fullterm infants in maternity wards. Acta Paediatr Scand. 1985;74(6):861–6.
13. Leow JY, Platt MP. Sudden, unexpected and unexplained early neonatal deaths in the North of England. Arch Dis Child Fetal Neonatal Ed. 2011;96(6):F440–2.
14. Filippi L, Laudani E, Tubili F, Calvani M, Bartolini I, Donzelli G. Incidence of sudden unexpected postnatal collapse in the therapeutic hypothermia era. Am J Perinatol. 2017;34(13):1362–7.
15. Filiano JJ, Kinney HC. A perspective on neuropathologic findings in victims of the sudden infant death syndrome: the triple-risk model. Biol Neonate. 1994;65(3–4):194–7.
16. Spinelli J, Collins-Praino L, Van Den Heuvel C, Byard RW. Evolution and significance of the triple risk model in sudden infant death syndrome. J Paediatr Child Health. 2017;53(2):112–5.
17. Blair PS, Sidebotham P, Berry PJ, Evans M, Fleming PJ. Major epidemiological changes in sudden infant death syndrome: a 20-year population-based study in the UK. Lancet. 2006;367(9507):314–9.
18. Weber MA, Ashworth MT, Risdon RA, Brooke I, Malone M, Sebire NJ. Sudden unexpected neonatal death in the first week of life: autopsy findings from a specialist centre. J Matern Fetal Neonatal Med. 2009;22(5):398–404.
19. Piumelli R, Davanzo R, Nassi N, Salvatore S, Arzilli C, Peruzzi M, et al. Apparent life-threatening events (ALTE): Italian guidelines. Ital J Pediatr. 2017;43:111.
20. Reyes JA, Somers GR, Chiasson DA. Sudden unexpected death in neonates: a clinico-pathological study. Pediatr Dev Pathol. 2018;21(6):528–36.
21. Hays S, Feit P, Barre P, Cottin X, Huin N, Fichtner C, et al. [Respiratory arrest in the delivery room while lying in the prone position on the mothers' chest in 11 full term healthy neonates]. Arch Pediatr. 2006;13(7):1067–8.
22. Rodriguez-Alarcon J, Melchor JC, Linares A, Aranguren G, Quintanilla M, Fernandez-Llebrez L, et al. Early neonatal sudden death or near death syndrome. An epidemiological study of 29 cases. Acta Paediatr. 1994;83(7):704–8.
23. Rodriguez-Alarcón Gómez J, Elorriaga IA, Fernández-Llebrez L, Fernández AP, Avellanal CU, Sierra CO. Episodios aparentemente letales en las primeras dos horas de vida durante el contacto piel con piel. Incidencia y factores de riesgo. Progresos de obstetricia y ginecología. 2011;54(2):55–9.
24. Schrewe B, Janvier A, Barrington K. Life-threatening event during skin-to-skin contact in the delivery room. BMJ Case Rep. 2010;2010.

25. Thach BT. Deaths and near deaths of healthy newborn infants while bed sharing on maternity wards. J Perinatol. 2014;34(4):275–9.
26. Friedman F Jr, Adrouche-Amrani L, Holzman IR. Breastfeeding and delivery room neonatal collapse. J Hum Lact. 2015;31(2):230–2.
27. Gatti II, Castel C, Andrini P, Durand P, Carlus C, Chabernaud J, et al. Cardiorespiratory arrest in full term newborn infants: six case reports. Arch Pediatr. 2004;11(5):432–5.
28. Foran A, Cinnante C, Groves A, Azzopardi DV, Rutherford MA, Cowan FM. Patterns of brain injury and outcome in term neonates presenting with postnatal collapse. Arch Dis Child Fetal Neonatal Ed. 2009;94(3):F168–77.
29. Peters C, Becher JC, Lyon AJ, Midgley PC. Who is blaming the baby? Arch Dis Child Fetal Neonatal Ed. 2009;94(5):F377–8.
30. Ludington-Hoe SM, Morgan K. Infant assessment and reduction of sudden unexpected postnatal collapse risk during skin-to-skin contact. Newborn Infant Nurs Rev. 2014;14(1):28–33.
31. Feldman-Winter L, Goldsmith JP. Safe sleep and skin-to-skin care in the neonatal period for healthy term newborns. Pediatrics. 2016;138(3).
32. Colson S. Does the mothers posture have a protective role to play during skin to skin contact. Clin Lactat. 2014;5(2):41–50.
33. Toker-Maimon O, Joseph LJ, Bromiker R, Schimmel MS. Neonatal cardiopulmonary arrest in the delivery room. Pediatrics. 2006;118(2):847–8.
34. Espagne S, Hamon I, Thiebaugeorges O, Hascoet J. Sudden death of neonates in the delivery room. Arch Pediatr. 2004;11(5):436–9.
35. Strayer DL, Drews FA, Johnston WA. Cell phone-induced failures of visual attention during simulated driving. J Exp Psychol Appl. 2003;9(1):23–32.
36. WHO. Baby-friendly hospital initiative: revised, updated and expanded for integrated care. Geneva: World Health Organization and UNICEF; 2009.
37. World Health Organisation. Evidence for the ten steps to successful breastfeeding. Geneva: WHO; 1998.
38. Section on Breastfeeding. Breastfeeding and the use of human milk. Pediatrics. 2012;129(3):e827–41.
39. Davanzo R, De Cunto A, Paviotti G, Travan L, Inglese S, Brovedani P, et al. Making the first days of life safer: preventing sudden unexpected postnatal collapse while promoting breastfeeding. J Hum Lact. 2015;31(1):47–52.
40. Moore ER, Bergman N, Anderson GC, Medley N. Early skin-to-skin contact for mothers and their healthy newborn infants. Cochrane Database Syst Rev. 2016;(11):CD003519.
41. Andres V, Garcia P, Rimet Y, Nicaise C, Simeoni U. Apparent life-threatening events in presumably healthy newborns during early skin-to-skin contact. Pediatrics. 2011;127(4):e1073–e6.
42. Matthijsse PR, Semmekrot BA, Liem KD. [Skin to skin contact and breast-feeding after birth: not always without risk!]. Ned Tijdschr Geneeskd. 2016;160:D171.
43. Dwyer T, Ponsonby AL, Newman NM, Gibbons LE. Prospective cohort study of prone sleeping position and sudden infant death syndrome. Lancet. 1991;337(8752):1244–7.
44. Stanley FJ, Byard RW. The association between the prone sleeping position and sudden infant death syndrome (SIDS): an editorial overview. J Paediatr Child Health. 1991;27(6):325–8.
45. Simson LR Jr, Brantley RE. Postural asphyxia as a cause of death in sudden infant death syndrome. J Forensic Sci. 1977;22(1):178–87.
46. AAP. The changing concept of sudden infant death syndrome: diagnostic coding shifts, controversies regarding the sleeping environment, and new variables to consider in reducing risk. Pediatrics. 2005;116(5):1245–55.
47. Moon RY. SIDS and other sleep-related infant deaths: expansion of recommendations for a safe infant sleeping environment. Pediatrics. 2011;128(5):1030–9.
48. Entwistle F. The evidence and rationale for the UNICEF UK baby friendly initiative standards. London: UNICEF; 2013.

49. Rinaldo P, Yoon HR, Yu C, Raymond K, Tiozzo C, Giordano G. Sudden and unexpected neonatal death: a protocol for the postmortem diagnosis of fatty acid oxidation disorders. Semin
Perinatol. 1999;23(2):204–10.

50. Marin N, Valverde E, Cabanas F. [Severe apparent life-threatening event during "skin-to-skin":
treatment with hypothermia]. An Pediatr (Barc). 2013;79(4):253–6.

51. Cornet MC, Maton P, Langhendries JP, Marion W, Marguglio A, Smeets S, et al. [Use
of therapeutic hypothermia in sudden unexpected postnatal collapse]. Arch Pediatr.
2014;21(9):1006–10.

52. Smit E, Liu X, Jary S, Cowan F, Thoresen M. Cooling neonates who do not fulfil the standard
cooling criteria—short- and long-term outcomes. Acta Paediatr. 2015;104(2):138–45.

53. Thoresen M. Who should we cool after perinatal asphyxia? Semin Fetal Neonatal Med.
2015;20(2):66–71.

54. Osredkar D, Thoresen M, Maes E, Flatebo T, Elstad M, Sabir H. Hypothermia is not neuroprotective after infection-sensitized neonatal hypoxic-ischemic brain injury. Resuscitation.
2014;85(4):567–72.

55. Mourvillier B, Tubach F, van de Beek D, Garot D, Pichon N, Georges H, et al. Induced hypothermia in severe bacterial meningitis: a randomized clinical trial. JAMA. 2013;310(20):2174–83.

56. Thayyil S, Oliveira V, Lally PJ, Swamy R, Bassett P, Chandrasekaran M, et al. Hypothermia
for encephalopathy in low and middle-income countries (HELIX): study protocol for a randomised controlled trial. Trials. 2017;18(1):432.

57. Thayyil S, Shankaran S, Wade A, Cowan FM, Ayer M, Satheesan K, et al. Whole-body cooling
in neonatal encephalopathy using phase changing material. Arch Dis Child Fetal Neonatal Ed.
2013;98(3):F280–1.

58. Robertson NJ, Nakakeeto M, Hagmann C, Cowan FM, Acolet D, Iwata O, et al. Therapeutic
hypothermia for birth asphyxia in low-resource settings: a pilot randomised controlled trial.
Lancet. 2008;372(9641):801–3.

59. Goldsmith JP. Hospitals should balance skin-to-skin contact with safe sleep policies. AAP
News; 2015.

60. British Association of Perinatal Medicine. Newborn early warning trigger and track (NEWTT):
a framework for practice. 2015.

61. Ministry of Health New Zealand. Observation of mother and baby in the immediate postnatal
period: consensus statements guiding practice. 2012.

62. Janiszewski H. Reducing the risk of baby falls in maternity units. Nurs Times.
2015;111(28–29):21–3.

63. Moon RY, Hauck FR, Colson ER, Kellams AL, Geller NL, Heeren T, et al. The effect of nursing quality improvement and mobile health interventions on infant sleep practices: a randomized clinical trial. JAMA. 2017;318(4):351–9.

Part III
The Very Preterm Infant: Controversies in Postnatal Management

Chapter 11
Mechanical Ventilation of the Preterm Infant

Kate Hodgson, Peter Davis, and Louise Owen

Introduction

With the advent of neonatal intensive care in the 1960s, survival of very preterm infants became a possibility. However, complications such as pneumothorax and pulmonary interstitial emphysema were common. Bronchopulmonary dysplasia (BPD) was described in survivors [1] and subsequently recognised as resulting from prolonged exposure to oxygen toxicity and ventilator induced lung injury [2]. The widespread implementation of exogenous surfactant therapy in the 1980s revolutionised neonatal intensive care, reducing mortality and decreasing the incidence of pulmonary air leak [3, 4], however the incidence of BPD remained high. Early non-invasive support with nasal continuous positive airway pressure (CPAP) is now the support mode of choice in the majority of preterm infants requiring primary respiratory support for respiratory distress syndrome (RDS). The novel alternative, nasal high flow (nHF), has increased in popularity in recent years.

Although using non-invasive support is the best approach to minimise ventilator-associated lung injury, many babies require mechanical ventilation due to respiratory failure or apnoea despite non-invasive support. In the large trials of CPAP versus intubation at birth for very preterm infants, intubation was frequently required for infants randomised to CPAP. In the Continuous Positive Airway Pressure or Intubation at birth (COIN) trial, 46% of the 25–28 week gestational age infants randomised to CPAP required intubation within the first 5 days of life [5]. Finer *et al.* found 83% of the 24–27 + 6 week gestation infants randomised to CPAP were intubated at some point during the trial [6]; and in the Vermont Oxford Network study, 52% of babies born at 26–29 + 6 weeks of gestation, commencing on CPAP without prior surfactant therapy, ultimately required intubation [7]. While

K. Hodgson (✉) · P. Davis · L. Owen
Newborn Research Centre, The Royal Women's Hospital, Melbourne, VIC, Australia
e-mail: pgd@unimelb.edu.au; louise.owen@thewomens.org.au;
kate.hodgson@thewomens.org.au

© Springer Nature Switzerland AG 2020
E. M. Boyle, J. Cusack (eds.), *Emerging Topics and Controversies in Neonatology*, https://doi.org/10.1007/978-3-030-28829-7_11

endotracheal ventilation remains necessary, the use of lung-protective ventilation strategies to mitigate the risk of BPD is essential.

The evidence for many aspects of mechanical ventilation of the preterm neonate is limited. This chapter examines the principles governing which babies should be ventilated, modes of ventilation, lung-protective strategies, surfactant provision, intubation and extubation practices, and future directions in research and clinical care.

Indications for Mechanical Ventilation

Early use of non-invasive support reduces the need for intubation and mechanical ventilation. Nasal CPAP prevents alveolar collapse, reduces work of breathing and decreases ventilation-perfusion mismatch [8]. Meta-analysis of available trials suggests that the use of nasal CPAP from birth reduces the combined outcome of death or BPD at 36 weeks' corrected gestation (relative risk 0.91 (95% confidence interval 0.84, 0.99), risk difference −0.04 (−0.07, 0.00)) [9]. However, mechanical ventilation is almost always required for the smallest and most immature infants. Data from the National Institute of Child Health and Human Development (NICHD) in the United States showed that at 24 h of life, 94% of infants born at 23 weeks of gestation were receiving mechanical ventilation [10]. This figure decreased to 40% for those born at 28 weeks of gestation.

There are no universally accepted indications for intubation and mechanical ventilation of the very preterm infant; this decision will depend upon individual patient circumstances, clinician practice, the clinical trajectory of the infant's respiratory distress syndrome, and unit-related factors such as the approach to minimally-invasive surfactant therapy and need to transfer ventilated babies. Indications for mechanical ventilation of the very preterm infant generally fall into three categories: hypoxia, respiratory acidosis and recurrent or refractory apnoea. Less common are the need for cardiovascular support, such as during cardiac failure, and the need for airway protection, such as with seizures.

The early randomised trials of non-invasive support had similar criteria for determining nasal CPAP failure and for initiating mechanical ventilation: hypoxia (FiO_2 >0.6), respiratory acidosis (pH <7.25 and pCO_2 >60–65 mmHg), or apnoea (more than 6–12 episodes requiring stimulation in 6 h) [5–7]. More recent trials of non-invasive support have generally had a lower FiO_2 threshold for intubation (0.4–0.5) [11–14]. The most common indication for intubation in very preterm neonates is high oxygen requirement [5, 15–17]. In an Australian cohort of infants <32 weeks of gestation in whom nasal CPAP failed, the median FiO_2 at the time of intubation was 0.5. High FiO_2 requirement within the first 2–6 h of life predicts subsequent need for intubation [15–17], in contrast to hypercapnia, which is a poor predictor [15–17].

Studies have not compared the short or long-term outcomes for infants who receive mechanical ventilation at lower versus higher threshold criteria for failure of non-invasive support. Mechanical ventilation should be reserved for those very preterm infants who have significant hypoxia, respiratory acidosis or apnoea, taking into consideration other patient-related factors.

Ventilation Modes

Modern ventilators have a myriad of available modes, with differing terminology and overlap between devices. The most commonly used modes allow synchronisation of the ventilator inflation with the patient's spontaneous breathing. Conventional mechanical ventilation modes differ in various ways. The ventilator can support all the patient's spontaneous breaths, or it can be set to deliver a predetermined number of inflations per minute. The inflation time can be determined by the infant's own efforts, or pre-set on the ventilator. Modes can be pressure-limited, with the positive inspiratory pressure (PIP) and positive end expiratory pressure (PEEP) set. Alternatively, with volume-targeted ventilation, the clinician sets a tidal volume and the ventilator will generate the PIP required to deliver this, up to a set maximum PIP. In the event of increased compliance, the PIP will reduce, and vice versa, so that a constant set tidal volume is maintained. The wide array of ventilator technologies can potentially lead to confusion for the clinician and make it challenging to select the best strategy for a particular patient and disease state.

Volume-Targeted Ventilation

Pressure-limited ventilation was the mainstay of neonatal mechanical ventilation for many years. Technological limitations meant it was not possible to measure the small tidal volumes required by very preterm infants. This has now been overcome, with the availability of sensitive flow meters with a very small dead space. Traditional pressure-limited ventilation requires a PIP and PEEP to be set; the tidal volume (determined by the difference between PIP and PEEP) may vary significantly from breath to breath and with changes in compliance. Given the changing compliance of the preterm infant lung, this may result in tidal volumes that are higher or lower than optimal.

However, with volume-targeted ventilation the clinician sets the desired tidal volume, which is delivered using variable PIP. Changes in lung compliance therefore have no effect on the tidal volume delivered, and volutrauma is reduced. Whilst the use of volume-targeted ventilation has increased, only 50% of tertiary neonatal units in a 2010 multi-national survey routinely used volume-targeted ventilation for preterm infants with RDS [18].

A Cochrane review meta-analysis compared the use of volume-targeted ventilation for neonates with pressure-limited ventilation modes [19]. Pooled data, from 20 trials involving 1065 neonates, demonstrated a significant reduction in pneumothorax (typical RR 0.52, 95% CI 0.31, 0.87), lower combined outcome of death or BPD (typical RR 0.73, 95% CI 0.59, 0.89), less periventricular leucomalacia (typical RR 0.45, 95% CI 0.21, 0.98), and fewer grade III/IV intraventricular haemorrhages (typical RR 0.53, 95% CI 0.37, 0.77) with the use of volume-targeted ventilation.

Evidence is limited regarding the ideal set tidal volume for preterm infants. Tidal volumes of greater than 8 mL/kg can cause volutrauma [20]; conversely, low tidal volumes of 3–3.5 mL/kg may result in atelectasis and increased release of pro-inflammatory cytokines [21]. Based on studies of spontaneously breathing preterm infants with RDS whilst on CPAP, a tidal volume of 4–6 mL/kg is suggested [22]. The smallest preterm babies may require tidal volumes in the higher end of that range, owing to the relatively larger dead space of the endotracheal tube for their weight [22]. Older infants may also require higher tidal volumes (5–8 mL/kg) to maintain normo-capnoea due to airway dilatation and increased dead space [18].

High Frequency Oscillatory Ventilation

High frequency oscillatory ventilation (HFOV) is a form of mechanical ventilation that uses a constant distending pressure, small tidal volumes, often smaller than dead space, and rapid ventilator rates. Proposed advantages over conventional ventilation include the use of lower peak airway pressures, and the ability to control oxygenation and ventilation independently [23]. A high volume strategy, with optimal lung recruitment and weaning of FiO_2 before mean airway pressure, is now regarded as the most appropriate strategy for HFOV in preterm infants [24]. Animal studies have shown that maintenance of lung volume prevents lung injury [25]. Using HFOV as a lung protective strategy may theoretically reduce the risk of lung injury and hence BPD. However, a 2015 Cochrane review pooled the available data (19 trials, 2096 patients) comparing elective HFOV with conventional ventilation for preterm infants and concluded that there was no difference in mortality or most short-term outcomes [24]. Furthermore, the risk of acute air leak was increased compared with conventional ventilation. Although elective use of HFOV resulted in a slightly reduced risk of BPD, the effect was inconsistent across trials.

Two early trials reported a higher incidence of severe intracranial ultrasound abnormalities in infants managed with HFOV [26, 27]. Subsequent studies have not shown the same trend and the Cochrane meta-analysis concluded that there was no difference in severe IVH rates [24]. Furthermore, long-term neurodevelopmental follow up data did not show any difference in outcomes. Eight RCTs reporting neurodevelopmental follow up data were included in the pooled analysis. One study found higher rates of moderate-severe neurodevelopmental impairment in infants managed with HFOV, two studies found lower rates, and five found no difference. Therefore HFOV does not appear to either adversely affect neurodevelopmental outcomes or offer significant advantages over conventional ventilation. Overall, there was no significant difference in the rates of more severe grades of IVH between the HFOV and CV groups (summary RR 1.10, 95% CI 0.95–1.27).

A ventilation strategy with HFOV aiming at optimal alveolar recruitment is now widely considered as being the most appropriate strategy for the use of HFOV in preterm infants in order to avoid lung injury. Some newer ventilators have the ability to deliver a set tidal volume during HFOV. Two prospective observational studies [28, 29], and one randomised crossover trial [30] have evaluated the use of volume guarantee with HFOV in preterm infants. It was found to be feasible and to result in more stable CO_2 levels than standard HFOV. Given the small sample sizes of these studies, further research is required.

Elective HFOV from birth has no clear advantage over conventional mechanical ventilation, particularly given the increased use of, and improvement in, volume-targeted ventilation. Given no clear advantage of one mode over another, it seems reasonable for individual units to develop and maintain expertise in one technique. For units choosing conventional ventilation, HFOV may be reserved for rescue therapy in those infants with severe respiratory failure.

Positive End Expiratory Pressure and 'Open Lung' Ventilation

PEEP is now almost universally utilised in mechanical ventilation of preterm infants. Short-term physiological benefits of PEEP include increased functional residual capacity, alveolar recruitment, reduced work of breathing and improved ventilation-perfusion matching [31, 32]. However, very little research has investigated the efficacy and risks of different PEEP levels.

Although evidence in neonates is scarce, excessive PEEP may cause air leak and hypercarbia, and may impede systemic venous return compromising cardiac function [32, 33]. Studies in preterm lambs show that mechanical ventilation at birth without PEEP causes increased levels of pro-inflammatory cytokines and lung injury [20]. Concurrent use of high tidal volume ventilation exacerbates this damage. The Cochrane review of PEEP for mechanically ventilated preterm infants identified only one eligible study comparing higher and lower levels of PEEP in preterm infants [32], with no statistically significant results. Despite this paucity of evidence, there is general consensus that PEEP is beneficial and surveys suggest it is universally applied [34–36].

The concept of an 'open lung' strategy for neonatal mechanical ventilation builds on the importance of PEEP. This approach involves optimal alveolar recruitment to avoid over-distension or atelectasis, allowing even distribution of tidal volume to the neonatal lung [37] and minimising damage to underinflated lung units ('atelectrauma') [38]. Animal studies have demonstrated the negative effects of atelectrauma: alveolar injury secondary to repeated collapse and re-opening, with resultant release of inflammatory mediators [39]. This injury can occur to both atelectatic and aerated sections of lung [40]. Whilst accepted as an evidence-based strategy in high-frequency ventilation [24], the clinical evidence for the use of an open-lung strategy during conventional ventilation is still developing [38].

An open-lung strategy is recommended during neonatal mechanical ventilation, with PEEP tailored to the individual patient and disease state.

Neurally Adjusted Ventilatory Assist

Synchronisation is an important component of mechanical ventilation; compared with the time-cycled ventilation mode, triggered ventilation is associated with a shorter duration of intubation [41]. Currently, most neonatal ventilators use a small, hot wire anemometer flow-sensor at the proximal airway to detect patient respiratory effort and subsequently initiate a ventilator breath [42, 43]. Neurally adjusted ventilatory assist (NAVA) is a new method of synchronisation, which can be used as an adjunct to either invasive or non-invasive ventilation. NAVA detects diaphragmatic electrical activity via electrodes on a nasogastric tube, and synchronises ventilator inflations with the infant's own respiratory effort. Delivered inflation pressure is then proportional to the infant's respiratory effort, potentially reducing the risk of lung injury due to volutrauma [44]. NAVA improves synchrony and reduces work of breathing in neonates, lowering PIP [45] and FiO_2 compared with conventional triggered ventilation [46–48].

Three randomised crossover trials have examined the short-term respiratory effects of NAVA. Two studies found that NAVA reduced PIP compared with conventionally triggered ventilation in preterm infants [45, 49]. This finding was reproduced in infants with evolving or established BPD. Shetty et al. randomised nine extremely preterm infants to NAVA or conventionally triggered ventilation and found improved oxygenation, with a lower oxygenation index, FiO_2 and MAP in those infants on NAVA [50]. Whilst a promising new technology, no studies have evaluated the safety and long-term outcomes of NAVA [44] and further research in this area is warranted before widespread implementation.

Surfactant

The availability of exogenous surfactant therapy transformed neonatal intensive care. Surfactant therapy reduces rates of mechanical ventilation, pneumothorax, death and the combined outcome of death or BPD [51]. However, the use of prophylactic surfactant (mandatory intubation and surfactant administration immediately after birth) has now been shown to have no benefit over selective surfactant therapy (administering to those infants with established respiratory distress syndrome) [51]. Meta-analyses suggest that the risk of death or BPD is actually lower with an approach using early stabilisation on CPAP and selective surfactant administration to those infants requiring intubation, compared with prophylactic administration [51]. This is likely due to higher rates of antenatal corticosteroid administration and non-invasive support provided in the modern era.

However, between 10 and 17% of infants cannot be immediately extubated after surfactant administration [7, 14]. Even in those infants who can be extubated quickly, some positive pressure ventilation, with associated volutrauma, is inevitable. Premedication for INSURE is also a controversial issue, balancing the risk of respiratory depression and potential unsuccessful extubation with the discomfort of laryngoscopy and surfactant administration. The INSURE (intubation, surfactant, extubation) method has become widely used over recent years, with inconclusive evidence regarding its efficacy. Several clinical trials [52, 53] and a meta-analysis [54] suggest that INSURE reduces the need for subsequent mechanical ventilation and pneumothorax.

There is emerging evidence supporting the use of minimally invasive surfactant therapy (MIST) or less-invasive surfactant administration (LISA) to avoid mechanical ventilation. During these techniques, surfactant is delivered using a feeding tube or catheter whilst the infant receives CPAP [55]. Current evidence suggests that MIST/LISA may reduce the need for intubation and ventilation and improve short-term respiratory outcomes, without any adverse effects [56]. There are several methods of MIST/LISA delivery.

Kribs *et al.* described surfactant administration via a feeding tube introduced into the trachea under direct vision using Magill forceps [57]. They randomised 220 infants between 26 and 28 weeks of gestation to either continue on nasal CPAP or receive surfactant via this method [58]. The intervention group had a lower rate of mechanical ventilation at day 3 (28% versus 46% in the control group, $p = 0.008$). Dargaville *et al.* have evaluated an alternative method of surfactant delivery, the Hobart method, which uses a vascular catheter without the need for Magill forceps [59]. Compared with historical controls, fewer 25–28 week gestation infants were mechanically ventilated within 72 h following MIST/LISA (32% vs. 68%, $p = 0.001$). Both methods require laryngoscopy and are typically performed without sedation, but this is controversial and practice varies. Data from animal models suggest that surfactant distribution is more uniform, and lung compliance is improved when surfactant is administered during spontaneous breathing, compared with during mechanical endotracheal ventilation [60].

A large multicentre randomised controlled trial of MIST using the Hobart method for preterm infants 25–28 weeks' gestation is underway [56]. Infants are randomised to receive surfactant via vascular catheter, or have a sham treatment, the primary outcome being death or BPD. The results are awaited.

In summary, selective surfactant administration reduces death or BPD in preterm infants; MIST/LISA may be an effective way of delivering surfactant and reducing BPD via the avoidance of mechanical ventilation.

Medications for Neonatal Intubation

In contrast to paediatric and adult anaesthesia and intensive care settings, emergency neonatal intubation is almost universally performed without induction medications [61]. However, disagreement exists with respect to the use of premedication for non-emergent neonatal intubation, and practice varies widely. The physiological benefits of premedication for endotracheal intubation are clear; vagolytics, analgesics and muscle relaxants reduce adverse physiological effects such as bradycardia, hypertension and hypoxia [62]. Furthermore, discomfort for the infant is minimised by the use of appropriate analgesic medications.

Current consensus recommendations from the American Academy of Paediatrics (AAP) and the Canadian Paediatric Society are that neonates should receive analgesic premedication for non-urgent endotracheal intubations [63, 64]. Despite this, rates of premedication use are low. A 2015 survey of 693 United States neonatologists found only 34% frequently use premedication before intubation [65]. Other studies of European and North American practices have found similar results [66–69]. In the United Kingdom, self-reported rates of premedication use were 37% in 1998, 93% in 2007 and 100% in 2015 [70], alongside an increased use of written guidelines on premedication [70].

Limited evidence exists with respect to the choice of medications for neonatal intubation and again practice varies considerably [65, 69]. Pharmacokinetic and pharmacodynamic data for analgesic drugs are limited for neonates and almost non-existent for preterm neonates; most data are extrapolated from data in older infants.

Fentanyl is preferable to morphine due to its more rapid onset of action [71, 72] and greater cardiovascular stability [64]. Adverse effects of fentanyl include respiratory depression and chest wall rigidity, which can be minimised by slow intravenous administration, and can be rapidly reversed with muscle relaxant. Other less commonly used agents include remifentanil, which has a quicker onset of action and shorter duration of action than fentanyl. Remifentanil has been trialled as an analgesic agent for INSURE (intubation-surfactant-extubation) [73], however it can cause hypotension and bradycardia in adults [71] and children [72]. One randomised controlled trial has compared the use of propofol with the use of morphine, atropine and suxamethonium for intubation of very preterm infants and found the time to successful intubation was quicker with propofol (120 s versus 260 s) [74]. However, limitations of the use of propofol include the need to combine with an opioid for analgesic effect, and the adverse effect of hypotension. Sedatives such as midazolam have no analgesic effect and are not recommended as a single pharmacologic agent for intubation.

The use of premedication (vagolytic, analgesic and muscle relaxant) should be standard practice for non-emergency neonatal intubation, in order to improve patient comfort, physiological stability and likelihood of successful intubation. Further research regarding pharmacokinetics and long-term effects of existing and new medications is required.

Videolaryngoscopy for Teaching Neonatal Intubation

Opportunities for junior medical staff to acquire proficiency in neonatal endotracheal intubation have decreased over time. The increased use of non-invasive support and the change from routine endotracheal suctioning of babies born through meconium-stained liquor have contributed to this trend. Videolaryngoscopy has emerged in recent years as a potential solution to this problem. This technology may improve teaching of neonatal intubation, and increase success rates for clinicians when opportunities for practice may be limited [75–77]. Videolaryngoscopy is addressed further in the chapters on education and management of the difficult airway.

Extubating Preterm Infants

Clinicians aim to extubate as early as possible to ventilation and optimise the chances of the first extubation being successful. Use of non-invasive support and caffeine treatment have been demonstrated to improve extubation success and should be standard care for the very preterm infant.

Post-extubation nasal high-flow therapy results in similar rates of treatment failure, compared with CPAP, though there are few published data for infants <28 weeks of gestation [78]. Compared with head box oxygen, CPAP significantly reduces respiratory failure within seven days of extubation [79], with some evidence that using higher CPAP pressures (7–9 cm H_2O versus 4–6 cm H_2O) further improves success [80].

Peri-extubation methylxanthine administration increases the chances of successful extubation compared with placebo or no treatment [81]. The optimal dosage of caffeine to facilitate extubation is yet to be determined; one study has reported increased success with high dose (80 mg/kg/day loading dose followed by 20 mg/kg/day maintenance) versus standard dose (20 mg/kg loading dose followed by 5 mg/kg/day maintenance) [82]. Whilst effective in facilitating extubation, postnatal corticosteroids, particularly when used early and in high doses, have deleterious effects on neurodevelopment. Thus they are generally only considered for infants who are difficult to wean from the ventilator, in whom the risks of continued mechanical ventilation and BPD may outweigh those of corticosteroid use (see Chap. 16).

Accurately identifying those infants likely to successfully transition to non-invasive support is of paramount importance. There are a number of patient-related factors associated with successful extubation, which may influence clinical decision-making regarding readiness for extubation.

Despite these measures, extubation failure is common, occurring in up to 40% of very preterm infants [83–85], with potential associated morbidities of physiological instability and airway trauma upon reintubation.

Chawla *et al.* conducted a secondary analysis of data from the Surfactant, Positive Pressure and Pulse Oximetry Randomised Trial (SUPPORT) [86]. They found higher 5-min Apgar score, higher pH, lower peak FiO_2 and pCO_2 prior to extubation and non-small for gestational age (SGA) status were associated with successful extubation in extremely preterm infants. Manley *et al.* [87] found similar predictors; both studies showed extubation failure was associated with long-term morbidity, including BPD, and mortality. In essence, the smallest, sickest babies are those most likely to 'fail' extubation, and to have a poor outcome.

Spontaneous breathing tests (SBTs) are widely used in the paediatric intensive care setting, with high sensitivity for predicting extubation success [88]. However, data regarding the utility of spontaneous breathing tests for neonates are sparse. Two neonatal studies have examined a brief (3–5 min) period of ETT CPAP in preterm infants and found high positive predictive values for extubation success [86, 89], but with conflicting negative predictive values. An SBT is simple to perform but, depending on how it is applied, it may aid the decision to extubate, or conversely, become a barrier to extubation. A recent meta-analysis examining tests of neonatal extubation readiness as predictors of successful extubation found significant heterogeneity, including for the definition of extubation success (1–5 days), concluding that there is a lack of strong evidence and further research is needed [90].

Several physiological parameters show promise in predicting extubation success, and are worthy of further evaluation. Reduced heart rate variability (HRV) and reduced respiratory variability (RV) have been investigated as potential predictors of extubation failure in neonates; both are useful predictors in adult patients [90]. Prospective observational studies have shown that HRV is decreased in preterm infants who fail extubation [91] and that the addition of RV to an SBT improves prediction of successful extubation [92]. A multicentre observational study is in progress to assess these parameters in 250 extremely preterm infants immediately prior to extubation, with the aim of developing an automated system to predict extubation readiness [93].

Conclusions

Judicious use of mechanical ventilation using a lung protective strategy can minimise the risk of bronchopulmonary dysplasia and long-term morbidity. Synchronised, volume-targeted ventilation and concomitant avoidance of high tidal volumes, appropriate positive end expiratory pressure and selective surfactant administration are all evidence-based strategies for limiting lung injury via volutrauma and atelectotrauma. Novel uses of existing therapies, such as minimally invasive surfactant therapy, and new technologies, such as physiological extubation readiness prediction and neurally adjusted ventilatory assist, are promising therapies, which may become standard care for very preterm infants in the future.

> **Box 11.1 Lung Protective Strategies for Neonatal Ventilation**
> - CPAP is appropriate first-line therapy for many preterm infants with RDS
> - Volume-targeted ventilation improves outcomes, compared with pressure-limited modes
> - Appropriate, patient-specific use of PEEP and an 'open lung' strategy can limit lung injury
> - Minimally invasive surfactant therapy has been adopted by many units as standard of care, though more evidence is required
> - Measures to improve extubation success include prophylactic caffeine administration and the immediate use of non-invasive respiratory support (to avoid de-recruitment)

References

1. Northway WH Jr, Rosan RC, Porter DY. Pulmonary disease following respiratory therapy of hyaline-membrane disease. Bronchopulmonary dysplasia. N Engl J Med. 1967;276(7):357–68.
2. Philip AG. Oxygen plus pressure plus time: the etiology of bronchopulmonary dysplasia. Pediatrics. 1975;55(1):44–50.
3. Fujiwara T, Maeta H, Chida S, Morita T, Watabe Y, Abe T. Artificial surfactant therapy in hyaline-membrane disease. Lancet. 1980;1(8159):55–9.
4. Merritt TA, Hallman M, Bloom BT, Berry C, Benirschke K, Sahn D, et al. Prophylactic treatment of very premature infants with human surfactant. N Engl J Med. 1986;315(13):785–90.
5. Morley CJ, Davis PG, Doyle LW, Brion LP, Hascoet JM, Carlin JB. Nasal CPAP or intubation at birth for very preterm infants. N Engl J Med. 2008;358(7):700–8.
6. Finer NN, Carlo WA, Walsh MC, Rich W, Gantz MG, Laptook AR, et al. Early CPAP versus surfactant in extremely preterm infants. N Engl J Med. 2010;362(21):1970–9.
7. Dunn MS, Kaempf J, de Klerk A, de Klerk R, Reilly M, Howard D, et al. Randomized trial comparing 3 approaches to the initial respiratory management of preterm neonates. Pediatrics. 2011;128(5):e1069–76.
8. Diblasi RM. Nasal continuous positive airway pressure (CPAP) for the respiratory care of the newborn infant. Respir Care. 2009;54(9):1209–35.
9. Schmolzer GM, Kumar M, Pichler G, Aziz K, O'Reilly M, Cheung PY. Non-invasive versus invasive respiratory support in preterm infants at birth: systematic review and meta-analysis. BMJ. 2013;347:f5980.
10. Stoll BJ, Hansen NI, Bell EF, Shankaran S, Laptook AR, Walsh MC, et al. Neonatal outcomes of extremely preterm infants from the NICHD Neonatal Research Network. Pediatrics. 2010;126(3):443–56.
11. Roberts CT, Owen LS, Manley BJ, Froisland DH, Donath SM, Dalziel KM, et al. Nasal high-flow therapy for primary respiratory support in preterm infants. N Engl J Med. 2016;375(12):1142–51.
12. Meneses J, Bhandari V, Alves JG, Herrmann D. Noninvasive ventilation for respiratory distress syndrome: a randomized controlled trial. Pediatrics. 2011;127(2):300–7.
13. Salvo V, Lista G, Lupo E, Ricotti A, Zimmermann LJ, Gavilanes AW, et al. Noninvasive ventilation strategies for early treatment of RDS in preterm infants: an RCT. Pediatrics. 2015;135(3):444–51.

14. Sandri F, Plavka R, Ancora G, Simeoni U, Stranak Z, Martinelli S, et al. Prophylactic or early selective surfactant combined with nCPAP in very preterm infants. Pediatrics. 2010;125(6):e1402–9.
15. Dargaville PA, Aiyappan A, De Paoli AG, Dalton RG, Kuschel CA, Kamlin CO, et al. Continuous positive airway pressure failure in preterm infants: incidence, predictors and consequences. Neonatology. 2013;104(1):8–14.
16. De Jaegere AP, van der Lee JH, Cante C, van Kaam AH. Early prediction of nasal continuous positive airway pressure failure in preterm infants less than 30 weeks gestation. Acta Paediatr. 2012;101(4):374–9.
17. Fuchs H, Lindner W, Leiprecht A, Mendler MR, Hummler HD. Predictors of early nasal CPAP failure and effects of various intubation criteria on the rate of mechanical ventilation in preterm infants of <29 weeks gestational age. Arch Dis Child Fetal Neonatal Ed. 2011;96(5):F343–7.
18. Klingenberg C, Wheeler KI, Owen LS, Kaaresen PI, Davis PG. An international survey of volume-targeted neonatal ventilation. Arch Dis Child Fetal Neonatal Ed. 2011;96(2):F146–8.
19. Klingenberg C, Wheeler KI, McCallion N, Morley CJ, Davis PG. Volume-targeted versus pressure-limited ventilation in neonates. Cochrane Database Syst Rev. 2017;10:CD003666.
20. Wallace MJ, Probyn ME, Zahra VA, Crossley K, Cole TJ, Davis PG, et al. Early biomarkers and potential mediators of ventilation-induced lung injury in very preterm lambs. Respir Res. 2009;10:19.
21. Lista G, Castoldi F, Bianchi S, Battaglioli M, Cavigioli F, Bosoni MA. Volume guarantee versus high-frequency ventilation: lung inflammation in preterm infants. Arch Dis Child Fetal Neonatal Ed. 2008;93(4):F252–6.
22. Klingenberg C, Wheeler KI, Davis PG, Morley CJ. A practical guide to neonatal volume guarantee ventilation. J Perinatol. 2011;31(9):575–85.
23. Hupp SR, Turner DA, Rehder KJ. Is there still a role for high-frequency oscillatory ventilation in neonates, children and adults? Expert Rev Respir Med. 2015;9(5):603–18.
24. Cools F, Offringa M, Askie LM. Elective high frequency oscillatory ventilation versus conventional ventilation for acute pulmonary dysfunction in preterm infants. Cochrane Database Syst Rev. 2015;(3):CD000104.
25. McCulloch PR, Forkert PG, Froese AB. Lung volume maintenance prevents lung injury during high frequency oscillatory ventilation in surfactant-deficient rabbits. Am Rev Respir Dis. 1988;137(5):1185–92.
26. High-frequency oscillatory ventilation compared with conventional mechanical ventilation in the treatment of respiratory failure in preterm infants. The HIFI Study Group. N Engl J Med. 1989;320(2):88–93.
27. Moriette G, Paris-Llado J, Walti H, Escande B, Magny JF, Cambonie G, et al. Prospective randomized multicenter comparison of high-frequency oscillatory ventilation and conventional ventilation in preterm infants of less than 30 weeks with respiratory distress syndrome. Pediatrics. 2001;107(2):363–72.
28. Enomoto M, Keszler M, Sakuma M, Kikuchi S, Katayama Y, Takei A, et al. Effect of volume guarantee in preterm infants on high-frequency oscillatory ventilation: a pilot study. Am J Perinatol. 2017;34(1):26–30.
29. Gonzalez-Pacheco N, Sanchez-Luna M, Ramos-Navarro C, Navarro-Patino N, de la Blanca AR. Using very high frequencies with very low lung volumes during high-frequency oscillatory ventilation to protect the immature lung. A pilot study. J Perinatol. 2016;36(4):306–10.
30. Iscan B, Duman N, Tuzun F, Kumral A, Ozkan H. Impact of volume guarantee on high-frequency oscillatory ventilation in preterm infants: a randomized crossover clinical trial. Neonatology. 2015;108(4):277–82.
31. Morley C. Continuous distending pressure. Arch Dis Child Fetal Neonatal Ed. 1999;81(2):F152–6.
32. Bamat N, Millar D, Suh S, Kirpalani H. Positive end expiratory pressure for preterm infants requiring conventional mechanical ventilation for respiratory distress syndrome or bronchopulmonary dysplasia. Cochrane Database Syst Rev. 2012;1:CD004500.
33. Shekerdemian L, Bohn D. Cardiovascular effects of mechanical ventilation. Arch Dis Child. 1999;80(5):475–80.

34. Alander M, Peltoniemi O, Saarela T, Anttila E, Pokka T, Kontiokari T. Current trends in paediatric and neonatal ventilatory care—a nationwide survey. Acta Paediatr. 2013;102(2):123–8.
35. Shalish W, Anna GM. The use of mechanical ventilation protocols in Canadian neonatal intensive care units. Paediatr Child Health. 2015;20(4):e13–9.
36. van Kaam AH, Rimensberger PC, Borensztajn D, De Jaegere AP, Neovent Study Group. Ventilation practices in the neonatal intensive care unit: a cross-sectional study. J Pediatr. 2010;157(5):767–71.e1–3.
37. van Kaam AH, de Jaegere A, Haitsma JJ, Van Aalderen WM, Kok JH, Lachmann B. Positive pressure ventilation with the open lung concept optimizes gas exchange and reduces ventilator-induced lung injury in newborn piglets. Pediatr Res. 2003;53(2):245–53.
38. van Kaam AH, Rimensberger PC. Lung-protective ventilation strategies in neonatology: what do we know—what do we need to know? Crit Care Med. 2007;35(3):925–31.
39. de Prost N, Ricard JD, Saumon G, Dreyfuss D. Ventilator-induced lung injury: historical perspectives and clinical implications. Ann Intensive Care. 2011;1(1):28.
40. Tsuchida S, Engelberts D, Peltekova V, Hopkins N, Frndova H, Babyn P, et al. Atelectasis causes alveolar injury in nonatelectatic lung regions. Am J Respir Crit Care Med. 2006;174(3):279–89.
41. Greenough A, Rossor TE, Sundaresan A, Murthy V, Milner AD. Synchronized mechanical ventilation for respiratory support in newborn infants. Cochrane Database Syst Rev. 2016;9:CD000456.
42. Keszler M. State of the art in conventional mechanical ventilation. J Perinatol. 2009;29(4):262–75.
43. Brown MK, DiBlasi RM. Mechanical ventilation of the premature neonate. Respir Care. 2011;56(9):1298–311; discussion 311–3
44. Rossor TE, Hunt KA, Shetty S, Greenough A. Neurally adjusted ventilatory assist compared to other forms of triggered ventilation for neonatal respiratory support. Cochrane Database Syst Rev. 2017;10:CD012251.
45. Kallio M, Koskela U, Peltoniemi O, Kontiokari T, Pokka T, Suo-Palosaari M, et al. Neurally adjusted ventilatory assist (NAVA) in preterm newborn infants with respiratory distress syndrome-a randomized controlled trial. Eur J Pediatr. 2016;175(9):1175–83.
46. Alander M, Peltoniemi O, Pokka T, Kontiokari T. Comparison of pressure-, flow-, and NAVA-triggering in pediatric and neonatal ventilatory care. Pediatr Pulmonol. 2012;47(1):76–83.
47. Stein H, Alosh H, Ethington P, White DB. Prospective crossover comparison between NAVA and pressure control ventilation in premature neonates less than 1500 grams. J Perinatol. 2013;33(6):452–6.
48. Stein H, Howard D. Neurally adjusted ventilatory assist in neonates weighing <1500 grams: a retrospective analysis. J Pediatr. 2012;160(5):786–9.e1.
49. Lee J, Kim HS, Sohn JA, Lee JA, Choi CW, Kim EK, et al. Randomized crossover study of neurally adjusted ventilatory assist in preterm infants. J Pediatr. 2012;161(5):808–13.
50. Shetty S, Hunt K, Peacock J, Ali K, Greenough A. Crossover study of assist control ventilation and neurally adjusted ventilatory assist. Eur J Pediatr. 2017;176(4):509–13.
51. Rojas-Reyes MX, Morley CJ, Soll R. Prophylactic versus selective use of surfactant in preventing morbidity and mortality in preterm infants. Cochrane Database Syst Rev. 2012;(3):CD000510.
52. Escobedo MB, Gunkel JH, Kennedy KA, Shattuck KE, Sanchez PJ, Seidner S, et al. Early surfactant for neonates with mild to moderate respiratory distress syndrome: a multicenter, randomized trial. J Pediatr. 2004;144(6):804–8.
53. Verder H, Albertsen P, Ebbesen F, Greisen G, Robertson B, Bertelsen A, et al. Nasal continuous positive airway pressure and early surfactant therapy for respiratory distress syndrome in newborns of less than 30 weeks' gestation. Pediatrics. 1999;103(2):E24.
54. Stevens TP, Harrington EW, Blennow M, Soll RF. Early surfactant administration with brief ventilation vs selective surfactant and continued mechanical ventilation for preterm infants with or at risk for respiratory distress syndrome. Cochrane Database Syst Rev. 2007;(4):CD003063.
55. Aguar M, Vento M, Dargaville PA. Minimally invasive surfactant therapy: an update. NeoReviews. 2014;15(7):e275–85.

56. Dargaville PA, Kamlin CO, De Paoli AG, Carlin JB, Orsini F, Soll RF, et al. The OPTIMIST-A trial: evaluation of minimally-invasive surfactant therapy in preterm infants 25–28 weeks gestation. BMC Pediatr. 2014;14:213.

57. Kribs A, Roll C, Gopel W, Wieg C, Groneck P, Laux R, et al. Nonintubated surfactant application vs conventional therapy in extremely preterm infants: a randomized clinical trial. JAMA Pediatr. 2015;169(8):723–30.

58. Gopel W, Kribs A, Ziegler A, Laux R, Hoehn T, Wieg C, et al. Avoidance of mechanical ventilation by surfactant treatment of spontaneously breathing preterm infants (AMV): an open-label, randomised, controlled trial. Lancet. 2011;378(9803):1627–34.

59. Dargaville PA, Aiyappan A, Cornelius A, Williams C, De Paoli AG. Preliminary evaluation of a new technique of minimally invasive surfactant therapy. Arch Dis Child Fetal Neonatal Ed. 2011;96(4):F243–8.

60. Bohlin K, Bouhafs RK, Jarstrand C, Curstedt T, Blennow M, Robertson B. Spontaneous breathing or mechanical ventilation alters lung compliance and tissue association of exogenous surfactant in preterm newborn rabbits. Pediatr Res. 2005;57(5 Pt 1):624–30.

61. Whyte S, Birrell G, Wyllie J. Premedication before intubation in UK neonatal units. Arch Dis Child Fetal Neonatal Ed. 2000;82:F38–41.

62. Barrington KJ, Byrne PJ. Premedication for neonatal intubation. Am J Perinatol. 1998;15(4):213–6.

63. Kumar P, Denson SE, Mancuso TJ. Premedication for nonemergency endotracheal intubation in the neonate. Pediatrics. 2010;125:608–15.

64. Barrington K. Premedication for endotracheal intubation in the newborn infant. Paediatr Child Health. 2011;16(3):159–71.

65. Muniraman HK, Yaari J, Hand I. Premedication use before nonemergent intubation in the newborn infant. Am J Perinatol. 2015;32(9):821–4.

66. Paola L, Elisabetta G, Giovanna B, Daniele M, Anna P, Luisa P, et al. Procedural pain in neonates: the state of the art in the implementation of national guidelines in Italy. Pediatr Anesth. 2013;23(5):407–14.

67. Johnston C, Barrington KJ, Taddio A, Carbajal R, Filion F. Pain in Canadian NICUs: have we improved over the past 12 years? Clin J Pain. 2011;27(3):225–32.

68. Sarkar S, Schumacher RE, Baumgart S, Donn SM. Are newborns receiving premedication before elective intubation? J Perinatol. 2006;26(5):286–9.

69. Durrmeyer X, Daoud P, Decobert F, Boileau P, Renolleau S, Zana-Taieb E, et al. Premedication for neonatal endotracheal intubation: results from the epidemiology of procedural pain in neonates study. Pediatr Crit Care Med. 2013;14(4):e169–75.

70. <8c72ed5cd5bc8f8c222127ee2c42a37101b8.pdf>.

71. <0000542-199710000-00061.pdf>.

72. Chanavaz C, Tirel O, Wodey E, Bansard JY, Senhadji L, Robert JC, et al. Haemodynamic effects of remifentanil in children with and without intravenous atropine. An echocardiographic study. Br J Anaesth. 2005;94(1):74–9.

73. Badiee Z, Vakiliamini M, Mohammadizadeh M. Remifentanil for endotracheal intubation in premature infants: a randomized controlled trial. J Res Pharm Pract. 2013;2(2):75–82.

74. Ghanta S, Abdel-Latif ME, Lui K, Ravindranathan H, Awad J, Oei J. Propofol compared with the morphine, atropine, and suxamethonium regimen as induction agents for neonatal endotracheal intubation: a randomized, controlled trial. Pediatrics. 2007;119(6):e1248–55.

75. Moussa A, Luangxay Y, Tremblay S, Lavoie J, Aube G, Savoie E, et al. Videolaryngoscope for teaching neonatal endotracheal intubation: a randomized controlled trial. Pediatrics. 2016;137(3):e20152156.

76. Nair S, Thomas EJ, Katakam L. Video laryngoscopy vs. direct laryngoscopy in teaching neonatal endotracheal intubation: a simulation-based study. Cureus. 2017;9(1):e962.

77. O'Shea JE, Thio M, Kamlin CO, McGrory L, Wong C, John J, et al. Videolaryngoscopy to teach neonatal intubation: a randomized Trial. Pediatrics. 2015;136(5):912–9.

78. Roberts CT, Hodgson KA. Nasal high flow treatment in preterm infants. Matern Health Neonatol Perinatol. 2017;3:15.

79. Ferguson KN, Roberts CT, Manley BJ, Davis PG. Interventions to improve rates of successful extubation in preterm infants: a systematic review and meta-analysis. JAMA Pediatr. 2017;171(2):165–74.
80. Buzzella B, Claure N, D'Ugard C, Bancalari E. A randomized controlled trial of two nasal continuous positive airway pressure levels after extubation in preterm infants. J Pediatr. 2014;164(1):46–51.
81. Henderson-Smart DJ, Davis PG. Prophylactic methylxanthines for endotracheal extubation in preterm infants. Cochrane Database Syst Rev. 2010;(12):CD000139.
82. Steer P, Flenady V, Shearman A, Charles B, Gray PH, Henderson-Smart D, et al. High dose caffeine citrate for extubation of preterm infants: a randomised controlled trial. Arch Dis Child Fetal Neonatal Ed. 2004;89(6):F499–503.
83. Carvalho CG, Silveira RC, Procianoy RS. Ventilator-induced lung injury in preterm infants. Rev Bras Ter Intensiva. 2013;25(4):319–26.
84. Kamlin CO, Davis PG, Argus B, Mills B, Morley CJ. A trial of spontaneous breathing to determine the readiness for extubation in very low birth weight infants: a prospective evaluation. Arch Dis Child Fetal Neonatal Ed. 2008;93(4):F305–6.
85. Stefanescu BM, Murphy WP, Hansell BJ, Fuloria M, Morgan TM, Aschner JL. A randomized, controlled trial comparing two different continuous positive airway pressure systems for the successful extubation of extremely low birth weight infants. Pediatrics. 2003;112(5):1031–8.
86. Chawla S, Natarajan G, Shankaran S, Carper B, Brion LP, Keszler M, et al. Markers of successful extubation in extremely preterm infants, and morbidity after failed extubation. J Pediatr. 2017;189:113–9.e2.
87. Manley BJ, Doyle LW, Owen LS, Davis PG. Extubating extremely preterm infants: predictors of success and outcomes following failure. J Pediatr. 2016;173:45–9.
88. Chavez A, dela Cruz R, Zaritsky A. Spontaneous breathing trial predicts successful extubation in infants and children. Pediatr Crit Care Med. 2006;7(4):324–8.
89. Kamlin CO, Davis PG, Morley CJ. Predicting successful extubation of very low birthweight infants. Arch Dis Child Fetal Neonatal Ed. 2006;91(3):F180–3.
90. Shalish W, Latremouille S, Papenburg J, Sant'Anna GM. Predictors of extubation readiness in preterm infants: a systematic review and meta-analysis. Arch Dis Child Fetal Neonatal Ed. 2019;104(1):F89–97.
91. Kaczmarek J, Chawla S, Marchica C, Dwaihy M, Grundy L, Sant'Anna GM. Heart rate variability and extubation readiness in extremely preterm infants. Neonatology. 2013;104(1):42–8.
92. Kaczmarek J, Kamlin CO, Morley CJ, Davis PG, Sant'anna GM. Variability of respiratory parameters and extubation readiness in ventilated neonates. Arch Dis Child Fetal Neonatal Ed. 2013;98(1):F70–3.
93. Shalish W, Kanbar LJ, Rao S, Robles-Rubio CA, Kovacs L, Chawla S, et al. Prediction of extubation readiness in extremely preterm infants by the automated analysis of cardiorespiratory behavior: study protocol. BMC Pediatr. 2017;17(1):167.

Chapter 12
Non-invasive Respiratory Support

Charles Christoph Roehr

This review presents the currently best available evidence on techniques for providing non-invasive respiratory support for preterm infants. It includes a summary of the current understanding of the complex changes in pulmonary physiology at birth and discusses the value of offering continuous distending pressure to infants undergoing fetal-to-neonatal transition. The review encompasses the changing needs for respiratory support of preterm infants during their disease progression from acute respiratory distress at birth to the more longstanding need for support during ongoing respiratory maturation. These may include nasal continuous positive airways pressure (nCPAP), nasal high-flow cannula therapy (nHFT), nasal non-invasive intermittent positive airway pressure (NIPPV) and nasal high-frequency oscillation ventilation (nHFOV). The various modes are discussed and a staged support strategy, stratified by disease stage, is proposed.

Establishing the most suitable form of non-invasive respiratory support remains one of the "hot topics" in neonatal medicine. By reviewing the current literature, this review highlights strengths and weaknesses of the various forms of non-invasive respiratory support available for newborn infants. A cautious attempt is made in advising on the most suitable mode of non-invasive respiratory support at particular gestational and chronological ages, disease entity and progression as well as clinical settings.

The current most extensively researched technique is nCPAP [1, 2]. However, several other forms of respiratory support have been trialed with very good results and enjoy eager adaptation into clinical practice. Looking into the future, much more research is needed to advise healthcare providers regarding choice of the most suitable modality for patients, the clinical care setting, and the needs and expectations

C. C. Roehr (✉)
Medical Sciences Division, Nuffield Department of Population Health, University of Oxford, Oxford, UK

Newborn Care, John Radcliffe Hospital, Oxford University Hospitals NHS Foundation Trust, Oxford, UK
e-mail: charles.roehr@paediatrics.ox.ac.uk

© Springer Nature Switzerland AG 2020   211
E. M. Boyle, J. Cusack (eds.), *Emerging Topics and Controversies in Neonatology*, https://doi.org/10.1007/978-3-030-28829-7_12

of the patients' family. A balance will need to be struck between the most effective care to ensure not only survival but also intact survival, aiming at obtaining the best possible long term outcomes. Thus, increased attention will need to be paid to the combination of optimising the means and timing of applying non-invasive respiratory support techniques in alignment with other supportive medical and ancillary therapies.

Non-invasive Respiratory Support for Neonates

Perinatal Transition: From Breathing Liquid to Air

The fetus breathes. Pulmonary fluid secreted by alveolar cells is shifted with breath like motions from the lungs to the amniotic cavity [3]. The presence of positive intra-pulmonary pressure is a physiologic stimulus, essential for normal fetal lung development [4, 5]. Likewise, fetal breathing movements are essential for preparing the respiratory musculature and the pulmonary tissue for their functions after birth [3, 6, 7].

Pulmonary Aeration: The Significance of Establishing the Functional Residual Capacity and Tidal Volume at Birth

Hooper and co-authors, in a seminal paper, summarise the current understanding of cardiopulmonary transition at birth: The lung, starting out as a liquid-filled organ with low pulmonary blood flow transitions into the organ of gas exchange. In order to establish gas exchange after birth, the fluid-filled airways immediately need to be cleared of lung fluid [5]. Pulmonary expansion is achieved by creating sub-atmospheric inspiratory pressures during the first diaphragmatic contractions [6]. Thus, the first breaths facilitate airway fluid clearance, primarily as a result from trans-epithelial pressure gradients generated during inspiration [8]. When breathing is established successfully, sufficient functional residual capacity (FRC) has been generated and regular breathing commences. However, failure to clear the terminal gas exchange units of fluid can lead to transient or persistently low arterial oxygen tension. Likewise, as the fluid cleared from the airways remains in the pulmonary interstitium it leads to an increase in interstitial tissue pressure [8]. This increases the chances of pulmonary liquid re-entering the larger airways on expiration. As liquid clearance from the lung tissue takes longer than from the airways, a raised intra-parenchymal pressure can be observed, lasting for several hours after birth [9]. Failure to establish lung liquid clearance results in a functional reduction of alveolar surface area, insufficient gas exchange, low oxygen saturations and carbon dioxide retention, increased work of breathing, and, ultimately, respiratory failure [9, 10].

The application of positive end-expiratory pressure (PEEP) reduces the pressure gradient for airway liquid re-entry and helps establish and maintain FRC [10]. Term infants generate an FRC of approximately 30 mL/kg and a tidal volume (V_t) of approximately 5 mL/kg within minutes of birth [6].

Respiratory Distress Syndrome in the Very Preterm Infant

The term "respiratory distress" characterizes an infant with laboured breathing, who may present with cyanosis and marked tachypnoea together with subcostal and intercostal, as well as tracheal recessions, nasal flaring and marked, audible grunting. These signs of respiratory distress are commonly seen in infants with pneumothorax, neonatal pneumonia, or congenital pulmonary disease (incl. congenital diaphragmatic hernia and pulmonary hypoplasia), to name only a few. Most frequently, however, respiratory distress syndrome (RDS) relates to respiratory compromise caused by surfactant deficiency and an immature respiratory system, which is most prevalent in the lower gestational age group infants (24–28 weeks of gestation).

The preterm infant's respiratory system differs from that of the term infant: Their pulmonary architecture at birth is at a much more immature, saccular developmental stage, their chest wall and larger airways are predominantly cartilaginous, providing comparatively less resistance against atmospheric pressure than the term born infants' [11]. Further, their surfactant system is still maturing and not yet fully functional [12]. The very preterm infant's respiratory drive is poorly controlled by the immature respiratory centre, which is less sensitive to carbon dioxide and provides a less coordinated respiratory pattern [13, 14]. These factors predispose very preterm infants to insufficient generation of V_t and FRC. Thus, very premature birth is associated with an increased risk for significant RDS [15, 16].

Mechanical Ventilation As a Risk Factor for Bronchopulmonary Dysplasia

The introduction of mechanical ventilation (MV) into neonatal care in the 1960s hallmarked the beginning of improved survival in babies with respiratory distress [17]. However, due to technological limitations of the early neonatal ventilators with regard to tidal volume delivery, MV was associated with many challenges. Not long after MV became available for use in preterm care, Northway and co-workers described the histopathological entity of "hyaline membrane disease", from which survivors suffered a debilitating disease distinct to ventilated newborns, characterised by prolonged respiratory distress, oxygen dependency and reduced exercise tolerance, now known as "bronchopulmonary dysplasia" (BPD) [18].

The discovery of the pulmonary compliance enhancing properties of exogenous surfactant replacement therapy in the 1990s markedly changed the outcome of respiratory distress syndrome (RDS) for many very preterm infants [19]. However, irrespective of many significant medical and technical advances in the care of preterm infants, and in keeping with the concept of "alveolar arrest" in the aetiology of BPD, MV remains a significant contributing factor for BPD, due to the inflicted volutrauma, barotrauma, atelectotrauma and biotrauma on the developing lungs [20].

Developing the Concept of Nasal Continuous Positive Airway Pressure in Preterm Infants

In 1971, Gregory and co-workers introduced the concept of continuous positive airway pressure for treating newborn infants with RDS [1]. In their seminal study, Gregory et al. documented a significant reduction in mortality from RDS in 20 infants with respiratory distress (birth weights between 930 and 3830 g), treated with CPAP which at the time was applied via a head box apparatus [1]. From then on, nasal CPAP proved a viable option to avoid the unwanted effects of MV on the preterm lung.

Though, whilst a multitude of nasal CPAP devices were quickly introduced to clinical care, by the mid 1980s the advent of more refined technology for MV and the success of exogenous surfactant replacement therapy marked almost the end of the CPAP era.

Important research by Avery and co-workers who described the lowest BPD rate in neonatal care centres where MV was largely avoided, was initially underrecognised [21]. Intubation and MV remained the standard treatment for RDS for almost another two decades until the use of CPAP was studied in larger randomised controlled trials [22–25]. Through these studies the paradigm of invasive respiratory support changed to offering non-invasive support for newborn infants with signs of RDS [26, 27].

Different Modes of Non-invasive Respiratory Support

Continuous Positive Airway Pressure

Since the first description of the so called "Gregory Box", the components of CPAP systems have followed a common principle: Devices for CPAP therapy include a patient interface (nowadays usually nasal prongs or masks), a set of pipes for positive airway pressure delivery, a heater and humidifier system and a CPAP-generator. The traditional water-lock CPAP-generator, commonly referred to as *Bubble CPAP*", has become the mainstay of CPAP therapy over the past decade [2, 28] More recent developments include variable flow CPAP and bi-phasic CPAP

(Bi-Level-CPAP or Si-PaP) [29]. Both modes aim to support spontaneous respiration through a reduction of the infant's work of breathing.

Water-Lock, or "Bubble-CPAP"

Early on, a relatively simple set-up with a water-locked circuit was used as a CPAP generator and a cut down endotracheal tube as the patient interface [30, 31]. By employing a constant gas flow towards the patient who was rested in a head-box, these devices had the expiratory limb immersed in a basin of water, thereby generating a constant, set expiratory pressure. Soon, these custom-made devices referred to as "Bubble-CPAP" were commonplace in many NICUs, until the slightly more sophisticated commercial "Bubble CPAP" systems became available [32].

CPAP Devices with Variable Gas Flow

Often based on the Beneviste principle, variable-flow CPAP has a special nasal interface which utilises a fluidic-flip mechanism which employs the Coanda-effect [33], to guide the direction of gas flow during inspiration and expiration. The Beneviste principle is thought to reduce the infant's work of breathing [33]. Several commercially available, standalone CPAP-devices as well as ventilators now offer this mode of non-invasive support.

Comparison of Constant Flow CPAP and Variable Flow CPAP

The many positive effects of CPAP are summarised in Table 12.1. Pillow and colleagues found that bubble CPAP, when compared to constant flow CPAP, reduced the work of breathing, improved gas exchange and increased lung volume [34]. Preceding these findings, Lee et al., in an earlier clinical study were able to show that infants on bubble CPAP, compared to respirator generated constant flow CPAP had statistically lower minute volumes and improved gas exchange [35]. Other authors have confirmed the positive effect of Bubble CPAP on oxygenation, which appears to be superior to that achieved using variable-flow [36, 37].

Early Nasal CPAP from Birth

O'Donnell et al., using video recordings of preterm infants at birth, proved that approximately 80% of extremely low gestational age newborn (ELGAN, birth weight <1000 g) infants show spontaneous breathing [38]. Thus, routine intubation

Table 12.1 Advantages and disadvantages of CPAP therapy

Advantages	Disadvantages
Increases functional residual capacity and tidal volume	Skin excoriation and nasal damage is commonly encountered, may give rise to bacterial infection, in particular by coagulase-negative staphylococci
Stabilises upper airway and chest wall stability and aids alveolar distension	Air may escape into the stomach, causing gaseous distension ("CPAP Belly")
Improves pulmonary compliance and reduces work of breathing	Increased intra-thoracic pressure may reduce venous return to the right heart and reduce cardiac output
Reduces the alveolar-arterial oxygen pressure gradient	Lung over-inflation decreases tidal volume and may increase p_{CO2} and the dead-space fraction
Reduces intrapulmonary shunting	High CPAP can lead to lung over-inflation, decreased compliance, and increased work of breathing
Reduces apnoea	

Modified from Ref. [2]

of even the most immature infants would interfere with their physiological fetal-neonatal transition. Since 2008, several large scale clinical trials have compared the use of invasive to non-invasive respiratory support of breathing very low birth weight (VLBW) and ELGANs from birth. Meta-analyses of these studies have shown significant positive impact on survival and overall pulmonary outcomes with no added negative effects in the non-pulmonary outcomes in the non-invasively managed patients [39, 40].

Depending on the author, the number needed to treat to save one VLBW infants from death or BPD lies between 25 and 35 (Fig. 12.1) [39]. Further, follow-up studies of VLBW infants treated with CPAP from birth compared to those routinely ventilated showed that pulmonary function was significantly improved at term equivalent age. Non-ventilated infants had significantly higher respiratory compliance, lower elastic work of breathing and, consequently, improved respiratory rate and minute ventilation [41]. In consequence of the compelling evidence for a non-invasive approach to stabilising preterm infants at birth, the American Academy of Pediatrics, as well as a European Consensus advise for preterm infants to be initially managed with CPAP, rather than intubation and ventilation [26, 27].

Nasal High-Flow Nasal Cannula Therapy

The application of medical gases at high flow rates via small nasal cannulae as another form of non-invasive, continuous distending pressure has steadily found its way into the respiratory management of neonates [42]. This form of respiratory therapy, in which small nasal cannulae are used to apply heated and humidified gas at flow rates of between 3 and 8 L/min, is commonly referred to as nasal high-flow therapy (nHFT) or high-flow nasal cannula therapy (HFNC). Different to the nasal

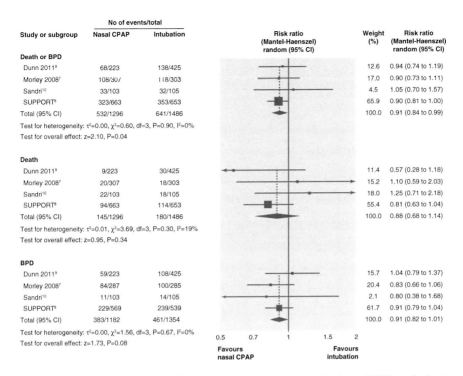

Fig. 12.1 Forest plot comparison of death or bronchopulmonary dysplasia (BPD), or both, at 36 weeks corrected gestation; death; and BPD at 36 weeks corrected gestation. *Nasal CPAP* continuous positive airway pressure. (Extracted from Ref. [39])

interfaces used with CPAP, which can be applied through masks, tight fitted binasal prongs or pharyngeal tubes, the cannulae used in nHFT are much smaller and, possibly for this reason, appear to be tolerated much better than conventional CPAP applications [43]. Bench top and controlled clinical studies suggest that both nCPAP and nHFT might exert comparable distending pressures [44, 45]. Other positive effects of nHFT include increased carbon dioxide washout, attenuation of the inspiratory resistance in the nasopharynx, improvement in conductance and pulmonary compliance, and reduced metabolic work of breathing [45, 46].

Data from observational and smaller controlled clinical trials pointed also towards equivalent efficacy of initial nHFT and nasal CPAP at similar distending pressures at birth [47, 48]. However, evidence from a large scale, randomised clinical trial did not confirm nHFT as an equally efficacious means to manage neonates at birth [49]. Conversely, according to recent meta-analyses and the Cochrane review by Wilkinson et al., nHFT is of equal efficacy to nasal CPAP when used for secondary respiratory support, following extubation, in preventing infants from re-intubation. Plus, nHFT further was found to have the added benefit of being associated with far less nasal trauma and fewer pneumothoraces [50].There is currently insufficient evidence from research to support nHFT use as primary therapy for

infants with RDS from birth [50]. However, some neonatal units with long experience in the use of nHFT have reported satisfactory results when employing nHFT as
both primary and secondary respiratory support, as recently demonstrated by
Zivanovic et al. [51].

Rationale for Alternative Modes of Non-invasive Respiratory Support

Although studies of early CPAP use in VLBW infants found that a significant proportion of VLBW and extremely low gestational age infants can be successfully
stabilised with CPAP [24, 25, 40], a fraction of these infants may require mechanical ventilation [52, 53]. Once intubated, timely extubation within 72 h occurs in
only about 33% of intubated infants. Of these, many will require reintubation due to
irregular respiratory effort, apnoea and profound desaturations. Therefore, various
alternative modes of non-invasive respiratory support have been introduced.

Definition of Non-invasive Positive Pressure Ventilation

Non-invasive positive pressure ventilation (NIPPV) describes the nasal or pharyngeal application of intermittent peak inspiratory pressure (PIP) inflations at pressures similar to those used during conventional ventilation on a baseline support of
positive end-expiratory pressure [54]. The assumption is that the PIP applied to the
nasopharynx travels down the distal airways and into the gas exchange units, similarly to invasive MV. Consequently, the result would be an elevated mean alveolar
distending pressure, which augments and maintains the tidal volume and supports
spontaneous breathing while protecting the airways from collapse during apnoea
[55, 56]. Recent evidence suggests that NIPPV, in particular when synchronised
(SNIPPV) with the infant's spontaneous breaths, reduces inspiratory effort, opti-
mises tidal volume and improves carbon dioxide exchange in prematurely born
infants [57].

Clinical Applications of Non-invasive Positive Pressure Ventilation

Indications for using neonatal NIPPV include primary and secondary respiratory
support, scenarios where higher mean airway pressure than CPAP or nHFT may be
required, or where significant apnoea of prematurity (AOP) places the infant at risk
for mechanical ventilation [57]. At present, there is a not a lot of data to recommend

the optimal PIP level, optimal difference between PIP and PEEP, inspiratory time or respiratory rate [58]. Studies differ regarding the level of applied PEEP (5–8 cmH$_2$O) and PIP (10–20 cmH$_2$O), the delta P between pressures (0–3 cmH$_2$O), inspiratory time (0.3–1 s) and any given backup rate [29, 59–61]. In practice, an invasive ventilation mode is chosen on the ventilator (IMV, SIMV, etc.) and intermittent positive airway pressure (IPPV) is applied via the patient interface (nasal or pharyngeal prong or face mask) or special commercial devices with bilevel positive airway pressure (BiPAP) modes can be chosen to achieve the same effect [62]. However, the largest, pragmatic, multinational, randomised controlled trial to date, by Kirpalani and co-workers, comparing NIPPV to nCPAP, with respect to the outcomes of reducing death before 36 weeks postmenstrual age or survival with bronchopulmonary dysplasia, found NIPPV not to be superior over nCPAP, when used as the primary form of respiratory support [63]. Further research of an equally large scale is pending.

Non-synchronised and Synchronised NIPPV

Investigating whether using NIPPV for treating AOP was superior over other forms of non-invasive respiratory support, Pantalitschka and coworkers performed a randomised crossover trial, comparing non-synchronised NIPPV with alternations of variable flow CPAP and bubble CPAP in VLBWI. The authors found that variable flow nCPAP was more effective in treating AOP in preterm infants than a conventional ventilator generated NIPPV, and refer to future studies to elucidate the value of synchronised NIPPV [64]. More recently, Gizzi et al. investigated the effects of flow-SNIPPV, NIPPV and nCPAP on the rate of AOP, bradycardia and gas exchange in preterm infants. In their study, SNIPPV seemed more effective than non-synchronised NIPPV and nCPAP in reducing the incidence of AOP, bradycardia and desaturation episodes in preterm infants [65]. As many of the latest generation of mechanical ventilators now offer synchronisation of NIPPV, results from further studies on the efficacy of synchronised NIPPV, preferably performed with comparable protocols and devices, are awaited. Despite initial promising data, according to recent surveys NIPPV has not yet been widely embraced in clinical practice as the method of first choice [66].

Nasal High-Frequency Oscillation Ventilation

Similar to NIPPV, pharyngeal or nasal application of high-frequency oscillation ventilation (nHFOV) has found its way in to neonatal care and is employed in around 20% of European NICUs [67]. First reports by Colaizy and colleagues highlighted the positive effects of nHFOV on, in particular, carbon dioxide clearance [68]. In light of this, DeLuca and co-workers performed an in-vitro study to examine the effect of applied nHFOV amplitude and recorded tidal volume and found a quasi-linear relationship ($r^2 = 0.99$) [69]. Other authors have reported individual cases or small case series on the clinical application of nHFOV, proving its feasibility and demonstrating adequate CO_2 elimination [65]. Only one medium scale ($n = 76$), prospective clinical trial of nHFOV has been published so far [70]. Whilst the results from Zhu et al. indicate that nHFOV, compared to nCPAP, effectively reduced the need for MV in preterm infants with moderate to severe RDS without an increase in adverse effects and had positive effects on CO_2 clearance [70], the study's methodology has also been criticised for comparing medium level CPAP pressures (6 cmH$_2$O) to higher pressures of nHFOV (mean distending pressures 6–10 cmH$_2$O) [71]. Further trials will need to clarify whether nHFOV is indeed superior to nCPAP.

Chronological and Disease Specific Considerations

Currently, by far the best researched non-invasive respiratory support technique remains nCPAP, followed by NIPPV and nHFT [72]. However, the other discussed forms of respiratory support may have their place in the treatment of neonatal lung disease over time. Starting from the early hours of life, where continuous distending pressure evidently aids lung liquid clearance and establishment of FRC [10], nCPAP has been proven to be beneficial for infants of all gestational ages, whether extremely preterm or term [26, 27, 39, 40]. Recently, nHFT and NIPPV were trialed as primary respiratory support with reasonably good results; however so far, evidence from large scale trials renders nHFT and NIPPV inferior to nCPAP [49, 63]. Importantly, for all modes of respiratory support other than nCPAP, sufficient data for infants of all gestational ages is clearly lacking. However, for the phase of respiratory support following extubation, convincing evidence exists to advocate both NIPPV and nHFT alongside nCPAP as secondary modes of respiratory support [50, 73]. For the often-times longstanding phase of ongoing respiratory support, nHFT, together with nCPAP, has found its place as a very well tolerated mode of non-invasive respiratory support. What is more, several investigations describe nHFT as the better tolerated form of support and one which is generally preferred over nCPAP by caregivers and parents [74, 75].

What Could Be Next? A Glimpse at the Future

Looking into the future, much more research is needed to advise health care providers regarding choice of the most suitable modality for individual patients, the clinical care setting, and the needs and expectations of the patients' family. Whilst nCPAP is well researched and accepted, simpler forms of non-invasive respiratory support such as nHFT might be easier to employ in areas of limited resources, both as primary and as secondary forms of non-invasive respiratory support. Conversely, support modes involving higher levels of technology, like NIPPV or SNIPPV, wherever feasible and affordable, may offer significant advantages over nCPAP alone.

A balance will need to be struck between the most effective care package to ensure not only survival but also intact survival, aiming at obtaining the best possible long-term outcomes [76]. Thus, more research in to these modes is required to prevent ventilation, minimise oxygen exposure and consequently, reduce death and BPD. More needs to be learnt regarding which would be the most suitable mode of support for infants of specific gestational ages, for specific disease entities and stages of disease progression. The use of non-invasive respiratory support techniques and surfactant replacement therapy has so far only been investigated for nCPAP [77]. The combination of ancillary treatments, such as Caffeine, Vitamin A, systemic, topical or inhaled corticosteroids or physiotherapy with non-invasive respiratory support is also widely under-researched and warrants more attention in future research.

To conclude, whilst non-invasive respiratory support has very much become the first choice of respiratory support of newborn infants, increased attention will need to be paid to identify the optimal mode of non-invasive support for individual patients, recognising their disease entity and progression, as well as towards researching the concomitant inclusion of further supportive medical and ancillary therapies.

References

1. Gregory GA, Kitterman JA, Phibbs RH, Tooley WH, Hamilton WK. Treatment of the idiopathic respiratory-distress syndrome with continuous positive airway pressure. N Engl J Med. 1971;284:1333–40.
2. Mahmoud RA, Roehr CC, Schmalisch G. Current methods of non-invasive ventilatory support for neonates. Paediatr Respir Rev. 2011;12:196–205.
3. Polglase GR, Wallace MJ, Grant DA, Hooper SB. Influence of fetal breathing movements on pulmonary hemodynamics in fetal sheep. Pediatr Res. 2004;56:932–8.
4. Jani JC, Flemmer AW, Bergmann F, Gallot D, Roubliova X, Muensterer OJ, Hajek K, Deprest JA. The effect of fetal tracheal occlusion on lung tissue mechanics and tissue composition. Pediatr Pulmonol. 2009;44:112–21.
5. Hooper SB, Te Pas AB, Kitchen MJ. Respiratory transition in the newborn: a three-phase process. Arch Dis Child Fetal Neonatal Ed. 2016;101:F266–71.
6. Vyas H, Field D, Milner AD, Hopkin IE. Determinants of the first inspiratory volume and functional residual capacity at birth. Pediatr Pulmonol. 1986;2:189–93.
7. Hooper SB, Harding R. Fetal lung liquid: a major determinant of the growth and functional development of the fetal lung. Clin Exp Pharmacol Physiol. 1995;22:235–47.
8. Siew ML, Wallace MJ, Allison BJ, Kitchen MJ, te Pas AB, Islam MS, Lewis RA, Fouras A, Yagi N, Uesugi K, Hooper SB. The role of lung inflation and sodium transport in airway liquid clearance during lung aeration in newborn rabbits. Pediatr Res. 2013;73:443–9.
9. Karlberg P. The adaptive changes in the immediate postnatal period, with particular reference to respiration. J Pediatr. 1960;56:585–604.
10. Siew ML, Te Pas AB, Wallace MJ, Kitchen MJ, Lewis RA, Fouras A, Morley CJ, Davis PG, Yagi N, Uesugi K, Hooper SB. Positive end-expiratory pressure enhances development of a

functional residual capacity in preterm rabbits ventilated from birth. J Appl Physiol (1985). 2009;106:1487–93.

11. Jobe AH. Lung maturation: the survival miracle of very low birth weight infants. Pediatr Neonatol. 2010;51:7–13.

12. Jobe AH. Lung maturational agents and surfactant treatments: are they complementary in preterm infants? J Perinatol. 1989;9:14–8.

13. Trippenbach T. Pulmonary reflexes and control of breathing during development. Biol Neonate. 1994;65:205–10.

14. Engoren M, Courtney SE, Habib RH. Effect of weight and age on respiratory complexity in premature neonates. J Appl Physiol. 2009;106:766–73.

15. Stoll BJ, Hansen NI, Bell EF, et al. Trends in care practices, morbidity, and mortality of extremely preterm neonates, 1993-2012. JAMA. 2015;314:1039–51.

16. Edwards MO, Kotecha SJ, Kotecha S. Respiratory distress of the term newborn infant. Paediatr Respir Rev. 2013;14:29–36.

17. Speer CP, Sweet DG, Halliday HL. Surfactant therapy: past, present and future. Early Hum Dev. 2013;89(Suppl 1):S22–4.

18. Baraldi E, Filippone M. Chronic lung disease after premature birth. N Engl J Med. 2007;357:1946–55.

19. Curstedt T, Halliday HL, Hallman M, Saugstad OD, Speer CP. 30 years of surfactant research—from basic science to new clinical treatments for the preterm infant. Neonatology. 2015;107:314–6.

20. Jobe AH, Ikegami M. Prevention of bronchopulmonary dysplasia. Curr Opin Pediatr. 2001;13:124–9.

21. Avery ME, Tooley WH, Keller JB, Hurd SS, Bryan MH, Cotton RB, Epstein MF, Fitzhardinge PM, Hansen CB, Hansen TN, et al. Is chronic lung disease in low birth weight infants preventable? A survey of eight centers. Pediatrics. 1987;79:26–30.

22. Dunn MS, Kaempf J, de Klerk A, de Klerk R, Reilly M, Howard D, Ferrelli K, O'Conor J, Soll RF, Vermont Oxford Network DRM Study Group. Randomized trial comparing 3 approaches to the initial respiratory management of preterm neonates. Pediatrics. 2011;128:e1069–76.

23. Finer NN, Carlo WA, Walsh MC, et al. Early CPAP versus surfactant in extremely preterm infants. N Engl J Med. 2010;362:1970–9.

24. Morley CJ, Davis PG, Doyle LW, Brion LP, Hascoet JM, Carlin JB, COIN Trial Investigators. Nasal CPAP or intubation at birth for very preterm infants. N Engl J Med. 2008;358:700–8.

25. Rojas MA, Lozano JM, Rojas MX, Laughon M, Bose CL, Rondon MA, Charry L, Bastidas JA, Perez LA, Rojas C, Ovalle O, Celis LA, Garcia-Harker J, Jaramillo ML, Colombian Neonatal Research Network. Very early surfactant without mandatory ventilation in premature infants treated with early continuous positive airway pressure: a randomized, controlled trial. Pediatrics. 2009;123:137–42.

26. Polin R, Committee on Fetus and Newborn; American Academy of Pediatrics. Respiratory support in preterm infants at birth. Pediatrics. 2014;133:171–4.

27. Sweet DG, Carnielli V, Greisen G, Hallman M, Ozek E, Te Pas A, Plavka R, Roehr CC, Saugstad OD, Simeoni U, Speer CP, Vento M, GHA V, Halliday HL. European consensus guidelines on the management of respiratory distress syndrome – 2019 update. Neonatology. 2019;115:432–51.

28. Morley CJ, Davis PG. Continuous positive airway pressure: scientific and clinical rationale. Curr Opin Pediatr. 2008;20:119–24.

29. Migliori C, Motta M, Angeli A, et al. Nasal bilevel vs. continuous positive airway pressure in preterm infants. Pediatr Pulmonol. 2005;40:426–30.

30. Speidel BD, Dunn PM. Effect of continuous positive airway pressure on breathing pattern of infants with respiratory-distress syndrome. Lancet. 1975;1:302–4.

31. Vogtmann C, Böttcher H, Raue W. [Problems of ventilation disorders in newborn and therapy possibilities]. Z Arztl Fortbild (Jena). 1974;68:77–82.

32. Roehr CC, Schmalisch G, Khakban A, Proquitté H, Wauer RR. Use of continuous positive airway pressure (CPAP) in neonatal units—a survey of current preferences and practice in Germany. Eur J Med Res. 2007;12:139–44.

33. Coman IM. The bright minds beyond our machines: Henry Coanda and his ideas. J Cardiovasc Med. 2007;8:251–2.

34. Pillow JJ, Hillman N, Moss TJ, Polglase G, Bold G, Beaumont C, Ikegami M, Jobe AH. Bubble continuous positive airway pressure enhances lung volume and gas exchange in preterm lambs. Am J Respir Crit Care Med. 2007;176:63–9.

35. Lee KS, Dunn MS, Fenwick M, Shennan AT. A comparison of underwater bubble continuous positive airway pressure with ventilator-derived continuous positive airway pressure in premature neonates ready for extubation. Biol Neonate. 1998;73:69–75.

36. Courtney SE, Kahn DJ, Singh R, Habib RH. Bubble and ventilator-derived nasal continuous positive airway pressure in premature infants: work of breathing and gas exchange. J Perinatol. 2011;31:44–50.

37. Pandit PB, Courtney SE, Pyon KH, Saslow JG, Habib RH. Work of breathing during constant- and variable-flow nasal continuous positive airway pressure in preterm neonates. Pediatrics. 2001;108:682–5.

38. O'Donnell CP, Kamlin CO, Davis PG, Morley CJ. Crying and breathing by extremely preterm infants immediately after birth. J Pediatr. 2010;156:846–7.

39. Schmölzer GM, Kumar M, Pichler G, Aziz K, O'Reilly M, Cheung PY. Non-invasive versus invasive respiratory support in preterm infants at birth: systematic review and meta-analysis. BMJ. 2013;347:f5980.

40. Fischer HS, Bührer C. Avoiding endotracheal ventilation to prevent bronchopulmonary dysplasia: a meta-analysis. Pediatrics. 2013;132:e1351–60.

41. Roehr CC, Proquitté H, Hammer H, Wauer RR, Morley CJ, Schmalisch G. Positive effects of early continuous positive airway pressure on pulmonary function in extremely premature infants: results of a subgroup analysis of the COIN trial. Arch Dis Child Fetal Neonatal Ed. 2011;96:F371–3.

42. Roehr CC, Yoder BA, Davis PG, Ives K. Evidence support and guidelines for using heated, humidified, high-flow nasal cannulae in neonatology: Oxford nasal high-flow therapy meeting, 2015. Clin Perinatol. 2016;43:693–705.

43. Wilkinson DJ, Andersen CC, Smith K, Holberton J. Pharyngeal pressure with high-flow nasal cannulae in premature infants. J Perinatol. 2008;28:42–7.

44. Lavizzari A, Veneroni C, Colnaghi M, Ciuffini F, Zannin E, Fumagalli M, Mosca F, Dellacà RL. Respiratory mechanics during NCPAP and HHHFNC at equal distending pressures. Arch Dis Child Fetal Neonatal Ed. 2014;99:F315–20.

45. Sivieri EM, Foglia EE, Abbasi S. Carbon dioxide washout during high flow nasal cannula versus nasal CPAP support: An in vitro study. Pediatr Pulmonol. 2017;52:792–8.

46. Dysart K, Miller TL, Wolfson MR, Shaffer TH. Research in high flow therapy: mechanisms of action. Respir Med. 2009;103:1400–5.

47. Reynolds P, Leontiadi S, Lawson T, Otunla T, Ejiwumi O, Holland N. Stabilisation of premature infants in the delivery room with nasal high flow. Arch Dis Child Fetal Neonatal Ed. 2016;101:F284–7.

48. Lavizzari A, Colnaghi M, Ciuffini F, Veneroni C, Musumeci S, Cortinovis I, Mosca F. Heated, humidified high-flow nasal cannula vs nasal continuous positive airway pressure for respiratory distress syndrome of prematurity: a randomized clinical noninferiority trial. JAMA Pediatr. 2016;170:1228.

49. Roberts CT, Owen LS, Manley BJ, Frøisland DH, Donath SM, Dalziel KM, Pritchard MA, Cartwright DW, Collins CL, Malhotra A, Davis PG, HIPSTER Trial Investigators. Nasal high-flow therapy for primary respiratory support in preterm infants. N Engl J Med. 2016;375:1142–51.

50. Wilkinson D, Andersen C, O'Donnell CP, De Paoli AG, Manley BJ. High flow nasal cannula for respiratory support in preterm infants. Cochrane Database Syst Rev. 2016;(2):CD006405.

51. Zivanovic S, Scrivens A, Panza R, Reynolds P, Laforgia N, Ives KN, Roehr CC. Nasal high-flow therapy as primary respiratory support for preterm infants without the need for rescue with nasal continuous positive airway pressure. Neonatology. 2019;115:175–81.

52. Fuchs H, Lindner W, Leiprecht A, Mendler MR, Hummler HD. Predictors of early nasal CPAP failure and effects of various intubation criteria on the rate of mechanical ventilation in preterm infants of <29 weeks gestational age. Arch Dis Child Fetal Neonatal Ed. 2011;96:F343–7.

53. Dargaville PA, Aiyappan A, De Paoli AG, Dalton RG, Kuschel CA, Kamlin CO, Orsini F, Carlin JB, Davis PG. Continuous positive airway pressure failure in preterm infants: incidence, predictors and consequences. Neonatology. 2013;104:8–14.

54. Roberts CT, Davis PG, Owen LS. Neonatal non-invasive respiratory support: synchronised NIPPV, non-synchronised NIPPV or bi-level CPAP: what is the evidence in 2013? Neonatology. 2013;104:203–9.

55. Barrington KJ, Bull D, Finer NN. Randomized trial of nasal synchronized intermittent mandatory ventilation compared with continuous positive airway pressure after extubation of very low birth weight infants. Pediatrics. 2001;107:638–41.

56. Owen LS, Manley BJ. Nasal intermittent positive pressure ventilation in preterm infants: equipment, evidence, and synchronization. Semin Fetal Neonatal Med. 2016;21:146–53.

57. Charles E, Hunt KA, Rafferty GF, Peacock JL, Greenough A. Work of breathing during HHHFNC and synchronised NIPPV following extubation. Eur J Pediatr. 2019;178:105–10.

58. Claure N, Bancalari E. Non-invasive ventilation in premature infants. Arch Dis Child Fetal Neonatal Ed. 2015;100:F2–3.

59. Kuhle S, Urschitz MS, Eitner S, Poets CF. Interventions for obstructive sleep apnea in children: a systematic review. Sleep Med Rev. 2009;13:123–31.

60. Kugelman A, Riskin A, Said W, Shoris I, Mor F, Bader D. A randomized pilot study comparing heated humidified high-flow nasal cannulae with NIPPV for RDS. Pediatr Pulmonol. 2015;50:576–83.

61. Owen LS, Morley CJ, Davis PG. Effects of synchronisation during SiPAP-generated nasal intermittent positive pressure ventilation (NIPPV) in preterm infants. Arch Dis Child Fetal Neonatal Ed. 2015;100:F24–30.

62. Ferguson KN, Roberts CT, Manley BJ, Davis PG. Interventions to improve rates of successful extubation in preterm infants: a systematic review and meta-analysis. JAMA Pediatr. 2017;171:165–74.

63. Kirpalani H, Millar D, Lemyre B, Yoder BA, Chiu A, Roberts RS, NIPPV Study Group. A trial comparing noninvasive ventilation strategies in preterm infants. N Engl J Med. 2013;369:611–20.

64. Pantalitschka T, Sievers J, Urschitz MS, Herberts T, Reher C, Poets CF. Randomised crossover trial of four nasal respiratory support systems for apnoea of prematurity in very low birthweight infants. Arch Dis Child Fetal Neonatal Ed. 2009;94:F245–8.

65. Czernik C, Schmalisch G, Bührer C, Proquitté H. Weaning of neonates from mechanical ventilation by use of nasopharyngeal high-frequency oscillatory ventilation: a preliminary study. J Matern Fetal Neonatal Med. 2012;25:374–8.

66. Mukerji A, Shah PS, Shivananda S, Yee W, Read B, Minski J, Alvaro R, Fusch C, Canadian Neonatal Network Investigators. Survey of noninvasive respiratory support practices in Canadian neonatal intensive care units. Acta Paediatr. 2017;106:387–93.

67. Fischer HS, Bohlin K, Bührer C, Schmalisch G, Cremer M, Reiss I, Czernik C. Nasal high-frequency oscillation ventilation in neonates: a survey in five European countries. Eur J Pediatr. 2015;174:465–71.

68. Colaizy TT, Younis UM, Bell EF, Klein JM. Nasal high-frequency ventilation for premature infants. Acta Paediatr. 2008;97:1518–22.

69. De Luca D, Carnielli VP, Conti G, Piastra M. Noninvasive high frequency oscillatory ventilation through nasal prongs: bench evaluation of efficacy and mechanics. Intensive Care Med. 2010;36:2094–100.

70. Zhu XW, Zhao JN, Tang SF, Yan J, Shi Y. Noninvasive high-frequency oscillatory ventilation versus nasal continuous positive airway pressure in preterm infants with moderate-severe respiratory distress syndrome: a preliminary report. Pediatr Pulmonol. 2017;52:1038–42.

71. Fischer HS, Rimensberger PC. Early noninvasive high-frequency oscillatory ventilation in the primary treatment of respiratory distress syndrome. Pediatr Pulmonol. 2018;53:126–7.

72. Owen LS, Manley BJ, Davis PG, Doyle LW. The evolution of modern respiratory care for preterm infants. Lancet. 2017;389:1649–59.

73. Lemyre B, Davis PG, De Paoli AG, Kirpalani H. Nasal intermittent positive pressure ventilation (NIPPV) versus nasal continuous positive airway pressure (NCPAP) for preterm neonates after extubation. Cochrane Database Syst Rev. 2014;(9):CD003212.

74. Klingenberg C, Pettersen M, Hansen EA, Gustavsen LJ, Dahl IA, Leknessund A, Kaaresen PI, Nordhov M. Patient comfort during treatment with heated humidified high flow nasal cannulae versus nasal continuous positive airway pressure: a randomised cross-over trial. Arch Dis Child Fetal Neonatal Ed. 2014;99:F134–7.

75. Roberts CT, Dawson JA, Alquoka E, Carew PJ, Donath SM, Davis PG, Manley BJ. Are high flow nasal cannulae noisier than bubble CPAP for preterm infants? Arch Dis Child Fetal Neonatal Ed. 2014;99:F291–5.

76. Zivanovic S, Roehr CC. One step further toward defining the optimal respiratory care package for neonates: interventions to successfully extubate preterm infants. JAMA Pediatr. 2017;171:120–1.

77. Dargaville PA. CPAP, surfactant, or both for the preterm infant: resolving the dilemma. JAMA Pediatr. 2015;169:715–7.

Chapter 13
Oxygen Management in Neonatal Care

Ben Stenson

History

When oxygen therapy for preterm infants first became widespread more than 60 years ago there were no pulse oximeters or blood gas machines. It was usual to prescribe oxygen in high concentrations to spontaneously breathing preterm infants for many weeks and this was associated with a new epidemic of blindness due to severe retinopathy of prematurity (ROP). Clinical trials in the 1950s compared this unrestricted oxygen treatment to a more curtailed approach, where the maximum oxygen concentration allowed was reduced and the duration of oxygen exposure was limited to a few days. There was a significant reduction in the risk of ROP.

It is worth reflecting on the scale of the difference in oxygen exposure between groups in these early trials that pre-dated mechanical ventilation because it greatly exceeded anything likely to occur today. At sea level, the partial pressure of oxygen (kPa) in the atmosphere is approximately equal to the inspired oxygen percentage. A healthy newborn infant breathing 80% oxygen is breathing oxygen at around 80 kPa and develops an arterial oxygen tension greater than 50 kPa within a few minutes [1]. Infants given unrestricted oxygen in the 1950s probably had extremely high PO_2 values for many weeks. Control infants were given oxygen limited to that required to eliminate cyanosis and received therapy for less than a week. There was not a statistically significant difference in risk of mortality between these exposures, although there were slightly more deaths with curtailed oxygen therapy. An era of oxygen restriction followed during which there were fewer cases of blindness, but mortality and cerebral palsy increased. It was estimated later that there might have

B. Stenson (✉)
Neonatal Unit, Royal Infirmary of Edinburgh, Little France Crescent, Edinburgh, Scotland

Neonatal Medicine, University of Edinburgh, Edinburgh, Scotland
e-mail: ben.stenson@nhslothian.scot.nhs.uk

© Springer Nature Switzerland AG 2020
E. M. Boyle, J. Cusack (eds.), *Emerging Topics and Controversies in Neonatology*, https://doi.org/10.1007/978-3-030-28829-7_13

been as many as 16 additional deaths from hypoxia for each case of blindness that was prevented during this period [2].

The arrival of blood gas analysers gave rise to the possibility of controlled oxygen therapy, adjusting inspired oxygen to achieve a desired oxygen level or range to minimise the competing risks of blindness from hyperoxia and death from hypoxia. There were not trials to determine the optimal PO_2 range. This approach was further limited by the need for frequent arterial punctures. The arrival of transcutaneous oxygen tension ($TcPO_2$) monitoring offered continuous non-invasive measurements. A randomised controlled trial published in 1987 compared oxygen therapy guided by intermittent arterial blood gases alone with the addition of continuous $TcPO_2$ monitoring [3]. Both study groups were targeted to maintain oxygen tensions of 50–70 mmHg (6.7–9.3 kPa). It was hoped that the availability of continuous feedback would lead to a reduction in ROP. Amongst the 296 infants studied, there were 8% fewer cases of ROP with the addition of continuous $TcPO_2$ monitoring but there were also 8% more deaths. Neither outcome was statistically significant. Although this was inconclusive, with the benefit of hindsight it may have been the first trial evidence in the context of controlled oxygen therapy to suggest that reducing oxygen exposure in the hope of diminishing ROP may increase the risk of mortality. Observational data from this trial suggested that cumulative exposure to oxygen tensions above 80 mmHg (10.7 kPa) may increase the risk of ROP [4]. Subsequent professional guidelines recommended that arterial oxygen tension (PaO_2) should be maintained between 50 and 80 mmHg (6.7–10.7 kPa) [5].

When pulse oximeter saturation (SpO_2) monitors became available they rapidly replaced $TcPO_2$ monitors because of their ease of use. There were no trials done to demonstrate that this improved outcome or to determine what the ideal SpO_2 range should be. There were legitimate concerns initially that saturation monitoring might not prevent hyperoxia because, with the shape of the haemoglobin/oxygen dissociation curve flattening at higher SpO_2, there could be unrecognised exposure to high PO_2. Professional guidelines recommended that SpO_2 should be targeted to 85–95% [6]. Later data from arterial blood samples from oxygen dependent preterm infants show that the arterial PaO_2 range observed with concurrent SpO_2 readings of 85–95% is 28.5–67 mmHg (3.8–8.9 kPa) [7]. Far from allowing more hyperoxia, the switch from $TcPO_2$ monitoring to SpO_2 monitoring aiming for SpO_2 85–95% shifted the target PO_2 range of preterm infants downwards by almost 3 kPa (more than 20 mmHg) to values well below the earlier lower limit of 50 mmHg and arguably began a second era of oxygen restriction that went unrecognised. Because these changes in practice occurred gradually and during a period when the use of antenatal steroids and surfactant dramatically reduced mortality, any effect on mortality from this reduction in oxygen levels may have been obscured.

With improving neonatal survival, the focus returned to morbidities such as retinopathy of prematurity. Persuasive observational data suggested that targeting lower SpO_2 might reduce the risk of retinopathy of prematurity without affecting the risk of mortality or cerebral palsy [8–10] encouraging a further trend in oxygen reduction. Silverman called for trials, arguing that there had never been a shred of convincing evidence to guide limits for the rational use of supplemental oxygen in the care of extremely premature infants. He described oxygen therapy as the albatross of neonatal medicine [11].

Evidence from More Recent Trials

Although there are many questions left to answer there have now been seven high quality randomised controlled trials of oxygen saturation targeting in very preterm infants that can be used to guide routine practice from neonatal unit admission until discharge, pending new evidence.

Oxygen Therapy in the Later Weeks of the Clinical Course

The first two important trials related to the later part of the clinical course, beyond the early weeks after birth and were conducted to see if there was benefit from higher SpO_2. The STOP ROP trial [12] randomised preterm infants who had survived until 35 weeks of gestation and had developed pre-threshold retinopathy of prematurity to lower (89–94%) versus higher (96–99%) SpO_2 targets. It was testing whether higher oxygen levels would diminish the progression of established ROP. There was not a clinically important effect on the eye disease, but the infants treated with the higher SpO_2 target range experienced more adverse pulmonary events and were more likely to be receiving oxygen or diuretics or still hospitalised at 3 months of corrected age. The intervention was provided until ophthalmic endpoints were reached and was not required to be continued beyond hospital discharge.

The first BOOST Trial [13] studied infants who had been born before 30 weeks of gestation and had survived to 32 weeks of gestation but were still receiving supplemental oxygen. The aim was to see whether maintaining higher SpO_2 levels would improve their growth and neurodevelopment. The infants were randomised to lower SpO_2 targets of 91–94% versus higher SpO_2 targets of 95–98%. The intervention was continued beyond hospital discharge. Growth and neurodevelopment to a year of corrected age were not improved in infants who were treated with the higher target range; targeting the higher range prolonged the duration of oxygen supplementation and increased resource usage.

Between them these two trials randomised over 1000 convalescent preterm infants during the weeks approaching hospital discharge and followed them until 3–12 months beyond term. Deaths were few in number in both trials, with more deaths in the infants randomised to higher targets rather than lower targets.

Although healthy infants born at term have SpO_2 readings in the high 90s, these trials show that, once an extremely preterm infant survives to beyond around 32 weeks, there is presently no well-evidenced advantage to targeting SpO_2 higher than 94%. Doing so will prolong their hospitalisation and make them more likely to require home oxygen, without important health benefits or reduced risk of death. There have not been further high-quality studies to determine the safest criteria for deciding whether or not an infant requires to be discharged home on supplemental oxygen. Consistent with this evidence, British Thoracic Society guidance in 2009 recommended that infants should be able to maintain their SpO_2 at 93% or above at the time of discharge home [14]. There is not new high quality evidence to support a higher target than this.

Oxygen Therapy in the Early Weeks of the Clinical Course

There have been five randomised controlled trials of different SpO_2 target ranges for extremely preterm infants in which the intervention commenced on the day of birth and was continued through the early weeks [15–20]. These trials were conducted independently, but were designed as part of an international collaboration called the Neonatal Oxygen Prospective Meta-analysis (NeOProM) collaboration [21]. This ensured that the trials had similar designs, interventions and outcome measures so that, although each could be considered individually, the individual participant data from the five trials could be combined in an individual participant data prospective meta-analysis including around 5000 infants. With this large sample size, quite small differences in important outcomes could be studied reliably and there would be a far greater capacity to investigate whether there were important sub-groups with different results.

All five trials randomised preterm infants born before 28 weeks of gestation to lower (85–89%) versus higher (91–95%) SpO_2 target ranges. The intervention began on the day of birth and continued until the infants reached 36 weeks corrected gestational age if they were still considered to require supplemental oxygen. The first trial results came from the SUPPORT Trial in 2010 [15] and the last from the BOOST-II UK and BOOST-II Australia trials in 2016 [20]. The NeOProM individual participant data meta-analysis was published in 2018 [22] and this included outcome information for 4965 infants and represents the most up to data and comprehensive analysis of data from the trials.

The primary outcome of the NeOProM meta-analysis was a composite of death or disability (defined as blindness, deafness, cognitive impairment or cerebral palsy). This was not significantly different between groups (Table 13.1). There was a highly significant difference between groups in the risk of mortality. There was no difference in the number of infants with one or more of the measures of disability. Survival analysis was used to look at when in the clinical course the difference in mortality between groups in the trials arose. The randomisation groups began to separate in terms of mortality risk around 2 weeks after birth and continued to diverge until around 3 months after birth.

Secondary outcomes included the individual elements of the disability definition, treatment for retinopathy of prematurity, necrotising enterocolitis (NEC), and oxygen supplementation at 36 weeks (Table 13.2). Infants randomised to the lower

Table 13.1 Results of the neonatal oxygen prospective meta-analysis (primary outcome and its components)

Outcome	Lower SpO$_2$	Higher SpO$_2$	Risk difference (%)	Relative risk (95% CI)	P value	I^2 (%)
Death or neurodevelopmental impairment[a]	1191/2228 (54%)	1150/2229 (52%)	1.7	1.04 (0.98–1.09)	0.21	14
Death	484/2433 (20%)	418/2440 (17%)	2.8	1.17 (1.04–1.31)	0.01	0
Neurodevelopmental impairment[a]	707/1744 (41%)	732/1811 (40%)	0.03	1.00 (0.93–1.08)	0.95	6

[a]Bayley Scales of Infant and Toddler Development version 3 (Bayley-III) cognitive or language score of less than 85; or severe visual loss (cannot fixate or is legally blind with visual acuity<6/60 in both eyes; or cerebral palsy with the Gross Motor Function Classification System level 2 or higher; or deafness requiring hearing aids

Table 13.2 Results of the neonatal oxygen prospective meta-analysis (selected secondary outcomes)

Outcome	Lower SpO$_2$	Higher SpO$_2$	Risk difference (%)	Relative risk (95% CI)	P value	I^2 (%)
Bayley-III score <85	647/1713 (38%)	672/1782 (38%)	−0.2	1.00 (0.92–1.08)	0.92	0
Cerebral palsy	106/1910 (6%)	107/1966 (5%)	0.1	1.02 (0.78–1.33)	0.88	19
Deafness	60/1905 (3%)	60/1959 (3%)	0.2	1.05 (0.74–1.49)	0.79	0
Severe visual impairment	25/1910 (1%)	23/1967 (1%)	0.1	1.12 (0.60–2.08)	0.73	0
Necrotising enterocolitis	227/2464 (9%)	170/2465 (7%)	2.3	1.33 (1.10–1.61)	0.003	0
Treatment for ROP	220/2020 (11)	308/2065 (15)	−4.0	0.74 (0.63–0.86	<0.001	80
Supplemental O$_2$ at 36 weeks	459/1846 (25%)	578/1910 (30%)	−5.6	0.81 (0.74–0.90)	<0.001	0

(85–89%) SpO$_2$ target range had significantly increased risk of NEC. Infants randomised to the higher (91–95%) SpO$_2$ targets had a higher risk of retinopathy of prematurity requiring treatment. There was no significant difference between groups in any of the individual measures of disability, including blindness. In fact, the number of infants with blindness was marginally greater in infants treated with the lower SpO$_2$ target. There was little heterogeneity in these results between trials when compared with the heterogeneity observed in other meta-analyses in the neonatal literature. This reflects the relatively large sample sizes and the fact that the trials were designed prospectively to be very similar.

The individual study protocols required high target group infants to achieve higher SpO$_2$ until 36 weeks. This means that it is not surprising that 5.6% more of the higher target group infants required supplemental oxygen at 36 weeks of gestation. This is biased by the protocols, and over-estimates differences between groups in risk of bronchopulmonary dysplasia. Physiological tests [23, 24] were used to determine this outcome in the SUPPORT [15] and BOOST-II UK [18] trials and the differences between groups in the risk of bronchopulmonary dysplasia in these individual trials were smaller and were not statistically significant (3.7% and 1.8% respectively).

Sub-group analyses from the NeOProM meta-analysis show that the finding of increased risk of mortality in infants randomised to SpO_2 targets of 85–89 are not significantly influenced by gestation at birth, gender, or whether or not infants were appropriately grown or small for gestational age. This is important because an earlier sub-group analysis from the SUPPORT trial had raised a hypothesis that the increased risk of mortality from targeting lower SpO_2 may be limited to infants born small for gestational age [25]. The pre-specified subgroup analysis of the NeOProM dataset using a common definition of SGA [26] and a further *post-hoc* analysis using the same definition used in the SUPPORT trial [27] did not show a significant difference between small for gestational age and appropriate for gestational age infants in the effects of SpO_2 targets on risk of mortality at 18–24 months.

Blind to any outcome data, an important sub-group analysis was proposed when an issue with the calibration of the Masimo Radical oximeters used in all five trials was identified, after the trials commenced [28]. The oximeter was found to return fewer SpO_2 values than expected in the range 87–90% and to shift displayed SpO_2 values above 87% upwards by 1–2%. This narrowed the lower SpO_2 target range. It also pushed the trial groups together and lowered the SpO_2 range under study because SpO_2 values in the high target range of 91–95% were being falsely elevated by up to 2%. The oximeter manufacturers provided new calibration software and revised oximeters were introduced into the UK and Australian BOOST-II trials [18, 20] and the Canadian Oxygen Trial [17]. These three trials therefore have sub-groups of infants treated with the original and the revised oximeters. After the revised oximeters were introduced, there was clearer separation between groups in SpO_2 distribution in the UK and Australian BOOST-II trials and the infants allocated to lower SpO_2 spent more time in their intended target range [18, 29]. Consequently the data gathered using the revised oximeters are worth separate consideration.

In the 1716 infants treated with revised oximeters in BOOST-II UK, BOOST-II Australia and the Canadian Oxygen Trial the difference in mortality between infants randomised to lower versus higher SpO_2 targets was 6.1% (risk ratio 1.38, 95% CI 1.13–1.68, $P = 0.001$ [30]. Pooling all data from the five trials before and after the oximeter change may therefore underestimate the mortality risk of targeting lower SpO_2.

Implications for Patients

Although the primary composite outcome of death or disability was not significantly different between groups, this does not mean that the significant effect on mortality was balanced by an opposite effect on disability. Targeting higher saturations increased the chances of an infant surviving by 2.8% (all data) to 6.1% (revised oximeters). One or more of the measures of disability was identified in 40.5% of low target group survivors and in 40.4% of high target group survivors. The relative risk for the composite of death or disability is not significant because it was dominated by the disability outcome which was more than twice as common [31].

Disability in the NeOProM trials was defined as any of, or a combination of deafness, blindness, cerebral palsy or cognitive impairment. The disability that results from these impairments may vary in severity and would not, in most cases, be considered equivalent to, or worse than death. The trials show that targeting higher SpO_2 will result in more infants requiring treatment for ROP. This treatment is highly effective and there was no increase in the number of blind infants in the trials. Treatment for retinopathy of prematurity is still an undesirable outcome because the condition and treatment have permanent structural and functional effects on the eye. Although retinopathy of prematurity has been associated epidemiologically with other adverse outcomes of prematurity [32], in the NeOProM trials infants randomised to higher SpO_2 were not at increased risk of other adverse outcomes. The increased risk of mortality with lower SpO_2 was not offset by any other outcome of similar importance. When these trials were planned, contemporary observational data did not predict that lower SpO_2 targets would be associated with increased risk of mortality. This reinforces the importance of randomised trials over observational data.

Achieved SpO_2 Patterns

In the BOOST-II trials, histograms of the percentage of time that infants spent at each SpO_2 were generated (Fig. 13.1). High target group infants had a distribution with its peak within the intended target range. Low target group infants had higher than intended SpO_2s. The peak of their achieved SpO_2 distribution was above their intended range. Observational data suggest that compliance with targets is more readily achieved with higher SpO_2 upper limits [33]. Lower SpO_2 values are on the steeper part of the haemoglobin-oxygen dissociation curve, where small changes in alveolar oxygen tension will produce bigger swings in saturation and are therefore intrinsically more unstable [34]. With manual oxygen adjustment, time spent in range is greater when a higher range is targeted [18, 35]. Significant differences in mortality, NEC and need for ROP treatment were seen between groups in the trials despite the low target groups achieving higher than intended SpO_2. This should raise a caution that the mortality risk of achieving a distribution of SpO_2 in the intended lower SpO_2 target range may be being underestimated and that new interventions that modify achieved SpO_2 such as servo control, should be researched vary carefully before they are introduced into routine practice. Post-hoc analyses of achieved SpO_2 in the SUPPORT trial shows that the risk of mortality was highest in infants with median SpO_2 less than 92% [36].

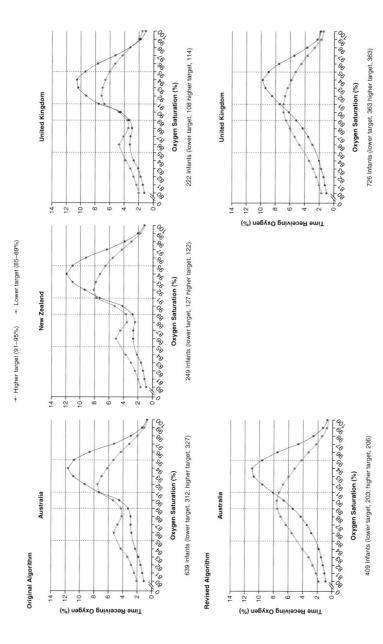

Fig. 13.1 Achieved SpO₂ distributions in the BOOST-II trials. Average frequency distributions of the time spent by each infant at each oxygen-saturation level from 80 to 100% while receiving supplemental oxygen. For trials in the United Kingdom and Australia, separate distributions are provided for infants managed using the original oximeter-calibration algorithm and those managed using the revised algorithm, according to whether they were assigned to receive a higher target of oxygen saturation (91–95%) or a lower target (85–89%). Revised oximeters were not used in the New Zealand trial. Vertical dotted lines indicate the intended target SpO₂ ranges of the randomization groups. (From: N Engl J Med, The BOOST II United Kingdom, Australia, and New Zealand Collaborative Groups, Oxygen Saturation and Outcomes in Preterm Infants. Volume 368 Page 2096. Copyright © (2013) Massachusetts Medical Society. Reprinted with permission)

International Guidelines

The Committee on Fetus and Newborn of the American Academy of Pediatrics released guidance on oxygen targeting in preterm infants in 2016 [37] The report pre-dated the publication of the NeOProM individual patient data meta-analysis. The report concluded that the ideal physiologic target range for oxygen saturation for infants of extremely low birth weight is likely patient-specific and dynamic and depends on various factors, including gestational age, chronologic age, underlying disease, and transfusion status. These are all important but untested hypotheses for future research. Present evidence does not support individualised care in relation to SpO_2 targeting in relation to these factors. The report identifies that SpO_2 limits of 90–95% may be safer for some infants than 85–89%. An upper alarm limit of 95% is supported. An appropriate lower alarm limit is not identified. European consensus guidelines, also published in 2016, recommend a SpO_2 target range of 90–94% with alarm limits of 89 and 95% [38]. In the NeOProM trials the upper alarm limit used in the higher SpO_2 groups was 95% and the lower alarm limits (where specified) were 89 or 90% [39].

Conclusions

There is now high quality evidence to inform oxygen saturation targeting in extremely preterm infants throughout their clinical course from neonatal unit admission to discharge. It has been demonstrated that restricting oxygen supplementation in the hope of reducing morbidity has no important benefit and carries an unacceptable mortality risk. These findings emerged from large trials that were spread widely across the developed world and are likely to be generalisable in similar resource settings in terms of nurse staffing and timely availability of ROP screening and treatment. It is possible that further trials might yet yield additional survival advantage. The oxygen tensions associated with SpO_2 values of 90–95% are still low relative to previously recommended PO_2 ranges. The fact that the mortality finding was unexpected even though highly consistent between trials demonstrates the crucial importance of participation in trials.

These trials have shown that oxygen saturation target ranges are important but they may not have have chanced upon the ideal range. Although they should inform current practice, further trials will be needed to investigate alternative SpO_2 ranges in comparison with the range 91–95%. Newer monitoring technologies that incorporate automated oxygen adjustment will facilitate this. Further analysis of the achieved SpO_2 distributions associated with adverse outcomes from the existing trials may help to inform the safety of researching different target ranges at different postnatal ages.

SpO_2 target ranges should be evidence based and no longer determined by individual clinician preference.

References

1. Huch A, Huch R, Rooth G. Monitoring the intravascular PO2 in newborn infants. J Perinat Med. 1973;1:53–9.
2. Bolton DP, Cross KW. Further observations on cost of preventing retrolental fibroplasia. Lancet. 1974;1:445–8.
3. Bancalari E, Flynn J, Goldberg RN, et al. Influence of transcutaneous oxygen monitoring on the incidence of retinopathy of prematurity. Pediatrics. 1987;79:663–9.
4. Flynn JT, Bancalari E, Snyder ES, et al. A cohort study of transcutaneous oxygen tension and the incidence and severity of retinopathy of prematurity. N Engl J Med. 1992;326(16):1050–4.
5. American Academy of Pediatrics. Committee on Fetus and Newborn, ACOG Committee on Obstetrics. Maternal and fetal medicine. Guidelines for perinatal care. 2nd ed. American Academy of Pediatrics: Elk Grove Village; 1988.
6. American Academy of Pediatrics and the American College of Obstetricians and Gynecologists. Guidelines for perinatal care. 6th ed. American Academy of Pediatrics: Elk Grove Village; 2007.
7. Quine D, Stenson BJ. Arterial oxygen tension (PaO_2) values in infants <29 weeks of gestation at currently targeted saturations. Arch Dis Child Fetal Neonatal Ed. 2009;94:F51–3.
8. Tin W, Milligan DW, Pennefather P, Hey E. Pulse oximetry, severe retinopathy, and outcome at one year in babies of less than 28 weeks gestation. Archives of Disease in Childhood. Arch Dis Child Fetal Neonatal Ed. 2001;84:F106–10.
9. Chow LC, Wright KW, Sola A, CSMC Oxygen Administration Study Group. Can changes in clinical practice decrease the incidence of severe retinopathy of prematurity in very low birth weight infants? Pediatrics. 2003;111:339–45.
10. Anderson CG, Benitz WE, Madan A. Retinopathy of prematurity and pulse oximetry: a national survey of recent practices. J Perinatol. 2004;24:164–8.
11. Silverman WA. A cautionary tale about supplemental oxygen: the albatross of neonatal medicine. Pediatrics. 2004;113:394–6.
12. Supplemental therapeutic oxygen for prethreshold retinopathy of prematurity (STOP-ROP), a randomized, controlled trial. I: primary outcomes. Pediatrics. 2000;105:295–310.
13. Askie LM, Henderson-Smart DJ, Irwig L, Simpson JM. Oxygen-saturation targets and outcomes in extremely preterm infants. N Engl J Med. 2003;349:959–67.
14. Balfour-Lynn IM, Field DJ, Gringras P, et al.; Paediatric Section of the Home Oxygen Guideline Development Group of the BTS Standards of Care Committee. BTS guidelines for home oxygen in children. Thorax. 2009;64 Suppl 2:ii1–26.
15. Carlo WA, Finer NN, Walsh MC, et al.; SUPPORT Study Group of the Eunice Kennedy Shriver NICHD Neonatal Research Network. Target ranges of oxygen saturation in extremely preterm infants. N Engl J Med. 2010;362:1959–69.
16. Vaucher YE, Peralta-Carcelen M, Finer NN, et al.; SUPPORT Study Group of the Eunice Kennedy Shriver NICHD Neonatal Research Network. Neurodevelopmental outcomes in the early CPAP and pulse oximetry trial. N Engl J Med. 2012;367:2495–2504.
17. Schmidt B, Whyte RK, Asztalos EV, et al.; Canadian Oxygen Trial (COT) Group. Effects of targeting higher vs lower arterial oxygen saturations on death or disability in extremely preterm infants: a randomized clinical trial. JAMA. 2013;309:2111–20.
18. BOOST II United Kingdom Collaborative Group, BOOST II Australia Collaborative Group, BOOST II New Zealand Collaborative Group, Stenson BJ, Tarnow-Mordi WO, Darlow BA, et al. Oxygen saturation and outcomes in preterm infants. N Engl J Med. 2013;368:2094–104.
19. Darlow BA, Marschner SL, Donoghoe M, et al. Randomized controlled trial of oxygen saturation targets in very preterm infants: two year outcomes. J Pediatr. 2014;165:30–35.e2.
20. BOOST-II Australia and United Kingdom Collaborative Groups, Tarnow-Mordi W, Stenson B, Kirby A, et al. Outcomes of two trials of oxygen-saturation targets in preterm infants. N Engl J Med. 2016;374:749–60.

21. Askie LM, Brocklehurst P, Darlow BA, et al. NeOProM: Neonatal Oxygenation Prospective Meta-analysis Collaboration study protocol. BMC Pediatr. 2011;11:6.
22. Askie LM, Darlow BA, Finer N, et al.; for the NeOProM Collaborators. Association between oxygen saturation targeting and death or disability in extremely preterm infants in the Neonatal Oxygenation Prospective Meta analysis Collaboration. JAMA. 2018;319(21):2190–2201.
23. Walsh MC, Yao Q, Gettner P, et al. Impact of a physiologic definition on bronchopulmonary dysplasia rates. Pediatrics. 2004;114:1305–11.
24. Quine D, Wong CM, Boyle EM, Jones JG, Stenson BJ. Non-invasive measurement of reduced ventilation: perfusion ratio and shunt in infants with bronchopulmonary dysplasia: a physiological definition of the disease. Arch Dis Child Fetal Neonatal Ed. 2006;91:F409–14.
25. Walsh MC, Di Fiore JM, Martin RJ, Gantz M, Carlo WA, Finer N. Association of oxygen target and growth status with increased mortality in small for gestational age infants: further analysis of the surfactant, positive pressure and pulse oximetry randomized trial. JAMA Pediatr. 2016;170:292–4.
26. Kramer MS, Platt RW, Wen SW, et al. A new and improved population-based Canadian reference for birth weight for gestational age. Pediatrics. 2001;108(2):E35.
27. Alexander GR, Himes JH, Kaufman RB, Mor J, Kogan M. A United States national reference for fetal growth. Obstet Gynecol. 1996;87(2):163–8.
28. Johnston ED, Boyle B, Juszczak E, King A, Brocklehurst P, Stenson BJ. Oxygen targeting in preterm infants using the Masimo SET radical pulse oximeter. Arch Dis Child Fetal Neonatal Ed. 2011;96:F429–33.
29. Stenson BJ, Donoghoe M, Brocklehurst P, et al. SpO_2 targeting and oximeter changes in the BOOST-II Australia and BOOST-II UK oxygen trials. J Pediatr. 2019;204:301–304.e2.
30. Askie LM, Darlow BA, Davis PG, et al. Effects of targeting lower versus higher arterial oxygen saturations on death or disability in preterm infants. Cochrane Database Syst Rev. 2017;4:CD011190.
31. Freemantle N, Calvert M, Wood J, Eastaugh J, Griffin C. Composite outcomes in randomized trials: greater precision but with greater uncertainty? JAMA. 2003;289:2554–9.
32. Schmidt B, Roberts RS, Davis PG, et al. Prediction of late death or disability at age 5 years using a count of 3 neonatal morbidities in very low birth weight infants. J Pediatr. 2015;167:982–6.e2.
33. Hagadorn JI, Furey AM, Nghiem TH, et al.; AVIOx Study Group. Achieved versus intended pulse oximeter saturation in infants born less than 28 weeks' gestation: the AVIOx study. Pediatrics. 2006;118:1574–82.
34. Jones JG, Lockwood GG, Fung N, et al. Influence of pulmonary factors on pulse oximeter saturation in preterm infants. Arch Dis Child Fetal Neonatal Ed. 2016;101:F319–22.
35. van Kaam AH, Hummler HD, Wilinska M, et al. Automated versus manual oxygen control with different saturation targets and modes of respiratory support in preterm infants. J Pediatr. 2015;167:545–50.e1–2.
36. Di Fiore JM, Martin RJ, Li H, et al; SUPPORT Study Group of the Eunice Kennedy Shriver National Institute of Child Health, and Human Development Neonatal Research Network. Patterns of oxygenation, mortality, and growth status in the surfactant positive pressure and oxygen trial cohort. J Pediatr. 2017;186:49–56.e1.
37. Cummings JJ, Polin RA; Committee on Fetus And Newborn. Oxygen targeting in extremely low birth weight infants. Pediatrics. 2016;138. pii: e20161576.
38. Sweet DG, Carnielli V, Greisen G, et al. European consensus guidelines on the management of respiratory distress syndrome—2016 update. Neonatology. 2017;111:107–25.
39. Stenson B, Saugstad OD. Oxygen treatment for immature infants beyond the delivery room: lessons from randomized studies. J Pediatr. 2018;200:12–8.

Chapter 14
Patent Ductus Arteriosus: The Conundrum and Management Options

Kiran More and Samir Gupta

Introduction

The ductus arteriosus (DA) is an essential component of fetal circulation, the patency of which constitutes the most common cardiovascular problem contributing to morbidity in preterm infants. The reported incidence of patent ductus arteriosus (PDA) in very preterm babies varies with the gestation and age of babies at assessment and the characteristics of the population included in the trial, but the figures can be as high as 50% [1]. Overall, the prevalence of PDA is inversely proportional to gestational age.

The presence of a PDA may not be benign in a premature infant. It has been reported that a significant PDA is associated with an increase in morbidity in preterm infants. A large PDA on day 3 in babies born before 28 weeks of gestation increases the odds of death or severe morbidity, intraventricular haemorrhage (IVH) and bronchopulmonary dysplasia (BPD), compared with neonates without a PDA [2]. There are also systemic complications such as increase in incidence of necrotising enterocolitis (NEC), and an eight-fold rise in neonatal mortality [3]. Janz-Robinson et al. [4], however, have shown that there is an increased risk of adverse neurodevelopmental outcomes at 2–3 years of age in infants with a medically or surgically treated PDA; so it is not clear if it is the PDA or intervention for PDA that is harmful. Although, the prevalence of PDA is associated with adverse outcomes, the evidence so far does not report any reduction in these outcomes after treatment of PDA [5, 6].

K. More
Division of Neonatology, Sidra Medicine, Doha, Qatar

S. Gupta (✉)
Division of Neonatology, Sidra Medicine, Doha, Qatar

Durham University, Stockton-on-Tees, UK
e-mail: samir.gupta@durham.ac.uk

© Springer Nature Switzerland AG 2020
E. M. Boyle, J. Cusack (eds.), *Emerging Topics and Controversies in Neonatology*, https://doi.org/10.1007/978-3-030-28829-7_14

As evidence is evolving, the approach to PDA is changing. A large observational trial revealed that, over the years, diagnosis of PDA declined from 51% to 38% (P < 0.001), the use of indomethacin or ibuprofen decreased from 32% to 18% and PDA ligation decreased from 8.4% to 2.9% (p < 0.01) [7]. During the study period, mortality decreased with no increase in any measured morbidity. The EPICE (Effective Perinatal Intensive Care in Europe) study, a large European population-based cohort study [8] raised concern that infants treated for PDA may be at higher risk of BPD or death; however, survival without significant neonatal morbidity was not related to PDA treatment in their cohort.

There has been a paradigm shift in the management of PDA in preterm newborns from early and aggressive closure to a more conservative approach of watchful waiting and spontaneous closure. This shift has resulted mainly from a lack of evidence from randomised controlled trials (RCTs) supporting treatment of a PDA and improving long-term outcomes. This is because most studies conducted to date have enrolled more mature preterm babies (over 1000 g or >28 weeks of gestation) whose PDA is more likely to close spontaneously. The studies were also primarily designed to assess PDA closure rates rather than clinically relevant outcomes. The high contamination rates of open treatment in placebo arm of RCTs, ranging from 23 to 83%, further makes it difficult to evaluate the outcomes after conservative (placebo) treatment. Well-designed large trials are urgently required to dispel the myth of adopting an approach of 'wait and see' due to lack of evidence, despite knowing the high morbidity and mortality rates associated with a persistent PDA. In this chapter, we will discuss the various controversies surrounding diagnosis and management options for PDA.

Natural History of Closure of the PDA

Controversy exists in defining persistent PDA because there are no physiological determinants to guide at what age the persistence of DA becomes pathological. PDA plays a pivotal role in fetal and transitional circulation. Closure, however, varies depending on gestation at birth and the underlying severity of lung disease, and persistently open DA beyond a certain age may pose haemodynamic effects in a premature infant. If the DA fails to close functionally beyond 48–72 h, then it usually starts showing haemodynamic effects especially in extremely preterm population.

The DA closes functionally in few hours to a couple of days after birth in term babies. In a small observational study by Jain et al. [9], no transductal flow was seen in 28 (56%) patients at 12–18 h and 48 (96%) neonates at 30–40 h of age respectively. In preterm infants of >30 weeks of gestation or >1500 g, the DA usually closes by day 4 in healthy infants, with or without evidence of respiratory distress [10]. For infants born at <30 weeks of gestation or birth weight <1500 g, Semberova et al. [11] reported that out of 280 infants, the PDA closed spontaneously before hospital discharge in 237 (85%). The median time to ductal closure was 71, 13, 8, and 6 days in <26 + 0, 26 + 0 to 27 + 6, 28 + 0 to 29 + 6, and >/=30 weeks, respectively. In preterm infants of <28 weeks, the DA closes spontaneously in approximately 73% of infants if untreated. In the largest multicentre RCT, Schmidt et al. [1] reported that in ELBW infants, the PDA closes spontaneously without treatment in up to 50% of cases. There is, however, a variable period of time for which the baby is exposed to the hemodynamic effects of a PDA. The clinical dilemma persists- is it reasonable to expose immature myocardium to physiological effects of untreated PDA? However, the clinical challenge of predicting which PDA will close spontaneously remains, as does the fact that the hemodynamic consequences of a PDA become clinically evident only days after birth.

PDA Diagnosis

Echocardiography Assessment

Controversy exists for a standardised definition of a hemodynamically significant (hsPDA) which will define the cut off limits for the size of a pathological DA, volume overload of heart and the exhaustion of compensatory mechanisms leading to pulmonary oedema and systemic hypoperfusion [9]. Timing of performing echocardiography (ECHO) screening is also debated and is guided by treatment approach. The general trend is to screen when clinical symptoms or signs of PDA are present, or in the first 24–72 h if the approach of early targeted treatment of PDA is practiced in the absence of clinical signs and symptoms. It is essential to perform echocardiography before commencing any medical treatment for PDA, as congenital heart disease with a ductal dependent circulation needs to be ruled out.

Conventional Echocardiography

Detailed echocardiography offers a more comprehensive assessment and could provide a more accurate method of grading PDA severity and selecting which PDAs warrant treatment. However, treatment of a PDA should be related to the clinical context of the infant to ascertain potential benefit.

PDA screening can be broadly grouped into

- Assessment of ductal characteristics
- Assessment of pulmonary over-circulation & left heart volume loading
- Assessment of ductal steal

Assessment of PDA on conventional ECHO as shown in Fig. 14.1. There are various flow patterns identified across PDA as shown in Fig. 14.2.

Table 14.1 gives a summary of guidance to help define the PDA significance for the treatment of a PDA (in the first 72 h of life) [12].

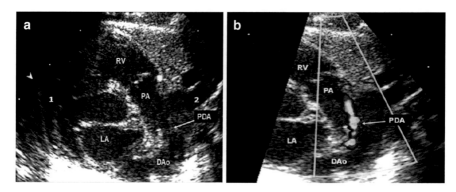

Fig. 14.1 2D and Colour Doppler of ductal flow

Tissue Doppler Imaging and Speckled Tracking

Tissue Doppler imaging (TDI) as a diagnostic modality has limitations, but it can complement routine echocardiography for assessing hsPDA. Evaluation of the heart within the first 24 h suggested that, at 5 h of age, babies with hsPDA had significantly higher systolic and diastolic velocities in both ventricles than those with a non-significant PDA [10]. Cardiac function assessment in preterm infants by measuring speckled tracking derived peak systolic strain (PSS) and strain rate (PSSR) in the first 28 days of life revealed that hsPDA resulted in a significantly lower PSS in the LV (left ventricle) free wall as of day 14 ($P < 0.01$) suggesting increased preload and some LV dysfunction [11]. After medical or surgical (day 28) intervention, LV PSS remained significantly lower ($P < 0.05$), but showed a tendency to increase ($P = 0.18$). Speckled tracking is also utilised in assessing PDA induced early and significant remodeling of the left heart in a long-standing PDA [13].

The role of TDI has been more investigated for determining myocardial performance and to help in early diagnosis of post-ligation cardiac syndrome [14, 15].

The Utility of Electrical Velocimetry: Non-invasive Cardiac Output Monitoring. (ICON(™) Monitor/NICOM) [16]

Cardiac output and cardiac index (CI) vary during various haemodynamic phases of PDA. A prospective observational study in preterm infants <28 weeks with hsPDA, managed with either intravenous ibuprofen or surgical closure reported use of electrical velocimetry with a non invasive cardiac monitor, the ICON(™) monitor [16]. The cardiac output index (CI) value was 0.29 L/kg/min (0.24–0.34). Among the patients with confirmed ductus closure (50%), a significant CI decline was shown (0.29 vs 0.24 L/kg/min, $P = 0.03$) after 72 h of ibuprofen therapy. A statistically

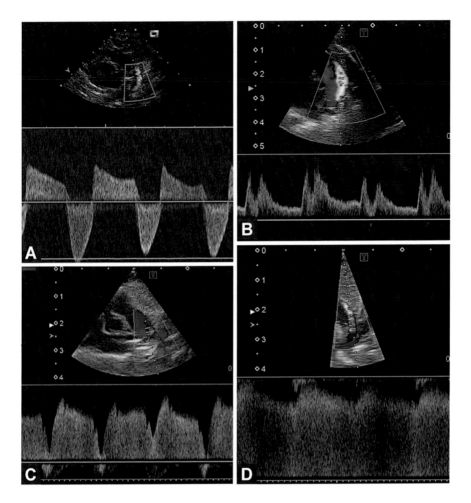

Doppler patterns

A. Bidirectional shunting in pulmonary hypertension

B. Pulsatile pattern in unrestrictive haemodynamically significant duct

C. Growing pattern in transitional circulation

D. Closing or continuous pattern in constricting ductus

Fig. 14.2 Various ductal flow patterns

Table 14.1 ECHO parameters determining clinical significance of a PDA: below is a guide to help define the PDA significance for the early treatment of a PDA (in the first 72 h of life) [12]

Measurement	Moderate PDA	Large PDA
Ductus arteriosus		
Diameter (mm)	1.5–3.0	>3.0
Ductal Velocity (m/s)	1.5–2.0	<1.5
Flow pattern	Pulsatile un-restrictive	Pulsatile un-restrictive
Direction of flow	Depends on relative Qp:Qs, generally left to right (If complete right to left flow then congenital heart should be ruled out)	
Pulmonary overcirculation		
LA:Ao ratio	1.5–1.7	>1.7
E wave to A wave ratio	1.0	>1.0
IVRT (ms)	35–45	<35
LVO (mL/kg/min)	300–400	>400
Pulmonary vein Doppler (m/s)	0.3–0.5	>0.5
PA diastolic flow (m/s)	0.3–0.5	>0.5
Systemic hypoperfusion		
Descending aorta diastolic flow	Absent	Reversed
Celiac artery diastolic flow	Absent	Reversed
Middle cerebral artery diastolic flow	Absent	Reversed

Qp:Qs ratio Ratio of systemic and pulmonary flow, *LA:Ao* left atrial to aortic root ratio, *IVRT* isovolumic relaxation time, *LVO* left ventricular output

significant decrease in stroke volume index (SVI) was found: 1.88 vs 1.62 mL/kg, P = 0.03 with a diminished index of contractility (ICON), 85 vs 140, (P = 0.02). All patients in this group showed a decline in the immediate postoperative CI (1 h after surgery) 0.24 vs 0.30 L/kg/min, P = 0.05, and a significant decrease in contractility (ICON 77 vs 147, P = 0.03).

Near Infra-Red Spectroscopy

Near infra-red spectroscopy (NIRS) monitoring has been used to predict the haemodynamic effects of PDA on tissue perfusion in various organs with some success. Chock et al. [17] studied preterm infants <29 weeks of gestation who underwent routine NIRS monitoring measuring cerebral saturations (Csat) and renal saturation (Rsat) levels. Their findings revealed that Rsat <66% identified an hsPDA with a sensitivity of 81% and specificity of 77%. They also looked at cerebral autoregulation post medical versus surgical treatment of hsPDA and demonstrated that autoregulation was better preserved after indometacin treatment of an hsPDA compared with surgical ligation [18].

Utility of Perfusion Index

Perfusion index (PI) was investigated as a bedside measurement to identify PDA in preterm infants [19]. PI was significantly lower in the hsPDA group compared to the no-PDA group on day 1 and 2 [20]. Also, it was observed that mean changes in PI (delta PI) and DeltaPI variability, may be able to detect PDA in preterm infants, remembering the fact that PI is dynamic and should be assessed continuously.

Feasibility of Biomarkers at the Point of Care

Various point of care biomarkers have been investigated for differentiating between infants with and without a PDA at various postnatal ages; however, there are many limitations for their routine clinical use [21].

Table 14.2 summarises utility of these biomarkers for assessing hsPDA.

The Conundrum of PDA Management [32]

The approach to the management of PDA in the preterm infant remains the most debated topic with the dilemma of whether to treat a PDA, and if so, when and how to intervene to improve short- and long-term outcomes. Various approaches have been reported including conservative or non-pharmacologic treatment, prophylactic treatment, early targeted treatment or late (symptomatic) therapy (Fig. 14.3).

Is Conservative Approach Always Safe?

Conservative management refers to management of PDA without medical/surgical closure, but utilising strategies to decrease the shunt volume and or the haemodynamics effects of PDA. This includes increasing positive end-expiratory pressure (PEEP) in a ventilated baby to limit left to right shunting and judicious use of diuretics [33]. This approach has evolved due to uncertainties surrounding treatment for PDA closure, concerns about side effects of treatment and lack of benefits of treatment reported from RCTs. However, the evidence so far has limitations, because the open treatment rates in placebo arms vary from 23 to 87% [5]. The study groups included babies up to 33 weeks of gestation who would now not be considered subjects for active treatment and the primary outcomes were assessing the closure of the PDA rather than clinical outcomes of interest.

Delayed commencement of medical treatment beyond the first week, however, showed a trend towards a reduced likelihood of successfully closing a PDA, especially at extremely preterm gestations [34]. This approach does not offer any benefits in the prevention of haemorrhagic complications such as IVH and pulmonary haemorrhage in extremely preterm infants who are at the highest risks for these complications.

Table 14.2 Utility of biomarkers assisting diagnosis of PDA

Biomarkers	Time of testing	Studies	Relevance	Limitations
Plasma N-terminal pro-B type natriuretic peptide (NT-proBNP)	Day 3 and 7	Kalra et al. [22] N = 51, <1259 g birth weight	Correlate with size	– Heterogeneity in NT-proB levels timing – Different methods of assays – Different reference ranges – Lack of normative data
	24 h	El-Khuffash et al. [23] Infants <32 weeks, <1500 g; N = 60; median gestation 27.7 weeks	Correlate BPD & death in prem	
	Day 3	Harris et al. [24] Infants <30 weeks, N = 51	Predicts hsPDA	
Urinary NT-proBNP	Day 2	Czernik et al. [25] N = 136, preterm infants (median (IQR): Gestational age 28 (26–30) weeks; birth weight 1030 (780–1270) g	Correlate with ductal patency	
Serum troponin T	48 h	El-Khuffash et al. [26] Median gestation of 28 weeks (IQR = 26.1–29.5 weeks) and median birth weight of 1.06 kg (IQR = 0.87–1.21 kg) N = 80	Correlate with patency, diameter, left atrial-to-aortic diameter ratio, & descending aortic end-diastolic velocity	Limited data Not readily available
C-reactive protein (CRP)	<3 days	Meinarde et al. [27] Birth weight </=1500 g & gestational age </=30 weeks; N = 88 infants	High CRP associated with PDA	Not consistent Marker of illness severity
Neutrophil to lymphocyte (N/L) ratio	<3 days	Temel et al. [28] N = 97; preterm gestation	Correlated with body weight in PDA group	Limited data
Platelet indices -platelet count and platelet mass	First days	Simon et al. [29] (systematic review) <32 weeks gest; 11 studies, N = 3479 Demir et al. [30] Preterm, N = 235	– Low platelet counts correlates with hsPDA – Platelet mass may be significant indicator of PDA closure	Association needs to be confirmed
Absolute nucleated red blood cell (aNRBC) counts	Day 1	Bin-Nun et al. [31] Gestational age ≤ 30 weeks N = 111	aNRBC levels were 3770 (728, 6015) hsPDA vs 865 (483, 2528) closed ductus	Limited data

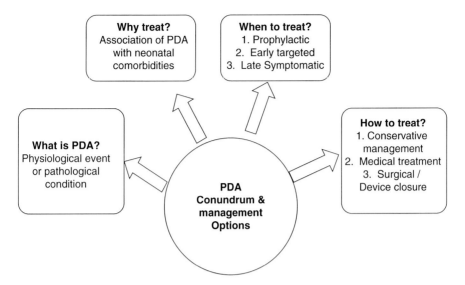

Fig. 14.3 PDA conundrum and Management Options

Restrictive Versus Liberal Fluids?

The evidence does not suggest that judicious restriction of fluids reduces the risk of PDA in a premature infant [35]. De Buyst et al. [36] reported that fluid restriction had no effect on PDA dimension but did decrease superior vena cava (SVC) flow significantly, so should be carefully followed. Fluid restriction before commencing medical treatment is not advised but it may help in the presence of oliguria associated with cox-inhibitor therapy, which can occur in over 50% of treated preterm infants [37]. Additionally, fluid restriction before surgical closure of PDA could increase the post-surgical complications due to decreased end diastolic volume.

Does Furosemide Cause Any Benefits or Harm?

Loop diuretics such as Furosemide have been routinely used by many clinicians to treat fluid overload secondary to hsPDA. However, in the early days of life, the use of diuretics may, in fact, cause intravascular fluid depletion which could worsen the ductal steal [38]. The concurrent use of Frusemide (IV) with indometacin has been shown to cause a significant rise in serum creatinine and the fractional excretion of sodium, resulting in hyponatremia and increased incidence of acute renal failure (ARF) [39]. The use of Frusemide has an effect on increasing prostaglandin responsiveness of the duct and could delay its spontaneous closure. Diuretic use is only justified in the presence of longstanding hsPDA with evidence of cardiomegaly with cor pulmonale, or co-existing with BPD. A recent Finnish cohort study, however, reported that exposure to furosemide was associated with decreased odds of PDA treatment (OR 0.72: 95% CI 0.65–0.79) [40].

Does Choice of Respiratory Support Have Any Effect on the PDA?

The use of continuous positive airways pressure (CPAP) on the first day of life in very low birth weight (VLBW) infants is increasing. Although the evidence so far does not suggest that non-invasive respiratory support reduces the incidence of PDA, the treatment of PDA has reduced with increasing use of non-invasive respiratory support [41]. This could be due to the change in clinical practice not substantiated by evidence.

Does Use of Caffeine Affect PDA?

Secondary outcome data from use of caffeine in very preterm infants reported a reduction in the rates of death or BPD and PDA [42]. The largest trial of caffeine in premature infants by Schmidt et al. [43] also reported a significant reduction in PDA requiring medical or surgical closure before discharge. It is, however, not clear whether this beneficial effect on PDA was due to a direct effect of caffeine on PDA haemodynamics or was due to improvements in the complications of prematurity on the whole.

Does Phototherapy Affect PDA?

There was a concern about delayed closure of PDA among babies exposed to phototherapy [44]. However, this has not been shown in other prospective trials [45]. There is little evidence that chest shielding during phototherapy may be associated with a decreased incidence of PDA among premature infants [46].

Prophylactic Approach: Should We Still Consider This?

The largest published trial of indometacin prophylaxis (IP) by Schmidt et al. [1] did not show any improvement in the rate of survival without neurosensory impairment at 18 months. However, there was a reduction in the frequency of PDA and severe periventricular and intraventricular haemorrhage (IVH) before discharge. Another recent observational study by Nelin et al. [47] demonstrated that infants receiving IP had a significantly lower relative risk (RR) of mortality 0.52 (95% CI 0.37–0.73,

P = 0.0001) and lower RR of developing the combined outcome of death or BPD (RR 0.91, 95% CI 0.85–0.98, P = 0.012) when compared with the control group. However, they failed to see an effect on the incidence of severe IVH or PDA ligation. Mirza et al. [48] reported that giving IP at ≤6 h of age is not associated with a reduction in IVH or death but is associated with a reduction in the treatment/ligation of PDA or death. Oral ibuprofen prophylaxis is also reported to have similar effect as low dose indometacin but with fewer side effects [49].

The prophylactic approach might reduce PDA requiring later treatment and IVH with no long term benefits but has the disadvantage of unnecessarily treating many preterm infants who would have otherwise closed their ductus spontaneously. This makes the prophylactic approach controversial and it is now rarely used. In the future babies may be selectively given prophylaxis based on genetic background and utilising metabolomics, which essentially is selective and individualised treatment rather than prophylactic treatment per se [50].

Early Targeted Approach for PDA Closure

Literature for every approach remains controversial, so an early targeted approach (ETA) by selecting preterm neonates who are more likely to develop complications of a hsPDA is likely to be justifiable, and might lead to improvement in both short and long term outcomes. This approach has the potential of having some benefits of the prophylactic approach, while minimising the risk of exposing a large number of babies to the side effects of drug treatment. Some supportive evidence for this approach comes from the limited observations in the randomised trial by Kluckow et al. [5] including extreme premature infant less than 29 weeks of gestation. This study reported that this approach is feasible and safe, and demonstrated a reduction in early pulmonary haemorrhage and the need for later medical treatment. Echocardiography screening for PDA in extremely preterm newborn infants, compared to the 'symptomatic' approach reduces the time to detect the PDA and allows treatment of babies before the haemodynamic effects of PDA cause any symptoms or signs [51].

In preclinical trials, pharmacological PDA closure was reported to improve alveolarisation and minimise the impairment of postnatal alveolar development that is the pathologic hallmark of "new bronchopulmonary dysplasia' (BPD) [52]. An early selective treatment approach for closure of a PDA was suggested to trial its effect on BPD. Currently, there are ongoing trials including a large RCT-Baby OSCAR trial in the United Kingdom, which is studying the short term outcomes to discharge and the long term outcomes of neurodevelopment and respiratory morbidity. The other trials utilizing this approach with different methodology include the French TRIOCAPI trial, the Dutch BeNEDuCTUS trial (and the Australian U-PDA trial [53].

Symptomatic Approach

Babies may not be symptomatic in first 72 h of life. Between day 4–7, if the PDA is still open, almost 67% preterm infants are symptomatic, with an audible murmur in 100% [54]. This approach, where medical treatment is offered when the baby is clinically symptomatic for the presence of hsPDA, has primarily compared different pharmacologic agents rather than treatment versus no treatment. The interpretation of results is further compounded by the high rates of open treatment in the reported trials. The Cochrane review by Malviya et al. suggests no difference between medical and surgical management for symptomatic PDAs [55].

Which Drug to Choose Amongst the Pharmacological Options?

Indometacin Therapy

The non-steroidal anti-inflammatory drug (NSAID), indometacin, was introduced as the preferred drug for ductal closure in the late 1970s [56], and remained the drug of choice until recently, in spite of its side effect profile. Indometacin facilitates DA closure by inhibiting cyclooxygenase COX-1(PTGS1) and COX-2(PTGS2) enzymes that are required for prostaglandin PGE2 synthesis. Medical treatment with indometacin compared to surgical ligation is preferred as the initial treatment for symptomatic PDA [55]. Indometacin has similar efficacy for ductal closure compared to ibuprofen [57]. However, it has not been shown to impact long term outcomes such as BPD or mortality.

Treatment Regimens

Standard: Initial dose of 0.2 mg/kg followed by two 0.1 mg/kg daily for 3 days, slow infusion. Faster infusion rates and dosing frequency, and also multiple courses have been tried with better results but increase the risk of developing periventricular leucomalacia.

Prophylaxis: 0.1 mg/kg once a day for up to 5 days.

Oral indometacin has been tried in developing countries due to lack of easy availability of an intravenous formulation which suggested equal efficacy; however, data is insufficient to recommend its routine use [58].

Ibuprofen Therapy

Ibuprofen, acting with a similar mechanism, emerged as a substitute for indometacin in the mid-1990s, [59] exhibiting equal efficacy, but with a reduced risk profile especially of NEC. Ibuprofen has become the drug of choice for PDA closure as described in the most recent Cochrane review by Ohlsson et al. [60] including 33 studies enrolling 2190 infants. They reported comparable failure rates for PDA closure with ibuprofen (oral or IV) and indometacin (oral or iv) and a significant reduction in failure to close a PDA (RR 0.26, 95% CI 0.11–0.62; RD −0.44, 95% CI −0.65 to −0.23) when compared with placebo. The risk of developing NEC was reduced for ibuprofen (16 studies, 948 infants; typical RR 0.64, 95% CI 0.45–0.93), as were transient renal insufficiency and duration of ventilatory support.

Dose regimens commonly followed; high dose (20-10-10 mg/kg/dose) and low dose (10-5-5 mg/kg/dose). Direct comparison between these two regimens has shown no difference [61]. However there is growing evidence that a higher dose might improve ductal closure rates with increasing postnatal age as compared to the standard doses.

Oral ibuprofen: The most recent meta-analysis by Mitra et al. [62] included 68 randomised clinical trials of 4802 infants with 14 different variations of indometacin, ibuprofen, or paracetamol (acetaminophen) treatment modalities. A high dose of oral ibuprofen was associated with a higher likelihood of PDA closure vs standard doses of intravenous ibuprofen or indomethacin, placebo or no treatment. It did not, however, change the likelihood of mortality, NEC, or IVH. This data is again from very preterm babies above 28 weeks of gestation rather than from extremely preterm babies.

Intravenous (IV) ibuprofen has been tried earlier with good efficacy, [63] but the side effect profile of the oral formulation is comparable to IV with less chance of hypernatremia [63]. IV Ibuprofen is reported to have increased side effects, including serious gastrointestinal bleeding [64] compared to the oral preparation, but the data is low quality and in infants above 28 weeks gestational age.

Paracetamol Therapy

Paracetamol was observed incidentally as an effective pharmacological agent for PDA closure [65]. Paracetamol acts at a different pathway by directly inhibiting the activity of prostaglandin synthase at the peroxidase region of the enzyme.

Dose regimen: 15 mg/kg/dose, every 6 h.

A recent Cochrane review by Ohlsson et al. [66] included eight studies (N = 916). Five moderate quality studies compared treatment of PDA with paracetamol versus ibuprofen, and enrolled 559 infants and reported similar efficacy (typical risk ratio (RR) 0.95, 95% confidence interval (CI) 0.75–1.21). Four moderate quality studies (n = 537) reported on gastrointestinal bleeding, which was lower in the paracetamol group compared to the ibuprofen group (typical RR 0.28, 95% CI 0.12–0.69). There is low-quality evidence that suggests paracetamol is as effective as indometacin in closing a PDA. Currently, numerous RCTs are ongoing for studying the efficacy of IV and oral paracetamol. There have been concerns about long term and neurological outcomes after paracetamol use in animal studies, including an increased risk of autism and cognitive impairment.

Oral paracetamol has mainly been used as rescue therapy after failed standard therapy or as a safer approach in the presence of contraindications to medical therapy such as intestinal perforation, renal failure, and thrombocytopenia. The neurodevelopmental outcomes at 18–24 months' corrected age did not differ among the preterm infants who received either paracetamol or ibuprofen [67]. Current evidence is therefore not adequate for recommending it for routine in the absence of more convincing data about safety.

How Safe Are NSAIDS?

Both cyclooxygenase inhibitors indometacin and ibuprofen are associated with vasoconstriction leading to renal dysfunction and gastrointestinal side effects such as feed intolerance, spontaneous intestinal perforation, and NEC. Enteral feeds are often discontinued or reduced during indometacin treatment, but this is controversial and has not been shown to make any difference [68].

Ibuprofen has fewer renal side effects, causes significantly less NEC and is associated with shorter duration of ventilation, making it the preferred drug of choice. The gastro-intestinal complications, including perforation, increase with the concomitant use of corticosteroids.

Surgical Ligation: Is This Still an Option?

PDA ligation provides an immediate and definitive option for ductal closure and is considered for hsPDA shunts when pharmacological treatment is either contraindicated or has failed to successfully close or reduce significant shunts in infants, especially those who remain dependent on mechanical ventilation.

Over the years, the approach to ligation has changed from a more aggressive to a very conservative approach. Prophylactic surgical ligation on the first day of life reduced rate of necrotising enterocolitis (30% versus 8%; $P = 0.002$) among extremely low birth weight (ELBW) infants compared with no treatment, but may lead to an increase in moderate to severe BPD among the surgically treated infants so this is not practised anymore [34]. In a large cohort of 3500 Canadian preterm infants born at <32 weeks of gestation with a symptomatic PDA, infants undergoing surgical ligation had reduced mortality but increased odds of BPD and ROP compared with infants medically treated, after adjustment for antenatal and perinatal confounders [69]. Early ligation at ≤2 weeks of life was associated with increased morbidity and mortality in VLBW infants and did not show benefit [70]. Sung et al. [71] compared mandatory closure versus non-intervention in 78 ELBW infants of 23–26 weeks of gestation requiring ventilator treatment with hsPDA. Their observation was that, despite longer PDA exposure, non-intervention was associated with significantly less BPD (38% versus 58%; $P < 0.05$). Ligation has not offered any improvement in rates of in mortality and long term neurodevelopmental impairment [72, 73].

Ligation is however, seriously questioned as it is associated with significant anaesthetic complications and immediate post-operative haemodynamic instability needing inotropic support [74]. In addition, there are surgical complications such as vocal fold paralysis, accidental recurrent laryngeal nerve ligation, [75] diaphragmatic paralysis, [76] and accidental pulmonary artery ligation [77].

Although the decision regarding PDA ligation remains controversial, defining the target population by careful patient selection and triaging is the way to go [78].

Do Newer Surgical Techniques Offer Any Promise?

The traditional ligation method is invasive and associated with complications, hence newer techniques are being explored. The trans-arterial and trans-venous approaches have been used and less complications are reported with trans-venous approach. Table 14.3 shows newer options available for surgical ductal closure.

The Influence of Genetics on Ductal Patency and Management

Clinical response and toxicity from drugs used to treat PDA are highly variable. Developmental and genetic aspects of pharmacokinetics and pharmacodynamics influence exposure and response to pharmacological therapies. Patel et al. [85] studied genetic modifiers of PDA in term infants and suggested the importance of the transforming growth factor-beta pathway in the closure of the term ductus arteriosus which in turn may help identify currently unknown targets for future therapeutic manipulation. New therapeutic targets and genetic studies will promote the practice of precision medicine.

Table 14.3 Newer surgical techniques

Surgical approach	Device used	Population used	Comment
Percutaneous / Transcatheter occlusion	Amplatzer duct Occluder II additional size (ADOIIAS) [79, 80]	VLBW infants (<1200 g)	– Surgical success depends on perfect patient selection and placement of the occluder
	Occlutech PDA(R) occluder (ODO) [81]	Older preterm infants	– Used for closure of larger ducts, tubular, or window-type ducts – Needs bigger studies and longer follow-ups
	Nit-Occlud coil in retrograde closure [82, 83]	Older infants beyond 1 year of age	– Good for small to moderate PDAs – Not tried in newborns yet
Transcatheter occlusion	Medtronic micro vascular plug (MVP) [84, 85]	– Small children – Extreme preterm	Large-diameter vascular embolisation device for the PDA occlusion

Conclusions

The controversy about the choice of drug and dose, route of administration and timing of treatment remains open to debate. The prophylactic approach has gone out of favour due to the unnecessary exposure to side effects of treatment in a large proportion of babies. The uncertainty of treatment benefits in babies with a symptomatic PDA has led to the emergence of a 'wait and watch' policy with an increasing number of babies discharged with persistent PDA, which is allowed to follow its natural course. The long term outcomes are not yet well evaluated or reported in well designed trials. Similarly, the surgical approach is being used less due to concerns about long term outcomes and increased risk of BPD.

The approach of selective, early targeted treatment holds promise and the ongoing trials should show if this approach has benefits in improving short and long term outcomes. Similarly, transcatheter surgical closure is an emerging technique that could potentially reduce the side effects of surgical closure and offer definitive closure of persistent PDA. The genetics studies, and better understanding of pharmacodynamics of drugs would help in dose optimisation to determine the most effective treatment dose while minimising the side effect profile. Until then, 'the jury is out' and the variation in practice for managing PDA remain as hot topics in neonatology.

Conflict of Interest Professor Samir Gupta is recipient of NIHR-HTA award for the Baby-OSCAR trial as chief investigator assessing early targeted treatment of PDA using ibuprofen.

References

1. Schmidt B, Davis P, Moddemann D, Ohlsson A, Roberts RS, Saigal S, et al. Long-term effects of indomethacin prophylaxis in extremely-low-birth-weight infants. N Engl J Med. 2001;344(26):1966–72.
2. Sellmer A, Bjerre JV, Schmidt MR, McNamara PJ, Hjortdal VE, Host B, et al. Morbidity and mortality in preterm neonates with patent ductus arteriosus on day 3. Arch Dis Child Fetal Neonatal Ed. 2013;98(6):F505–10.
3. Noori S, McCoy M, Friedlich P, Bright B, Gottipati V, Seri I, et al. Failure of ductus arteriosus closure is associated with increased mortality in preterm infants. Pediatrics. 2009;123(1):e138–44.
4. Janz-Robinson EM, Badawi N, Walker K, Bajuk B, Abdel-Latif ME. Neurodevelopmental outcomes of premature infants treated for patent ductus arteriosus: a population-based cohort study. J Pediatr. 2015;167(5):1025–32.e3.
5. Kluckow M, Jeffery M, Gill A, Evans N. A randomised placebo-controlled trial of early treatment of the patent ductus arteriosus. Arch Dis Child Fetal Neonatal Ed. 2014;99(2):F99–F104.
6. Aranda JV, Clyman R, Cox B, Van Overmeire B, Wozniak P, Sosenko I, et al. A randomized, double-blind, placebo-controlled trial on intravenous ibuprofen L-lysine for the early closure of nonsymptomatic patent ductus arteriosus within 72 hours of birth in extremely low-birth-weight infants. Am J Perinatol. 2009;26(3):235–45.
7. Bixler GM, Powers GC, Clark RH, Walker MW, Tolia VN. Changes in the diagnosis and management of patent ductus arteriosus from 2006 to 2015 in United States neonatal intensive care units. J Pediatr. 2017;189:105–12.

8. Edstedt Bonamy AK, Gudmundsdottir A, Maier RF, Toome L, Zeitlin J, Bonet M, et al. Patent ductus arteriosus treatment in very preterm infants: a European Population-Based Cohort Study (EPICE) on variation and outcomes. Neonatology. 2017;111(4):367–75.

9. Polat TB, Celik IH, Erdeve O. Early predictive echocardiographic features of hemodynamically significant patent ductus arteriosus in preterm VLBW infants. Pediatr Int. 2016;58(7):589–94.

10. Lee A, Nestaas E, Liestol K, Brunvand L, Lindemann R, Fugelseth D. Tissue Doppler imaging in very preterm infants during the first 24 h of life: an observational study. Arch Dis Child Fetal Neonatal Ed. 2014;99(1):F64–9.

11. Helfer S, Schmitz L, Buhrer C, Czernik C. Tissue Doppler-derived strain and strain rate during the first 28 days of life in very low birth weight infants. Echocardiography. 2014;31(6):765–72.

12. van Laere D, van Overmeire B, Gupta S, El Khuffash A, Savoia M, McNamara PJ, et al. Application of NPE in the assessment of a patent ductus arteriosus. Pediatr Res. 2018;84(Suppl 1):46–56.

13. de Waal K, Phad N, Collins N, Boyle A. Cardiac remodeling in preterm infants with prolonged exposure to a patent ductus arteriosus. Congenit Heart Dis. 2017;12(3):364–72.

14. El-Khuffash AF, Jain A, Weisz D, Mertens L, McNamara PJ. Assessment and treatment of post patent ductus arteriosus ligation syndrome. J Pediatr. 2014;165(1):46–52.e1.

15. El-Khuffash AF, Jain A, Dragulescu A, McNamara PJ, Mertens L. Acute changes in myocardial systolic function in preterm infants undergoing patent ductus arteriosus ligation: a tissue Doppler and myocardial deformation study. J Am Soc Echocardiogr. 2012;25(10):1058–67.

16. Rodriguez Sanchez de la Blanca A, Sanchez Luna M, Gonzalez Pacheco N, Arriaga Redondo M, Navarro Patino N. Electrical velocimetry for non-invasive monitoring of the closure of the ductus arteriosus in preterm infants. Eur J Pediatr. 2018;177(2):229–35.

17. Chock VY, Rose LA, Mante JV, Punn R. Near-infrared spectroscopy for detection of a significant patent ductus arteriosus. Pediatr Res. 2016;80(5):675–80.

18. Chock VY, Ramamoorthy C, Van Meurs KP. Cerebral oxygenation during different treatment strategies for a patent ductus arteriosus. Neonatology. 2011;100(3):233–40.

19. Gomez-Pomar E, Makhoul M, Westgate PM, Ibonia KT, Patwardhan A, Giannone PJ, et al. Relationship between perfusion index and patent ductus arteriosus in preterm infants. Pediatr Res. 2017;81(5):775–9.

20. Terek D, Altun Koroglu O, Ulger Z, Yalaz M, Kultursay N. The serial changes of perfusion index in preterm infants with patent ductus arteriosus: is perfusion index clinically significant? Minerva Pediatr. 2016;68(4):250–5.

21. Weisz DE, McNamara PJ, El-Khuffash A. Cardiac biomarkers and haemodynamically significant patent ductus arteriosus in preterm infants. Early Hum Dev. 2017;105:41–7.

22. Kalra VK, DeBari VA, Zauk A, Kataria P, Myridakis D, Kiblawi F. Point-of-care testing for B-type natriuretic peptide in premature neonates with patent ductus arteriosus. Ann Clin Lab Sci. 2011;41(2):131–7.

23. El-Khuffash AF, Slevin M, McNamara PJ, Molloy EJ. Troponin T, N-terminal pro natriuretic peptide and a patent ductus arteriosus scoring system predict death before discharge or neurodevelopmental outcome at 2 years in preterm infants. Arch Dis Child Fetal Neonatal Ed. 2011;96(2):F133–7.

24. Harris SL, More K, Dixon B, Troughton R, Pemberton C, Horwood J, et al. Factors affecting N-terminal pro-B-type natriuretic peptide levels in preterm infants and use in determination of haemodynamic significance of patent ductus arteriosus. Eur J Pediatr. 2018;177(4):521–32.

25. Czernik C, Metze B, Muller C, Buhrer C. Urinary NT-proBNP and ductal closure in preterm infants. J Perinatol. 2013;33(3):212–7.

26. El-Khuffash A, Barry D, Walsh K, Davis PG, Molloy EJ. Biochemical markers may identify preterm infants with a patent ductus arteriosus at high risk of death or severe intraventricular haemorrhage. Arch Dis Child Fetal Neonatal Ed. 2008;93(6):F407–12.

27. Meinarde L, Hillman M, Rizzotti A, Basquiera AL, Tabares A, Cuestas E. C-reactive protein, platelets, and patent ductus arteriosus. Platelets. 2016;27(8):821–3.

28. Temel MT, Coskun ME, Akbayram S, Demiryurek AT. Association between neutrophil/lymphocyte ratio with ductus arteriosus patency in preterm newborns. Bratisl Lek Listy. 2017;118(8):491–4.

29. Simon SR, van Zogchel L, Bas-Suarez MP, Cavallaro G, Clyman RI, Villamor E. Platelet counts and patent ductus arteriosus in preterm infants: a systematic review and meta-analysis. Neonatology. 2015;108(2):143–51.
30. Demir N, Peker E, Ece I, Agengin K, Bulan KA, Tuncer O. Is platelet mass a more significant indicator than platelet count of closure of patent ductus arteriosus? J Matern Fetal Neonatal Med. 2016;29(12):1915–8.
31. Bin-Nun A, Mimouni FB, Fink D, Sela H, Hammerman C. Elevated nucleated red blood cells at birth predict hemodynamically significant patent ductus arteriosus. J Pediatr. 2016;177:313–5.
32. Evans N. Preterm patent ductus arteriosus: a continuing conundrum for the neonatologist? Semin Fetal Neonatal Med. 2015;20(4):272–7.
33. Letshwiti JB, Semberova J, Pichova K, Dempsey EM, Franklin OM, Miletin J. A conservative treatment of patent ductus arteriosus in very low birth weight infants. Early Hum Dev. 2017;104:45–9.
34. Cassady G, Crouse DT, Kirklin JW, Strange MJ, Joiner CH, Godoy G, et al. A randomized, controlled trial of very early prophylactic ligation of the ductus arteriosus in babies who weighed 1000 g or less at birth. N Engl J Med. 1989;320(23):1511–6.
35. Bell EF, Acarregui MJ. Restricted versus liberal water intake for preventing morbidity and mortality in preterm infants. Cochrane Database Syst Rev. 2014;(12):CD000503.
36. De Buyst J, Rakza T, Pennaforte T, Johansson AB, Storme L. Hemodynamic effects of fluid restriction in preterm infants with significant patent ductus arteriosus. J Pediatr. 2012;161(3):404–8.
37. Takami T, Yoda H, Ishida T, Morichi S, Kondo A, Sunohara D, et al. Effects of indomethacin on patent ductus arteriosus in neonates with genetic disorders and/or congenital anomalies. Am J Perinatol. 2013;30(7):551–6.
38. Brion LP, Campbell DE. Furosemide for symptomatic patent ductus arteriosus in indomethacin-treated infants. Cochrane Database Syst Rev. 2001;(3):CD001148.
39. Lee BS, Byun SY, Chung ML, Chang JY, Kim HY, Kim EA, et al. Effect of furosemide on ductal closure and renal function in indomethacin-treated preterm infants during the early neonatal period. Neonatology. 2010;98(2):191–9.
40. Thomson EJ, Greenberg RG, Kumar K, Laughon M, Smith PB, Clark RH, et al. Association between furosemide exposure and patent ductus arteriosus in hospitalized infants of very low birth weight. J Pediatr. 2018;199:231–6.
41. Flannery DD, O'Donnell E, Kornhauser M, Dysart K, Greenspan J, Aghai ZH. Continuous positive airway pressure versus mechanical ventilation on the first day of life in very-low-birth-weight infants. Am J Perinatol. 2016;33(10):939–44.
42. Lodha A, Seshia M, McMillan DD, Barrington K, Yang J, Lee SK, et al. Association of early caffeine administration and neonatal outcomes in very preterm neonates. JAMA Pediatr. 2015;169(1):33–8.
43. Schmidt B, Roberts RS, Davis P, Doyle LW, Barrington KJ, Ohlsson A, et al. Caffeine therapy for apnea of prematurity. N Engl J Med. 2006;354(20):2112–21.
44. Barefield ES, Dwyer MD, Cassady G. Association of patent ductus arteriosus and phototherapy in infants weighing less than 1000 grams. J Perinatol. 1993;13(5):376–80.
45. Surmeli-Onay O, Yurdakok M, Karagoz T, Erkekoglu P, Ertugrul I, Takci S, et al. A new approach to an old hypothesis; phototherapy does not affect ductal patency via PGE2 and PGI2. J Matern Fetal Neonatal Med. 2015;28(1):16–22.
46. Mannan J, Amin SB. Meta-analysis of the effect of chest shielding on preventing patent ductus arteriosus in premature infants. Am J Perinatol. 2017;34(4):359–63.
47. Nelin TD, Pena E, Giacomazzi T, Lee S, Logan JW, Moallem M, et al. Outcomes following indomethacin prophylaxis in extremely preterm infants in an all-referral NICU. J Perinatol. 2017;37(8):932–7.
48. Mirza H, Laptook AR, Oh W, Vohr BR, Stoll BJ, Kandefer S, et al. Effects of indomethacin prophylaxis timing on intraventricular haemorrhage and patent ductus arteriosus in extremely low birth weight infants. Arch Dis Child Fetal Neonatal Ed. 2016;101(5):F418–22.

49. Kalani M, Shariat M, Khalesi N, Farahani Z, Ahmadi S. A comparison of early ibuprofen and indomethacin administration to prevent Intraventricular hemorrhage among preterm infants. Acta Med Iran. 2016;54(12):788–92.
50. Fanos V, Pusceddu M, Dessi A, Marcialis MA. Should we definitively abandon prophylaxis for patent ductus arteriosus in preterm new-borns? Clinics (Sao Paulo). 2011;66(12):2141–9.
51. Juarez-Dominguez G, Iglesias-Leboreiro J, Rendon-Macias ME, Bernardez-Zapata I, Patino-Bahena EJ, Agami-Micha S, et al. [Echocardiographic screening vs. symptomatic diagnosis for patent ductus arteriosus in preterms]. Rev Med Inst Mex Seguro Soc. 2015;53(2):136–41.
52. Clyman RI. The role of patent ductus arteriosus and its treatments in the development of bronchopulmonary dysplasia. Semin Perinatol. 2013;37(2):102–7.
53. Gupta S, McNamara P. Contemporary approach to the patent ductus arteriosus and future considerations. Semin Fetal Neonatal Med. 2018;23(4):223–4.
54. Pourarian S, Sharma D, Farahbakhsh N, Cheriki S, Bijanzadeh F. To evaluate the prevalence of symptomatic and non-symptomatic ductus arteriosus and accuracy of physical signs in diagnosing PDA in preterm infants using blinded comparison of clinical and echocardiographic findings during the first week of life: a prospective observational study from Iran. J Matern Fetal Neonatal Med. 2017;30(14):1666–70.
55. Malviya MN, Ohlsson A, Shah SS. Surgical versus medical treatment with cyclooxygenase inhibitors for symptomatic patent ductus arteriosus in preterm infants. Cochrane Database Syst Rev. 2013;(3):CD003951.
56. Friedman WF, Hirschklau MJ, Printz MP, Pitlick PT, Kirkpatrick SE. Pharmacologic closure of patent ductus arteriosus in the premature infant. N Engl J Med. 1976;295(10):526–9.
57. Malikiwi A, Roufaeil C, Tan K, Sehgal A. Indomethacin vs ibuprofen: comparison of efficacy in the setting of conservative therapeutic approach. Eur J Pediatr. 2015;174(5):615–20.
58. Yadav S, Agarwal S, Maria A, Dudeja A, Dubey NK, Anand P, et al. Comparison of oral ibuprofen with oral indomethacin for PDA closure in Indian preterm neonates: a randomized controlled trial. Pediatr Cardiol. 2014;35(5):824–30.
59. Van Overmeire B, Follens I, Hartmann S, Creten WL, Van Acker KJ. Treatment of patent ductus arteriosus with ibuprofen. Arch Dis Child Fetal Neonatal Ed. 1997;76(3):F179–84.
60. Ohlsson A, Walia R, Shah SS. Ibuprofen for the treatment of patent ductus arteriosus in preterm or low birth weight (or both) infants. Cochrane Database Syst Rev. 2015;(2):CD003481.
61. Dornelles LV, Corso AL, Silveira Rde C, Procianoy RS. Comparison of two dose regimens of ibuprofen for the closure of patent ductus arteriosus in preterm newborns. J Pediatr. 2016;92(3):314–8.
62. Mitra S, Florez ID, Tamayo ME, Mbuagbaw L, Vanniyasingam T, Veroniki AA, et al. Association of placebo, indomethacin, ibuprofen, and acetaminophen with closure of hemodynamically significant patent ductus arteriosus in preterm infants: a systematic review and meta-analysis. JAMA. 2018;319(12):1221–38.
63. Olukman O, Calkavur S, Ercan G, Atlihan F, Oner T, Tavli V, et al. Comparison of oral and intravenous ibuprofen for medical closure of patent ductus arteriosus: which one is better? Congenit Heart Dis. 2012;7(6):534–43.
64. Sarici SU, Dabak O, Erdinc K, Okutan V, Lenk MK. An unreported complication of intravenously administered ibuprofen: gastrointestinal bleeding. Eur Rev Med Pharmacol Sci. 2012;16(3):325–7.
65. Hammerman C, Bin-Nun A, Markovitch E, Schimmel MS, Kaplan M, Fink D. Ductal closure with paracetamol: a surprising new approach to patent ductus arteriosus treatment. Pediatrics. 2011;128(6):e1618–21.
66. Ohlsson A, Shah PS. Paracetamol (acetaminophen) for patent ductus arteriosus in preterm or low birth weight infants. Cochrane Database Syst Rev. 2018;4:CD010061.
67. Oncel MY, Eras Z, Uras N, Canpolat FE, Erdeve O, Oguz SS. Neurodevelopmental outcomes of preterm infants treated with oral paracetamol versus ibuprofen for patent ductus arteriosus. Am J Perinatol. 2017;34(12):1185–9.

68. Louis D, Torgalkar R, Shah J, Shah PS, Jain A. Enteral feeding during indomethacin treatment for patent ductus arteriosus: association with gastrointestinal outcomes. J Perinatol. 2016;36(7):544–8.

69. Mirea L, Sankaran K, Seshia M, Ohlsson A, Allen AC, Aziz K, et al. Treatment of patent ductus arteriosus and neonatal mortality/morbidities: adjustment for treatment selection bias. J Pediatr. 2012;161(4):689–94.e1.

70. Youn Y, Moon CJ, Lee JY, Lee C, Sung IK. Timing of surgical ligation and morbidities in very low birth weight infants. Medicine. 2017;96(14):e6557.

71. Sung SI, Chang YS, Chun JY, Yoon SA, Yoo HS, Ahn SY, et al. Mandatory closure versus non-intervention for patent ductus arteriosus in very preterm infants. J Pediatr. 2016;177:66–71.e1.

72. Weisz DE, Mirea L, Rosenberg E, Jang M, Ly L, Church PT, et al. Association of patent ductus arteriosus ligation with death or neurodevelopmental impairment among extremely preterm infants. JAMA Pediatr. 2017;171(5):443–9.

73. Weisz DE, More K, McNamara PJ, Shah PS. PDA ligation and health outcomes: a meta-analysis. Pediatrics. 2014;133(4):e1024–46.

74. Hallik M, Tasa T, Starkopf J, Metsvaht T. Dosing of milrinone in preterm neonates to prevent postligation cardiac syndrome: simulation study suggests need for bolus infusion. Neonatology. 2017;111(1):8–11.

75. Jabbour J, Uhing M, Robey T. Vocal fold paralysis in preterm infants: prevalence and analysis of risk factors. J Perinatol. 2017;37(5):585–90.

76. Hsu KH, Chiang MC, Lien R, Chu JJ, Chang YS, Chu SM, et al. Diaphragmatic paralysis among very low birth weight infants following ligation for patent ductus arteriosus. Eur J Pediatr. 2012;171(11):1639–44.

77. Kim D, Kim SW, Shin HJ, Hong JM, Lee JH, Han HS. Unintended pulmonary artery ligation during PDA ligation. Heart Surg Forum. 2016;19(4):E187–8.

78. Resende MH, More K, Nicholls D, Ting J, Jain A, McNamara PJ. The impact of a dedicated patent ductus arteriosus ligation team on neonatal health-care outcomes. J Perinatol. 2016;36(6):463–8.

79. Morville P, Akhavi A. Transcatheter closure of hemodynamic significant patent ductus arteriosus in 32 premature infants by amplatzer ductal occluder additional size-ADOIIAS. Catheter Cardiovasc Interv. 2017;90(4):612–7.

80. Morville P, Douchin S, Bouvaist H, Dauphin C. Transcatheter occlusion of the patent ductus arteriosus in premature infants weighing less than 1200 g. Arch Dis Child Fetal Neonatal Ed. 2018;103(3):F198–f201.

81. Dedeoglu R, Bilici M, Demir F, Demir F, Acar OC, Hallioglu O, et al. Short-term outcomes of patent ductus arteriosus closure with new Occlutech(R) duct occluder: a multicenter study. J Interv Cardiol. 2016;29(3):325–31.

82. Zanjani KS, Sobhy R, El-Kaffas R, El-Sisi A. Multicenter off-label use of nit-occlud coil in retrograde closure of small patent ductus arteriosus. Pediatr Cardiol. 2017;38(4):828–32.

83. Wang-Giuffre EW, Breinholt JP. Novel use of the medtronic micro vascular plug for PDA closure in preterm infants. Catheter Cardiovasc Interv. 2017;89(6):1059–65.

84. Sathanandam S, Justino H, Waller BR 3rd, Radtke W, Qureshi AM. Initial clinical experience with the Medtronic micro vascular plug in transcatheter occlusion of PDAs in extremely premature infants. Catheter Cardiovasc Interv. 2017;89(6):1051–8.

85. Patel PM, Momany AM, Schaa KL, Romitti PA, Druschel C, Cooper ME, et al. Genetic modifiers of patent ductus arteriosus in term infants. J Pediatr. 2016;176:57–61.e1.

Chapter 15
Glucocorticoid Treatment for Bronchopulmonary Dysplasia

Tanja Restin and Dirk Bassler

Abbreviations

ACTH	Adrenocorticotropic hormone
aOR	Adjusted odds ratio
BPD	Bronchopulmonary dysplasia
BSID	Bayley Scales of Infant Development
CI	Confidence interval
CP	Cerebral palsy
HPA	Hypothalamic-pituitary-adrenal
NNT	Number needed to treat
PMA	Postmenstrual age
RCT	Randomised controlled trial
RD	Risk difference
ROP	Retinopathy of prematurity
RR	Risk reduction

Introduction

Cortisone is a steroid hormone which has been characterized by Kendall in 1949 as "compound E" extracted from adrenal glands [1]. Due to its broad effects concerning the stress response, circadian rhythm and immunity, it became heavily used in very different medical fields ranging from allergies to cancer, from autoimmune diseases to circulatory support. However, the exact mechanism of action is still unclear. In newborns, corticosteroids are effective in the prevention of bronchopulmonary dysplasia, might help to speed up the extubation procedure but also have

T. Restin · D. Bassler (✉)
Department of Neonatology, University Hospital Zurich, University of Zurich, Zurich, Switzerland
e-mail: tanja.restin@usz.ch; dirk.bassler@usz.ch

© Springer Nature Switzerland AG 2020
E. M. Boyle, J. Cusack (eds.), *Emerging Topics and Controversies in Neonatology*, https://doi.org/10.1007/978-3-030-28829-7_15

relevant negative side effects, especially long-term. Beside the physiological background, we will highlight the current evidence concerning systemic, inhaled and instilled glucocorticoids with a special focus on very preterm infants.

Corticosteroids: Mechanism of Action

The hypothalamic-pituitary-adrenal (HPA) axis is activated when an organism is under stress such that survival is prioritised over less essential physiological functions. When activated, the hypothalamus releases corticotropin releasing factor and arginine vasopressin via the pituitary glands. Subsequent secretion of adrenocorticotropic hormone (ACTH) then stimulates the adrenal glands to produce corticosteroids as an adaptive stress response. It has been shown that invasive procedures can lead to increased cortisol levels in fetuses starting at about 20 weeks of gestational age, independent from the maternal stress response [2]. However, stress response matures with gestational age. Overall fetal basal levels of cortisol are low, ranging from 20 to 50 nmol/L [3], which is five- to ten-fold lower compared to maternal levels [4]. The activity of placental 11-β-hydroxysteroid dehydrogenase-type 2, which converts active cortisol into inactive cortisone, was recently identified as contributing to placental cortisol clearance. This placental enzyme activity explains the difference between basal maternal and fetal cortisol levels [5].

Corticosteroids affect all organ systems, change body metabolism and regulate water balance [6]. In fetuses, these hormones promote organ maturation and significantly increase postnatal viability [7, 8]. Corticosteroids induce the breakdown of fats [9], carbohydrates [10] and proteins [11] and thereby rapidly mobilise energy. Additionally, they interfere with the action of insulin, contributing to hyperglycaemia [12]. These catabolic effects, summarised as "fight to flight response" have been attributed to the glucocorticoid activity of steroids [13]. Additionally, corticosteroids contribute to the retention of salt and water, an effect attributed to the mineralocorticoid activity [14]. The molecular mechanisms behind all these findings are still not fully elucidated.

Corticosteroids and Inflammation

Corticosteroids suppress inflammation and immune response [13]. The anti-inflammatory effect of corticosteroids has partially been explained by the inhibition of the promoter region of pro-inflammatory cytokines [15, 16], their post-translational modification [17], the trapping of activated NFκB (nuclear factor kappa-light-chain-enhancer of activated B cells) [18], and the activation of anti-inflammatory cytokines such as TGFβ (transforming growth factor β) [16].

Corticosteroid activity correlates with the regulation of protein synthesis [19]. Moreover, corticosteroids reduce the production and release of prostaglandins [20,

21]. Studies of the inhalation of the corticosteroid budesonide, demonstrated that sphingosine-1 phosphate-induced secretion of the pro-inflammatory mediator interleukin 6 was decreased with corticosteroid application [22].

Critically ill patients, especially preterm infants, display lower levels of total serum cortisol, which may contribute to an overwhelming pro-inflammatory septic response [23]. On the other hand, corticosteroid treatment induces a neutrophilic leukocytosis after about 24 h [24]. In contrast to acute infections, corticosteroids do not induce a characteristic "left shift" with significant (more than 5%) amounts of immature neutrophils [25]. The main reason for the increased levels of neutrophils in the blood has shown to be the detachment of neutrophils from the endothelium [26]. The suppression of apoptosis and delayed tissue migration also contribute to increased neutrophil levels, with about 10% of the increase due to the release of neutrophils from the bone marrow [27]. Because inflammation decisively contributes to the pathogenesis of bronchopulmonary dysplasia (BPD) in preterm infants, corticosteroids are an anti-inflammatory therapeutic option [28].

Corticosteroids and the Lung

Postnatally, corticosteroids accelerate lung maturation, induce the thinning of double capillary loops and increase the levels of anti-oxidant enzymes [29]. They seem to induce surfactant production. However, postnatal corticosteroid concentration is not associated with improved survival [30, 31]. In animal studies, corticosteroid treatment led to impaired saccular septation and to a decreased final number of alveoli compared to untreated controls [29, 32]. Consequently, it remains unknown if corticosteroids might also reduce the final alveolar surface area in humans. A cross-sectional study of 105 children born between 1992 and 1994 demonstrated that those treated with postnatal glucocorticoids displayed worse expiratory flows in spirometry tests 10 years later [33]. However, the cohort of children who received postnatal glucocorticoids was born at a significantly lower gestational age and had longer treatment periods for both mechanical ventilation and oxygen. Nevertheless, especially ventilator dependent newborns often showed remarkable short term-improvement of lung-function [34].

Natural and Synthetic Corticosteroids

Natural Corticosteroids

Natural corticosteroids have both glucocorticoid and mineralocorticoid activity, with varying relative activities [35]. For example, cortisol has almost no mineralocorticoid activity whereas aldosterone has nearly exclusive mineralocorticoid activity [36, 37]. In cases of adrenal insufficiency, children display signs of fatigue and weakness, hypoglycaemia and gastrointestinal complaints. Excess cortisol also activates type I mineralocorticoid receptors to induce mineralocorticoid activity [38]. The majority of serum cortisol is bound to proteins, namely albumin and corticosteroid-binding protein, facilitating the transport of this lipophilic agent via the blood stream [39]. Physiological maintenance dose of hydrocortisone is 6–12 mg/m²/day. After correction for surface area, the doses in infants and children are comparable [40, 41]. Corticosteroids generally display a physiological pulsatile secretion which leads to an ultradian rhythm in all studied species [42]. In extremely low birthweight infants, these pulsations show lower variations compared to mature newborns [43]. The cortisol response may be changed by polymorphisms in the glucocorticoid receptor [44]. Moreover, several drugs, such as phenobarbital, phenytoin and rifampin induce the P450 enzyme system and thereby induce corticosteroid clearance [45, 46].

Synthetic Corticosteroids

Synthetic corticosteroids, namely hydrocortisone (synthetic cortisone), mimic the action of the naturally occurring corticosteroids and can be substituted in case of adrenal gland insufficiency. However, unlike cortisol they have little or no affinity to plasma proteins but circulate freely. High doses of synthetic corticosteroids have been used in a broad range of indications from acute allergic reactions, immunological diseases, acute leukaemia and treatment of post-operative nausea to lung maturation in preterm infants. Interestingly, two doses of either dexamethasone (6 mg) or betamethasone (12 mg) given maternally 24 h before birth significantly improve the overall mortality and morbidity of a preterm baby [47]. Chemical modification of corticosteroids, such as 6-alpha or 9-alpha fluorination in dexamethasone, fludrocortisone and betamethasone, or 6-alpha methylation in methylprednisolone or methyloxazoline addition at positions 16 or 17 in delfazacort, can protect from oxidation by 11-β-hydroxysteroid dehydrogenase-type 2 in the placenta. Postnatally, corticosteroid metabolism occurs primarily in the liver, and both the active compound and inactive metabolites are excreted into the urine [48, 49]. In the following sections we will focus on the current pulmonary indications of corticosteroid use in newborn care, which mainly refers to the application of glucocorticoids.

Application of Glucocorticoids in Neonates

In contrast to the huge benefits of prenatal corticosteroids, the application of postnatal glucocorticoids to newborns is controversial. Currently, postnatal glucocorticoids are administered to the preterm infant in three different ways, most commonly through systemic administration, but alternative promising delivery methods through inhalation or direct tracheal instillation mixed with surfactant are also utilized.

Systemic Glucocorticoids

The American Pediatric Society [50], the Canadian Pediatric Society [51] and the European Association of Perinatal Medicine currently do not advocate the general use of systemic glucocorticoids [52]. Although there was a significant decline in usage since the late 1990s, recent studies found that 8–9% of newborns born with very low birth weight are treated with glucocorticoids postnatally [53–55]. Some studies even demonstrated that among children weighing below 750 g, more than 20% were treated with glucocorticoids [54], although only two thirds were on significant respiratory support [55]. The most commonly prescribed synthetic corticosteroid for newborns was dexamethasone, which shows both the greatest efficacy and the most side effects [30].

Historically, this drug was chosen for neonatal application because of its predominant glucocorticoid activity and long half-life [34]. In extremely low birth weight infants, the half-life of dexamethasone is approximately 9 ± 3 h, which is longer than in children and adults [56]. Dexamethasone is lipophilic and easily crosses the blood brain barrier. While the effects of glucocorticoids on the brain have not been studied in detail in humans, animal studies suggest that dexamethasone negatively affects neuronal, especially hippocampal function [57, 58]. The timing of the glucocorticoid treatment seems to play an important role for both efficacy and potential harm.

Early Systemic Dexamethasone

A systematic review from the Cochrane Collaboration looked at neonates receiving early postnatal dexamethasone treatment, defined as treatment during the first 7 days of life. It yielded the following results: dexamethasone treatment did not influence mortality assessed at 36 weeks of postmenstrual age (PMA) (Relative risk (RR) 1.08, 95% Confidence Interval (CI) 0.94–1.25 in 2487 newborns recruited in 14 studies). At the same PMA, it significantly reduced the rate of BPD (RR 0.71, 95% CI 0.62–0.81; $p < 0.001$ in 2584 infants in 16 studies). The composite outcome of death or BPD both after 28 days (RR 0.91 95% CI 0.86–0.96, $p < 0.001$) and at 36 weeks of PMA (RR 0.87, 95% CI 0.8–0.94, $p < 0.001$) was significantly better after dexamethasone treatment. Moreover, it significantly reduced the rate of extubation failure by day 3, 7, and 28 by 16–29% (3 days, RR 0.73, 95% CI 0.62–0.86; 7 days: RR 0.71, 95% CI 0.61–0.84, 28 days: RR 0.84, 95% CI 0.72–0.98). Interestingly, the rate of retinopathy of prematurity (ROP), including severe ROP, was reduced (RR 0.84, 95% CI 0.72–0.99, $p = 0.03$ including 359 infants in seven studies). However, it was observed that the application of dexamethasone increased the risks of hypertension (RR 1.84, 95% CI 1.53–2.21, RD 0.1), hyperglycaemia (RR 1.35, 95% CI 1.21–1.49, $p < 0.001$), gastrointestinal haemorrhage (1.87 95% CI 1.35–2.58, $p < 0.001$), gastrointestinal perforation (RD 0.03, 95% CI 0.01–0.05), growth failure (RR 6.67, 95% CI 2.27–19.62) and hypertrophic cardiomyopathy (HOCM) (RR 4.33, 95% CI 1.4–13.37). The data on growth failure and HOCM are based on a single study with 50 patients [59].

The risk for gastrointestinal perforation seems to be aggravated in combination with the use of indomethacin [60]. Notably, the rate of children with cerebral palsy (CP) was significantly increased (RR 1.75, 95% CI 1.20–2.55; RD 0.02 in seven studies including 921 infants). Shinwell et al. reported a significantly increased rate of CP or neurodevelopmental delay after a three-day course of dexamethasone treatment in the early postnatal period (Odds Ratio (OR) 4.62, 95% CI 2.38–8.98) [61].

Early Systemic Hydrocortisone

Hydrocortisone increases blood pressure and reduces vasopressor requirements [62]. Consequently, it is often primarily employed for neonatal refractory hypotension. The Cochrane review assessing the effects of treatment with early postnatal glucocorticoids for chronic lung disease also included studies in which low hydrocortisone doses were given for blood pressure management [31].

The half-life of hydrocortisone is relatively short, approximately 100 minutes [63]. It should be noted that while side effects of hydrocortisone have been shown to be reduced compared to dexamethasone, there is less demonstrated efficacy with this regimen. However, the subgroup analyses by the applied type of glucocorticoid revealed that early hydrocortisone treatment significantly reduced mortality to discharge (RR 0.8, 95% CI 0.65–0.98) [31]. This analysis included 1433 infants enrolled in 11 different studies ($p = 0.04$). Moreover, the combined outcome of death or BPD was significantly reduced at 36 weeks of PMA (RR 0.9, 95% CI 0.82–0.99 including the data of 1379 infants in 9 trials).

The dose of hydrocortisone varied considerably between 15 mg/kg/dose given twice within 24 h [64] and 1 mg/kg loading dose followed by 0.5 mg/kg maintenance treatment for varying periods. Side effects such as hypertension (RR 3, 95% CI 0.33–26.9 in 1 study with 50 infants [65]) and gastrointestinal perforation (RR 1.7, 95% CI 1.07–2.7 in seven studies including 1104 infants, $p = 0.02$) were noted. One multicentre randomised trial of hydrocortisone to prevent early adrenal insufficiency was stopped because of an increase in spontaneous gastrointestinal perforation in the hydrocortisone group [66]. This study concluded that the combination of hydrocortisone and indomethacin should be avoided.

Concerning long term effects, there has been no reported association with the development of CP (RR 1.05, 95% CI 0.66–1.66 in six studies including 1052 infants, $p = 0.84$). The PREMILOC study, a multicenter French randomised controlled trial (RCT), demonstrated that early low dose hydrocortisone with

0.5 mg/kg of hydrocortisone hemisuccinate twice a day for 7 days, followed by 0.5 mg/kg once a day for a further 3 days significantly increased the survival rate without BPD at 36 weeks PMA (adjusted OR 1.48, 95% CI 1.02–2.16, $p = 0.04$) [67]. However, this trial was closed early due to a lack of funding [68].

A subgroup analysis of children between 24 and 25 weeks of PMA age detected a significantly increased rate of sepsis. At 2-year follow-up, there was no statistically significant difference in neurodevelopmental outcomes [69]. As the original study was not powered for detection of neurodevelopmental differences, this secondary analysis should be interpreted with caution. Future international studies with a neurological follow up later than 2 years of age would enable detection of subtle neurological differences between the different treatment groups and increase the confidence in the early administration of low dose hydrocortisone for the prevention of BPD.

Late Systemic Glucocorticoids

The Cochrane review on late treatment with glucocorticoids did not clearly differentiate between studies giving dexamethasone (about two third) and those with hydrocortisone (about one third) [30]. Taken together, neonatal mortality within the first 28 days was significantly reduced (RR 0.49, 95% CI 0.28–0.85, $p = 0.011$). Late postnatal glucocorticoid treatment reduces the rate of BPD at 36 weeks of PMA (RR 0.77, 95% CI 0.67–0.88, $p < 0.001$). Moreover, the rate of extubation failure is reduced by the third day (RR 0.76, 95% CI 0.69–0.84, $p > 0.001$), seventh day (RR 0.65, 95% CI 0.59–0.72, $p < 0.001$), and 28th day (RR 0.58, 95% CI 0.37–0.89, $p = 0.013$).

Late postnatal glucocorticoid treatment reduces the rate of children who have to be discharged with home oxygen therapy by 29% (RR 0.71, 95% CI 0.54–0.94, $p = 0.018$). Despite these benefits, the authors of the review concluded that the lower risk of BPD "may not outweigh" the actual or potential adverse effects of late systemic glucocorticoid therapy.

Short-term adverse effects include hyperglycaemia (RR 1.51, 95% CI 1.26–1.81), glycosuria (RR 8.03 95% CI 2.43–26.52, $p < 0.001$), and hypertension (RR 2.12, 95% CI 1.45–3.1, $p < 0.001$). Additionally, late postnatal glucocorticoid administration increases the rate of children with HOCM (RR 2.76, 95% CI 1.33–5.74, $p = 0.0064$). The risk of severe ROP is increased (RR 1.38, 95% CI 1.07–1.79, $p = 0.014$, 12 studies including 558 infants).

The risk of CP at 1–3 years of age was not significantly increased among infants who were treated with systemic glucocorticoids when they were more than 7 days old (RR 1.1, 95% CI 0.79–1.54, $p = 0.57$). However, when assessing four studies reporting an "abnormal neurological exam" with variable criteria for long-term follow up, those with late dexamethasone treatment had a significantly worse outcome (RR 1.81, 95% CI 1.05–3.11, $p = 0.033$, comprising 200 patients).

The highest effect in this meta-analysis can be attributed to the study of Kothadia, which used a 42 day course of dexamethasone treatment [70]. The European Consensus Guideline on the Management of Respiratory Distress Syndrome 2016 suggested "low dose dexamethasone <0.2 mg/kg/day" for babies who remain ventilator dependent after 1–2 weeks [52] and the update of the current guideline 2019 still advises "the smallest effective dose" for "babies at highest risk of BPD" [71].

Valid data on the use of alternative glucocorticoids such as hydrocortisone is lacking. The recently completed SToP-BPD study will address whether hydrocortisone treatment applied between day 7 and 14 is indicated in neonates and if so, under which conditions [72, 73].

Inhaled Glucocorticoids

Administration of inhaled glucocorticoids could theoretically suppress pulmonary inflammation, while having fewer side effects than systemic application of glucocorticoids. This hypothesis was addressed in a meta-analysis published by Shinwell et al., which includes 16 randomised controlled trials [74]. These trials investigated the role of various inhaled glucocorticoids. The intervention initiation varied from day 1 to 60 days of life. The primary composite outcome of mortality or BPD was significantly reduced in the glucocorticoid treatment group (RR 0.86, 95% CI 0.75–0.99; $p = 0.03$, $n = 1285$ in 6 trials). The incidence of BPD at 36 weeks of PMA was also significantly reduced with a number needed to treat (NNT) of 14 (RR 0.77, 95% CI 0.65–0.91, $p = 0.003$, $n = 1168$ in 7 trials) [74]. Inhaled glucocorticoids did not show any significant effect on the occurrence of sepsis, intraventricular hemorrhage, persistent ductus arteriosus, ophthalmic morbidities or necrotising enterocolitis.

The largest RCT included in the meta-analysis is the placebo-controlled NEuroSIS trial, which evaluated treatment with 400 mcg budesonide every 12 h in the first 14 days of life, and then 200 mcg every 12 h until the infants no longer needed supplemental oxygen or reached a PMA of 32 weeks [75].

In this trial, the composite outcome of death or BPD was reduced with borderline significance (RR stratified according to gestational age 0.86, 95% CI 0.75–1; $p = 0.05$). This treatment effect was due to a significant decrease in BPD (RR 0.74; 95% CI 0.6–0.91, $p = 0.004$). However, mortality rates were higher in the budesonide group, although this effect was not significant (RR 1.23; 95% CI 0.91–0.69, $p = 0.17$). Neither death certificates and autopsy reports nor post-hoc analyses could unravel reasons for this finding [76, 77].

Follow-up of patients enrolled in NEuroSIS did not show any significant difference in the only predefined secondary long term outcome, neurodevelopmental disability, which was defined as the composite of CP, cognitive delay (Bayley Mental Development Index score <85, BSID, second version), deafness or blindness between corrected age of 18–22 months (RR 0.93; 95% CI 0.80–1.09; $p = 0.40$). However, exploratory post-hoc analysis suggested more deaths in the budesonide group (RR 1.37; 95% CI 1.01–1.86, $p = 0.04$) [78]. The analyses were not adjusted for multiple testing and the difference in mortality largely reflected the difference in mortality before hospital discharge, so chance may have had an effect on these findings.

Intratracheal Glucocorticoids

Delivery of glucocorticoids to the periphery of the lungs may be facilitated by the aid of surfactant as a vehicle. With this approach, the beneficial properties of the surfactant therapy are not affected [79]. Additionally, the solubility and the absorption of budesonide may be enhanced with the addition of surfactants [80].

In a pilot trial with 116 newborns, Yeh and colleagues treated the neonates every 8 h with either 0.25 mg/kg of budesonide mixed with 100 mg/kg of surfactant (Survanta®) or surfactant alone. This therapy was performed every 8 h until the required fraction of inspired oxygen (FiO_2) was below 30% or until extubation. Inclusion criteria were very low birth weight (less than 1500 g) and severe respiratory distress, which was defined as mechanical ventilation with a FiO_2 of more than 0.6 shortly after birth [81]. This research group could demonstrate that the combined therapy with budesonide and surfactant improved the combined outcome of death and chronic lung disease. A follow up trial with 265 infants was performed [82]. The meta-analysis of these two RCTs demonstrated that the budesonide/surfactant combination reduced the composite outcome of death and BPD (RR 0.6; 95% CI 0.49–0.74, $p < 0.001$, NNT 3), and BPD alone (RR 0.57, 95% CI 0.43–0.76; $p < 0.001$, NNT 5) [83]. With the exception of elevated blood pressure in the treatment group, both groups were comparable in somatic growth and in the number of adverse events including intraventricular haemorrhage or sepsis. The current data on instilled glucocorticoids is promising, but in our view, the results need to be replicated in larger RCTs before this approach can be safely adapted.

Issues that May Be Important when Considering Glucocorticoids in Newborn Care

In addition to the choice of drug (dexamethasone versus hydrocortisone), the time point of initiation ("early" versus "late") and the application route (systemic versus inhaled or instilled), the cumulative dose may play a role when it comes to safety and efficacy issues. Onland and colleagues evaluated the effects of different dosing regimens on rates of BPD and long-term neurodevelopment in another systematic review from the Cochrane Collaboration [84].

Some of the included studies reported a modulating effect of treatment regimens in favour of higher-dosage regimens on the incidence of BPD and neurodevelopmental impairment. Despite this, they concluded that recommendations on the optimal type, dosage, or timing of initiation of corticosteroid for the prevention of BPD in preterm infants cannot be made based on the available data with a high level of credibility [84]. It remains to be resolved whether the short-term improvements of pulmonary function also translate into the reduction of long-term pulmonary complications.

An alternative way to interpret the available clinical trial data was suggested by Doyle et al. in an innovative meta-regression originally published in 2005 and updated in 2014 [85, 86]. The authors plotted net benefit or net harm (death or CP at 2 years) against the baseline BPD event rate (in control groups of infants) in the published RCTs. In this analysis, an excess risk associated with glucocorticoid use was evident when there was a low baseline risk of BPD. This shifts to a net benefit when the therapy is initiated at a higher event rate. The BPD risk at which dexamethasone treatment could be considered beneficial with more than 95% chance was determined to be above 60%. Although several prediction models have been proposed [87], the individual prediction of BPD risk remains difficult. In addition to calculation by available online tools (https://neonatal.rti.org/index.cfm), the regional BPD risk should be considered. Future studies on evaluation of glucocorticoids may thus focus on infants with a very high risk of developing BPD [88].

Conclusions

Synthetic systemic glucocorticoids are powerful drugs, which significantly reduce the risk for BPD and extubation failure in the short term. However, current recommendations suggest restricting the use to infants who can otherwise not be weaned from the ventilator, because systemic dexamethasone treatment is associated with impaired neurological outcomes.

Administration especially during the first week of life is associated with an increased rate of CP in the long term. Treatment with hydrocortisone during the first 7 days of life may be less beneficial for the lung compared with dexamethasone but improves the composite outcome of BPD and death at 36 weeks PMA. One concern is that early hydrocortisone treatment increases the risk of gastrointestinal perforation.

Late systemic glucocorticoid treatment (after 7 days) reduces the risk for BPD, but may also negatively affect neurological function. However, large studies powered for long term evaluation of neurological outcomes after glucocorticoid treatment are still missing. The inhalation with glucocorticoids, especially budesonide treatment reduces the rate of BPD at 36 weeks PMA, but the association with increased mortality in the largest trial is of potential concern. Another promising approach is the instillation of a mixture of glucocorticoids and surfactant, which has been shown to reduce the rate of BPD at 36 weeks PMA. Certainly, larger RCTs are needed to fully evaluate both useful and adverse effects of this treatment approach. For a summary of the main beneficial and harmful effects of various regimen of glucocorticoid application for BPD, see Table 15.1.

Table 15.1 Main benefits and harms of various corticosteroid regimens for BPD

Treatment	Benefit	Harm
Systemic early dexamethasone treatment (<8 days of life)	Reduction in BPD at 36 weeks PMA (RR 0.71, 95% CI 0.62–0.81; $p < 0.001$) [31]	Increase in CP at 2 years of age (RR 1.75, 95% CI 1.20–2.55; $p = 0.0038$) [31]
Systemic early hydrocortisone treatment (<8 days of life)	Reduction in BPD at 36 weeks not significant (RR 0.91, 95% CI 0.80–1.05; $p = 0.19$) but significant reduction in mortality to discharge (RR 0.8, 95% CI 0.65–0.98; $p = 0.035$) [31]	Increase in CP not significant (RR 1.05, 95% CI 0.66–1.66, $p = 0.84$) but significant increase in gastrointestinal perforation (RR 1.7, 95% CI 1.07–2.7, $p = 0.02$) [31]
Systemic late glucocorticoid treatment (>7 days of life)	Significant reduction in BPD at 36 weeks of PMA (RR 0.77, 95% CI 0.67–0.88, $p < 0.001$) [30]	Increase in CP not significant (RR 1.10, 95% CI 0.79–1.54, $p = 0.57$) but evidence for increase in abnormal neurological exam (RR 1.81, 95% CI 1.05–3.11, $p = 0.033$) [30]
Inhaled glucocorticoids	Significant reduction in BPD at 36 weeks of PMA (RR 0.74; 95% CI 0.6–0.91, $p = 0.004$) [74]	No effect on neurosensory impairment but suggested increase in mortality (RR 1.37; 95% CI 1.01–1.86, $p = 0.04$) [78]
Instilled glucocorticoids	Significant reduction in BPD (RR 0.57, 95% CI 0.43–0.76; $p < 0.001$) [83]	Besides increase in blood pressure, no detected side effects, but tested in a small number of patients

References

1. Kendall EC. Some observations on the hormone of the adrenal cortex designated compound E. Proc Staff Meet Mayo Clin. 1949;24(11):298–301.
2. Gitau R, et al. Fetal hypothalamic-pituitary-adrenal stress responses to invasive procedures are independent of maternal responses. J Clin Endocrinol Metab. 2001;86(1):104–9.
3. Nahoul K, et al. Plasma corticosteroid patterns in the fetus. J Steroid Biochem. 1988;29(6):635–40.
4. Beitins IZ, et al. The metabolic clearance rate, blood production, interconversion and transplacental passage of cortisol and cortisone in pregnancy near term. Pediatr Res. 1973;7(5):509–19.
5. Stirrat LI, et al. Transfer and metabolism of cortisol by the isolated perfused human placenta. J Clin Endocrinol Metab. 2018;103(2):640–8.
6. Liu D, et al. A practical guide to the monitoring and management of the complications of systemic corticosteroid therapy. Allergy Asthma Clin Immunol. 2013;9(1):30.
7. Liggins GC, Howie RN. A controlled trial of antepartum glucocorticoid treatment for prevention of the respiratory distress syndrome in premature infants. Pediatrics. 1972;50(4):515–25.
8. Liggins GC. Adrenocortical-related maturational events in the fetus. Am J Obstet Gynecol. 1976;126(7):931–41.
9. Rimsza ME. Complications of corticosteroid therapy. Am J Dis Child. 1978;132(8):806–10.
10. Lecocq FR, Mebane D, Madison LL. The acute effect of hydrocortisone on hepatic glucose output and peripheral glucose utilization. J Clin Invest. 1964;43:237–46.
11. Kaplan SA, Shimizu CS. Effects of cortisol on amino acids in skeletal muscle and plasma. Endocrinology. 1963;72:267–72.

12. van Raalte DH, Ouwens DM, Diamant M. Novel insights into glucocorticoid-mediated diabetogenic effects: towards expansion of therapeutic options? Eur J Clin Invest. 2009;39(2):81–93.
13. Coutinho AE, Chapman KE. The anti-inflammatory and immunosuppressive effects of glucocorticoids, recent developments and mechanistic insights. Mol Cell Endocrinol. 2011;335(1):2–13.
14. Mulrow PJ, Forman BH. The tissue effects of mineralocorticoids. Am J Med. 1972;53(5):561–72.
15. Zhang G, Zhang L, Duff GW. A negative regulatory region containing a glucocorticosteroid response element (nGRE) in the human interleukin-1beta gene. DNA Cell Biol. 1997;16(2):145–52.
16. Almawi WY, et al. Regulation of cytokine and cytokine receptor expression by glucocorticoids. J Leukoc Biol. 1996;60(5):563–72.
17. Rhen T, Cidlowski JA. Antiinflammatory action of glucocorticoids—new mechanisms for old drugs. N Engl J Med. 2005;353(16):1711–23.
18. Auphan N, et al. Immunosuppression by glucocorticoids: inhibition of NF-kappa B activity through induction of I kappa B synthesis. Science. 1995;270(5234):286–90.
19. O'Malley BW. Mechanisms of action of steroid hormones. N Engl J Med. 1971;284(7):370–7.
20. Perretti M, D'Acquisto F. Annexin A1 and glucocorticoids as effectors of the resolution of inflammation. Nat Rev Immunol. 2009;9(1):62–70.
21. Lewis GP, Piper PJ. Inhibition of release of prostaglandins as an explanation of some of the actions of anti-inflammatory corticosteroids. Nature. 1975;254(5498):308–11.
22. Che W, et al. Corticosteroids inhibit sphingosine 1-phosphate-induced interleukin-6 secretion from human airway smooth muscle via mitogen-activated protein kinase phosphatase 1-mediated repression of mitogen and stress-activated protein kinase 1. Am J Respir Cell Mol Biol. 2014;50(2):358–68.
23. Marik PE, et al. Recommendations for the diagnosis and management of corticosteroid insufficiency in critically ill adult patients: consensus statements from an international task force by the American College of Critical Care Medicine. Crit Care Med. 2008;36(6):1937–49.
24. Shoenfeld Y, et al. Prednisone-induced leukocytosis. Influence of dosage, method and duration of administration on the degree of leukocytosis. Am J Med. 1981;71(5):773–8.
25. Calhoun DA, Kirk JF, Christensen RD. Incidence, significance, and kinetic mechanism responsible for leukemoid reactions in patients in the neonatal intensive care unit: a prospective evaluation. J Pediatr. 1996;129(3):403–9.
26. Juul SE, Haynes JW, McPherson RJ. Evaluation of neutropenia and neutrophilia in hospitalized preterm infants. J Perinatol. 2004;24(3):150–7.
27. Akgul C, Moulding DA, Edwards SW. Molecular control of neutrophil apoptosis. FEBS Lett. 2001;487(3):318–22.
28. Ghanta S, Leeman KT, Christou H. An update on pharmacologic approaches to bronchopulmonary dysplasia. Semin Perinatol. 2013;37(2):115–23.
29. Vyas J, Kotecha S. Effects of antenatal and postnatal corticosteroids on the preterm lung. Arch Dis Child Fetal Neonatal Ed. 1997;77(2):F147–50.
30. Doyle LW, et al. Late (>7 days) systemic postnatal corticosteroids for prevention of bronchopulmonary dysplasia in preterm infants. Cochrane Database Syst Rev. 2017;10:CD001145.
31. Doyle LW, et al. Early (<8 days) systemic postnatal corticosteroids for prevention of bronchopulmonary dysplasia in preterm infants. Cochrane Database Syst Rev. 2017;10:CD001146.
32. Massaro D, et al. Postnatal development of alveoli. Regulation and evidence for a critical period in rats. J Clin Invest. 1985;76(4):1297–305.
33. Smith LJ, et al. Post-natal corticosteroids are associated with reduced expiratory flows in children born very preterm. J Paediatr Child Health. 2011;47(7):448–54.
34. Mammel MC, et al. Controlled trial of dexamethasone therapy in infants with bronchopulmonary dysplasia. Lancet. 1983;1(8338):1356–8.
35. Stewart PM, Mason JI. Cortisol to cortisone: glucocorticoid to mineralocorticoid. Steroids. 1995;60(1):143–6.

36. Meikle AW, Tyler FH. Potency and duration of action of glucocorticoids. Effects of hydrocortisone, prednisone and dexamethasone on human pituitary-adrenal function. Am J Med. 1977;63(2):200–7.
37. Munoz-Durango N, et al. Modulation of immunity and inflammation by the mineralocorticoid receptor and aldosterone. Biomed Res Int. 2015;2015:652738.
38. Clore J, Schoolwerth A, Watlington CO. When is cortisol a mineralocorticoid? Kidney Int. 1992;42(6):1297–308.
39. Sandberg AA, Slaunwhite WR Jr, Antoniades HN. The binding of steroids and steroid conjugates to human plasma proteins. Recent Prog Horm Res. 1957;13:209–60; discussion 260–7
40. Linder BL, et al. Cortisol production rate in childhood and adolescence. J Pediatr. 1990;117(6):892–6.
41. Kenny FM, Malvaux P, Migeon CJ. Cortisol production rate in newborn babies, older infants, and children. Pediatrics. 1963;31:360–73.
42. Lightman SL, et al. The significance of glucocorticoid pulsatility. Eur J Pharmacol. 2008;583(2–3):255–62.
43. Jett PL, et al. Variability of plasma cortisol levels in extremely low birth weight infants. J Clin Endocrinol Metab. 1997;82(9):2921–5.
44. Cvijanovich NZ, et al. Glucocorticoid receptor polymorphisms and outcomes in pediatric septic shock. Pediatr Crit Care Med. 2017;18(4):299–303.
45. Putignano P, et al. The effects of anti-convulsant drugs on adrenal function. Horm Metab Res. 1998;30(6–7):389–97.
46. McAllister WA, et al. Rifampicin reduces effectiveness and bioavailability of prednisolone. Br Med J (Clin Res Ed). 1983;286(6369):923–5.
47. Roberts D, et al. Antenatal corticosteroids for accelerating fetal lung maturation for women at risk of preterm birth. Cochrane Database Syst Rev. 2017;3:CD004454.
48. Mahesh VB, Ulrich F. Metabolism of cortisol and cortisone by various tissues and subcellular particles. J Biol Chem. 1960;235:356–60.
49. Shackleton CH. Mass spectrometry in the diagnosis of steroid-related disorders and in hypertension research. J Steroid Biochem Mol Biol. 1993;45(1–3):127–40.
50. Committee on Fetus and Newborn. Postnatal corticosteroids to treat or prevent chronic lung disease in preterm infants. Pediatrics. 2002;109(2):330–8.
51. Postnatal corticosteroids to treat or prevent chronic lung disease in preterm infants. Paediatr Child Health. 2002;7(1):20–46.
52. Sweet DG, et al. European consensus guidelines on the management of respiratory distress syndrome—2016 update. Neonatology. 2017;111(2):107–25.
53. Walsh MC, et al. Changes in the use of postnatal steroids for bronchopulmonary dysplasia in 3 large neonatal networks. Pediatrics. 2006;118(5):e1328–35.
54. Soll RF, et al. Obstetric and neonatal care practices for infants 501 to 1500 g from 2000 to 2009. Pediatrics. 2013;132(2):222–8.
55. Virkud YV, et al. Respiratory support for very low birth weight infants receiving dexamethasone. J Pediatr. 2017;183:26–30.e3.
56. Charles B, et al. Pharmacokinetics of dexamethasone following single-dose intravenous administration to extremely low birth weight infants. Dev Pharmacol Ther. 1993;20(3–4):205–10.
57. Cotterrell M, Balazs R, Johnson AL. Effects of corticosteroids on the biochemical maturation of rat brain: postnatal cell formation. J Neurochem. 1972;19(9):2151–67.
58. Huang CC, et al. Effects of neonatal corticosteroid treatment on hippocampal synaptic function. Pediatr Res. 2007;62(3):267–70.
59. Romagnoli C, et al. Effect on growth of two different dexamethasone courses for preterm infants at risk of chronic lung disease. A randomized trial. Pharmacology. 1999;59(5):266–74.
60. Stark AR, et al. Adverse effects of early dexamethasone treatment in extremely-low-birth-weight infants. National Institute of Child Health and Human Development Neonatal Research Network. N Engl J Med. 2001;344(2):95–101.

61. Shinwell ES, et al. Early postnatal dexamethasone treatment and increased incidence of cerebral palsy. Arch Dis Child Fetal Neonatal Ed. 2000;83(3):F177–81.
62. Higgins S, Friedlich P, Seri I. Hydrocortisone for hypotension and vasopressor dependence in preterm neonates: a meta-analysis. J Perinatol. 2010;30(6):373–8.
63. Cranny RL, Kirschvink JF, Kelley VC. The half-life of hydrocortisone in normal newborn infants. AMA J Dis Child. 1960;99:437–43.
64. Baden M, et al. A controlled trial of hydrocortisone therapy in infants with respiratory distress syndrome. Pediatrics. 1972;50(4):526–34.
65. Bonsante F, et al. Early low-dose hydrocortisone in very preterm infants: a randomized, placebo-controlled trial. Neonatology. 2007;91(4):217–21.
66. Watterberg KL, et al. Prophylaxis of early adrenal insufficiency to prevent bronchopulmonary dysplasia: a multicenter trial. Pediatrics. 2004;114(6):1649–57.
67. Baud O, et al. Effect of early low-dose hydrocortisone on survival without bronchopulmonary dysplasia in extremely preterm infants (PREMILOC): a double-blind, placebo-controlled, multicentre, randomised trial. Lancet. 2016;387(10030):1827–36.
68. Wang H, Rosner GL, Goodman SN. Quantifying over-estimation in early stopped clinical trials and the "freezing effect" on subsequent research. Clin Trials. 2016;13(6):621–31.
69. Baud O, et al. Association between early low-dose hydrocortisone therapy in extremely preterm neonates and neurodevelopmental outcomes at 2 years of age. JAMA. 2017;317(13):1329–37.
70. Kothadia JM, et al. Randomized placebo-controlled trial of a 42-day tapering course of dexamethasone to reduce the duration of ventilator dependency in very low birth weight infants. Pediatrics. 1999;104(1 Pt 1):22–7.
71. Sweet DG, et al. European consensus guidelines on the management of respiratory distress syndrome—2019 update. Neonatology. 2019;115(4):432–50.
72. Onland W, et al. Systemic hydrocortisone to prevent bronchopulmonary dysplasia in preterm infants (the SToP-BPD study): statistical analysis plan. Trials. 2018;19(1):178.
73. Onland W, et al. Systemic hydrocortisone to prevent bronchopulmonary dysplasia in preterm infants (the SToP-BPD study); a multicenter randomized placebo controlled trial. BMC Pediatr. 2011;11:102.
74. Shinwell ES, et al. Inhaled corticosteroids for bronchopulmonary dysplasia: a meta-analysis. Pediatrics. 2016;138(6).
75. Bassler D. Inhalation or instillation of steroids for the prevention of bronchopulmonary dysplasia. Neonatology. 2015;107(4):358–9.
76. Bassler D, et al. Early inhaled budesonide for the prevention of bronchopulmonary dysplasia. N Engl J Med. 2015;373(16):1497–506.
77. Koch A, et al. Inhaled glucocorticoids and pneumonia in preterm infants: post hoc results from the NEuroSIS trial. Neonatology. 2017;112(2):110–3.
78. Bassler D, et al. Long-term effects of inhaled budesonide for bronchopulmonary dysplasia. N Engl J Med. 2018;378(2):148–57.
79. Nimmo AJ, et al. Intratracheal administration of glucocorticoids using surfactant as a vehicle. Clin Exp Pharmacol Physiol. 2002;29(8):661–5.
80. Wiedmann TS, Bhatia R, Wattenberg LW. Drug solubilization in lung surfactant. J Control Release. 2000;65(1–2):43–7.
81. Yeh TF, et al. Early intratracheal instillation of budesonide using surfactant as a vehicle to prevent chronic lung disease in preterm infants: a pilot study. Pediatrics. 2008;121(5):e1310–8.
82. Yeh TF, et al. Intratracheal administration of budesonide/surfactant to prevent bronchopulmonary dysplasia. Am J Respir Crit Care Med. 2016;193(1):86–95.
83. Venkataraman R, et al. Intratracheal administration of budesonide-surfactant in prevention of bronchopulmonary dysplasia in very low birth weight infants: a systematic review and meta-analysis. Pediatr Pulmonol. 2017;52(7):968–75.
84. Onland W, et al. Systemic corticosteroid regimens for prevention of bronchopulmonary dysplasia in preterm infants. Cochrane Database Syst Rev. 2017;1:CD010941.

85. Doyle LW, et al. Impact of postnatal systemic corticosteroids on mortality and cerebral palsy in preterm infants: effect modification by risk for chronic lung disease. Pediatrics. 2005;115(3):655–61.
86. Doyle LW, et al. An update on the impact of postnatal systemic corticosteroids on mortality and cerebral palsy in preterm infants: effect modification by risk of bronchopulmonary dysplasia. J Pediatr. 2014;165(6):1258–60.
87. Laughon MM, et al. Prediction of bronchopulmonary dysplasia by postnatal age in extremely premature infants. Am J Respir Crit Care Med. 2011;183(12):1715–22.
88. Doyle LW, Cheong JLY. Postnatal corticosteroids to prevent or treat bronchopulmonary dysplasia—who might benefit? Semin Fetal Neonatal Med. 2017;22(5):290–5.

Chapter 16
Feeding and Nutrition

Nicholas D. Embleton

Introduction: The Nutritional Vulnerability of Preterm Infants

Dietary nutrients not only provide the building blocks for new tissue, but also promote growth and development by increasing the levels of endogenous growth factors such as IGF-1 [1] which in turn are critical for the growth of neural tissue including the brain and retina [2]. The multiple mechanisms that link poor nutrition to worse longer term neurocognitive outcomes are listed in Table 16.1. The nutrient requirements of preterm infants are staggering: a preterm infant requires more energy (per kcal/kg/day) than an elite rider in the Tour de France, and needs a protein intake (in g/kg/day) equivalent to an adult eating a large beef burger every 2 h. This requirement exists in the context of a baby who, at 1 kg, is composed of only 100 g lean tissue with virtually no fat stores. The birth of a preterm infant deserves to be seen as a nutritional emergency requiring the immediate commencement of parenteral nutrition (PN) [3].

Necrotising enterocolitis (NEC) remains the most feared complication of neonatal medicine, and the role of probiotics and donor human milk (DHM) are discussed in later sections. Support for mothers to provide their own breast milk must be seen as a key priority of nutrition and feeding practice on every NICU, and providing early colostrum within 12–24 h of life directly into the cheek ('buccal colostrum') is now widely practised, despite the lack of large scale randomised controlled trials (RCTs).

Considerable data over the last few years show a dose-response relationship between mother's own milk (MOM) intake and improvements in almost every key neonatal morbidity including NEC, retinopathy of prematurity (ROP), late onset

N. D. Embleton (✉)
Newcastle Hospitals NHS Foundation Trust, Newcastle upon Tyne, UK
e-mail: Nicholas.embleton@ncl.ac.uk

© Springer Nature Switzerland AG 2020
E. M. Boyle, J. Cusack (eds.), *Emerging Topics and Controversies in Neonatology*, https://doi.org/10.1007/978-3-030-28829-7_16

Table 16.1 Mechanisms linking early nutrition and later brain outcome in preterm infants

Nutrient mechanism affecting brain	Example or explanation
Nutrient accretion into new tissue	Diets with insufficient macronutrient and micronutrient intakes will impair brain growth
Diet must contain nutrients providing energy for basal metabolism and new tissue synthesis	Dietary or stored carbohydrate and lipid provide energy, but tissue protein will be catabolised if diet does not meet energy needs
Nutrient impacts on growth factors and signaling molecules	Energy and protein (or amino acid) intakes affect IGF-1 concentrations which control neuronal processes of growth and differentiation
Nutrients affecting gene expression	B12, folate and choline (acting as methyl donors) and iron directly affect gene expression of neural tissues
Nutritional (food) sources affecting diseases that damage the developing brain	Lack of mother's own breast milk increases the incidence of NEC and other diseases associated with a 'cytokine storm' that damages white matter
Nutrient-microbe interactions	Increasing data show bi-directional connections as part of the Gut-Brain axes involving neural tissue, peptides and signaling molecules

sepsis (LOS) and chronic lung disease (CLD) as well as decreasing length of stay [4–6]. Indeed, it could be argued that one of the most important priorities in neonatal nutrition research is not to better understand how human milk exerts these amazing benefits, but simply how we best support mothers to increase the amount of MOM they are able to provide [7]. A recent community-based study in term infants showed that financial incentives improve breast-feeding rates: [8] given the time required for mothers to express MOM, and the associated opportunity costs (i.e. time that cannot be spent caring for the family, travelling or working), exploration of how we might improve MOM provision through the use of appropriate remuneration or incentives would appear to be an important research question on many NICUs.

Starting and Increasing Milk Feeds: What's New?

There are few recent high quality data on when best to start orogastric or nasogastric (OG/NG) milk feeds, although most NICUs now commence milk as soon as MOM is available often as 'buccal colostrum' [9]. The large Abnormal Doppler Enteral Prescription Trial (ADEPT) showed there was no benefit in delaying the start of enteral feeds for several days in high risk infants [10], and most units now start milk feeds in the first 48–72 h of life in the vast majority of preterm infants as soon as MOM is available. It is unlikely that future RCTs comparing the precise start date (e.g. day 1 or day 3) will be sufficiently large to show impacts on important outcomes such as NEC, sepsis, or length of stay.

A recently completed large RCT, the Speed of Increases in milk Feeds Trial (SIFT), looked at the effect of 'slow' or 'fast' increases in feeding rates on long-term developmental outcome at 2 years of age [11]. Whilst pre-discharge data showed little impact on rates of sepsis or NEC, and there was no overall impact on neurodevelopment at 2 years age, sub-group analysis has generated controversy [12]. Sub-group analyses suggests a slightly higher rate of moderate or severe motor impairment in the faster feed group, an effect that appears in the sub-group who were solely formulae fed (un-published data presented at European Academy of Pediatric Societies meeting, Paris, November 2018). The study includes multiple pre-specific secondary and sub-group analyses so this result may simply be due to chance, but no doubt will generate further debate on the optimal rate of speed increases.

However, given the size of SIFT (n = 2804) this RCT will dominate the Cochrane meta-analysis (MA) for the immediate future given that no other comparable large trials are registered as "in progress" [12]. In summary, many NICUs routinely use buccal colostrum, most will start milk feeds as soon as sufficient MOM becomes available, and most will use the results of the SIFT trial to guide feeding speed increases. If MOM is not available, we do not know whether it is better to start DHM in the first 1–2 days or whether we should wait longer for MOM to become available. Neonatal medicine is a global specialty and so it is also important to consider whether the evidence base is equally applicable in other contexts. For example, in low and middle-income countries (LMICs) where parenteral nutrition (PN) is not routinely available, the balance of risks and benefits of early milk feeds may differ, as might the effect of probiotics or other interventions.

Parenteral Nutrition

Early provision of parenteral energy and protein reduces postnatal weight loss, the risks of BPD and ROP, and in observational studies is associated with improved cognitive outcome at 2 years of age [2, 13, 14]. However, no RCT or meta-analysis has shown clear evidence of benefit on cognitive outcomes in infancy or childhood. Whilst most NICUs routinely provide PN to very low birthweight (VLBW, below 32 weeks of gestation) infants on admission, practice varies and some use birthweight cut-offs e.g. below 1500 g as an indication for provision. There has been little recent research to determine if more mature babies might also benefit, for example those born 32–34 weeks of gestation or weighing more than 1500 g, in whom the balance of risks and potential benefits may differ.

Recent guidelines (2018) for paediatric PN from a working group representing the European Society of Pediatric Gastroenterology, Hepatology and Nutrition (ESPGHAN), the European Society of Pediatric Research (ESPR) and the European Society of Parenteral and Enteral Nutrition (ESPEN) have been published [15–20] and a summary of the recommendations for preterm infants is provided in Table 16.2. These are, however, in part 'expert opinion' and, for most nutrients, adequately powered RCTs are lacking, and there are very few with long term functional outcomes. Whilst there is general agreement over the recommended ranges for most micronutrients, the optimal macronutrient regime remains uncertain.

Table 16.2 Summary of recent EPSGHAN 2018 parenteral nutrition guidelines for preterm infants

Nutrient	Recommendation per kg/day	Comments
Amino acids	>1.5 g (first 24 h) 2.5–3.5 g (day 2–3 & growing)	Start on admission Accompany with >65 kcal/kg of *non-protein* energy (growing)
Total energy	45–55 kcal (first 24 h) 90–120 kcal (growing)	Amount includes all energy sources including amino acids
Carbohydrate	5.8–11.5 g (first 24 h) 5.8–17.3 g (growing)	Equivalent to 4–8 mg/kg/min of glucose Usual target (11.5–14.4 g)
Lipid	0–2 g (first 24 h) Up to 4 g (maximum amount)	Can start on admission and always before day 2
Sodium	0–2 mmol (first 2–3 days) 2–5 mmol (growing)	Higher amounts may be needed longer term
Calcium	0.8–2 mmol (first few days) 1.6–3.5 mmol (growing)	Use Ca:P ratio of 0.8–1.0 in first few days
Phosphorus	1.0–2.0 mmol (first few days) 1.6–3.5 mmol (growing)	Monitor plasma phosphate closely in first few days

Provision of PN is complex and may cause harm; always check calculations against reference texts

PN energy intakes and hyperglycaemia. Numerous observational studies show that preterm infants, and those born extremely low birthweight (ELBW) in particular, tend to be relatively intolerant of high intakes of carbohydrate in the first few days and many develop hyperglycaemia. This is due to multiple factors including relative insulin resistance, inadequate insulin secretion, stress, sepsis, and vasopressor or corticosteroid use. One study showed that adoption of a more 'enhanced' PN regime was associated with an increased incidence of hyperglycaemia and worse outcomes including death [21]. Neonatal intensive care units (NICUs) that use higher carbohydrate intakes will often need to give more than half of all ELBW infants insulin in order to control blood glucose levels [22] whereas other units tend to administer or reduce PN carbohydrate intakes before commencing insulin. There are some data to show that insulin use increases IGF-1 levels and decreases key morbidities [23], but there are no adequately powered RCTs with longer term outcomes to determine the best strategy. There is therefore an important need for a large pragmatic trial that compares a 'high energy intake' PN strategy using insulin to maintain blood glucose (for example, less than 10–12 mmol/L) with a strategy that first decreases energy intakes in order to avoid or limit insulin use.

Early PN lipid intakes. Current data suggest it is safe to provide intravenous lipid intakes of up to 2 g/kg/day on day 0, although RCTs and meta-analyses do not show any longer term benefit compared with lower starting intakes [24]. Consensus opinion suggests ELBW can receive PN lipid intakes of 3–4 g/kg/day after the first few days but no RCTs exist to help determine the optimal intake, and lower parenteral intakes will be required where enteral milk is tolerated.

There are no recent data to determine whether routine measurement of serum cholesterol or triglyceride is useful and clinical practice varies widely between NICUs. Whilst use of multi-component lipid emulsions containing for example, fish oil, is increasing, there is no evidence that routine use (compared to soy bean emulsions) is beneficial [24]. A recent RCT showed no differences in body composition including levels of intra-hepatic lipid accumulation when comparing multi-component to soy bean oil based lipids [25]. Limited evidence in children suggests that multi-component fish oil emulsions may decrease bilirubin levels in those receiving prolonged PN, but there is no high quality evidence in preterm infants.

PN amino acid intakes. In the 1970s and 1980s, when PN was first used in preterm infants, amino acids (AA) were often not started until day 2–3 and were then only increased gradually. However, over the last 20 years data has shown widespread growth failure in preterm infants [26, 27] and this has led many NICUs to start and increase AA more rapidly. This 'enhanced' approach was supported by several short-term physiological studies showing this was not associated with abnormal plasma AA profiles [28]. Whilst there are several RCTs of higher AA intakes, most are under-powered for longer term brain outcomes, although some small trials show apparent neurological advantages for enhanced regimes [29–32]. In recent years, several RCTs and observational studies showed that higher AA intakes need to be accompanied by higher intakes of phosphate to avoid hypophosphatemia [33–35]. This may be associated with impaired muscle function, but might be, largely, prevented by providing equimolar amounts of calcium and phosphate in PN solutions.

In the UK, the Standardised, Concentrated, Additional Macronutrients Parenteral Nutrition Study (SCAMP) study showed that providing higher AA intakes, that aimed to provide up to 3.8 g/kg/day after the first few days, was associated with improved head growth [36]. In contrast, another large RCT, the Nutritional Evaluation and Optimisation in Neonates (NEON) trial, showed no advantage of commencing 3 g/kg/day on day 1, compared with a regime that increased more gradually and only to a maximum of 2.7 g/kg/day after a few days [25]. Neither trial has reported cognitive outcomes in infancy, and a recent review was unable to find consistent evidence of longer term brain benefit for more 'aggressive' regimes [32]. Importantly, a recent large trial (n = 1440) in children and infants (including some who were newborn at full term), compared immediate commencement of PN with delayed introduction (after 6 days) and showed *increased* rates of sepsis and prolonged hospital stay in the immediate arm of the trial [37, 38]. Whilst that study did not include preterm infants, the study reinforces the concept that dietary intake of nutrients in excess of metabolic capacity may be harmful. Subsequent analysis of this study showed that the risk of adverse outcome was most strongly related to the AA component of PN rather than to carbohydrate or lipid intakes [39]. This suggests that further study is required before we can be sure of the best AA composition and regime for preterm infants. It is possible that commencing AA at a rate of 3–4 g/kg/day in unstable, septic or very growth restricted infants overloads metabolic capacity, and a more gradual introduction over 2–3 days is just as beneficial.

Milk Feeding and Necrotising Enterocolitis

There is no doubt that, for every clinician practising in high income countries (HICs), the most serious complication associated with feeding and nutrition is NEC, and this is now also an increasing problem in many low and middle income countries (LMICs) [40]. The 'fear of NEC' tends to dominate much of the day to day decision making on NICUs, including issues such as how fast to increase milk feeds, whether to withhold feeds during blood transfusion [41], if and when to start breast milk fortifier (BMF), as well as more strategic NICU decisions around the use of prophylactic probiotics and DHM [42]. The number of preterm infants developing NEC has increased as survival rates increase, and combined with late onset sepsis, NEC now represents the most common cause of death after the first week of life [43]. NEC has been recognised as a serious and common disease in preterm infants for the last 30 years, although research aimed at prevention is hampered by its unpredictable and sporadic occurrence, and the need for large scale research collaborations to test the efficacy of clinical interventions. Indeed, it seems that there has never been a well-designed RCT adequately powered to determine a meaningful (and realistic) reduction in NEC as a primary outcome.

Recent data show that around 150 infants die from NEC every year in England [44]: this is higher than that from all childhood leukaemia and lymphoma combined (based on national UK data [45]). A recent systematic review demonstrated that there was substantial variation in NEC rates in HIC settings with rates varying between 2 and 7% for infants born <32 weeks gestation, and between 5 and 22% in those born <1000 g birthweight [46]. This fourfold variation in incidence suggest that changes in clinical practice or interventions have the potential to modify the disease, although variations in reporting systems, study quality and NEC definitions make comparisons difficult. The majority of studies continue to base diagnosis on use of a modified Bell's stage, despite the widespread recognition of the limitations associated with this definition that was originally proposed to assist in clinical management decisions *after* a diagnosis of NEC was made, rather than to confirm a diagnosis.

Overall, the studies showed considerable inconsistency in the use of this and other definitions. This inconsistency not only makes inter-unit or international comparisons difficult, but may limit the generalisability of studies that aim to reduce the incidence or impact of NEC [46]. It remains to be seen whether attempts to provide workable case gestation specific case definitions for use in large scale epidemiological studies will be adopted more widely [47].

Donor Human Milk and NEC

There is now widespread acceptance that NEC represents the end result of multiple different aetio-pathologic processes, and no single intervention will abolish NEC. The use of DHM has increased substantially in the last few years and is now widespread in many countries.

A recent Cochrane meta-analysis shows that use of DHM does reduce NEC when given as sole diet compared to infant formula [48] although the benefits when used as a supplement to MOM may be less. Interestingly, another meta-analysis suggests that use of DHM does not significantly reduce the most serious forms of NEC [49] and a large database survey of 13,463 infants in England was unable to show clear differences in NEC rates between regions that did, and did not, use DHM [42]. The largest RCT of DHM to date showed no effects on a combined outcome of NEC, sepsis and death when DHM or formula was used to meet a shortfall in availability of MOM over the first 10 days. Whilst short term use in this study may appear to be a key limitation, it is worth noting that around two thirds of the key outcomes (including NEC) occurred during this early 10 day period [4]. In contrast, whilst a large Canadian trial determined there was no evidence of benefit from DHM use on cognitive outcome in infancy, NEC as a secondary outcome was significantly higher in those receiving formula to make up any shortfall in MOM availability [50].

However, there are no DHM versus formula trials that have been powered to show a reduction in NEC or all cause mortality as a primary outcome.

Whilst there are no controlled trial data to show that DHM improves survival without severe disability in infancy, there may be other advantages. Many view DHM as an important component of a strategy that aims to improve overall breast feeding rates, and there are some data to support this idea although the studies are also inconsistent [51]. Further large well designed RCTs in high risk infants are required to explore effects on NEC or sepsis, to better define which populations of infants may benefit, and to determine cost-effectiveness in reducing diseases such as NEC, or improving other health outcomes, for example breast feeding at discharge.

In addition, a better understanding of the impact of various 'technical' aspects of DHM including collection, storage, transport and pasteurisation may enable the development of alternative strategies, such as UV-light sterilisation [52, 53] that might better protect immuno-active components. Considerable recent work has also highlighted the complex roles of specific human milk oligosaccharides (HMOs) in promoting gut health. Recent data show that milk rich in specific individual HMOs, might provide the greatest reductions on NEC reduction. Whilst the individual HMO composition of MOM cannot be modified by maternal diet, it is possible that certain individual donors might provide milk that is especially efficacious [54, 55].

Probiotics and Risk of NEC or Sepsis

There are few areas in neonatal medicine that have caused more heated debate than the role of prophylactic probiotics for preterm infants [9, 56–62]. Numerous meta-analyses, controlled trials and systematic reviews have concluded that probiotics significantly reduce the risk of NEC and sepsis, and may have other benefits such as a reduction in time to full enteral feeds [63–65]. Although trials are inconsistent

Table 16.3 Clinical concerns or uncertainties surrounding routine use of prophylactic probiotics for preterm infants

1. Choice of optimal species or strains and/or combinations
2. Optimal dose, timing of start and stopping
3. Difference in effects depending on milk diet (breast versus formula)
4. Local/national availability of safe and consistent product
5. Product quality control (contamination) and quality assurance (taxonomy control)
6. Infant safety in short term e.g. sepsis and long-term e.g. allergy risk
7. NICU safety from cross-colonisation or carriage of antibiotic resistance genes
8. Interference with more 'natural' patterns of early microbial ecosystem acquisition
9. Lack of regulatory control as a food supplement
10. Lack of guidelines or support for use from professional organisations

[66], the evidence base to support the routine use of probiotics still appears considerably stronger than that for DHM. Probiotics are also generally cheap, easy to transport, store and administer, and are likely to be acceptable in settings where cultural restrictions limit the use of DHM, for example in certain Islamic countries due to concerns of milk-kinship [67, 68]. Despite this, probiotic practice varies, and many NICUs in Europe and North America do not support routine use. Many consider that these uncertainties and other concerns outweigh potential benefits at present (see Table 16.3).

Notwithstanding the concerns listed, many find it difficult to ignore the considerable evidence in favour of routine use from more than 25 RCTs, and the overwhelming data suggesting they are 'safe'.

Despite being administered to 100,000 s of infants there is only a limited number of case-reports of invasive probiotic sepsis exist and, in addition, the RCT data show reductions in late onset sepsis from other organisms and reductions in 'all cause' mortality suggesting that overall they do more good than harm. Emerging data also suggest they may be effective in LMICs although further large scale studies are warranted, given the differing balance of risks and benefits to HICs where most trials have been conducted [40]. However, making firm recommendations is difficult because most RCTs used different products. As it is currently impossible to identify the optimal species or strains with the strongest functional benefits, novel meta-analytic techniques have been employed. A recent paper from ESPGHAN adopted a network meta-analytic approach to show the combinations and types of species (or strains) with the strongest evidence of benefit to reduce the risk of NEC or LOS, or improve feed tolerance [69]. Further data are clearly needed but there are few large scale probiotic RCTs in planning listed on trial registries. Clinicians must review the available data and base their approach on this, consider generalisability to their setting, population and practice rather than expect this complex decision to be made for them.

Conclusions

The last few years have seen an increased focus on the need to provide good nutrition to preterm infants, and a greater understanding of how this may translate to longer term benefits. Improvements in care have been made that are due to advances in our mechanistic understanding of disease processes, newborn physiology and the mechanisms of actions of key interventions such as breast milk and other immunonutrients. The next 10 years will be really exciting. We will see a greater integration of 'omics' (genomics, microbiomics, and metabolomics etc.) into research and clinical practice, and new biomarkers will be developed. Biomarkers will include genes, microbes, proteins, metabolites or RNA gene transcripts, and we will 'find' them in stool, urine and other non-invasive specimens [70, 71]. These will allow us to 'fine-tune' our interventions to the individual, identify infants at highest risk of disease to enrol into RCTs, provide early warning of disease so clinical management can be adapted and make our diagnoses more robust. However, improvements in clinical management will require research collaboration on a national and international level if we are to develop nutritional practices to improve health and reduce disease. High quality prospective RCTs are essential.

References

1. Yumani DFJ, Lafeber HN, van Weissenbruch MM. Dietary proteins and IGF I levels in preterm infants: determinants of growth, body composition, and neurodevelopment. Pediatr Res. 2014;77(1–2):156–63. http://www.nature.com/doifinder/10.1038/pr.2014.172.
2. Stoltz Sjöström E, Lundgren P, Öhlund I, Holmström G, Hellström A, Domellöf M. Low energy intake during the first 4 weeks of life increases the risk for severe retinopathy of prematurity in extremely preterm infants. Arch Dis Child Fetal Neonatal Ed. 2016;101(2):F108–13. http://www.ncbi.nlm.nih.gov/pubmed/25678632.
3. Embleton ND, Cleminson J, Zalewski S. What growth should we aim for in preterm neonates? Paediatr Child Health (Oxford). 2017;27(1):18–22. http://linkinghub.elsevier.com/retrieve/pii/S1751722216301767.
4. Corpeleijn WE, de Waard M, Christmann V, van Goudoever JB, Jansen-van der Weide MC, Kooi EMW, et al. Effect of donor milk on severe infections and mortality in very low-birth-weight infants: the early nutrition study randomized clinical trial. JAMA Pediatr. 2016;170(7):654–61. http://archpedi.jamanetwork.com/article.aspx?doi=10.1001/jamapediatrics.2016.0183%5Cn. http://www.ncbi.nlm.nih.gov/pubmed/27135598.
5. Zhou J, Shukla VV, John D, Chen C. Human milk feeding as a protective factor for retinopathy of prematurity: a meta-analysis. Pediatrics. 2015;136(6):e1576–86. http://pediatrics.aappublications.org/cgi/doi/10.1542/peds.2015-2372.
6. Patel AL, Johnson TJ, Engstrom JL, Fogg LF, Jegier BJ, Bigger HR, et al. Impact of early human milk on sepsis and health-care costs in very low birth weight infants. J Perinatol. 2013;33(7):514–9. https://doi.org/10.1038/jp.2013.2.
7. Renfrew MJ, Craig D, Dyson L, McCormick F, Rice S, King SE, et al. Breastfeeding promotion for infants in neonatal units: a systematic review and economic analysis. Health Technol Assess. 2009;13(40):1–146, iii–iv. http://www.ncbi.nlm.nih.gov/pubmed/19728934. [cited 2015 Jan 2]

8. Relton C, Strong M, Thomas KJ, Whelan B, Walters SJ, Burrows J, et al. Effect of financial incentives on breastfeeding: a cluster randomized clinical trial. JAMA Pediatr. 2018;172(2):1–7.

9. Cleminson JS, Zalewski SP, Embleton ND. Nutrition in the preterm infant: what's new? Curr Opin Clin Nutr Metab Care. 2016;19(3):220–5.

10. Leaf A, Dorling J, Kempley S, McCormick K, Mannix P, Linsell L, et al. Early or delayed enteral feeding for preterm growth-restricted infants: a randomized trial. Pediatrics. 2012;129(5):e1260–8. http://www.ncbi.nlm.nih.gov/pubmed/22492770.

11. Abbott J, Berrington J, Bowler U, Boyle EM, Dorling J, Embleton N, et al. The speed of increasing milk feeds: a randomised controlled trial. BMC Pediatr. 2017;17(1):39. http://bmc-pediatr.biomedcentral.com/articles/10.1186/s12887-017-0794-z.

12. Oddie S, Young L, McGuire W. Slow advancement of enteral feed volumes to prevent necrotising enterocolitis in very low birth weight infants. Cochrane Database Syst Rev. 2017;(8):CD001241. https://doi.org/10.1002/14651858.CD001241.pub7. http://onlinelibrary. wiley.com/doi/10.1002/14651858.CD005249.pub2/pdf/standard%5Cn. http://www.ncbi.nlm. nih.gov/pubmed/23152230.

13. Klevebro S, Westin V, Stoltz Sjöström E, Norman M, Domellöf M, Edstedt Bonamy AK, et al. Early energy and protein intakes and associations with growth, BPD, and ROP in extremely preterm infants. Clin Nutr. 2019;38(3):1289–95.

14. Stephens BE, Walden RV, Gargus RA, Tucker R, McKinley L, Mance M, Julie Nye BRV. First-week protein and energy intakes are associated with 18-month developmental outcomes in extremely low birth weight infants. Paediatrics. 2009;123(5):1337–43.

15. Joosten K, Embleton N, Yan W, Senterre T, Espr E. ESPGHAN/ESPEN/ESPR guidelines on pediatric parenteral nutrition: Energy. Clin Nutr. 2018;37(6 Pt B):2309–14.

16. Mihatsch W, Shamir R, van Goudoever JB, Fewtrell M, Lapillonne A. ESPEN/ESPEN/ESPR/CSPEN guidelines on pediatric parenteral nutrition: guideline development process for the updated guidelines. Clin Nutr. 2018;37(6 Pt B):2306–8.

17. van Goudoever JB, Carnielli V, Darmaun D, Sainz de Pipaon M. ESPGHAN/ESPEN/ESPR guidelines on pediatric parenteral nutrition: amino acids. Clin Nutr. 2018;37(6 Pt B):2315–23.

18. Mihatsch W, Fewtrell M, Goulet O, Molgaard C, Picaud J, Senterre T. ESPGHAN/ESPEN/ESPR guidelines on pediatric parenteral nutrition: calcium, phosphorus and magnesium. Clin Nutr. 2018;37(6 Pt B):2360–5.

19. Mesotten D, Joosten K, van Kempen A, Verbruggen S, Espen E. ESPGHAN/ESPEN/ESPR guidelines on pediatric parenteral nutrition: carbohydrates. Clin Nutr. 2018;37(6 Pt B):2337–43.

20. Jochum F, Moltu SJ, Senterre T, Nomayo A, Iacobelli S, Espen E, et al. ESPGHAN/ESPEN/ESPR guidelines on pediatric parenteral nutrition: fluid and electrolytes. Clin Nutr. 2018;37(6 Pt B):2344–53.

21. Stensvold HJ, Strommen K, Lang AM, Abrahamsen TG, Steen EK, Pripp AH, et al. Early enhanced parenteral nutrition, hyperglycemia, and death among extremely low-birth-weight infants. JAMA Pediatr. 2015;169(11):1003–10. http://www.ncbi.nlm.nih.gov/pubmed/26348113.

22. Morgan C. The potential risks and benefits of insulin treatment in hyperglycaemic preterm neonates. Early Hum Dev. 2015;91(11):655–9.

23. Beardsall K, Vanhaesebrouck S, Frystyk J, Ogilvy-Stuart AL, Vanhole C, van Weissenbruch M, et al. Relationship between insulin-like growth factor I levels, early insulin treatment, and clinical outcomes of very low birth weight infants. J Pediatr. 2014;164(5):1038–1044.e1. http://www.ncbi.nlm.nih.gov/pubmed/24518169. [cited 2015 Jan 2]

24. Hojsak I, Colomb V, Braegger C, Bronsky J, Campoy C, Domellöf M, et al. ESPGHAN Committee on Nutrition Position Paper. Intravenous lipid emulsions and risk of hepatotoxicity in infants and children. J Pediatr Gastroenterol Nutr. 2016;62(5):776–92. http://content.wkhealth. com/linkback/openurl?sid=WKPTLP:landingpage&an=00005176-201605000-00019.

25. Uthaya S, Liu X, Modi N. Nutritional evaluation and optimisation in neonates trial: is the protein-to-energy ratio important? Reply. Am J Clin Nutr. 2016;103(6):1721–2.

26. Embleton NDE, Pang N, Cooke RJ, Background A. Postnatal malnutrition and growth retarda-
    tion: an inevitable consequence of current recommendations in preterm infants? Pediatrics.
    2001;107(2):270–3. http://pediatrics.aappublications.org/cgi/doi/10.1542/peds.107.2.270.
27. Ehrenkranz RA, Dusick AM, Vohr BR, Wright LL, Wrage LA, Poole WK. Growth in the
    neonatal intensive care unit influences neurodevelopmental and growth outcomes of extremely
    low birth weight infants. Pediatrics. 2006;117(4):1253–61. http://www.ncbi.nlm.nih.gov/
    pubmed/16585322. [cited 2015 Jan 2]
28. Thureen PJ, Hay WW. Early aggressive nutrition in preterm infants. Semin Neonatol.
    2001;6(5):403–15. http://www.ncbi.nlm.nih.gov/pubmed/11988030. [cited 2015 Jan 2]
29. Blakstad EW, Strømmen K, Moltu SJ, Wattam-Bell J, Nordheim T, Almaas AN, et al. Improved
    visual perception in very low birth weight infants on enhanced nutrient supply. Neonatology.
    2015;108(1):30–7.
30. Strommen K, Blakstad EW, Moltu SJ, Almaas AN, Westerberg AC, Amlien IK, et al. Enhanced
    nutrient supply to very low birth weight infants is associated with improved white matter matu-
    ration and head growth. Neonatology. 2015;107(1):68–75.
31. Strømmen K, Haag A, Moltu SJ, Veierød MB, Blakstad EW, Nakstad B, et al. Enhanced
    nutrient supply to very low birth weight infants is associated with higher blood amino acid
    concentrations and improved growth. Clin Nutr ESPEN. 2017;18(0424):16–22. https://doi.
    org/10.1016/j.clnesp.2017.01.003.
32. Embleton ND, Van Den Akker CHP. Early parenteral amino acid intakes in preterm babies:
    does NEON light the way? Arch Dis Child Fetal Neonatal Ed. 2018;103(2):F92–4.
33. Moltu SJ, Strømmen K, Blakstad EW, Almaas AN, Westerberg AC, Brække K, et al. Enhanced
    feeding in very-low-birth-weight infants may cause electrolyte disturbances and septice-
    mia - A randomized, controlled trial. Clin Nutr. 2013;32(2):207–12. https://doi.org/10.1016/j.
    clnu.2012.09.004.
34. Embleton ND, Morgan C, King C. Balancing the risks and benefits of parenteral nutrition for
    preterm infants: can we define the optimal composition? Arch Dis Child Fetal Neonatal Ed.
    2015;100(1):F72–5.
35. Mulla S, Stirling S, Cowey S, Close R, Pullan S, Howe R, et al. Severe hypercalcaemia and
    hypophosphataemia with an optimised preterm parenteral nutrition formulation in two epochs
    of differing phosphate supplementation. Arch Dis Child Fetal Neonatal Ed. 2017;102(5):F451–
    5. http://fn.bmj.com/lookup/doi/10.1136/archdischild-2016-311107.
36. Morgan C, McGowan P, Herwitker S, Hart AE, Turner MA. Postnatal head growth in preterm
    infants: a randomized controlled parenteral nutrition study. Pediatrics. 2014;133(1):e120–8.
    http://pediatrics.aappublications.org/cgi/doi/10.1542/peds.2013-2207.
37. Koletzko B, Goulet O, Jochum F, Shamir R. Use of parenteral nutrition in the pediatric ICU:
    should we panic because of PEPaNIC? Curr Opin Clin Nutr Metab Care. 2017;20(3):201–3.
    http://insights.ovid.com/crossref?an=00075197-201705000-00010
38. Fivez T, Kerklaan D, Mesotten D, Verbruggen S, Wouters PJ, Vanhorebeek I, et al. Early versus
    late parenteral nutrition in critically ill children. N Engl J Med. 2016;374(12):1111–22.
39. Vanhorebeek I, Verbruggen S, Casaer MP, Gunst J, Wouters PJ, Hanot J, et al. Effect of early
    supplemental parenteral nutrition in the paediatric ICU: a preplanned observational study of
    post-randomisation treatments in the PEPaNIC trial. Lancet Respir Med. 2017;2600(17):1–9.
    http://linkinghub.elsevier.com/retrieve/pii/S2213260017301868.
40. Deshpande G, Jape G, Rao S, Patole S. Benefits of probiotics in preterm neonates in low-income
    and medium-income countries: a systematic review of randomised controlled trials. BMJ Open.
    2017;7(12):e017638. http://bmjopen.bmj.com/lookup/doi/10.1136/bmjopen-2017-017638.
41. Gale C, Modi N, WHEAT Trial Development Group. Neonatal randomised point-of-
    care trials are feasible and acceptable in the UK: results from two national surveys. Arch
    Dis Child Fetal Neonatal Ed. 2016;101(1):86–7. http://fn.bmj.com/lookup/doi/10.1136/
    archdischild-2015-308882.
42. Battersby C, Marciano Alves Mousinho R, Longford N, Modi N. Use of pasteurised human
    donor milk across neonatal networks in England. Early Hum Dev. 2018;118:32–6. https://doi.
    org/10.1016/j.earlhumdev.2018.01.017.

43. Berrington JE, Hearn RI, Bythell M, Wright C, Embleton ND. Deaths in preterm infants: changing pathology over 2 decades. J Pediatr. 2012;160(1):49–53.e1.
44. Battersby C, Longford N, Mandalia S, Costeloe K, Modi N. Incidence and enteral feed antecedents of severe neonatal necrotising enterocolitis across neonatal networks in England, 2012–13: a whole-population surveillance study. Lancet Gastroenterol Hepatol. 2017;2(1):43–51. https://doi.org/10.1016/S2468-1253(16)30117-0.
45. Children's cancer mortality. http://www.cancerresearchuk.org/health-professional/cancer-statistics/.
46. Battersby C, Santhalingam T, Costeloe K, Modi N. Incidence of neonatal necrotising enterocolitis in high-income countries: a systematic review. Arch Dis Child Fetal Neonatal Ed. 2018;103(2):F182–9.
47. Battersby C, Longford N, Costeloe K, Modi N. Development of a gestational age–specific case definition for neonatal necrotizing enterocolitis. JAMA Pediatr. 2017;171(3):256–63. http://archpedi.jamanetwork.com/article.aspx?doi=10.1001/jamapediatrics.2016.3633.
48. Quigley M, Embleton ND, McGuire W. Formula versus donor breast milk for feeding preterm or low birth weight infants (review). Cochrane Database Syst Rev. 2018;6:CD002971.
49. Silano M, Milani GP, Fattore G, Agostoni C. Donor human milk and risk of surgical necrotizing enterocolitis: a meta-analysis. Clin Nutr. 2019;38(3):1061–6. https://doi.org/10.1016/j.clnu.2018.03.004.
50. O'Connor DL, Gibbins S, Kiss A, Bando N, Brennan-Donnan J, Ng E, et al. Effect of supplemental donor human milk compared with preterm formula on neurodevelopment of very low-birth-weight infants at 18 months. JAMA. 2016;316(18):1897. http://jama.jamanetwork.com/article.aspx?doi=10.1001/jama.2016.16144.
51. Williams T, Nair H, Simpson J, Embleton N. Use of donor human milk and maternal breastfeeding rates: a systematic review. J Hum Lact. 2016;32:212–20. http://jhl.sagepub.com/cgi/doi/10.1177/0890334416632203.
52. Li Y, Nguyen DN, de Waard M, Christensen L, Zhou P, Jiang P, et al. Pasteurization procedures for donor human milk affect body growth, intestinal structure, and resistance against bacterial infections in preterm pigs. J Nutr. 2017;147(6):1121–30. http://jn.nutrition.org/lookup/doi/10.3945/jn.116.244822.
53. Menon G, Williams TC. Human milk for preterm infants: why, what, when and how? Arch Dis Child Fetal Neonatal Ed. 2013;98(6):F559–62. http://www.ncbi.nlm.nih.gov/pubmed/23893267
54. Autran CA, Kellman B, bode L. Human milk oligosaccharide composition predicts risk of necrotizing enterocolitis in preterm infants. Gut. 2018;67(6):1064–70.
55. Autran CA, Schoterman MHC, Jantscher-Krenn E, Kamerling JP, Bode L. Sialylated galacto-oligosaccharides and 2′-fucosyllactose reduce necrotising enterocolitis in neonatal rats. Br J Nutr. 2016;116(02):294–9. http://www.journals.cambridge.org/abstract_S0007114516002038.
56. Manzoni P, Rizzollo S, Vain N, Mostert M, Stronati M, Tarnow-Mordi W, et al. Probiotics use in preterm neonates: what further evidence is needed? Early Hum Dev. 2011;87(Suppl 1):S3–4. http://www.ncbi.nlm.nih.gov/pubmed/21288665. [cited 2015 Jan 2].
57. Tarnow-Mordi W, Soll RF. Probiotic supplementation in preterm infants: it is time to change practice. J Pediatr. 2014;164(5):959–60. https://doi.org/10.1016/j.jpeds.2013.12.050.
58. Modi N. Probiotics and necrotising enterocolitis: the devil (as always) is in the detail. Commentary on N. Ofek Shlomai et al.: probiotics for preterm neonates: what will it take to change clinical practice? (Neonatology 2014;105:64-70). Neonatology. 2014;105(1):71–3. http://www.ncbi.nlm.nih.gov/pubmed/24296920. [cited 2015 Jan 2].
59. Deshpande G, Rao S, Patole S. Probiotics in neonatal intensive care—back to the future. Aust New Zeal J Obstet Gynaecol. 2015;55(3):210–7. http://doi.wiley.com/10.1111/ajo.12328.
60. Embleton ND, Zalewski S, Berrington JE. Probiotics for prevention of necrotizing enterocolitis and sepsis in preterm infants. Curr Opin Infect Dis. 2016;29(3):256–61.
61. Patel RM, Underwood MA. Probiotics and necrotizing enterocolitis. Semin Pediatr Surg. 2018;27(12):39–46. https://doi.org/10.1053/j.sempedsurg.2017.11.008.

62. Thomas J. Probiotics for the prevention of NEC in VLBW infants: a meta-analysis and systematic review. Acta Paediatr. 2016;38(1):42–9.
63. Indrio F, Riezzo G, Tafuri S, Ficarella M, Carlucci B, Bisceglia M, et al. Probiotic supplementation in preterm: feeding intolerance and hospital cost. Nutrients. 2017;9(9):1–8.
64. Rao SC, Athalye-jape GK, Deshpande GC. Probiotic supplementation and late-onset sepsis in preterm infants: a meta-analysis. Pediatrics. 2016;137(3):e20153684.
65. Alfaleh K, Anabrees J, Bassler D. Probiotics for prevention of necrotizing enterocolitis in preterm infants (review). Cochrane Database Syst Rev. 2011;(3):CD005496.
66. Costeloe K, Hardy P, Juszczak E, Wilks M, Millar MR. Bifidobacterium breve BBG-001 in very preterm infants: a randomised controlled phase 3 trial. Lancet. 2015;6736(15):1–12. https://doi.org/10.1016/S0140-6736(15)01027-2.
67. El-Khuffash A, Unger S. The concept of milk kinship in Islam: issues raised when offering preterm infants of Muslim families donor human milk. J Hum Lact. 2012;28(2):125–7. http://www.ncbi.nlm.nih.gov/pubmed/22311893. [cited 2015 Jan 2].
68. Ozdemir R, Ak M, Karatas M, Ozer A, Dogan DG, Karadag A. Human milk banking and milk kinship: perspectives of religious officers in a Muslim country. J Perinatol. 2015;35(2):137–41. http://www.nature.com/doifinder/10.1038/jp.2014.177.
69. van den Akker CHP, van Goudoever JB, Szajewska H, Embleton ND, Hojsak I, Reid D, et al. Probiotics for preterm infants: a strain specific systematic review and network meta-analysis. J Pediatr Gastroenterol Nutr. 2018;67(1):103–22. http://insights.ovid.com/crossref?an=00005176-900000000-96905%0A. http://www.ncbi.nlm.nih.gov/pubmed/29384838.
70. Embleton ND, Berrington JE, Dorling J, Ewer AK, Juszczak E, Kirby JA, et al. Mechanisms affecting the gut of preterm infants in enteral feeding trials. Front Nutr. 2017;4:14. http://journal.frontiersin.org/article/10.3389/fnut.2017.00014/full.
71. Schwartz S, Friedberg I, Ivanov IV, Davidson LA, Goldsby JS, Dahl DB, et al. A metagenomic study of diet-dependent interaction between gut microbiota and host in infants reveals differences in immune response. Genome Biol. 2012;13(4):r32. http://www.pubmedcentral.nih.gov/articlerender.fcgi?artid=3446306&tool=pmcentrez&rendertype=abstract.

Chapter 17
Blood Pressure Management in the Very Preterm Infant: More than Just Millimetres

Eugene M. Dempsey and Elisabeth M. W. Kooi

Introduction

Often one finds oneself standing at the bedside of a preterm infant in the first hours of life observing blood pressure values on the bedside monitor trying to decide whether one needs to worry or not. Will the consultant be upset that I did not start an inotrope as the mean blood pressure value was 1 mmHg below the gestational age for at least 1 h? A mean blood pressure below a certain predefined value can begin a cascade of interventions commencing with volume administration, inotrope and sometimes corticosteroid treatment with little evidence to support such therapeutic interventions [1].

Significant uncertainty remains in this area of newborn care, but as a community, after years of managing preterm infants with low blood pressure, there are a few areas of certainty. Firstly the more immature the preterm infant, the greater the likelihood they will have a low blood pressure and receive volume and inotropes [2].

E. M. Dempsey (✉)
Department of Paediatrics and Child Health, Cork University Maternity Hospital, Cork, Ireland

Irish Centre for Fetal and Neonatal Translational Research, University College Cork, Cork, Ireland

INFANT Research Centre, Cork University Maternity Hospital, University College Cork, Cork, Ireland
e-mail: g.dempsey@ucc.ie

E. M. W. Kooi
Department of Paediatrics and Child Health, Cork University Maternity Hospital, Cork, Ireland

Division of Neonatology, University of Groningen, University Medical Center Groningen, Beatrix Children's Hospital, Groningen, The Netherlands
e-mail: e.kooi@umcg.nl

© Springer Nature Switzerland AG 2020
E. M. Boyle, J. Cusack (eds.), *Emerging Topics and Controversies in Neonatology*, https://doi.org/10.1007/978-3-030-28829-7_17

Secondly the majority of treated babies are treated within the first 24 h of life, regardless of gestational age [2]. This is an important point when one considers the underlying pathophysiology. Thirdly there is significant variability in treatment rates across centres, which is not explained by case mix alone, but rather by differing management strategies for the very same problem [2, 3].

One of the most commonly used criteria for intervening is based on the gestational age rule [4]. The decision to intervene based on mean blood pressure value 1 mmHg below the gestational age measured in mmHg is crude and lacks any scientific rigour [5]. Simple rules are sometimes just that: 'simple' and as often is the case, may be too good to be true. If the mean blood pressure is very low, e.g. less than 20 mmHg or less than 15 mmHg then there certainly is a greater risk of adverse outcome and intervention seems warranted [6]. If however the mean blood pressure is 1 or 2 mmHg below the gestational age in the first hours of life, does this warrant intervention? Or indeed if it is 1 or 2 mmHg above that intervention is not warranted? What is clear is the current evidence base does not answer these questions appropriately and there is an urgent need to explore other assessment tools that may provide greater clarity on the infant's overall cardiovascular status.

(Re)Defining shock in the preterm infant is an important first step in resolving the age old question of when one should intervene for a low blood pressure or clinical poor perfusion. In this chapter we explore the various aetiologies, definitions and assessment methods, and provide the most recent evidence on intervention strategies. We look towards how we might better manage the age old question of when and how to intervene for the preterm infant with low blood pressure.

Etiology of Low Blood Pressure and/or Circulatory Failure

During Transition

During normal term feto-neonatal transition, clamping of the umbilical cord removes the previous low resistance system of the placenta, resulting in a sudden and significant rise in systemic vascular resistance. The pulmonary vascular resistance (PVR) falls with lung aeration, and the intra-cardiac and extra-cardiac shunting changes from the intrauterine right to left, towards the postnatal left to right. With closure of the foramen ovale, and gradual closure of the ductus arteriosus, the left heart now ensures perfusion of the body and brain, whereas the right heart receives blood from body and brain, to subsequently pump it through the pulmonary vascular bed [7]. Oxygenation is now dependent on the lungs, and with normal lung function, arterial oxygen saturation quickly rises from a fetal level of approximately 60% to a neonatal level of up to 100%. This normal process can be altered with preterm delivery. Table 17.1 outlines a number of the potential factors that can impact upon cardiorespiratory wellbeing. The immature myocardium is equipped with fewer adrenoreceptors and more fibrous non contractile tissue [8] resulting in

Table 17.1 Etiology for disturbed hemodynamic transition in the very preterm infant

Causes for altered hemodynamics	Hemodynamic effects
Underdeveloped lungs, RDS, PPHN, no steroids	PVR remains high, shunt remains right to left, hypoxia
Immature myocardium	Reduced contractility, CO, and filling
Patent ductus arteriosus	Shunting either direction, depending on SVR and PVR
Placental dysfunction (PET, IUGR)	Redistribution blood to brain, altered cardiac function
Inflammation (sepsis, PROM)	Affects SVR and PVR
Hemorrhage/blood loss/immediate cord clamping	Reduced blood volume
Mechanical ventilation/pneumothorax	Impact on cardiac filling and cardiac output

impaired systolic and diastolic dysfunction, often manifest as decreased cardiac output and low blood pressure [9]. The immature ductus arteriosus tends to remain patent, and will facilitate either right to left shunting with high pulmonary vascular resistance, or left to right shunting in the setting of a normal reduction in pulmonary vascular resistance [10]. Placental dysfunction from pre-eclampsia, with or without intra-uterine growth restriction (IUGR) and brain sparing, affects normal development of systemic and brain vasculature and cardiac function [11]. Intrauterine inflammation from sepsis, and/or prolonged ruptured membranes, can result in high PVR [12]. Placental hemorrhage may change hemodynamics through blood loss and anemia. Mechanical ventilation can also significantly impact upon blood pressure and systemic blood flow [13, 14].

Each of the factors above may affect haemodynamic changes during transition. Anticipation is always key. The patients to be most concerned about are:

- The more immature newborns, typically 23–26 weeks gestation.
- Absence of antenatal corticosteroid administration.
- Multiple pregnancies.
- Placental abruption.
- Immediate cord clamping.
- Infants requiring mechanical ventilation.

Etiology of Circulatory Failure Beyond the Transitional Period

The incidence of hypotension beyond the first few days of life in preterm infants is unknown but it is significantly lower than in the first days of life. The clinical picture is generally more consistent with the typical stages of shock such as compensated, uncompensated and irreversible [15]. The etiology is variable, predominantly occurring in the setting of late onset sepsis and necrotising enterocolitis. The patent ductus arteriosus can be a contributing factor to potential poor perfusion in these circumstances. The assessment modalities described are the same. The choice of therapeutic agent may be similar, but it is important to note the maturational changes that occur may result in different doses of these agents to achieve similar efficacy.

Suggested Assessment Strategies

There are a few important basic bedside clinical assessments that should be performed. These include evaluation of heart rate, capillary refill time, blood pressure, level of activity and urinary output. When evaluating mean blood pressure invasively ensure the arterial trace is correct and, if non-invasive measurements are being performed, ensure that the cuff size and position is appropriate for the weight and size of the infant. Also remember that non-invasive measurements can vary between devices [16, 17], and tend to overestimate mean blood pressure values when the true invasive mean values are low. When assessing heart rate and mean blood pressure values evaluate the trend over the last hour or two. This is usually easily displayed on the bedside monitor and will allow you make a more informed decision. Point of care testing such as lactate values are also important and will be discussed. The role of ancillary tests are outlined and discussed. For many readers, some or all of these assessment modalities are now becoming standards of care. The pros and cons are outlined in the sections below.

Blood Pressure Intervention Standards

There are numerous blood pressure standards in existence [1], which in itself should raise some concerns. We are uncertain if there are other areas of care where such a large number of purported normative reference ranges exist. Some of these are weight based [18], some are gestation based [2, 19, 20] but are all are characterised by an increase in values with increasing gestational age, birth weight and increasing postnatal age. The most common 'range' utilised is the gestational age based rule [5], which neglects the natural rise in blood pressure over the first days of life. Thus, a newborn delivered at 25 weeks gestation may have a mean blood pressure at day 4 of 26 mmHg and be considered normotensive, which neglects the natural rise in blood pressure during this period of adaptation [21].

The reliance on blood pressure values to guide intervention is historic. Generally, blood pressure is easy to measure, either invasively or non-invasively. Invasive measurements not only allow one to continuously evaluate the systolic, diastolic and mean blood pressure values, but also to readily determine the effect of a particular intervention such as volume or inotrope administration. More recent reviews suggest differentiating between systolic and diastolic components of arterial blood pressure. These individual components may provide a more physiological basis to the underlying problem and thus enhance the therapeutic intervention [22]. Over-reliance on blood pressure values has been the hallmark of management to date, and it is now important to acknowledge that blood pressure is only one objective assessment of cardiovascular wellbeing. The relationship between cardiac output and blood pressure is complex, with a number of echocardiography studies highlighting the poor relationship between pressure and flow [23, 24]. Determination of cardiac output and end organ perfusion at the bedside would seem to be a more logical approach to the problem rather than intervention based on blood pressure values in isolation. However these modalities are not readily available at the bedside in the majority of neonatal units, especially out of hours when these problems can be perceived to occur most frequently! A complete clinical assessment is a good start.

Clinical Bedside Assessment

Conventional clinical assessment to determine organ perfusion typically consists of assessing the infant's general appearance (colour, activity, core and peripheral temperature), heart rate, capillary refill time, and urine output. Each of these individually may not be highly sensitive or specific, but when combinations are included the positive predictive values increase for detecting low flow states as determined by echocardiography [25]. Readily available point of care testing will provide pH and lactate values, and whilst these need to be interpreted carefully, their inclusion as diagnostic tools may be helpful. It would appear to be more logical to include each of these parameters in determining the overall cardiovascular status than solely relying on blood pressure values. A cap refill time >3 s had a negative predictive value (NPV) of 91% which is very good, but a positive predictive value (PPV) of only 33% [26]. This means that, in two thirds of cases, prolonged capillary refill times greater than 3 s are associated with normal flow states. Miletin in a similar study combined prolonged capillary refill times >4 s and lactate values >4.0 mmol/L and improved the PPV to 80% with a NPV of 88%. Thus, combining both parameters means that prolonged capillary refill times and elevated lactates were consistent with a low flow state in 80% of cases [23]. De Boode and colleagues highlight the importance of combining parameters in assessing cardiovascular instability [25]. The challenges arise when some parameters are consistent with clinical instability and others are not. Determining which is more relevant is where clinical decision making comes into play. However there can be variability and subjectivity, which ultimately means variation in practice. Tibby and colleagues previously evaluated clinicians' ability to determine cardiac output [27]. They asked 27 clinicians to assess whether cardiac index was high, normal, or low using bedside assessment (blood pressure, pulse volume, heart rate, central venous pressure [CVP]) and measures of organ perfusion (urine output, acid base, serum lactate, capillary refill time, mental status, core-peripheral temperature gradient) in a PICU setting. They identified a very poor relationship between clinicians' estimates and measured cardiac index (by echocardiography) in over 100 assessments. Whilst this study was performed 20 years ago and in the setting of a PICU including a mix of patients, there is no suggestion that this may be any different in the NICU setting. Thus other assessment tools are required to achieve diagnostic accuracy, and it is only then, that rational decision making can take place.

Ancillary Investigations

A variety of measures for the assessment of neonatal haemodynamic status have been developed over the last 20 years or so. More recently, focus has shifted to the assessment of macro-circulation and cardiac function using echocardiography, the utilisation of near infrared spectroscopy (NIRS) to assess the adequacy of cerebral end organ perfusion and more recently the use of continuous assessments of cardiac output. Below is a summary of a number of ancillary investigations.

Echocardiography

The ability to perform cardiac echocardiography (echo) in the NICU setting is now becoming an almost essential component of neonatal practice. Various training program recommendations are now available, with programs across Europe [28, 29], North America [30] and Australasia [31]. It is reassuring to know that the performance of bedside echo in the care of extremely preterm infants was not associated with any clinically relevant changes in peripheral and cerebral oxygenation during the study [32]. Undoubtedly echocardiography leads to changes in the management of individual patients, especially in the setting of the management of a patent ductus arteriosus (PDA) [33, 34] and in the management of persistent pulmonary hypertension in the newborn (PPHN) [35]. A time series study evaluating the introduction of an echo service in a tertiary level NICU in Canada found that in over 300 studies performed, approximately 45% resulted in 'direct management contributions'. The majority of these reflected ductal management with a minority reflecting management of low blood pressure [36]. This study was not designed to evaluate if this had any direct therapeutic benefit. In the setting of low blood pressure in the very preterm infant during the first days of life, can echocardiography make a difference to management? [22]. Whilst suggested treatment algorithms have been previously devised, which incorporated measures of cardiac output to guide intervention [37], this approach has not been evaluated in a prospective study. Utilising echocardiography assessments to prevent low flow states has not resulted in an improved outcome. In essence, usefulness probably depends somewhat on the underlying cause of low blood pressure or potentially low perfusion state. In cases of poor contractility patients may benefit from the administration of an inotrope; in cases where there may be a very large ductus potentially contributing to low systemic flow then treatment may make a difference, but in a large majority of cases where cardiac function may be normal is intervention warranted or careful observation sufficient? It may be that one benefit of echocardiography may be an absolute reduction in the number of patients administered potentially harmful medications. This question remains unanswered and clearly the need for such a targeted approach needs to be evaluated prospectively.

NIRS for the Assessment of Organ Oxygenation and Perfusion

NIRS is increasingly being used in daily clinical practice in the NICU, primarily to assess cerebral oxygenation. The different absorption and dispersion characteristics of light of various wavelengths can be used to separately evaluate biological tissue contents such as hemoglobin and oxygenated hemoglobin. Most NIRS devices currently used in neonatology have sensors which measure approximately 2–3 cm in depth [38]. By measuring cerebral tissue oxygen saturation in combination with peripheral arterial oxygen saturation fractional tissue oxygen extraction (FTOE) can be calculated and cerebral blood flow can be assessed indirectly [39]. NIRS monitoring helps to detect critically low tissue oxygen delivery in preterm infants with clinical sepsis, where clinical signs fail to do so [40], and may provide additional information to the decision making process around closure of the PDA [41, 42]. NIRS has been found to correlate with markers of cardiac output in preterm infants [43–45].

A seminal study evaluated the role of NIRS in preterm infants less than <28 weeks of gestation over the first 72 h of life [46]. Patients were randomised into either the treatment group with visible cerebral NIRS combined with a treatment guideline, or the control group with standard care, with non-visible NIRS measurements obtained [47]. The burden of cerebral hypoxia was significantly reduced in the monitoring group. In terms of clinical outcomes, mortality in the monitoring arm was 14% versus 25% in the standard of care group. There was no difference in adverse long term outcome measurements.

Measuring both cerebral oxygenation and blood pressure, and combining the values measured gives insight into the presence or absence of cerebrovascular auto-regulation [48, 49]. This may allow the clinician to find the optimal blood pressure range for a particular individual, and potentially prevent the harmful cerebral blood flow fluctuations in preterm infants. When cerebrovascular auto-regulation is intact, measuring mesenteric oxygenation by NIRS may help in detecting imminent hemodynamic failure. The role of NIRS in assessment of the hypotensive preterm infant certainly warrants further evaluation, and its use in neonatal care may represent a paradigm shift in how this particular problem is managed into the future. Targeting end organ specific tissue perfusion may be a more physiological approach than focusing on mean arterial blood pressure alone.

Non-invasive Cardiac Output Monitoring

Non-invasive cardiac output monitoring (NICOM) represents a potential monitoring modality that provides real time bedside information on stroke volume, heart rate and cardiac output and along with blood pressure monitoring can provide an estimate of the systemic vascular resistance. It is conceivable that the availability of such data may provide a more individualised and tailored approach to the management of low blood pressure or potentially altered systemic blood flow states. Two types of devices exist, incorporating either electrical velocimetry (EV) or transthoracic bioreactance (TBR) [50–52]. Comparative studies with echocardiography reveal a systemic underestimation of left ventricular output with both devices in preterm infants [53, 54]. Studies have documented changes pertaining to the medical and surgical treatment of the ductus arteriosus [55, 56], changes related to normal haemodynamic transition [50, 57], and alterations secondary to therapeutic hypothermia and rewarming [58]. Currently there are no data on the use of non-invasive cardiac output monitoring in preterm infants with low blood pressure or clinical evidence of poor perfusion. This is an area that clearly warrants further exploration.

Perfusion Index for the Assessment of Peripheral Arterial Perfusion

Perfusion index (PI) provides a relative assessment of the pulse strength obtained from the bedside pulse oximeter. Pulse oximeters generate a photoplethysmography (PPG) waveform using two light emitting diodes at infrared and red wavelengths (940 and 660 nm). The amplitude of the PPG waveform represents arterial pulsation and thus reduced amplitude represents reduced volume of arterial blood flow, manifest as altered altered light absorption of the pulsatile component compared to the non pulsatile component [59, 60]. It is easy to measure and it has shown to relate to various clinical circumstances making it a potential additive measure in hemodynamic assessment of the very preterm infant [61–63]. Cerebral regional tissue oxygen saturation and preductal perfusion index were strongly correlated with right cardiac output during low cardiac output states in preterm infants born at less than 28 weeks of gestation [64]. In a recent observation in very preterm infants, the preductal PI and PI-variability were able to identify a PDA; it was found that the preductal PI was significantly lower in infants with PDA compared to infants without PDA, possibly due to the higher compensatory cardiac output in the PDA patients, increasing the non-pulsatile component of PI [65]. In 99 very preterm infants, low values and reduced short-term variability of the PI on day one was associated with early mortality before 72 h of life, acquired severe periventricular-intraventricular haemorrhage, or severe cystic leukomalacia [66]. To date, no studies have been

Table 17.2 Suggested interventions for hypotension

BP	Clinical appearance	CO/cardiac function (echo/NICOM)	Organ perfusion (NIRS/SVC)	Suggested approach
Normal	Well	Normal	Normal	No treatment
Normal	Poor	Normal	Normal	Observation initially, may warrant early intervention
Low	Poor	Normal	Normal	Intervention required: Epinephrine or dopamine
Low	Well	Normal	Normal	Observation initially, may warrant intervention
Low	Well	Low	Normal	Intervention required: Consider epinephrine
Normal	Poor	Low	Low	Intervention required: Adrenaline or dobutamine
Low	Poor	Low	Low	Intervention required: Dopamine/adrenaline +/ dobutamine
Low	Poor	Normal	Low	Intervention required: Adrenaline or dopamine

performed to assess whether the use of PI benefits haemodynamic management of preterm infants in the first days of life.

It is easy to appreciate how each of the parameters listed above may provide additional information upon which to make a better decision around the underlying cause of circulatory instability or indeed underlying circulatory stability. The challenge is in deciphering which is more relevant to any particular patient at any particular point in time. However as difficult some of this assessment may be, it should be clear now that the utilisation of single blood pressure values or simple blood pressure rules upon which to intervene is too simplistic an approach. Table 17.2 provides a summary of assessment modalities currently available (Fig. 17.1).

Treatment Options

Volume Expansion

Several surveys performed in the last 5 years have shown that volume expansion with a fluid bolus remains the first choice in the management of the haemodynamically unstable preterm infant [4, 67], often followed by a second bolus, prior to the administration of dopamine. However, little evidence supports the use of volume in hypotensive preterm infants [68]. A meta-analysis of five studies concluded that there is insufficient evidence to determine whether infants with cardiovascular

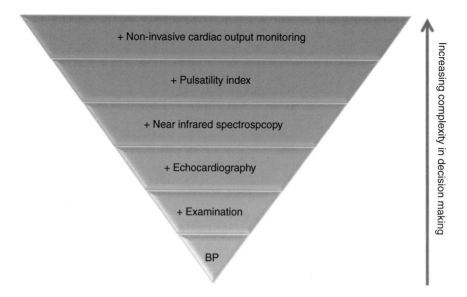

Fig. 17.1 Assessment modalities

compromise benefit from volume expansion, and they reported no benefit using albumin compared to saline [69].

In the majority of preterm infants, especially during the immediate postnatal period, hypotension is infrequently caused by true hypovolaemia, and volume resuscitation may indeed not be warranted and may be potentially harmful [68]. It is thought to increase preload and subsequently cardiac output, but it does not seem to improve cerebral oxygenation [40]. There have been no trials comparing volume versus no volume as the initial approach prior to commencing an inotrope, and it is unlikely that such a trial will take place. In the absence of supporting evidence, judicious use of volume as a first line intervention would be reasonable. The recent HIP trial compares volume and dopamine versus volume and placebo in preterm infants with low blood pressure in the first days of life. The trial attempts to limit volume administration to a single bolus of normal saline. It will be interesting to determine the instances where this was the case.

Inotropes, Vasopressors and Inodilators

The aim of these agents is to improve organ perfusion, primarily by increasing cardiac output, and/or decreasing peripheral systemic vascular resistance (SVR), and/or increasing SVR to increase blood pressure. It is important to recognise that very few studies regarding the efficacy of these drugs have been performed in this patient population, though some are planned [70].

Despite the fact that these vasoactive drugs have been used for preterm infants for almost half a century, evidence regarding end organ blood flow, specifically cerebral perfusion, and important short term outcome for both hypotension and low-flow states in preterm infants is still lacking [71]. From a number of small studies, it is safe to assume that most inotropes and vasopressors result in an increase in blood pressure values. Less is known however about their effect on end organ perfusion. For the different drugs used in preterm hypotension, end organ perfusion is probably mediated by alterations in systemic BP, pulmonary vascular resistance, cardiac output, a direct effect on organ vasculature, or a combination of these effects.

In clinical practice, to be able to choose the optimal treatment in an unwell infant with signs of poor perfusion is the new challenge, and one can no longer advise the 'cookbook approach' of the pre-set sequence of dopamine, dobutamine, adrenaline and steroids that is often used. Combining the knowledge on the etiology for the circulatory compromise, the theoretical modes of action of the various available drugs, and the ability for some to measure the effect of the chosen agent, using measures of micro- and macro perfusion will help guide our course of action. Unfortunately, little is known on the specific pharmacokinetics and pharmacodynamics in the very preterm infant, and the susceptibility for the agents in these patients [72], which are different from those in more mature patients [73]. Many recent publications provide excellent overviews of the various vasoactive agents, their mode of action, and proposed doses [74, 75].

Dopamine is the most studied inotrope in the newborn and the most used [4]. Numerous cohort studies have shown it to increase BP and cardiac output (CO) in hypotensive preterm infants [76–80]. However there is conflicting evidence from randomised controlled trials on the effects of dopamine. The inotrope/vasopressor imbalance may result in a reduction in cardiac output [81]. Compared to dobutamine, a beta adrenergic agent, dopamine seems to have more potential in increasing BP and heart rate [82], whereas *dobutamine* results in higher left ventricular output and SVC flow [83], probably by lowering SVR. Also, dopamine may result in increased PVR in infants with a PDA [84]. It has been suggested that dopamine may have negative effects on the cerebrovascular auto-regulatory capacity in very preterm infants [85] but this has not been identified by others [86]. In a follow up study neurodevelopmental outcome at 3 years may be worse in infants treated with dopamine versus dobutamine [87]. In a meta-analysis of observational studies dopamine did not only increase BP but also cerebral blood flow [82].

A potentially more potent adrenergic agent would be *adrenaline* (epinephrine). There have been a few randomised trials comparing dopamine to adrenaline [81, 88]. Adrenaline results in a more increased HR, and a higher incidence of hyperglycaemia, and a higher cardiac output. In the paediatric population with septic shock, adrenaline seems more effective and reduces mortality when compared with dopamine [89].

Noradrenaline (norepinephrine) has more potent alpha mediated effects compared to adrenaline, and results in vascular constriction, with a subsequent increased SVR and blood pressure. It may be useful in septic shock, in order to correct the low

SVR [90], A number of cohort studies have reported the effects of noradrenaline in the preterm infant [91, 92], though RCTs to confirm these findings in preterm infants are lacking.

Milrinone, a phosphodiesterase type III inhibitor, both enhances myocardial contractility and diastolic function, and results in after-load reduction. However, it did not prevent a low flow state in high risk preterm infants, compared to placebo [93, 94]. There is conflicting evidence for and against its use following duct ligation. Halliday and colleagues found no benefit for prophylactic milrinone administration following PDA ligation in premature infants although others suggest possible benefit [33, 95]. Further studies in preterm infants are warranted.

A pilot RCT in 2015 in 20 very preterm infants during the first 24 h of life compared vasopressin (arginine vasopressin) to dopamine. Both agents resulted in similar BP increase but less tachycardia in the vasopressin group [96]. It acts through renal water resorption and by regulating smooth muscle tone, with marked vasopressor effects (Barrett CCM 2007). More studies are needed before this potential drug can be recommended in the treatment of shock in the very preterm infant.

Corticosteroids

The Cochrane meta-analysis updated in 2011 on 123 infants with hypotension, concluded that hydrocortisone (HC) may be as effective as dopamine when used as a primary treatment for hypotension. HC also appeared effective in treatment of refractory hypotension in preterm infants without an increase in short term adverse consequences. The Cochrane group, however, do not recommend the routine use of steroids in hypotensive preterm infants because of the lack of long term benefit and safety data [97]. Previously, a random effects meta-analysis showed that HC results in an increased BP (seven studies; $N = 144$) and reduces vasopressor requirement (five studies; $N = 93$). It remains unclear from this analysis, however, if this effect also had clinically beneficial results [98].

There is some debate on whether endogenous cortisol levels should be taken into account in the decision to start steroid therapy in hypotensive infants: In a retrospective cohort study, in 106 infants <28 weeks of gestation in a timeframe when the HC dose for this indication was not standardised, both low (1–3 mg/kg/day) and high dose steroids (4 mg/kg/day) seemed to improve blood pressure. The other finding in this cohort was that treating infants with HC who have baseline cortisol levels >15 mcg dL − 1 was associated with increased hyperglycaemia and death without demonstrated benefit, suggesting that HC therapy should be avoided in that population. As acknowledged by the authors, this study is limited by its relatively small sample size and retrospective study design, adding the risk of treatment selection bias [99].

We would suggest that, if steroids are to be administered, hydrocortisone would be the agent of choice and that these would not be administered as a first line therapeutic agent.

Proposed Intervention Strategies

The following is a list of suggestions. There is limited evidence to support the approaches that are tabulated below. However the aim is to highlight the complexity of the problem rather than just blood pressure based interventions. The clinical assessment remains very important in the decision making process, albeit acknowledging the inherent subjective variation that may exist.

These can be summarised as follows:

- Normal BP, normal cardiac output, normal organ perfusion: no action required.
- Low BP, normal cardiac output, normal organ perfusion (OP): Probably good, continue to measure BP
- Low BP, low Cardiac output, normal OP (auto-regulation): Probably no harm yet, but intervention should be considered.
- Low BP, Low Cardiac output, Low OP: Need to act to improve cardiac output and improve organ perfusion
- Normal BP, normal Cardiac output, Low OP: Probably need to act to improve organ perfusion

Future Perspectives

Management of low blood pressure in the preterm infant is complicated. Simple rules to guide therapy are misleading. The future will bring a much more complex system of assessment which will guide individualised specific therapies. These assessment tools need rigorous evaluation, such as the recent Safeboosc trial of cerebral near infrared spectroscopy which places the end organ at the centre of the solution [47] and represents a paradigm shift in our current approach to haemodynamic instability. Therapies need more rigorous evaluation, and administration methods also need to be considered, especially in the smallest infants were infusion rates may be particularly low [100]. We are now entering a new era where we will move beyond one simple, albeit important parameter of haemodynamic status, where blood pressure monitoring will be augmented by other assessment modalities allowing a more individualised approach to the care of the haemodynamically unstable preterm infant.

Acknowledgements *Funding source:* This article was supported by a Science Foundation Ireland Research Centre Award (INFANT-12/RC/2272).

Conflict of interest: The authors have no actual or potential conflicts of interest relevant to this article to disclose.

References

1. Dempsey EM, Barrington KJ. Treating hypotension in the preterm infant: when and with what: a critical and systematic review. J Perinatol. 2007;27(8):469–78.
2. Laughon M, Bose C, Allred E, O'Shea TM, Van Marter LJ, Bednarek F, et al. Factors associated with treatment for hypotension in extremely low gestational age newborns during the first postnatal week. Pediatrics. 2007;119(2):273–80.
3. Batton B, Li L, Newman NS, Das A, Watterberg KL, Yoder BA, et al. Use of antihypotensive therapies in extremely preterm infants. Pediatrics. 2013;131(6):e1865–73.
4. Stranak Z, Semberova J, Barrington K, O'Donnell C, Marlow N, Naulaers G, et al. International survey on diagnosis and management of hypotension in extremely preterm babies. Eur J Pediatr. 2014;173(6):793–8.
5. Development of audit measures and guidelines for good practice in the management of neonatal respiratory distress syndrome. Report of a Joint Working Group of the British Association of Perinatal Medicine and the Research Unit of the Royal College of Physicians. Arch Dis Child. 1992;67(10 Spec No):1221–7.
6. Barrington KJ, Stewart S, Lee S. Differing blood pressure thresholds in preterm infants, effects on frequency of diagnosis of hypotension and intraventricular haemorrhage. Pediatr Res. 2002;51:455A.
7. Noori S, Stavroudis TA, Seri I. Systemic and cerebral hemodynamics during the transitional period after premature birth. Clin Perinatol. 2009;36(4):723–36, v.
8. Anderson PA. Maturation and cardiac contractility. Cardiol Clin. 1989;7:209–25.
9. Pladys P, Wodey E, Beuchee A, Branger B, Betremieux P. Left ventricle output and mean arterial blood pressure in preterm infants during the 1st day of life. Eur J Pediatr. 1999;158(10):817–24.
10. Kluckow M, Evans N. Ductal shunting, high pulmonary blood flow, and pulmonary hemorrhage. J Pediatr. 2000;137(1):68–72.
11. Mitchell T, MacDonald JW, Srinouanpranchanh S, Bammler TK, Merillat S, Boldenow E, et al. Evidence of cardiac involvement in the fetal inflammatory response syndrome: disruption of gene networks programming cardiac development in nonhuman primates. Am J Obstet Gynecol. 2018;218(4):438.e1–438.e16.
12. Galinsky R, Hooper SB, Wallace MJ, Westover AJ, Black MJ, Moss TJ, et al. Intrauterine inflammation alters cardiopulmonary and cerebral haemodynamics at birth in preterm lambs. J Physiol. 2013;591(8):2127–37.
13. de Waal KA, Evans N, Osborn DA, Kluckow M. Cardiorespiratory effects of changes in end expiratory pressure in ventilated newborns. Arch Dis Child Fetal Neonatal Ed. 2007;92(6):F444–8.
14. Lakkundi A, Wright I, de Waal K. Transitional hemodynamics in preterm infants with a respiratory management strategy directed at avoidance of mechanical ventilation. Early Hum Dev. 2014;90(8):409–12.
15. Seri I. Circulatory support of the sick preterm infant. Semin Neonatol. 2001;6(1):85–95.
16. Shimokaze T, Akaba K, Saito E. Oscillometric and intra-arterial blood pressure in preterm and term infants: extent of discrepancy and factors associated with inaccuracy. Am J Perinatol. 2015;32(3):277–82.
17. O'Shea J, Dempsey EM. A comparison of blood pressure measurements in newborns. Am J Perinatol. 2009;26(2):113–6.
18. Versmold HT, Kitterman JA, Phibbs RH, Gregory GA, Tooley WH. Aortic blood pressure during the first 12 hours of life in infants with birth weight 610 to 4,220 grams. Pediatrics. 1981;67(5):607–13.
19. Cunningham S, Symon AG, Elton RA, Zhu C, McIntosh N. Intra-arterial blood pressure reference ranges, death and morbidity in very low birthweight infants during the first seven days of life. Early Hum Dev. 1999;56(2–3):151–65.

20. Lee J, Rajadurai VS, Tan KW. Blood pressure standards for very low birthweight infants during the first day of life. Arch Dis Child Fetal Neonatal Ed. 1999;81(3):F168–70.
21. Batton B, Li L, Newman NS, Das A, Watterberg KL, Yoder BA, et al. Evolving blood pressure dynamics for extremely preterm infants. J Perinatol. 2014;34(4):301–5.
22. El-Khuffash A, McNamara PJ. Hemodynamic assessment and monitoring of premature infants. Clin Perinatol. 2017;44(2):377–93.
23. Miletin J, Pichova K, Dempsey EM. Bedside detection of low systemic flow in the very low birth weight infant on day 1 of life. Eur J Pediatr. 2009;168(7):809–13.
24. Kluckow M, Evans N. Relationship between blood pressure and cardiac output in preterm infants requiring mechanical ventilation. J Pediatr. 1996;129(4):506–12.
25. de Boode WP. Clinical monitoring of systemic hemodynamics in critically ill newborns. Early Hum Dev. 2010;86(3):137–41.
26. Osborn DA, Evans N, Kluckow M. Clinical detection of low upper body blood flow in very premature infants using blood pressure, capillary refill time, and central-peripheral temperature difference. Arch Dis Child Fetal Neonatal Ed. 2004;89(2):F168–73.
27. Tibby SM, Hatherill M, Marsh MJ, Morrison G, Anderson D, Murdoch IA. Clinical validation of cardiac output measurements using femoral artery thermodilution with direct Fick in ventilated children and infants. Intensive Care Med. 1997;23(9):987–91.
28. de Boode WP, Singh Y, Gupta S, Austin T, Bohlin K, Dempsey E, et al. Recommendations for neonatologist performed echocardiography in Europe: consensus statement endorsed by European Society for Paediatric Research (ESPR) and European Society for Neonatology (ESN). Pediatr Res. 2016;80(4):465–71.
29. Singh Y, Gupta S, Groves AM, Gandhi A, Thomson J, Qureshi S, et al. Expert consensus statement 'Neonatologist-performed Echocardiography (NoPE)'-training and accreditation in UK. Eur J Pediatr. 2016;175(2):281–7.
30. Mertens L, Seri I, Marek J, Arlettaz R, Barker P, McNamara P, et al. Targeted neonatal echocardiography in the neonatal intensive care unit: practice guidelines and recommendations for training. Writing Group of the American Society of Echocardiography (ASE) in collaboration with the European Association of Echocardiography (EAE) and the Association for European Pediatric Cardiologists (AEPC). J Am Soc Echocardiogr. 2011;24(10):1057–78.
31. Kluckow M, Seri I, Evans N. Functional echocardiography: an emerging clinical tool for the neonatologist. J Pediatr. 2007;150(2):125–30.
32. Noori S, Seri I. Does targeted neonatal echocardiography affect hemodynamics and cerebral oxygenation in extremely preterm infants? J Perinatol. 2014;34(11):847–9.
33. El-Khuffash AF, Jain A, Weisz D, Mertens L, McNamara PJ. Assessment and treatment of post patent ductus arteriosus ligation syndrome. J Pediatr. 2014;165(1):46–52.e1.
34. Sehgal A, Paul E, Menahem S. Functional echocardiography in staging for ductal disease severity: role in predicting outcomes. Eur J Pediatr. 2013;172(2):179–84.
35. Elsayed YN, Amer R, Seshia MM. The impact of integrated evaluation of hemodynamics using targeted neonatal echocardiography with indices of tissue oxygenation: a new approach. J Perinatol. 2017;37(5):527–35.
36. Harabor A, Soraisham AS. Utility of targeted neonatal echocardiography in the management of neonatal illness. J Ultrasound Med. 2015;34(7):1259–63.
37. Subhedar NV. Treatment of hypotension in newborns. Semin Neonatol. 2003;8(6):413–23.
38. van Bel F, Lemmers P, Naulaers G. Monitoring neonatal regional cerebral oxygen saturation in clinical practice: value and pitfalls. Neonatology. 2008;94(4):237–44.
39. Dix LM, van Bel F, Lemmers PM. Monitoring cerebral oxygenation in neonates: an update. Front Pediatr. 2017;5:46.
40. Kooi EM, van der Laan ME, Verhagen EA, Van Braeckel KN, Bos AF. Volume expansion does not alter cerebral tissue oxygen extraction in preterm infants with clinical signs of poor perfusion. Neonatology. 2013;103(4):308–14.
41. Underwood MA, Milstein JM, Sherman MP. Near-infrared spectroscopy as a screening tool for patent ductus arteriosus in extremely low birth weight infants. Neonatology. 2007;91(2):134–9.

42. Chock VY, Ramamoorthy C, Van Meurs KP. Cerebral oxygenation during different treatment strategies for a patent ductus arteriosus. Neonatology. 2011;100(3):233–40.

43. Moran M, Miletin J, Pichova K, Dempsey EM. Cerebral tissue oxygenation index and superior vena cava blood flow in the very low birth weight infant. Acta Paediatr. 2009;98(1):43–6.

44. Takami T, Suganami Y, Sunohara D, Kondo A, Mizukaki N, Fujioka T, et al. Umbilical cord milking stabilizes cerebral oxygenation and perfusion in infants born before 29 weeks of gestation. J Pediatr. 2012;161(4):742–7.

45. Garner RS, Burchfield DJ. Treatment of presumed hypotension in very low birthweight neonates: effects on regional cerebral oxygenation. Arch Dis Child Fetal Neonatal Ed. 2013;98(2):F117–21.

46. Hyttel-Sorensen S, Austin T, van Bel F, Benders M, Claris O, Dempsey E, et al. A phase II randomized clinical trial on cerebral near-infrared spectroscopy plus a treatment guideline versus treatment as usual for extremely preterm infants during the first three days of life (SafeBoosC): study protocol for a randomized controlled trial. Trials. 2013;14:120.

47. Hyttel-Sorensen S, Pellicer A, Alderliesten T, Austin T, van Bel F, Benders M, et al. Cerebral near infrared spectroscopy oximetry in extremely preterm infants: phase II randomised clinical trial. BMJ. 2015;350:g7635.

48. Verhagen EA, Hummel LA, Bos AF, Kooi EM. Near-infrared spectroscopy to detect absence of cerebrovascular autoregulation in preterm infants. Clin Neurophysiol. 2014;125(1):47–52.

49. Kooi EMW, Verhagen EA, Elting JWJ, Czosnyka M, Austin T, Wong FY, et al. Measuring cerebrovascular autoregulation in preterm infants using near-infrared spectroscopy: an overview of the literature. Expert Rev Neurother. 2017;17(8):801–18.

50. He SR, Zhang C, Liu YM, Sun YX, Zhuang J, Chen JM, et al. Accuracy of the ultrasonic cardiac output monitor in healthy term neonates during postnatal circulatory adaptation. Chin Med J. 2011;124(15):2284–9.

51. Ballestero Y, Lopez-Herce J, Urbano J, Solana MJ, Botran M, Bellon JM, et al. Measurement of cardiac output in children by bioreactance. Pediatr Cardiol. 2011;32(4):469–72.

52. Norozi K, Beck C, Osthaus WA, Wille I, Wessel A, Bertram H. Electrical velocimetry for measuring cardiac output in children with congenital heart disease. Br J Anaesth. 2008;100(1):88–94.

53. Song R, Rich W, Kim JH, Finer NN, Katheria AC. The use of electrical cardiometry for continuous cardiac output monitoring in preterm neonates: a validation study. Am J Perinatol. 2014;31(12):1105–10.

54. Weisz DE, Jain A, McNamara PJ, El-Khuffash A. Non-invasive cardiac output monitoring in neonates using bioreactance: a comparison with echocardiography. Neonatology. 2012;102(1):61–7.

55. Rodriguez Sanchez de la Blanca A, Sanchez Luna M, Gonzalez Pacheco N, Arriaga Redondo M, Navarro Patino N. Electrical velocimetry for non-invasive monitoring of the closure of the ductus arteriosus in preterm infants. Eur J Pediatr. 2018;177(2):229–35.

56. Torigoe T, Sato S, Nagayama Y, Sato T, Yamazaki H. Influence of patent ductus arteriosus and ventilators on electrical velocimetry for measuring cardiac output in very-low/low birth weight infants. J Perinatol. 2015;35(7):485–9.

57. Freidl T, Baik N, Pichler G, Schwaberger B, Zingerle B, Avian A, et al. Haemodynamic transition after birth: a new tool for non-invasive cardiac output monitoring. Neonatology. 2017;111(1):55–60.

58. Wu TW, Tamrazi B, Soleymani S, Seri I, Noori S. Hemodynamic changes during rewarming phase of whole-body hypothermia therapy in neonates with hypoxic-ischemic encephalopathy. J Pediatr. 2018;197:68–74.e2.

59. Alderliesten T, Lemmers PM, Baerts W, Groenendaal F, van Bel F. Perfusion index in preterm infants during the first 3 days of life: reference values and relation with clinical variables. Neonatology. 2015;107(4):258–65.

60. Kinoshita M, Hawkes CP, Ryan CA, Dempsey EM. Perfusion index in the very preterm infant. Acta Paediatr. 2013;102(9):e398–401.

61. De Felice C, Goldstein MR, Parrini S, Verrotti A, Criscuolo M, Latini G. Early dynamic changes in pulse oximetry signals in preterm newborns with histologic chorioamnionitis. Pediatr Crit Care Med. 2006;7(2):138–42.

62. Kroese JK, van Vonderen JJ, Narayen IC, Walther FJ, Hooper S, Te Pas AB. The perfusion index of healthy term infants during transition at birth. Eur J Pediatr. 2016;175(4):475–9.

63. Zaramella P, Freato F, Quaresima V, Secchieri S, Milan A, Grisafi D, et al. Early versus late cord clamping: effects on peripheral blood flow and cardiac function in term infants. Early Hum Dev. 2008;84(3):195–200.

64. Janaillac M, Beausoleil TP, Barrington KJ, Raboisson MJ, Karam O, Dehaes M, et al. Correlations between near-infrared spectroscopy, perfusion index, and cardiac outputs in extremely preterm infants in the first 72 h of life. Eur J Pediatr. 2018;177(4):541–50.

65. Gomez-Pomar E, Makhoul M, Westgate PM, Ibonia KT, Patwardhan A, Giannone PJ, et al. Relationship between perfusion index and patent ductus arteriosus in preterm infants. Pediatr Res. 2017;81(5):775–9.

66. Van Laere D, O'Toole JM, Voeten M, McKiernan J, Boylan GB, Dempsey E. Decreased variability and low values of perfusion index on day one are associated with adverse outcome in extremely preterm infants. J Pediatr. 2016;178:119–24.e1.

67. Sehgal A, Osborn D, McNamara PJ. Cardiovascular support in preterm infants: a survey of practices in Australia and New Zealand. J Paediatr Child Health. 2012;48(4):317–23.

68. Evans N. Volume expansion during neonatal intensive care: do we know what we are doing? Semin Neonatol. 2003;8(4):315–23.

69. Osborn DA, Evans N. Early volume expansion for prevention of morbidity and mortality in very preterm infants. Cochrane Database Syst Rev. 2004(2):CD002055.

70. Dempsey EM, Barrington KJ, Marlow N, O'Donnell CP, Miletin J, Naulaers G, et al. Management of hypotension in preterm infants (the HIP trial): a randomised controlled trial of hypotension management in extremely low gestational age newborns. Neonatology. 2014;105(4):275–81.

71. Garvey AA, Kooi EMW, Dempsey EM. Inotropes for preterm infants: 50 years on are we any wiser? Front Pediatr. 2018;6:88.

72. Ogasawara K, Sato M, Hashimoto K, Imamura T, Go H, Hosoya M. A polymorphism in the glucocorticoid receptor gene is associated with refractory hypotension in premature infants. Pediatr Neonatol. 2018;59(3):251–7.

73. Giaccone A, Zuppa AF, Sood B, Cohen MS, O'Byrne ML, Moorthy G, et al. Milrinone pharmacokinetics and pharmacodynamics in neonates with persistent pulmonary hypertension of the newborn. Am J Perinatol. 2017;34(8):749–58.

74. Joynt C, Cheung PY. Treating hypotension in preterm neonates with vasoactive medications. Front Pediatr. 2018;6:86.

75. Ergenekon E, Rojas-Anaya H, Bravo MC, Kotidis C, Mahoney L, Rabe H. Cardiovascular drug therapy for human newborn: review of pharmacodynamic data. Curr Pharm Des. 2017;23(38):5850–60.

76. Lundstrom K, Pryds O, Greisen G. The haemodynamic effects of dopamine and volume expansion in sick preterm infants. Early Hum Dev. 2000;57(2):157–63.

77. Cuevas L, Yeh TF, John EG, Cuevas D, Plides RS. The effect of low-dose dopamine infusion on cardiopulmonary and renal status in premature newborns with respiratory distress syndrome. Am J Dis Child. 1991;145(7):799–803.

78. Padbury JF. Neonatal dopamine pharmacodynamics: lessons from the bedside. J Pediatr. 1998;133(6):719–20.

79. Zhang J, Penny DJ, Kim NS, Yu VY, Smolich JJ. Mechanisms of blood pressure increase induced by dopamine in hypotensive preterm neonates. Arch Dis Child Fetal Neonatal Ed. 1999;81(2):F99–F104.

80. Evans N, Osborn D, Kluckow M. Mechanism of blood pressure increase induced by dopamine in hypotensive preterm neonates. Arch Dis Child Fetal Neonatal Ed. 2000;83(1):F75–6.

81. Phillipos EZ, Barrington KJ, Robertson MA. Dopamine versus epinephrine for inotropic support in the neonate: a randomised blinded trial. Peditr Res. 1996;39:A238.
82. Sassano-Higgins S, Friedlich P, Seri I. A meta-analysis of dopamine use in hypotensive preterm infants: blood pressure and cerebral hemodynamics. J Perinatol. 2011;31(10):647–55.
83. Osborn D, Evans N, Kluckow M. Randomized trial of dobutamine versus dopamine in preterm infants with low systemic blood flow. J Pediatr. 2002;140(2):183–91.
84. Liet JM, Boscher C, Gras-Leguen C, Gournay V, Debillon T, Roze JC. Dopamine effects on pulmonary artery pressure in hypotensive preterm infants with patent ductus arteriosus. J Pediatr. 2002;140(3):373–5.
85. Eriksen VR, Hahn GH, Greisen G. Dopamine therapy is associated with impaired cerebral autoregulation in preterm infants. Acta Paediatr. 2014;103(12):1221–6.
86. Wong FY, Barfield CP, Horne RS, Walker AM. Dopamine therapy promotes cerebral flow-metabolism coupling in preterm infants. Intensive Care Med. 2009;35(10):1777–82.
87. Osborn DA, Evans N, Kluckow M, Bowen JR, Rieger I. Low superior vena cava flow and effect of inotropes on neurodevelopment to 3 years in preterm infants. Pediatrics. 2007;120(2):372–80.
88. Pellicer A, Valverde E, Elorza MD, Madero R, Gaya F, Quero J, et al. Cardiovascular support for low birth weight infants and cerebral hemodynamics: a randomized, blinded, clinical trial. Pediatrics. 2005;115(6):1501–12.
89. Ventura AM, Shieh HH, Bousso A, Goes PF, de Cassia FOFI, de Souza DC, et al. Double-blind prospective randomized controlled trial of dopamine versus epinephrine as first-line vasoactive drugs in pediatric septic shock. Crit Care Med. 2015;43(11):2292–302.
90. Rizk MY, Lapointe A, Lefebvre F, Barrington KJ. Norepinephrine infusion improves haemodynamics in the preterm infants during septic shock. Acta Paediatr. 2018;107(3):408–13.
91. Tourneux P, Rakza T, Abazine A, Krim G, Storme L. Noradrenaline for management of septic shock refractory to fluid loading and dopamine or dobutamine in full-term newborn infants. Acta Paediatr. 2008;97(2):177–80.
92. Rowcliff K, de Waal K, Mohamed AL, Chaudhari T. Noradrenaline in preterm infants with cardiovascular compromise. Eur J Pediatr. 2016;175(12):1967–73.
93. Paradisis M, Evans N, Kluckow M, Osborn D, McLachlan AJ. Pilot study of milrinone for low systemic blood flow in very preterm infants. J Pediatr. 2006;148(3):306–13.
94. Paradisis M, Evans N, Kluckow M, Osborn D. Randomized trial of milrinone versus placebo for prevention of low systemic blood flow in very preterm infants. J Pediatr. 2009;154(2):189–95.
95. Sehgal A. Haemodynamically unstable preterm infant: an unresolved management conundrum. Eur J Pediatr. 2011;170(10):1237–45.
96. Rios DR, Kaiser JR. Vasopressin versus dopamine for treatment of hypotension in extremely low birth weight infants: a randomized, blinded pilot study. J Pediatr. 2015;166(4):850–5.
97. Ibrahim H, Sinha IP, Subhedar NV. Corticosteroids for treating hypotension in preterm infants. Cochrane Database Syst Rev. 2011(12):CD003662.
98. Higgins S, Friedlich P, Seri I. Hydrocortisone for hypotension and vasopressor dependence in preterm neonates: a meta-analysis. J Perinatol. 2010;30(6):373–8.
99. Peeples ES. An evaluation of hydrocortisone dosing for neonatal refractory hypotension. J Perinatol. 2017;37(8):943–6.
100. van der Eijk AC, van Rens RM, Dankelman J, Smit BJ. A literature review on flow-rate variability in neonatal IV therapy. Paediatr Anaesth. 2013;23(1):9–21.

Chapter 18
Retinopathy of Prematurity

Samira Anwar and Aarti Patel

Introduction

Retinopathy of prematurity (ROP) is a potentially treatable sight-threatening disorder that results from the abnormal development of intraretinal vasculature in preterm infants. ROP occurs worldwide [1] and, in the United States, it is the third most common cause of childhood blindness [2]. Visual impairment resulting from ROP varies, with rates of 2–12% in highly industrialised countries in Northern Europe and up to 38% in the low to middle income countries of Latin America and South East Asia [3]. Babies born before 32 weeks of gestation, or with birth weight below 1000 g are most likely to develop ROP that requires treatment, which is known as Type 1 ROP, according to the International Committee for the Classification of Retinopathy of Prematurity [4]. In less developed countries, Type 1 ROP can also occur in more mature infants [5], and it is recognised that the reported prevalence will be influenced by the availability of resources to allow screening for and treatment of the disease [6]. Although the prevalence has remained stable in the United States [7], the increasing problem of ROP on a global scale [8] has driven the need to target screening and assessment as well as explore opportunities for new treatment methods.

The retina is incompletely vascularised at birth and the high oxygen demands of the photoreceptor layer lead to local ischaemia and the release of intra-ocular vascular endothelial growth factors (VEGF). In preterm birth, the physiological ischaemia of

S. Anwar (✉)
University Hospitals of Leicester NHS Trust, Leicester, UK

Department of Neuroscience, Psychology and Behaviour, University of Leicester, Leicester, UK
e-mail: sa528@leicester.ac.uk

A. Patel
Ulverscroft Eye Unit, University of Leicester, Leicester, UK
e-mail: ap552@le.ac.uk

© Springer Nature Switzerland AG 2020
E. M. Boyle, J. Cusack (eds.), *Emerging Topics and Controversies in Neonatology*, https://doi.org/10.1007/978-3-030-28829-7_18

normal intra-retinal vascular growth is disrupted by the effects of oxygen [9, 10]. This leads to the release of abnormally elevated levels of intra-ocular VEGF and arrested angiogenesis of the intra-retinal vascular bed in the avascular portion of the incomplete immature retina. In higher risk infants, this process may result in intra-retinal haemorrhage, oedema and subsequent retinal detachment. Early identification and treatment using photoreceptor ablative laser therapy of the affected retina reduces the risk of sight loss [11]. Infants therefore undergo regular ocular screening performed by an ophthalmologist in the nursery to identify high risk babies. Identifying the infants that benefit most from ROP intervention is based on subjective assessment of the retinal appearance and can vary between specialists [12]. Furthermore, although up to 30% may have severe ROP [13, 14] less than 5% of all infants who are screened have Type 1 ROP [15] resulting in a proportion of unnecessary examinations. Consequently, recent developments in ROP study have sought to investigate newer methods of assessment through imaging and to explore early prognostic factors accurately identifying preterm infants with Type 1 ROP. The primary objective has been both to reduce unnecessary screening, and to maximise treatment outcome from judicious intervention without missing infants that require treatment.

ROP Imaging Modalities

Conventional ocular screening for ROP requires visualisation of the retina using a binocular indirect ophthalmoscope (BIO). Dilation of the pupil is achieved after instillation of drops prior to the examination which allows the ophthalmologist detailed views of the peripheral retina and the line of vascularisation between the developed and avascular retina. Improvements in imaging techniques have resulted in better identification of structures not visible with conventional examination.

Fluorescein Angiography

In the investigation of retinal disease, a widespread diagnostic tool is fluorescein angiography (FA). Sodium fluorescein is a dye that is stimulated by blue light (465–490 nm), showing yellow-green (520–530 nm) fluorescence. Fluorescein is administered through peripheral intravenous injection and is rapidly distributed throughout the body, appearing in the retinal tissues within a few seconds. The pattern of fluorescence outlining the retinal vessels is observed and recorded using a camera projecting blue light. This allows detection of the developing superficial intra-retinal microcirculation normally invisible to the ophthalmologist using conventional BIO examination. FA aids in determining the extent of the vascular abnormality and the areas of underperfused or ischaemic retina. FA also reveals subtle early disease undetectable with direct visualization [16, 17] that may develop and require treatment later. An example of FA with color image is shown below in Fig. 18.1:

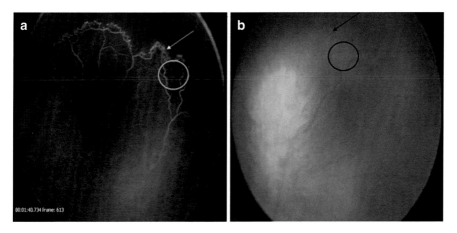

Fig. 18.1 Right eye. Superior and nasal retina. Fluorescein angiogram (FA) left image (**a**) with corresponding color image on the right (**b**). Arrows show the demarcation of vascular to non-vascular retina

In Fig. 18.1, FA highlights the hyperfluorescent vessel tips, which are bulbous, but no vessels exist beyond the demarcation. The circle on the FA image highlights the absence of vessels (dark area) within the retina which represents ischaemia. This is not evident on the corresponding color image.

Increased tortuosity and dilation of retinal vessels may signal the development of Type 1 ROP. This appearance is known as 'Plus' disease but the vascular changes preceding this appearance are not always easily recognised by conventional examination. Fluorescein angiography has been used in premature infants where the appearance of the retinal vessels begins to show increased tortuosity and dilation and also in those infants where further treatment is being contemplated but the timing of that intervention is unclear.

The application of imaging devices with FA facility has made use of FA increasingly practical in the nursery. Ng et al. [16] studied 23 consecutive premature infants born at gestational age (GA) 30 weeks or less and weighing 1500 g or less. This was during routine ROP screening with every patient undergoing FA at the first screening session. The youngest patient was 26.3 weeks GA, the lowest birth weight was 660 g. Between 1 and 5 angiograms were performed for each patient depending on need based on clinical observation and comparison of FA changes from the first screening session. A total of 51 sessions of FA were performed. There were no adverse effects reported in any of the babies at any of the sessions. The study commenced in 2003 and by 2006, over 200 such FA's had been performed safely.

The results showed clearly the distinction between vascular and non-vascular retina, regression of ROP where there was remodelling of vessels and cessation of fluorescein leakage in those areas that were improving. FA also demonstrated abnormalities in the capillary network adjacent to the demarcation (ridge) not visible on direct observation and subsequent progression to 'Plus' disease in a baby who then required treatment. The authors described arteriovenous abnormalities seen exclusively on FA that likely represented incompetent vessels within areas of ischaemia. This provided objective evidence for abnormal retinal areas indicating the extent and severity of ischaemia, key information in the decision-making process on whether to intervene or not.

A similar study in 2008 by Azad et al. [18] reported favourable results from the use of FA in detecting missed areas of active ROP in the peripheral retina particularly in those babies who had undergone at least one treatment. They were also able to identify earlier detection of new vessels in retinal zones associated with high risk disease (Zone1/Zone2) that were undetectable with direct visualisation.

Lepore et al. [19] retrospectively examined FA for severe acute phase ROP at the time of laser photocoagulation. Their FA findings showed extreme variability in both the type and number of retinal lesions. Within the ischaemic retina only some or all of the features described in severe ischaemic retinopathy were seen. The conclusion from this is that for each individual baby's FA, previous angiograms are necessary in order to demonstrate progression and worsening of ischaemic vascular signs in order to benefit from pre-treatment angiography and in particular where further intervention may be necessary.

A drawback of FA is that the typical appearance of premature retinal vessels, that are, by definition immature before significant ROP develops, is currently unknown. Consequently, the interpretation of FA when significant ROP develops cannot be used to absolutely affirm that there is increasing ischaemia in a particular baby's eye and therefore its role is limited as an adjunct in the decision-making process. However, FA allows objective assessment of the retina as it develops and the development of ROP in very high-risk infants so that timing of intervention is better targeted with greater clinical effectiveness. Further, it permits detection of early significant disease not visualized using indirect ophthalmoscopy or conventional color imaging devices so that treatment is timely, as better structural outcomes are associated with early intervention rather than late [10].

By quantifying the development of the immature vessels before the onset of disease, in those cases where further treatment is necessary, meaningful comparisons may be made with previously recorded angiograms so that treatment can be directed into those areas of ischaemia that are shown to have changed. This reduces the overall amount of surgical destruction and the time necessary to perform retreatment.

Ultra-Wide Field Imaging (UWFI)

A non-contact method of retinal examination known as ultra-wide field imaging (UWFI) has been developed using scanning laser technology. UWFI is advocated in the assessment of the retina due to the superior visualisation of the retinal periphery, using fewer images than those acquired from narrower field contact devices such as those that require the use of a probe resting on the infant's eye. There is an additional advantage in clarity of view for patients with media haze and small pupils since the technology does not require conventional light sources. This is particularly of benefit for patients who have undergone surgery or intravitreal injections for retinal disease. Its use has been limited to older children and adults who are co-operative or those that can physically use the instruments (i.e. sitting upright). However, this method is being utilised in the monitoring of ROP [20] and a technique to position preterm infants in the nursery into a UWFI device has been developed known as the 'flying baby' [21]. However, a major disadvantage of UWFI is the cost and size of the devices, and currently no portable machines are available.

Optical Coherence Tomography (OCT) in Prematurity

Optical coherence tomography (OCT) performs cross-sectional imaging of tissue structures using a technique similar to ultrasound. In the place of ultrasound waves, OCT utilises backscattered or back reflected light to create high resolution images (1–15 μm) of the retina [22]. Since inception in 1991, OCT has revolutionised clinical care for many adult ocular conditions influencing diagnostic criteria, screening guidelines and surgical intervention.

Conventional OCT imaging requires patients to sit up and position their head towards a chin rest, thereby limiting application to premature infants. Despite these challenges Patel et al. were able to successfully adapt a table-mounted device for supine imaging of a premature infant under general anaesthetic [23]. The authors demonstrated that OCT could provide additional valuable information to conventional BIO examination in preterm infants, leading to a more accurate diagnosis and change of subsequent management. In a similar case report, Vinekar et al. also adapted a table-mounted device to image supine premature infants; however the device was smaller and could be using in the neonatal unit without sedation [24]. The report describes changes to the retinal structure before and after laser treatment for two cases of severe ROP.

More recently, OCT specifically designed for handheld use has become commercially available. Subsequent papers have demonstrated excellent feasibility of imaging premature infants without sedation in the neonatal unit [25, 26].

During the preterm period, studies have shown that the hand held OCT device (HHOCT) can identify structures not visible with conventional BIO examination. Initial case reports describe presence of retinoschisis (splitting of the retinal layers), retinal detachment and pre-retinal structures such as fibrovascular tissue [27, 28]. Several studies also report the presence of macular edema. Macular edema consists of the accumulation of fluid filled spaces at the macula with resulting distortion of retinal structures. In older children and adults, this is typically associated with reduced function and subsequent visual loss, where it is described as cystoid macular edema (CME).

Although the appearance of fluid filled spaces at the macula in preterm infants shares some similarities to that of CME, the pathophysiology and clinical visual significance of the transient macular edema of preterm and term infants is currently unknown and remains speculative. Vinekar et al. report a prevalence of 29.1% amongst infants imaged after 35 weeks PMA with statistically significantly greater thickness for infants with more severe ROP [29]. In contrast Maldonado et al. report varying prevalence from 13% at 31 weeks PMA to 65% at 36 weeks PMA with no statistical differences between ROP groups [30]. The differences between study results may be due to ethnicity, age of participants and sample size. Interestingly, Vinekar et al. report resolution of macula edema by 52 weeks PMA demonstrating the dynamic nature of retinal development in the first few months of life [29].

The application of HHOCT for the diagnosis and management of ROP remains unclear at present. Maldonado et al. examined HHOCT images of ten premature infants who progressed to severe ROP requiring treatment [31]. Retinal vessel abnormalities were described and developed to a risk score. However, the analysis was based on a small cohort of participants and requires further study. A recent report by Anwar et al. [32] suggests that foveal width measured using HHOCT, is significantly different in early PMA, when screening begins, for infants with ROP in comparison with those where ROP is absent. This observation could distinguish between preterm infants that require screening from those that do not, thereby reducing the number of infants that require ocular examination. Although further investigation is required to determine prognostic capability, HHOCT and the newer modality of HHOCT with FA, demonstrate the future potential in understanding the development of ROP and early identification of Type 1 ROP utilising these imaging technologies.

Additional HHOCT studies have explored the development of retinal structures in vivo, In a study of fovea maturation using HHOCT Vajzovic et al. imaged a series of premature infants, children and an adult [33]. The authors were able to compare results to histology samples identifying the cellular structural basis of the HHOCT images. In a subsequent paper the group report infants born before 32 weeks GA to have delayed photoreceptor development compared to control group full term infants when imaged at 37–42 weeks postmenstrual age suggesting premature birth may affect retinal development later in life [34].

ROP Risk Algorithms and Tools

Screening programmes for ROP aim to identify all infants at risk of developing sight-threatening ROP. In the largest published study, The Multicentre Trial of Cryotherapy for ROP, 4099 infants with a birth weight less than 1251 g were monitored for developing ROP [35]. The study found the incidence and severity were higher for lower birth weight categories forming the basis for international screening programmes [36–38].

Globally approximately 845,000, and in the UK approximately 8100, preterm infants are screened for ROP annually [39]. Less than 5% screened infants require treatment resulting in many children undergoing multiple examinations unnecessarily and increasing the economic burden of screening programs [14, 15]. This has led many researchers to explore additional factors that may help determine which infants are at highest risk of severe ROP.

Postnatal weight gain is one such factor suggested as a predictor for severe ROP. Allergaert et al. compared 25 premature infants who reached threshold ROP with 25 'controls' defined as premature infants with statistically similar gestational age at birth [40]. The study found absolute weight gain (weight increase per day) to be statistically higher in 'control' infants as compared to those who reached threshold ROP; however relative weight gain (i.e. weight increase per day corrected for current weight) did not differ between groups. In a similar case-control larger study with 111 participants, Wallace et al. reported similar findings [41]. Using a multivariate regression model, the study found an association between rate of postnatal weight gain and severity of ROP, which in contrast to Allergaert et al. remained significant when corrected for current weight.

These studies have led to further exploration of postnatal weight gain in ROP and research groups across the world have attempted to incorporate this additional factor into prediction models for ROP (Table 18.1).

Löfqvist and Hellström et al. [42] were the first to describe an algorithm including weekly weight gain and serum insulin-like growth factor 1 (IGF-1, involved in regulating retinal neovascularisation in both animal and human models of ROP) [50]. Using a calculated threshold to determine infants at risk of developing severe ROP the group found all infants who required treatment and 84% of infants who did not develop severe ROP were identified. This has led to the WINROP (Weight, IGF, Neonatal Retinopathy of Prematurity) surveillance program available online where patient details can be entered and a risk score calculated weekly [51]. More recent larger studies using simplified WINROP algorithms without IGF-1 have found very high sensitivities for predicting severe ROP: 100% in a Swedish cohort or 353 infants [43], 95.7% in a Swedish cohort of extremely premature infants [44] and 98.6% in a large multicentre American/Canadian cohort of 1706 infants [52]. However further studies in different populations have found lower sensitivities e.g. 55% in a Mexican cohort of 352 infants, highlighting the potential differences between countries and subsequent application of any risk algorithm.

Eckert et al. have described a simpler model named ROPScore, which can be calculated at 6 weeks chronological age using an Excel spreadsheet [49]. The authors describe 96% and 94% sensitivity for identifying any ROP and Type 1 or type 2 ROP respectively in a Brazilian cohort of 474 infants. Although not at the target of 100% the results show the importance of weight gain even when calculated using relatively simple methods.

In the United States, Binenbaum et al. initially developed the PINT ROP (Premature Infants in Need of Transfusion) model from data collected from another study in premature infants [45]. Similar to WINROP, the model was based on BW, GA, and weight gain and utilised a threshold to identify infants at risk of severe ROP [45]. The algorithm demonstrated 99% sensitivity in a cohort of 451 American/Canadian/Australian participants. The model was updated with data from large multicentre ROP screening records to form CHOP ROP (Children's Hospital of Philadelphia). This model assessed different methods of weight gain as well as other potential factors that may influence ROP including ethnicity, co-morbidities and clinical course. In the most recent publication the group describe a 100% sensitivity for detecting type 1 or 2 ROP in a US/Canadian cohort of 7483 participants [47].

Overall these studies show potential for improving current screening guidelines for ROP. Further large-scale studies in different populations is required prior to a change in international screening guidelines.

Table 18.1 Summary of risk algorithms for predicting retinopathy of prematurity

Name, year of publication	Sample size	Country	Study design	Inclusion criteria	Outcome	Results % (95% CI)
WINROP, 2006 [42]	79	Sweden	Single centre, retrospective	GA < 32 weeks	ROP 0/1: none or stage 1 ROP 2: stage 2 ROP 3: stage 3 ROPT: treated	Predictive model includes GA, BW, IGF-1, weight gain
Updated WINROP, 2009 [43]	353	Sweden	Single centre, retrospective	GA < 32 weeks	Stage 3 ROP	Predictive model includes GA, BW, weight gain Sensitivity 100 (90–100) Specificity 84.5 (81–88) PPV 41 NPV 100
Updated WINROP, 2013 [44]	407	Sweden	Multicentre, retrospective	GA < 27 weeks	Type 1 ROP	Predictive model includes GA, BW, weight gain Sensitivity 95.7 (84.3–99.2) Specificity 23.9 (19.6–28.7) PPV 14.1 (10.5–18.5) NPV 97.7 (91.2–99.6)
PINT ROP, 2011 [45]	451	Canada, United States, Australia	Multicenter retrospective (ROP data collected from another study)	BW < 1000 g	Severe ROP defined as stage 3, 4, or 5, or treatment with laser or cryotherapy ablation	Predictive model includes BW, GA, and daily weight gain rate calculated from the current and previous weeks' weights Sensitivity 99 (94–100) Specificity 36 (32–41) PPV 26 (22–30) NPV 99 (96–100)

CHOP ROP, 2012 [46]	524	United States	Single centre, retrospective	BW $\leq$ 1500 g, or GA $\leq$ 30 weeks	Type 1 or Type 2 ROP	Predictive model includes BW, GA, and daily weight gain rate calculated using daily weight measurements Sensitivity 98 (89–100) Specificity 53 (49–58) PPV 17 (13–22) NPV 100 (98–100)
Updated CHOP ROP, 2017 [47]	7483	Canada, United States	Multicenter retrospective	BW $\leq$ 1500 g, or GA $\leq$ 30 weeks	Type 1 or Type 2 ROP	Updated predictive model Sensitivity 100 Specificity 12.0
CO ROP, 2016 [48]	499	United States	Single centre, retrospective	BW $\leq$ 1500 g, or GA $\leq$ 30 weeks, or unstable clinical course	Any ROP	Revised screening criteria to infants GA $\leq$ 30 weeks and BW $\leq$ 1500 g and weight gain $\leq$ 650 g in first month Sensitivity 96.4 (92.3–98.7) Specificity 33.7 (28.7–39.1)
ROP Score, 2012 [49]	474	Brazil	Single centre, prospective	BW $\leq$ 1500 g and/or GA $\leq$ 32 weeks	Type 1 or Type 2 ROP	Model utilises a point scoring system to be calculated at 6 weeks Sensitivity 96 Specificity 56 PPV 10.5 (7–15.1) NPV 99.6 (98.1–99.9)

Ocular Treatment Using Anti Vascular Endothelial Growth Factor

Newer therapies for the treatment of ROP include the use of intra-vitreal vascular endothelial growth factor (VEGF). Vascular endothelial factor A (VEGF-A) promotes the growth of vascular endothelial cells [53] and is a key molecule expressed during vascularisation [54, 55]. VEGF binds to receptor kinases that are upregulated or downregulated depending on local levels of ischaemia, stage of vascular development and location. Elevated VEGF is found in pathological intra ocular neovascularisation [56–58] and has led to the development of anti-VEGF receptor antibody therapies such as Bevacizumab (Avastin® Roche) and Ranibizumab (Lucentis® Novartis) for vascular retinopathies, notably age-related macular degeneration.

Intra-ocular vascularisation in ROP occurs in two phases from studies in mice. Phase 1 occurs before 31–32 weeks PMA [10] where extremely preterm animals received supplemental oxygen. The hyperoxia induces vaso-obliteration and loss of capillary beds [9]. Phase 2 begins when there is a reduction in the relative level of oxygen or a disparity between the increasing oxygen demands of the retina with a significant increase in tissue hypoxia which results in increased upregulation of VEGF production. This is often at around 32–34 weeks postmenstrual age. Subsequently, this leads to the creation of arteriolar-venular shunts bypassing the ischaemic capillary beds and changes in flow with tortuosity and dilation of retinal vessels in vulnerable individuals. Peripheral neorevascularisation at the demarcation between vascular and avascular retina occurs with the development of the vascular elevation or 'ridge', described as Stage 3 ROP.

Conventional treatment of sight threatening ROP has been from retinal photoablation using diode laser photocoagulation delivered through a binocular indirect ophthalmoscope. Absorption of light energy (810 nm) by the retinal pigment epithelium in the ischaemic vascular retina leads to destruction of photoreceptors. This leads to reduced oxygen demand and intra ocular VEGF, a change in the vascular flow within the inner retina and the normalisation of the vascular retina (regression of ROP). However, laser is destructive and the use of anti VEGF intra-vitreal injections to treat neovascularisation in aggressive ROP was advocated as a possible alternative/adjunctive therapy [59–62]. Mintz-Hittner et al. [62] suggested improved outcomes using anti-VEGF injections in Type 1 ROP confined to Zone 1 versus laser photocoagulation. Since then, investigators describe effective outcomes from minimal doses for therapeutic effect [63, 64] in light of growing concern regarding the effect of various anti-VEGF drugs [65] and the possible systemic [66] and ocular consequences. Ocular concerns have included late reactivation of ROP [67] severe fibrotic reaction and tractional retinal detachment [68], delay in full retinal vascularisation [69] and late retinal detachment [70]. Presently, anti-VEGF is increasingly being used [71, 72] but the consensus is that further study is still necessary to determine the optimal timing and dose, and to understand the long term ocular and systemic effects of its use in sight threatening ROP [73].

Summary

Retinopathy of prematurity remains a challenging problem in the management of premature infants. It is increasing worldwide and has a significant impact on neonates and caregivers as well as on the allocation of healthcare provision within nations. There have been notable improvements in the screening, assessment and treatment for ROP, but the rapid developments in ocular imaging technology, vascular drug therapies and neonatal care offer further opportunities to improve outcomes as well as deepen our understanding of this important disease.

References

1. Gilbert C. Retinopathy of prematurity: a global perspective of the epidemics, population of babies at risk and implications for control. Early Hum Dev. 2008;84:77–82.
2. Kong L, Fry M, Al-Samarraie M, Gilbert C, Steinkuller PG. An update on progress and the changing epidemiology of causes of childhood blindness worldwide. J AAPOS. 2012;16:501–7.
3. Gilbert C, Rahi J, Eckstein M, O'Sullivan J, Foster A. Retinopathy of prematurity in middle-income countries. Lancet. 1997;350:12–4.
4. International Committee for the Classification of Retinopathy of Prematurity. The international classification of retinopathy of prematurity revisited. Arch Ophthalmol. 2005;123:991–9.
5. Gilbert C. Characteristics of infants with severe retinopathy of prematurity in countries with low, moderate, and high levels of development: implications for screening programs. Pediatrics. 2005;115:e518–25.
6. Gergely K, Gerince A. Retinopathy of prematurity—epidemics, incidence, prevalence, blindness. Bratisl Lek List. 2010;111:514–7.
7. Quinn GE, Barr C, Bremer D, et al. Changes in course of retinopathy of prematurity from 1986 to 2013 comparison of three studies in the United States. Ophthalmology. 2016;123:1595–600.
8. Blencowe H, Lawn JE, Vazquez T, Fielder A, Gilbert C. Preterm-associated visual impairment and estimates of retinopathy of prematurity at regional and global levels for 2010. Pediatr Res. 2013;74(Suppl 1):35–49.
9. Claxton S, Fruttiger M. Role of arteries in oxygen induced vaso-obliteration. Exp Eye Res. 2003;77:305–11.
10. Hartnett ME, Penn JS. Mechanisms and management of retinopathy of prematurity. N Engl J Med. 2012;367:2515–26.
11. Good WV. Final results of the early treatment for retinopathy of prematurity (ETROP) randomized trial. Trans Am Ophthalmol Soc. 2004;102:233–48; discussion 248–50
12. Wallace DK, Quinn GE, Freedman SF, Chiang MF. Agreement among pediatric ophthalmologists in diagnosing plus and pre-plus disease in retinopathy of prematurity. J AAPOS. 2008;12:352–6.
13. Stoll BJ, Hansen NI, Bell EF, et al. Neonatal outcomes of extremely preterm infants from the NICHD neonatal research network. Pediatrics. 2010;126:443–56.
14. Good WV, Hardy RJ, Dobson V, Palmer EA, Phelps DL, Quintos M, Tung B, Early Treatment for Retinopathy of Prematurity Cooperative Group. The incidence and course of retinopathy of prematurity: findings from the early treatment for retinopathy of prematurity study. Pediatrics. 2005;116:15–23.
15. Adams GGW, Bunce C, Xing W, Butler L, Long V, Reddy A, Dahlmann-Noor AH. Treatment trends for retinopathy of prematurity in the UK: active surveillance study of infants at risk. BMJ Open. 2017;7:1–7.

16. Ng EYJ, Lanigan B, O'Keefe M. Fundus fluorescein angiography in the screening for and management of retinopathy of prematurity. J Pediatr Ophthalmol Strabismus. 2015;43:85–90.

17. Zepeda-Romero LC, Oregon-Miranda AA, Lizarraga-Barrón DS, Gutiérrez-Camarena O, Meza-Anguiano A, Gutiérrez-Padilla JA. Early retinopathy of prematurity findings identified with fluorescein angiography. Graefes Arch Clin Exp Ophthalmol. 2013;251:2093–7.

18. Azad R, Chandra P, Khan M, Darswal A. Role of intravenous fluorescein angiography in early detection and regression of retinopathy of prematurity. J Pediatr Ophthalmol Strabismus. 2008;45:36–9.

19. Lepore D, Molle F, Pagliara MM, Baldascino A, Angora C, Sammartino M, Quinn GE. Atlas of fluorescein angiographic findings in eyes undergoing laser for retinopathy of prematurity. Ophthalmology. 2011;118:168–75.

20. Theodoropoulou S, Ainsworth S, Blaikie A. Ultra-wide field imaging of retinopathy of prematurity (ROP) using Optomap-200TX. BMJ Case Rep. 2013;2:1–2.

21. Patel CK, Fung THM, Muqit MMK, Mordant DJ, Brett J, Smith L, Adams E. Non-contact ultra-widefield imaging of retinopathy of prematurity using the Optos dual wavelength scanning laser ophthalmoscope. Eye. 2013;27:589–96.

22. Huang D, Swanson EA, Lin CP, et al. Optical coherence tomography. Science. 1991;254:1178–81.

23. Patel CK. Optical coherence tomography in the management of acute retinopathy of prematurity. Am J Ophthalmol. 2006;141:582–4.

24. Vinekar A, Sivakumar M, Shetty R, Mahendradas P, Krishnan N, Mallipatna A, Shetty KB. A novel technique using spectral-domain optical coherence tomography (Spectralis, SD-OCT+HRA) to image supine non-anaesthetized infants: utility demonstrated in aggressive posterior retinopathy of prematurity. Eye (Lond). 2010;24:379–82.

25. Maldonado RS, J a I, Sarin N, Wallace DK, Freedman S, Cotten CM, Toth CA. Optimizing hand-held spectral domain optical coherence tomography imaging for neonates, infants, and children. Invest Ophthalmol Vis Sci. 2010;51:2678–85.

26. Mallipatna A, Vinekar A, Jayadev C, Dabir S, Sivakumar M, Krishnan N, Mehta P, Berendschot T, Yadav N. The use of handheld spectral domain optical coherence tomography in pediatric ophthalmology practice: our experience of 975 infants and children. Indian J Ophthalmol. 2015;63:586–93.

27. Chavala SH, Farsiu S, Maldonado R, Wallace DK, Freedman SF, Toth CA. Insights into advanced retinopathy of prematurity using handheld spectral domain optical coherence tomography imaging. Ophthalmology. 2009;116:2448–56.

28. Muni RH, Kohly RP, Charonis AC, Lee TC. Retinoschisis detected with handheld spectral-domain optical coherence tomography in neonates with advanced retinopathy of prematurity. Arch Ophthalmol. 2010;128:57–62.

29. Vinekar A, Avadhani K, Sivakumar M, Mahendradas P, Kurian M, Braganza S, Shetty R, Shetty BK. Understanding clinically undetected macular changes in early retinopathy of prematurity on spectral domain optical coherence tomography. Invest Ophthalmol Vis Sci. 2011;52:5183–8.

30. Maldonado RS, O'Connell R, Ascher SB, Sarin N, Freedman SF, Wallace DK, Chiu SJ, Farsiu S, Cotten M, Toth CA. Spectral-domain optical coherence tomographic assessment of severity of cystoid macular edema in retinopathy of prematurity. Arch Ophthalmol (Chicago, Ill 1960). 2012;130:569–78.

31. Maldonado RS, Yuan E, Tran-Viet D, Rothman AL, Tong AY, Wallace DK, Freedman SF, Toth CA. Three-dimensional assessment of vascular and perivascular characteristics in subjects with retinopathy of prematurity. Ophthalmology. 2014;121:1289–96.

32. Anwar SA, Nath M, Patel A, Lee H, Brown S, Gottlob T, Proudlock F. Potential utility of foveal morphology in preterm infants measured using hand-held optical coherence tomography in retinopathy of prematurity screening. Retina. 2019. https://doi.org/10.1097/IAE.0000000000002622. [Epub ahead of print].

33. Vajzovic L, Hendrickson AE, O'connell RV, Clark L, Tran-Viet D, Possin D, Chiu SJ, Farsiu S, Toth CA. Maturation of the human fovea: correlation of spectral-domain optical coherence tomography findings with histology. Am J Ophthalmol. 2012;154:779–789.e2.
34. Vajzovic L, Rothman AL, Tran-viet D, Cabrera MT, Freedman SF, Toth CA. Delay in retinal photoreceptor development in very preterm compared to term infants. Invest Ophthalmol Vis Sci. 2015;56(2):908–13.
35. Palmer EA, Flynn JT, Hardy RJ, Phelps DL, Phillips CL, Schaffer DB, Tung B. Incidence and early course of retinopathy of prematurity. The Cryotherapy for Retinopathy of Prematurity Cooperative Group. Ophthalmology. 1991;98:1628–40.
36. Royal College of Paediatrics and Child Health RC of OBA of PM, BLISS. Guideline for the screening and treatment of retinopathy of prematurity UK retinopathy of prematurity guideline. 2008.
37. Jefferies AL, Canadian Paediatric Society, Fetus and Newborn Committee. Retinopathy of prematurity: an update on screening and management. Paediatr Child Health. 2016;21(2):101–8.
38. Fierson WM, American Academy of Pediatrics Section on Ophthalmology; American Academy of Ophthalmology; American Association for Pediatric Ophthalmology and Strabismus; American Association of Certified Orthoptists. Screening examination of premature infants for retinopathy of prematurity. Pediatrics. 2013;131:189–95.
39. Blencowe H, Lee ACC, Cousens S, et al. Preterm birth-associated neurodevelopmental impairment estimates at regional and global levels for 2010. Pediatr Res. 2013;74(Suppl 1):17–34.
40. Allegaert K, Vanhole C, Casteels I, Naulaers G, Debeer A, Cossey V, Devlieger H. Perinatal growth characteristics and associated risk of developing threshold retinopathy of prematurity. J Am Assoc Pediatr Ophthalmol Strabismus. 2003;7:34–7.
41. Wallace DK, Kylstra JA, Phillips SJ, Hall JG. Poor postnatal weight gain: a risk factor for severe retinopathy of prematurity. J AAPOS. 2000;4:343–7.
42. Löfqvist C, Andersson E, Sigurdsson J, Engström E, Hård A, Niklasson A, Smith L, Hellström A. Longitudinal postnatal weight and insulin-like growth factor I measurements in the prediction of retinopathy of prematurity. Arch Ophthalmol. 2006;124:1711–8.
43. Hellström A, Hard A-L, Engstrom E, Niklasson A, Andersson E, Smith L, Löfqvist C. Early weight gain predicts retinopathy in preterm infants: new, simple, efficient approach to screening. Pediatrics. 2009;123:e638–45.
44. Lundgren P, Stoltz Sjöström E, Domellöf M, Källen K, Holmström G, Hård AL, Smith LE, Löfqvist C, Hellström A. WINROP identifies severe retinopathy of prematurity at an early stage in a nation-based cohort of extremely preterm infants. PLoS One. 2013;8:1–6.
45. Binenbaum G, Ying GS, Quinn GE, Dreiseitl S, Karp K, Roberts RS, Kirpalani H. A clinical prediction model to stratify retinopathy of prematurity risk using postnatal weight gain. Pediatrics. 2011;127:e607–14.
46. Binenbaum G, Ying G-S, Quinn GE, Huang J, Dreiseitl S, Antigua J, Foroughi N, Abbasi S. The CHOP postnatal weight gain, birth weight, and gestational age retinopathy of prematurity risk model. Arch Ophthalmol (Chicago, Ill 1960). 2012;130:1560–5.
47. Binenbaum G, Ying GS, Tomlinson LA. Validation of the Children's Hospital of Philadelphia retinopathy of prematurity (CHOP ROP) model. JAMA Ophthalmol. 2017;135:871–7.
48. Cao JH, Wagner BD, McCourt EA, et al. The Colorado-retinopathy of prematurity model (CO-ROP): postnatal weight gain screening algorithm. J AAPOS. 2016;20:19–24.
49. Eckert GU, Fortes Filho JB, Maia M, Procianoy RS. A predictive score for retinopathy of prematurity in very low birth weight preterm infants. Eye. 2012;26:400–6.
50. Hellstrom A, Engstrom E, Hard A, et al. Postnatal serum insulin-like growth factor I deficiency is associated with retinopathy of prematurity and other complications of premature birth. Pediatrics. 2003;112:1016–20.
51. University of Gothenberg. https://www.winrop.com.
52. Wu C, Löfqvist C, Smith LEH, VanderVeen DK, Hellström A, WINROP Consortium. Importance of early postnatal weight gain for normal retinal angiogenesis in very preterm infants. Arch Ophthalmol. 2012;130:992–9.

53. Ferrara N. Vascular endothelial growth factor: basic science and clinical progress. Endocr Rev. 2004;25:581–611.
54. Carmeliet P, Ferreira V, Breier G, et al. Abnormal blood vessel development and lethality in embryos lacking a single VEGF allele. Nature. 1996;380:435–9.
55. Ferrara N. VEGF and intraocular neovascularization: from discovery to therapy. Transl Vis Sci Technol. 2016;5:10.
56. Malecaze F. Detection of vascular endothelial growth factor messenger RNA and vascular endothelial growth factor-like activity in proliferative diabetic retinopathy. Arch Ophthalmol. 1994;112:1476.
57. Kvanta A. Ocular angiogenesis: the role of growth factors. Acta Ophthalmol Scand. 2006;84:282–8.
58. Aiello LP, Avery RL, Arrigg PG, et al. Vascular endothelial growth factor in ocular fluid of patients with diabetic retinopathy and other retinal disorders. N Engl J Med. 1994;331:1480–7.
59. Chung EJ, Kim JH, Ahn HS, Koh HJ. Combination of laser photocoagulation and intravitreal bevacizumab (Avastin®) for aggressive zone I retinopathy of prematurity. Graefes Arch Clin Exp Ophthalmol. 2007;245:1727–30.
60. Travassos A, Teixeira S, Ferriera P, Regadas I, Travassos A, Esperancinha F, Prieto I, van Velze R, Valido A, Machado MC. Intravitreal bevacizumab in aggressive posterior retinopathy of prematurity. Ophthalmic Surg Lasers Imaging Retina. 2007;38:233–7.
61. Quiroz-Mercado H, Martinez-Castellanos MA, Hernandez-Rojas ML, Salazar-Teran N, Chan RVP. Antiangiogenic therapy with intravitreal bevacizumab for retinopathy of prematurity. Retina. 2008;28:S19–25.
62. Mintz-Hittner HA, Kuffel RR. Intravitreal injection of Bevacizumab (Avastin) for treatment of stage 3 retinopathy of prematurity in zone 1 or posterior zone II. Retina. 2008;28:831–8.
63. Wallace DK, Dean TW, Hartnett ME, et al. A dosing study of Bevacizumab for retinopathy of prematurity: late recurrences and additional treatments. Ophthalmology. 2018;125(12):1961–6.
64. Hillier RJ, Connor AJ, Shafiq AE. Ultra-low-dose intravitreal bevacizumab for the treatment of retinopathy of prematurity: a case series. Br J Ophthalmol. 2018;102(2):260–4.
65. Avery RL. Bevacizumab (Avastin) for retinopathy of prematurity: wrong dose, wrong drug, or both? J AAPOS. 2012;16:2–4.
66. Morin J, Luu TM, Superstein R, Ospina LH, Lefebvre F, Simard M-N, Shah V, Shah PS, Kelly EN. Neurodevelopmental outcomes following Bevacizumab injections for retinopathy of prematurity. Pediatrics. 2016;137:e20153218.
67. Hu J, Blair MP, Shapiro MJ, Lichtenstein SJ, Galasso JM, Kapur R. Reactivation of retinopathy of prematurity after bevacizumab injection. Arch Ophthalmol. 2012;130:1000–6.
68. Zepeda-Romero LC, Liera-Garcia JA, Gutiérrez-Padilla JA, Valtierra-Santiago CI, Cardenas-Lamas LJ. Paradoxical vascular-fibrotic reaction after intravitreal bevacizumab for retinopathy of prematurity. Eye. 2010;24:931–3.
69. Tahija SG, Hersetyati R, Lam GC, Kusaka S, McMenamin PG. Fluorescein angiographic observations of peripheral retinal vessel growth in infants after intravitreal injection of bevacizumab as sole therapy for zone I and posterior zone II retinopathy of prematurity. Br J Ophthalmol. 2014;98:507–12.
70. Jang SY, Choi KS, Lee SJ. Delayed-onset retinal detachment after an intravitreal injection of ranibizumab for zone 1 plus retinopathy of prematurity. J AAPOS. 2010;14:457–9.
71. Mintz-Hittner H, Geloneck MM, Chuang AZ. Clinical Management of recurrent retinopathy of prematurity after intravitreal Bevacizumab monotherapy. Ophthalmology. 2016;123:1845–55.
72. Yang X-M, Zhao Y-X, Wang Z-H, Liu L. Effect of anti-VEGF treatment on retinopathy of prematurity in zone II stage 3. Int J Ophthalmol. 2018;11:641–4.
73. Sankar MJ, Sankar J, Chandra P. Anti-vascular endothelial growth factor (VEGF) drugs for treatment of retinopathy of prematurity. Cochrane Database Syst Rev. 2018;1:CD009734. https://doi.org/10.1002/14651858.CD009734.pub3.

Part IV
Long Term Effects Following Extreme Prematurity

Chapter 19
Neurodevelopmental Problems

Joe Fawke and Rebecca Lancaster

Introduction

This chapter will consider:

- How do survival rates impact on neurodisability rates?
- What impact do factors other than prematurity, including major neonatal morbidities, have on developmental prognosis and how should this inform counselling?
- What is the relationship of cognitive problems to decreasing gestational age across the gestational age spectrum?
- What happens to early cognitive impairment as children grow up?
- How should we provide developmental follow up in order to optimise the chance of early recognition and intervention?
- Collection and use of neurodevelopmental outcome data

How Do Survival Rates Impact on Disability Rates?

When comparing survival rates over time or between different gestational ages it is important to consider the denominator used. Rates of disability free survival and survival without major disability will vary depending on whether these are reported as

J. Fawke (✉)
University Hospitals of Leicester NHS Trust, Leicester, UK

Health Education East Midlands, Leicester, UK
e-mail: joe.fawke@uhl-tr.nhs.uk

R. Lancaster
Department of Health Sciences, George Davies Centre, University of Leicester, Leicester, UK
e-mail: Rebecca.lancaster4@nhs.net

© Springer Nature Switzerland AG 2020
E. M. Boyle, J. Cusack (eds.), *Emerging Topics and Controversies in Neonatology*, https://doi.org/10.1007/978-3-030-28829-7_19

the proportion of all births, live births or admissions to the neonatal unit. This is particularly key for those of a lower gestational age who may be less likely to be offered active care in the delivery room. Work by Smith in 2019 adds a cautionary note about comparing rates of survival at very early gestations as a proportion of live births, due to wide variation in how signs of life at birth are reported across countries [1].

The approach a country takes to extremely preterm birth will have an impact on survival. For example, a policy of not providing intensive care to babies born <24 weeks of gestation would result in 100% mortality at 22/23 weeks. More subtly, differences in how interventional neonatal teams are for the very smallest babies will have less stark, but still important effects on survival and disability rates.

How Has Survival Changed over Time and What Impact Has This Had on Neurodevelopment?

Healthcare professionals have often worried that improved survival might come at the expense of increased neurodevelopmental problems. A review of the world literature in 1981 [62] showed the high mortality in the early years of neonatology had improved with survival for VLBW infants tripling and the prevalence of disability stabilised. Since then multiple studies have shown improved survival across time-based cohorts of infants born extremely preterm. This has been shown in several countries including the UK [2, 3], Canada [4], France [5], Sweden [6] and Japan [7] (Table 19.1). A 2019 meta-analysis of 65 cohort studies from 2000 to 2017 [11] for babies born at 22^{+0} to 26^{+6} weeks of gestation concluded that survival had improved, rates of severe impairment reduced and disability free survival increased.

Many healthcare professionals involved in neonatal care are concerned that, as rates of survival of extremely preterm infants improve, there will be an increase in rates of children with major disabilities. Longitudinal analysis of the UK EPICure

Table 19.1 Changes over time in longitudinal cohort studies

Study	Time period	Gestation	Survival	Major disability	No major disability
EPICure [2, 3] (UK)	1995 & 2006	≤25 + 6	↑	→	↑
EPIPage [5] (France)	1997 & 2011	25–26	↑	↓	↑
Sweden [6, 8]	2004–2007 & 2014–2016	22–26	↑	NR	↑
VICs (Australia) [9]	1991–1992, 1997 & 2005	<28	→	→	→
Japanese Neonatal Research Network [7]	2003–2012 1982–1991 vs 1992–2005	22–32 23–27	↑ ↑	↓/→[a] ↑	NR NR
US [10]	2011-2015	≤26	↑	↓	↑
Meta-analysis [11]	2000–2017	<27	↑	↓	↑

NR not reported
[a]CP, Visual & hearing impairment ↓, cognitive →

cohorts showed improved survival and improved disability free survival. However, survival with major disability remained static [3]. The Victorian Infant Collaborative (VIC) group in Australia had similar mortality and disability across three time epochs (1991–1992, 1997, 2005) [6]. The French cohort in the EPIPAGE study [5] showed increased survival without severe or moderate neuromotor or sensory disabilities between 1997 and 2011 for infants born at 25–26 weeks of gestation, but not for other gestations. The Japanese Neonatal Research Network reported reduced mortality from 2003 to 2012 and this was associated with reduced cerebral palsy (CP) rates, reduced visual and hearing impairments but no change in cognitive impairment [7]. Neurodevelopmental follow up data from the National Institute of Child Health and Human Development (NICHD) in America report improved survival rates with reduced moderate to severe neurodevelopmental impairment but increased mild impairment in a 2011–2015 cohort [10].

The trend towards earlier intervention continues across most countries with modern medical systems. A review of 70 hospitals in 10 European regions in 2003 and 2011/12 showed that both obstetricians and neonatologists had become more interventional in pregnancies <27 weeks of gestation. Over this time survival at <27 weeks increased from 50 to 58%; more interventional centres had better survival but developmental outcomes were not reported [12].

The 2019 British Association of Perinatal Medicine (BAPM) framework on perinatal management of extreme preterm birth before 27 weeks of gestation [13] suggested a risk based approach to active management. This involved using gestational age and a range of non-modifiable and modifiable fetal risk factors and considering maternal factors to suggest three levels of risk (extremely high, high and moderate) of a poor outcome. A poor outcome was taken as death or severe disability, although families may differ in what outcomes they consider 'poor'. The importance of counselling and involving families in decision making was emphasised and it was acknowledged that it is not possible to be completely objective in classifying level of risk. It suggested that, for those with an extremely high risk of a poor outcome, palliative care would usually be in the best interests of the child; moderately high risk should prompt careful counselling and discussion with the family and joint decisions about active care whilst lower risk babies would usually receive active management [13].

Countries that have looked at place of birth have found that babies born at larger centres have higher survival rates. In the UK, the EPICure study found that delivery in a tertiary neonatal unit not only improved the chance of survival but did so without worsening developmental outcomes [14].

How Does Survival Change with Increasing Gestational Age and What Impact Does This Have on Neurodevelopment?

The Australian Victorian Infant Collaboration evaluated survival, survival with major disability and survival without major disability in babies born below 28 weeks of gestation. They found increasing gestational age from 24 to 27 + 6 weeks improved survival and survival without disability but had less impact on the rate of survival with major disability with similar rates seen at 24, 25, 26 and 27 weeks [9]. In contrast EPICure-2 (22–26 weeks) showed increased gestation to be associated with reduced rates of moderate or severe disability [3].

2016 UK data [15] shows that 1 year survival for babies alive in labour at 22 weeks was 5%, 23 weeks 28%, 24 weeks 54%, 25 weeks 71% and 26 weeks 80%. The survival figures for babies offered active care were 35%, 38%, 60%, 74% and 82% respectively. The 2019 BAPM framework [13] estimated the prevalence of severe impairment based on 4 major studies [5, 8, 10, 16] as:

- $22 + 0$–$22 + 6$ weeks: 1-in-3 survivors
- $23 + 0$–$23 + 6$ weeks: 1-in-4 survivors
- $24 + 0$–$25 + 6$ weeks: 1-in-7 survivors
- $26 + 0$ and over: 1-in-10 survivors

In 2016, 16 US academic centres reported that in $22 + 0$ to $26 + 6$ week gestation liveborn infants, each week increase in gestational age decreases the risk of neurodevelopmental impairment (OR 0.69 (0.48–0.99)) and the combined risk of neurodevelopmental impairment or death (OR 0.6 (0.48–0.78)) [17]. Further US data on this cohort reported an improving trend for survivors of overall neurodevelopmental impairment, severe cognitive impairment, moderate cognitive impairment, motor impairment and hearing impairment. Composite outcomes of death or moderate-severe neurodevelopmental impairment decreased from 61 to 50% if a *Bayley Scales of Infant and Toddler Development, third edition* (Bayley-III) cognitive cut off of 70 was used. They did, however, find an increase in mild impairments for example whilst severe cerebral palsy (CP) rates dropped by 43% mild CP increased by 13%. They concluded there was a shift towards an increase in milder neurocognitive impairment among preterm survivors [10].

Studies looking at moderately preterm and late preterm infants report better outcomes than studies looking at extremely preterm cohorts. Across the whole gestational age range, increasing gestational age has a clear impact on both survival and neurodevelopmental outcomes.

What About Infants Born at 22/23 Weeks of Gestation and Infants Less Than 500 g Birthweight?

Each time we lower the gestational age at which intensive care is considered the same questions arise. 'Can we' and 'should we' provide that intensive care? Julius Hess in a 30 year review of neonatal outcomes in 1953 said [18]:

> *Much has been accomplished in our time in lowering mortality and morbidity among premature infants but it must be remembered that in these small infants, even with the best of nursing care and most modern equipment, the death rate cannot be cut beyond an irreducible minimum, largely because of their immature development at birth.*

He was quoting mortality of 87% for extremely low birth weight (ELBW), 58.5% for very low birthweight (VLBW) and 9.3% for low birth weight (LBW) infants [18]. Impressive figures for the time but very different from today's outcomes with modern neonatal intensive care.

Recently, more questions about offering intensive care to 22 week gestation infants have occurred. The numbers of infants involved are small which contributes to widely varied survival and developmental outcomes. For example, 2017 rates of survival to 28 days for all live births at 22 weeks of gestation are quoted as 57% (Japan), 47% (Sweden), 17% (Norway), 14% (US), 8% (UK), 6% (France) and 4% (Canada) [1]. Case studies, single centres reporting surprisingly good outcomes and sometimes overly optimistic media reports contribute to the discussion.

Small numbers of babies and different approaches to offering antenatal steroids, magnesium sulphate, resuscitation, centralisation of care and differences in the amount of intensive care provided at this extreme of prematurity affect survival and developmental outcomes and cloud the issue further. A study exploring selective intervention versus universal intervention for 22 week infants in a Swedish and an American centre did not show that selecting which of these babies to resuscitate improved survival, but it did show that having an 'ethos' of expected intervention increased rates of survival; neurodevelopmental outcomes were not reported [19].

Epicure-2 reported that 98% of 22 week gestation infants born in 2006 in England and Wales died and 0.7% survived without disability [2]. The Victorian Infant Cohort in Australia reported that 71% died and of the survivors, none were free of major disability. In both countries, active care was not routinely offered to 22 week gestation infants. The Japanese neonatal research network reported survival of 18% (<300 g), 41% (301–400 g) and 60% (401–500 g) in the period 2003–2012, with survival at <500 g improving from 40% in 2003 to 68% in 2012. However, they also reported that at least one severe morbidity was present in 81–89% of survivors [7].

In 2019 the National Institute for Child Health and Development (NICHD) neonatal research network in the US reported a retrospective analysis of live born babies born 22–26 weeks of gestation with a birth weight less than 400g [20]. Just under half of these babies received active resuscitation, 26% of which survived to discharge. In the subgroup of babies born at 22–23 weeks of gestation, 28% received active resuscitation and of those, 17% survived to discharge.

Of all those actively resuscitated, who did not die after neonatal discharge or get lost to follow up, 74% had moderate or severe neurodevelopmental impairment, most with multiple morbidities.

This chapter cannot decide whether resuscitation of babies born at 22 weeks or very severely growth restricted babies is appropriate; that is a decision for neonatal services and the populations they serve. There are complex issues around possible pain and suffering for the baby, future quality of life, the ability for parents to understand the outcomes and give informed consent when that information that is not completely clear to professionals at the moment.

Perception of quality of life may be different for professionals, parents and the extremely preterm survivors [21]. Principles of distributive justice and cost effectiveness also inform the debate in a finite resource health system.

Where resuscitation is offered the morbidity associated with survival should be considered and careful attention should be paid to postnatal trajectories. Regular re-evaluation of the appropriateness of ongoing intensive care should be informed by family and clinicians views.

Predicting Neurodevelopmental Problems: What Impact Do Factors Other Than Prematurity Have on Developmental Prognosis?

Whilst gestational age is an important risk factor for death or neurodevelopmental problems it is not the only significant risk factor. Other variables (Table 19.2), available at various time points in an infant's clinical course, can significantly increase or decrease the risk of neurodevelopmental problems.

Antenatal Factors

A number of studies [22, 26] and NICE guidance [23] have considered antenatal risk factors for neurodevelopmental problems. Consistent findings are that being male, not receiving antenatal steroids and having a lower birth weight are all risk factors that confer additional risk of neurodevelopmental problems in addition to the risk derived from gestational age.

Table 19.2 Risk factors beyond gestational age for neurodevelopmental problems

Antenatal	Postnatal
Male Sex [22, 23]	Grade 3 or 4 IVH [5, 11, 22]
Not receiving antenatal steroids [22, 23]	Cystic PVL [23, 24]
	Postnatal corticosteroid use [22, 23]
Multiple pregnancy [22]	Surgery [22]
Birth weight [22, 23]	Neonatal Sepsis [23]
	ROP [24]
	HIE [23]
	↑length of mechanical ventilation [24]
	Requiring chest compressions in the delivery room [17]
	Hypothermia on admission to NICU [25]

IVH intraventricular haemorrhage, *PVL* periventricular leucomalacia, *ROP* retinopathy of prematurity, *HIE* hypoxic ischaemic encephalopathy, *NICU* neonatal intensive care unit

Post-natal Factors

Postnatal factors become evident over time allowing a refinement of the original estimate of risk of death or neurodevelopmental problems which can inform serial counselling of parents and families. A range of studies have explored the impact of the presence or absence of neonatal co-morbidities on outcomes and tried to quantify the added risk or benefit conferred.

The phrase 'outcome trajectories' [27, 28] has been used to describe an increase or decrease in the estimated risk of a poor outcome informed by the passage of time and clinical events on the neonatal intensive care unit (NICU). A number of neonatal morbidities are consistently found to worsen neurodevelopmental outcomes and these include grade 3–4 intraventricular haemorrhage (IVH), cystic periventricular leucomalacia (PVL) and an association with receiving postnatal steroids.

It is unclear whether the relationship with postnatal steroids is causative, or by association with worse lung disease, especially as commonly used postnatal steroid treatment regimens have become shorter and lower doses have been used. This led the 2019 NICE guidance on Neonatal Specialist Respiratory [29] care to conclude that there was no good evidence of increased risk of adverse developmental outcomes with postnatal steroids if they were given after 8 days of age. This is discussed further in Chapter 16. US NICHD neonatal research network data [10] showed an association between a longer duration of mechanical ventilation and increased hearing impairment. Other neonatal morbidities that act as independent risk factors for poorer neurodevelopmental outcomes are neonatal surgery, sepsis, retinopathy of prematurity or hypoxic-ischaemic encephalopathy.

An accumulation of these independent risk factors has a cumulative effect on the risk of death or neurodisability [17, 22, 26, 28]. An exploration of the relative impact of various postnatal morbidities amongst the Victorian Infant Cohort studies found that the four postnatal morbidities that posed the greatest risk of death or major disability were grade 3–4 intraventricular haemorrhage (IVH), cystic periventricular leucomalacia (PVL), postnatal steroids for bronchopulmonary dysplasia (BPD) and neonatal surgery. Major disability was defined as having one or more of the following: Gross Motor Function Classification Score (GMFCS) of 2–5, Intelligence Quotient (IQ) Z score <−2, blindness, deafness. In these Australian cohorts of <28 week gestation infants, those with none of these postnatal morbidities had a 48% survival with 7% major disability whilst having ≥3 of these postnatal morbidities gave a 3% survival and 69% major disability [28].

Figure 19.1 is adapted from Cheong et al. [28] who discuss postnatal developmental trajectories. Ambalavanan et al. [27] describe a risk calculator developed using US NICHD data that uses postnatal morbidities to modify the risk of having neurodevelopmental problems. Various other risk factor models to predict neurodevelopmental outcome have been developed with differing methodologies and these have been systematically reviewed [30].

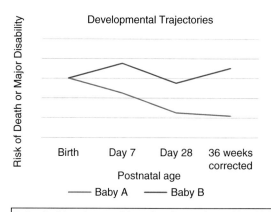

This graph shows the concept of differing developmental trajectories of two babies with identical risks of death or major disability at birth. The risk for death or disability changes for the two babies according to postnatal events.

Baby A: A boy born at 24 weeks of gestation, with a birth weight of 700g, was ventilated for 12 hours, he received one dose of surfactant and was extubated to CPAP successfully on day one. He received parenteral nutrition from day 1. He was weaning CPAP and establishing enteral feeds by day 7. By day 28 he did not need respiratory support, had established enteral feeds with expressed breast milk via a nasogastric tube and was gaining weight well. At 36 weeks corrected age he was breast feeding, had no respiratory support, had a normal cranial ultrasound, no ROP and was preparing for discharge.

Baby B: A boy born at 24 weeks of gestation, with a birth weight of 700g, intubated and given two doses surfactant. He had a pulmonary haemorrhage on day 2 and a left side grade four IVH on day 4. He was ventilated for 2 weeks then had CPAP for 6 weeks. He had one episode of medically managed NEC at four weeks of age requiring re-ventilation for four days. He received bilateral laser treatment for ROP. At 36 weeks he was preparing for discharge in home oxygen.

CPAP = continuous positive airway pressure   ROP = retinopathy of prematurity
NEC = necrotising enterocolitis   IVH = Intraventricular haemorrhage

Fig 19.1 Neurodevelopmental trajectories. (Adapted from Cheong et al. [28] Lancet Child and Adolescent Health)

Cerebral Palsy

Extremely preterm graduates are at risk of a spectrum of motor difficulties later in life. Cerebral palsy (CP) is the most commonly reported adverse motor outcome in neurodevelopmental follow up studies. Standard definitions for cerebral palsy exist [31] which makes comparison of CP rates between studies easier. The rates of other, more variably defined, motor problems vary according to the cut off scores on standardised testing that is taken to represent a problem. Several studies report the degree of functional impairment experienced by the child with CP. This is most commonly done using the Gross Motor Functions Classification Score [32] (GMFCS) although other measures such as the Manual Ability Classification Score [33] (MACS) which rates bimanual hand function can provide useful supplementary information.

Longitudinal national and regional cohort studies of extremely preterm infants have reported a drop in the prevalence of CP over time in the UK [2] (<25^{+6} weeks;

17–14%), France [5] (24–31 weeks; 9–5.4%), Japan [7] (≤32 weeks; 12.3–7.1%) and US [10] (Table 19.3). A large meta-analysis of 25 studies conducted after 2006 showed a pooled CP prevalence of 6.5% for ELBW and VLBW infants, with higher

Table 19.3 Cerebral palsy rates

Country	Study	Birth year	Gestation/ birth weight	CP rate (%)	95% CI	Comments
National cohort studies						
France [5, 34]	EPIPAGE 2	2011	24	15.4	(4.2–34.9)	
			25–26	7.9	(4.5–12.6)	
			27–31	4.9	(3.7–6.4)	
			32–34	0.2	(0.0–1.3)	
			24–31	5.4	(4.2–6.8)	
	EPIPAGE 1	1997	24	7.1	(0.1–38.8)	
			25–26	17.8	(11.4–25.9)	
			27–31	8.0	(6.6–9.70)	
			32–34	2.8	(1.5–4.7)	
			24–31	9.0	(7.5–10.6)	
UK [2]	EPICure 2	2006	22–25	14	nr	
	EPICure 1	1995	22–25	17	nr	
Sweden [8]	EXPRESS	2004–2007	<27	9.5	nr	60% mild CP (GMFCS 1) 14 cases after 2.5 years CP % 7.0 @2.5 years 9.5% @6.5 years
Belgium [35]	EPIBEL		≤26 weeks			
US [10]	NIHR	2011–2015	≤26 weeks			
Large database studies						
Finland [36]	National register study	1991–2008	<32	8.7	(8.0–9.4)	<32 n = 6347 32–33 n = 6799 34–36 n = 39,932 Hospital discharge & social insurance records, using ICD codes Followed up to 7 years
			32–33	2.4	2.0–2.7)	
			34–36	0.56	(0.49–0.64)	
			32–36	0.8	(0.7–0.9)	

(continued)

Table 19.3 (continued)

Country	Study	Birth year	Gestation/ birth weight	CP rate (%)	95% CI	Comments
Sweden [37]	National register study	2007– 2010	<28	5.9		n = 104,715 live births
			28–31	4.6		<28 n = 373
			32–36	0.6		28–31 n = 525
			<37	1.3		32–36 n = 5012
						CP verified at 4–8 years
UK [38]	Regional database study	1991– 2000	<28	6.7	(5.1– 8.6)	n = 846 < 28 weeks
			28–31	5.9	(4.9– 7.0)	n = 2070 at 28–31 weeks
						n = 15,881 32–36 weeks
			32–36	1.0	(0.8– 1.1)	Followed up to 8 years
Meta-analysis						
Multi- national [39]	25 studies	After 2006	28	10.0	(8.1– 12.2)	
			28–31	4.4	(3.3– 6.3)	
			<1000	8.4	(6.6– 10.7)	
			<1500	4.2	(2.9– 6.20)	

nr not reported

prevalence associated with lower birthweight (ELBW 8.4% 95% CI 6.6–10.7) versus (VLBW 4.2% 95% CI 2.9–6.2). The same meta-analysis showed a rate of 10% (95% CI 8.1–12.2) for <28 week gestation infants and a rate of 4.5% (95% CI 3.3–6.3) for 28–31 weeks [24].

The overall trend across time has been for CP prevalence to reduce with studies in the 1990s generally reporting higher prevalence of CP than studies since 2006 [2, 5, 7].

Large database studies and a pooled meta-analysis support the idea that CP prevalence is higher at lower gestations and birthweights. The meta-analysis suggested a linear relationship between increasing CP prevalence and decreasing gestational age [24]. Most studies assessed the presence of CP between 18 months and 3 years old. However, it is noted that CP can become evident after 3 years of age and the EXPRESS study [8] from Sweden reported higher CP rates at 6.5 year follow up (9.5%) than at 2.5 years (7%).

In addition to the risk of CP conferred by lower gestational ages other risk factors independently increase the chance of a premature baby having CP. These are grade 3–4 IVH, cystic PVL, sepsis, bronchopulmonary dysplasia (BPD) requiring mechanical ventilation at 36 weeks, not receiving antenatal steroids and requiring postnatal steroids before 32 weeks corrected gestation [9]. However, the evidence for postnatal steroids as a risk factor for CP is contradictory with the NICE neonatal specialist respiratory care guideline reporting no increase in risk if the steroids are given after 8 days of age.

Cognitive Outcomes

The largest proportion of disability following preterm birth is accounted for by cognitive deficit. Cognitive deficits have an impact on how a child progresses through school and subsequently impact upon adult prospects of employment and functioning in later life. Determining cognitive outcomes across populations is essential not only for reviewing the impact of early care but also for informing educational systems. On an individual level screening for cognitive issues allows for early intervention.

Rates of severe morbidity are often included in the discussion of and influence the approach to the initiation and continuation of active care at preterm birth. As the limits of proposed viability are being pushed further and rates of survival of extremely preterm babies have increased over time it is important to determine what effect this has had on trends in cognitive outcomes.

Challenges in Measuring Cognitive Outcomes in Preterm Birth

There are multiple challenges that complicate comparing cognitive outcomes between studies. Figure 19.2 gives an overview of outcomes from Europe [3, 8, 34, 40–43] Australia [9, 44, 45] and the US [10] in extremely preterm children born since 1990.

There are many factors that need to be taken into consideration when looking at the variation in outcomes reported in studies of preterm birth.

Moderate to severe cognitive impairment is fairly consistently reported across studies as scores >2 standard deviations below the normative mean. In some studies, the normative mean is the psychometric testing materials' mean in others this is a term born control group mean.

The nature of the Flynn effect, the natural trend upwards in IQ over time [47], impacts on results depending on which normative mean is used. In studies without a control group the rates of cognitive deficit are likely to be underestimated. EPICure at 6 years determined the rate of moderate to severe cognitive impairment to be 41% when using class norms but only 21% when using test norms [41]. Similarly, in the EXPRESS study, the rate of moderate to severe impairment was 32% using control norms but only 19% if using the test norms [43].

As time progresses psychometric testing materials are updated. Careful consideration needs to be given to whether results from new versions are comparable to those tested with the older version. For example, many have found that the *Bayley Scales of Infant and Toddler Development, third edition* (Bayley-III) underestimates cognitive impairment compared to the earlier edition of the assessment, *Bayley Scales of Infant Development, second edition* (BSID II) [48]. Therefore, it is important to note whether studies have accounted for this in their analysis when comparing changes in outcomes over time.

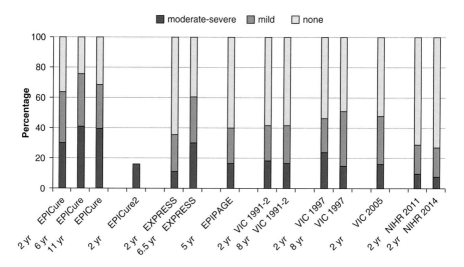

EPICure 2yr[40] 6yr[41] 11yr[42] EPICure2 2yr[2] EXPRESS 2yr[43] 6.5yr[8] EPIPAGE 2yr[50] VIC91-2 2yr[9] 8yr[45] VIC97 2yr[9] 8yr[45]
VIC05[9] NICHD[10]
*SD=standard deviation

Fig. 19.2 Percentage of cognitive impairment categorised into moderate-severe, mild, and none across ages and different countries

Some of the challenges of comparing cognitive outcomes across studies are demonstrated when considering the NICHD 2 year outcome data shown in Fig. 19.2. The rate of moderate-severe cognitive impairment seems improved compared to earlier European and Australian cohorts. Although encouraging it is hard to be certain if this is a genuine finding, as the authors of the study comment that it is unclear as to which cut off scores should be used in the Bayley -III to comparatively categorise levels of cognitive impairment [10]. The lack of a term born control group complicates interpretation further, as mentioned previously comparing preterm mean scores against the test mean scores often underestimates the rate of cognitive deficit.

Other important considerations when comparing cognitive outcomes across studies include; whether the study is based on birthweight categorisations, the proportion of each gestational age included, the substitution or omission of those with assigned low scores and whether the cohort is geographically or entire population based.

What Are the Rates of Cognitive Impairment?

Reported rates of moderate to severe cognitive impairment vary from 8% to 40% across studies as shown in Fig. 19.2. This variation, in part, is likely to be accounted for by some of the factors discussed in the previous section. It is apparent that many extreme preterm infants go onto to have significant cognitive deficits. But this is counterbalanced by the fact that there is a proportion who survive with no cognitive deficit (28–64%).

Whilst there will be some children born extremely preterm with a cognitive score equal to or greater than that of their term born peers, as a population, extremely preterm infants' mean cognitive scores are significantly lower. This varies from 0.8 to 1.5 of standard deviation [49].

Table 19.4 demonstrates mean point deficit ranges of 9–24 points lower than the mean scores of term born peers. Figure 19.7 illustrates that this lower mean score compared to term born classmates persists as the extreme preterm cohort ages.

What Is the Relationship Between Risk of Cognitive Deficit and Decreasing Gestational Age?

The origin of cognitive deficit in preterm survivors is likely to be multifactorial. The global effect of having all organs immature exposes these individuals to several complications of prematurity that are known to be associated with poorer cognitive outcomes. These include development of PVL, late onset sepsis and BPD requiring treatment with steroids. Low maternal IQ and low socioeconomic status also have a correlation with poorer cognitive outcome [23].

Several studies suggest that a lower gestational age at birth has some bearing on cognitive outcome. Retrospective analysis of outcomes in Neonatal Network centres in America [10] and Japan [7] report a reduction in mean cognitive score as gestational age decreases. National cohort studies in England [3], France [5] and Sweden [8] do not report a statistically significant difference in cognitive scores per gestational week age but do report a trend in mean score deficit as gestational age lowers (Fig. 19.3).

In Sweden, the EXPRESS study found that the mean Bayley-III scores increased with gestational age by 2.5 points per week (95% CI, 1.0–4.0) [43]. This continued to be demonstrated at the 6 years follow up where there was a 4.1 point increase in mean score per gestational age week (95% CI, 2.7–5.5) [8].

EPICure (UK) at 6 years [40] reported reducing mean scores with decreasing gestational age, but this was not found to be significant after correction for sex. At

Table 19.4 Preterm mean cognitive score and point deficit compared to term born control group

Country	Study	Year of birth	Gestational age range/ mean birth weight	Age of follow up	Test used	Mean cognitive score point deficit compared with term born control group		Mean cognitive score	
						Point deficit	95% CI*99%	Mean score	95% CI /(SD)
UK	EPICure	1995	22–25	2 years [40]	BSID-II	n/a	n/a	84	(12)
				6 years [50]	K-ABC	−24.2	−27.7 to −20.6	81.6	79–84.2
				11 years [50]	K-ABC	−20.7	−24.1 to −17.3	83.4	80.8–85.9
				19 years [50]	WASI-II	−18.1	−22.8 to −13.5	85.7	82.7–88.8
	EPICure2	2006	22–26	2 years [3]	Bayley-III	n/r	n/r	89	(19)
Sweden	EXPRESS	2004–7	22–26 783 g	2.5yr [43]	Bayley-III	−9.2	*−11.5 to −6.9	94	(12.3)
		2004–7	22–26 770 g	6.5 [8] years	WISC-IV	−14.2	−16.3 to −12.1	83.4	(14.8)
France	EPIPAGE	1997	22–32	2 years [5]	ASQ	n/a	n/a	n/a	n/a
				5 years [34]	K-ABC	−18 +22-26 weeks	n/r	n/r	n/r
	EPIPAGE 2	2011	22–32	2 years [5]	ASQ	n/a	n/a	n/a	n/a
Australia	VIC	1991–2	22–27 887 g	2 years [51]	BSID-II	−9.4	n/r	95.5	n/r
				8 years [52]	WISC-III	−9.6	−12.7 to −6.6	94.9	(16.5)
		1997	22–27 833 g	8 years [52]	WISC-IV	−11.8	−14.9 to −8.6	93.8	(14.7)
		2005	22–27	2 years [9]	Bayley-III	−11.4	−14.3 to −8.6	97.5	(12.6)
			22–27 867 g	8 years [52]	DAS-II	−12.7	−15.9 to −9.5	94.7	(15.7)
US	NIHR	2011–2014	22–26	2 years [10]	Bayley II	n/a	n/a	89.2	(15.4)

Bayley Scales of Infant Development—second edition = BSID II Bayley Scales of Infant and Toddler Development 3 = Bayley-III Mental Development Index Kaufman Assessment Battery for Children = KABC Mental Processing Score Wechsler Abbreviated Scale of Intelligence-Second/fourth Edition = WIAT- II/ IV Full Scale IQ Ages and Stages Questionnaire = ASQ Differential Ability Scales- second edition = DAS-II Global Conceptual Ability score
n/r not reported, *n/a* not applicable

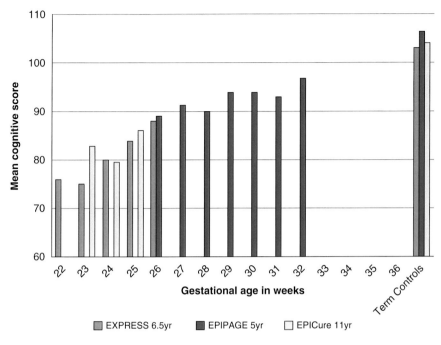

EXPRESS[8] EPIPAGE[50] EPICure[53]

Fig. 19.3 Mean cognitve score per gestational age week across three countries

11 years there was a 4.5 point increase in mean score per gestational age week (95% CI, 1.4–7.7) [42]. Epicure2 at 2 years showed a difference in mean cognitive scores per gestational age week. This ranged from a mean score of 80 (SD 21) at 23 weeks increasing to 91 (SD 18) at 26 weeks. Statistical significance was determined for increasing rates of severe/moderate impairment with decreasing gestational age [3].

Conversely EPIBEL (Belgium) in a national cohort of infants less than ≤26 weeks of gestation found no difference in overall cognitive outcome based on gestational age [35]. Additionally, in VIC (Australia) results from those born <28 weeks followed up at 8 years demonstrated little difference between mean cognitive scores between those born <26 weeks and those born >26 weeks (−1.7, CI −6.4 to 3) [44].

While a one or two point difference between weeks is not clinically significant if this continues over weeks (as indicated by Fig. 19.3) then it can be seen that extremely preterm birth confers a much greater risk for cognitive deficit than very preterm birth. This is reflected in the findings of a recent meta-analysis that reported a pooled prevalence of cognitive delay of 29.4% vs 14.3% for extreme preterm and very preterm children respectively [39].

The literature is not entirely conclusive on the matter of a gestational age-related cognitive decline. This may be in part due to small numbers at lower gestational ages making it difficult to reach statistical significance. However, those that report a trending decline as illustrated by Fig. 19.3 raise questions as to what can be done to better protect the preterm brain from ex utero insults in addition highlighting how extremely preterm infants are a vulnerable group for lower cognitive scores.

What Is the Effect of Sex on Cognitive Outcomes?

Sex not only appears to have an effect on survival but also on cognitive outcomes. Several studies report that males are much more likely to have lower scores than females, see Fig. 19.4.

EPICure (UK) found that at 6 years of age boys were 10 IQ points behind girls and at 11 years of age this effect continued. Boys on average had an 8 point deficit (95% CI 3–13) in IQ score when compared with girls [53]. Boys were more likely to have a serious cognitive impairment when compared with girls OR 2.1 (95% CI 1.2–3.7) [42].

In EXPRESS (Sweden) the mean adjusted FSIQ score for boys was 4.3 (95% CI 1.5–7.2) points lower than girls. The overall percentage of boys with a moderate or severe disability was higher than the overall percentage of girls with a moderate or severe disability (38.1% vs 28.3%) aOR, 1.6 (95% CI, 1.1–2.5 P < .05) [8]. Similarly, in the ELGAN (US) study more boys than girls had cognitive delay (42% vs 27%) at 18–24 months [46].

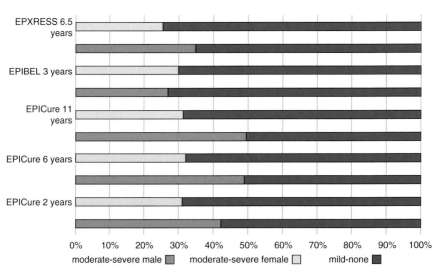

EXPRESS[8] EPIBEL[35] EPICure11years[42] 6years[41] 2years[40]

Fig. 19.4 Percentage of moderate-severe cognitive deficit (>2 SD below mean) versus mild-none by sex in children born extremely prematurely

It is important to note that this difference in gender score is not seen in term born controls [42]. This may explain why EPIPAGE (France) at 5 years reported no difference between sex, as their cohort included a much wider gestational age range of 24–32 weeks [34].

What Happens to the Cognitive Deficit as the Extreme Preterm Infant Gets Older?

Just as there are challenges in comparing outcomes across studies, there are challenges with comparing outcomes within studies. Attrition rates in longitudinal cohort studies are significant. Participants with more significant neuro motor/sensory impairment and lower socio-economic status are more likely to miss further follow up visits [42, 50, 54]. Adjustment needs to be made for this, otherwise results may falsely give the impression of improvement over time.

Longitudinal studies such as EPICure (UK) and VIC (Australia) have demonstrated overall trends in cognition as the child grows. EPICure have determined that there continues to be a clinically significant difference in mean IQ scores compared to term born controls as the child gets older [50] (Fig. 19.5). There is a marginal increase in mean score at each time point of assessment with a marginal decrease in cognitive score with the term born control groups [50]. Conversely the VIC have shown that the mean IQ scores for the extreme preterm stay relatively constant whilst the term born counterparts have a marginal increase in cognitive score as time passes [52]. Both groups conclude that for a population mean there is relative stability of cognitive scores.

However, on an individual basis there is some variation in cognitive outcome over time. The biggest changes are seen between assessments performed at preschool age and at school age. EPICure demonstrated a 24% shift from no disability to severe disability at age 6 years [41]. In part this may be due to the lack of a control group at 2 years of age. However EXPRESS (Sweden) found that less than half of children with moderate/severe disability at 6 years had been identified at 2 years [43]. Differing methods of assessments as participants get older may play into this change in individual scores.

EXPRESS comment that the *Wechsler Abbreviated Scale of Intelligence* (WISC) emphasises elements of executive function, which might explain worse outcomes at 6 years than in studies that do not use WISC [8]. It has also been noted that the Bayley-III used at the preschool assessment has poor sensitivity at lower scores [48].

Researchers involved in the VIC study discuss that the BSID-II is dependent on language skills whereas the WISC has a heavy emphasis on reasoning ability and working memory areas, which are vulnerable in preterm children. They surmise that this therefore may account for the findings of a higher proportion with mild cognitive impairment at 8 years than at 2 years [51].

A recent systematic review with meta-analysis concludes that pre-school developmental assessments have poor positive predictive value in detecting those who

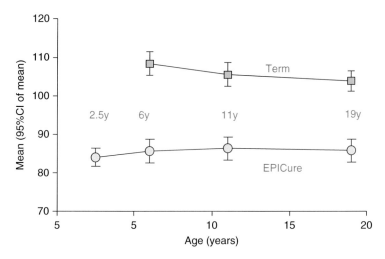

Fig. 19.5 Mean cognitive scores for extremely preterm and term control children from 2.5 to 19 years from the EPICure study [50] data are shown for participants who complete assessments at each age

have cognitive deficits at school age [55]. This has an important bearing on the need for developmental follow up past the age of 2 years in addition to increasing awareness amongst education professionals of the difficulties that ex preterm infants may face later in life. It also opens the opportunity for further research into implementing interventions to support learning [56].

Improvement over Time?

As discussed, there is variation in cognitive outcomes in extremely preterm infants reported across studies in several countries. The many advances in neonatal medicine do not appear to have conferred a significant cognitive advantage. Little difference has been seen in the rates of severe and moderate cognitive deficits between cohorts in longitudinal studies. In VICs (Australia) the mean IQ z score was similar across the three cohorts 1991–1992, −0.7, 1997, −0.8 and 2005–0.74 [44]. Additionally, EPICure (UK) found similar proportions of children with severe cognitive impairment across the two cohorts 1995 14% vs 2006 13% [3]. Retrospective analysis of outcomes across neonatal networks in America 2011–2014 [10] and Japan 2003–2012 [7] both conclude that there is little difference in the rate of moderate to severe cognitive impairment over the time periods studied.

   These studies have shown an improvement in rates of survival, particularly at lower gestations. The trend in improvement in neurodevelopmental outcomes discussed earlier in the chapter is accounted for by a reduction in CP rates and perhaps lower hearing and visual impairment rates rather than an improvement in cognitive outcomes. In the face of greater numbers of smaller and earlier gestational age babies surviving, while there does not seem to be an improvement there also does not seem to be an increase in the proportion of those surviving with severe cognitive impairment.

How Should We Screen for These Problems to Optimise the Chance of Early Recognition and Intervention?

Different countries have adopted differing approaches to screening preterm children for neurodevelopmental problems and some systems are more structured than others. The UK has a universal developmental screening program for all children and the NICE Developmental follow up of children and young people born preterm guideline [23] has recently recommended a structured follow up program for babies born preterm at higher risk of neurodevelopmental problems. This is summarised in Fig. 19.6.

This developmental follow up approach utilises validated parenteral questionnaires such as the Parent Report of Children's Abilities- revised for preterm infants (PARCA-R) to inform developmental follow up [57]. Once established, this may help streamline developmental assessments, but limitations include validation over restricted age ranges (e.g. 22–26 months for PARCA-R) and the fact that the tests are language dependant and so may not work for families whose first language is not English.

Neonatal neurodevelopmental follow up is commonly carried out at 2 years corrected age in the UK and this is audited under the UK national neonatal audit project (NNAP). The NICE guideline added a 4 year follow up for those at highest risk of neurodevelopmental problems recognising the limitations of developmental assessment at 2 years corrected age.

The purpose of screening targeted preterm populations for neurodevelopmental problems is to facilitate early intervention. The nature of the intervention would be related to the type of problem. Professional consensus is that early intervention is beneficial but finding solid evidence for early intervention programs has been challenging. Improved information sharing between health and education sectors may be helpful in supporting children born preterm with additional developmental needs [56].

Adult Outcomes

One of the challenges of assessing adult outcomes for survivors of extreme prematurity is that these outcomes, of necessity, reflect neonatal care from many years earlier. Longer term adult outcomes are unclear as extremely preterm survival was very rare 70 years ago.

Saigal [58] reported higher rates of functional limitations in adults with a mean age of 23 years born ELBW compared to term born controls with vision and hearing

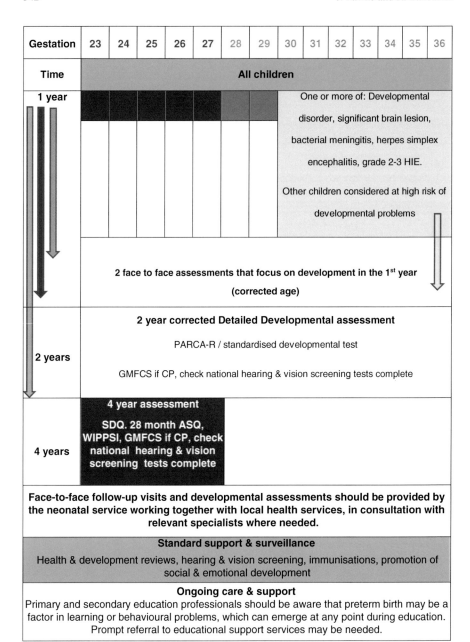

Fig. 19.6 Neurodevelopmental follow up of babies and Children born preterm in the UK as defined in NICE Guidance

impairments, learning difficulties, reduced dexterity, clumsiness and reduced self-care skills.

In Norway 68% of children born at 23–27 weeks gestation completed high school versus 72% at 31–33 weeks gestation and 75% at >37 weeks gestation [59]. Both Sweden [60] and Norway [59] report young adults born preterm are more likely to have a disability pension: Sweden, 13.2% at 24–28 weeks gestation versus 1.3% at term and in Norway 10.6% at 23–27 weeks gestation versus 1.7% at term.

Hack et al. [61] have studied those born preterm into adulthood and found that fewer VLBW than low birth weight (LBW) infants had graduated from high school 74% versus 83% and the mean IQ of VLBW versus LBW was 87 and 92 respectively.

Collection and Use of Neurodevelopmental Outcome Data

There are multiple reasons for assessing neurodevelopmental outcomes and collating that data. This can be considered at an individual/family level or from a healthcare system /commissioning perspective.

Individuals and Families

Neurodevelopmental follow up gives parents an opportunity to discuss concerns they may have about their baby's development. It serves to reassure about normal aspects of development, explain corrected gestational age and how this affects the time that developmental milestones may be achieved. Not correcting for prematurity is a common reason why parents are concerned about early developmental milestones and may artificially suggest either developmental delay where it is not present or greater delay than is present.

Where problems are becoming apparent it allows healthcare professions to discuss these problems and offers an opportunity to intervene. The interventions required will depend on the situation but may include early physiotherapy/occupational therapy or input from a speech and language therapist for either feeding or language development problems.

A developmental follow up service allows healthcare professions to build up expertise in the follow up of neonatal unit graduates and to become familiar with the range of problems that children and parents face and address common parental concerns. For example, personal experiences from the EPICure study [42] and running a developmental clinic suggest parental concerns vary over time.

Fig. 19.7 Parental
concerns over time
following extremely
preterm birth

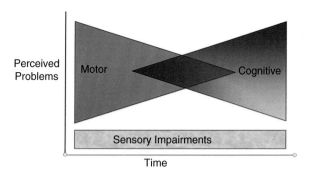

The schematic in Fig. 19.7 represents common parental concerns about the development of their baby who was born extremely preterm. Motor issues often predominate over the first few months with concerns over sitting, rolling, crawling, walking which evolve into worries about speech development and learning abilities. As the educational demands placed on a child increase concern over cognitive problems and the ability to integrate and synthesise information become common.

When children are old enough to attend a pre-school group or move into primary school education then identified problems can be flagged up to education professionals, so that they are aware of the issues. This creates the possibility of earlier educational intervention with the hope that this will improve educational attainment. Recently web-based resources have been developed in the UK to help educational professionals understand the developmental challenges some children born preterm face [56].

The identification of evolving developmental delay may act as a prompt for further investigations. This can lead to intervention pathways or diagnostic clarification which can help with focusing and accessing support. Parental support groups of various types exist in many areas and participating in a developmental follow up clinic allows these to be signposted to families.

Healthcare Systems

Collation of outcomes from structured neurodevelopmental follow up services informs clinical staff, has educational benefits for healthcare professionals and informs audit benchmarking of neonatal services. This is important for antenatal and postnatal counselling for parents facing extreme prematurity; particularly when they encounter events that are risk factors for adverse neurodevelopmental outcomes. It can help inform some degree of prognostication for babies on the NICU which may be an important component of decisions around the appropriateness of on-going intensive care.

Structured follow up acts as a safety check for new treatments or clinical management strategies. Longer term developmental follow up has influenced the use of antenatal and postnatal steroids, oxygen saturation targets and use of antenatal magnesium sulphate and is therefore it is central to how the speciality of neonatal medicine progresses.

Neurodevelopmental outcomes can be used to benchmark services. Although caution is needed when considering the lower numbers of extremely preterm babies as a small number of events can significantly change the outcome data. Audit of developmental follow up services and outcomes can act as markers of service configuration and organisation.

Commissioning

Healthcare costs associated with severe developmental delay are very high. Local health services need to have an idea of how much service provision is likely to be required in order to make resource allocation decisions. This includes service planning for both health care & education, for instance estimating of how many children may have special educational needs. Knowledge of preterm birth rates, prevalence and severity of developmental delay and resources that may assist those born preterm, helps with funding decisions. Information from structured neurodevelopmental follow up allows us to advocate for these children and highlights the needs that some of them have.

Conclusion

Neurodevelopmental outcomes following extremely preterm birth are critically important to patients and their families. Knowledge of these outcomes inform many aspects of neonatal intensive care and the counselling and prognostication given to families.

The overall picture is one of improved survival [2–7, 10–12] and dropping rates of CP [5, 7, 10, 24], improved neurosensory outcomes [7, 48] and reduced moderate- severe disability rates [2, 3, 11, 17, 48]. However, the evidence around cognitive outcome is less clear with rates of moderate to severe cognitive deficit remaining fairly static, albeit in the face of increased survival of more extremely preterm babies, including some at 22–23 weeks or <500 g. A child's cognitive score does not necessarily translate directly to a predicted level of functional outcome. Chapter 22 describes in further detail the impact of the educational and behavioural challenges that are encountered by many born extremely preterm.

Healthcare professionals and families need to be aware of the possibility of reduced rates of moderate-severe disability being accompanied by an increase in mild [48] disability.

The risk of neurodevelopmental problems for a baby is not a static risk [27, 28]. An initial risk defined by gestation, birthweight and antenatal factors is modified by postnatal events. It is therefore important for health care professionals to consider this in their ongoing discussions with families.

In order to identify neurodevelopmental problems in those babies at higher levels of risk structured follow up programmes are essential [23]. These programmes have the potential to facilitate early intervention, by informing families, clinical staff and education services of areas of additional need. Information gathered from such follow up programmes support the case for commissioning of services and helps to ensure that extremely preterm survivors get the additional support that they require as they mature into children and young adults.

References

1. Smith L. Comparing international survival rates of extremely preterm infants: the impact of variation in reporting signs of life. Infant. 2019;15:62–4.
2. Costeloe K, Hennessy E, Haider S, Stacey F, Marlow N, Draper E. Short term outcomes after extreme preterm birth in England: comparison of two birth cohorts in 1995 and 2006 (the EPICure studies). BMJ. 2012;345:e7976.
3. Moore T, Hennessy E, Myles J, Johnson S, Draper E, Costeloe K, Marlow N. Neurological and developmental outcome in extremely preterm children born in England in 1995 and 2006: the EPICure studies. BMJ. 2012;345:e7961.
4. Shah PS, Dunn M, Aziz K, et al. Sustained quality improvement in outcomes of preterm neonates with a gestational age less than 29 weeks: results from the evidence-based practice for improving quality phase 3. Can J Physiol Pharmacol. 2019;97:213–21.
5. Pierrat V, Marchand-Martin L, Arnaud C, et al.; EPIPAGE-2 Writing Group. Neurodevelopmental outcome at 2 years for preterm children born at 22 to 34 weeks' gestation in France in 2011: EPIPAGE-2 cohort study. BMJ. 2017;358:j3448.
6. Norman M, Hallberg B, Abrahamsson T, et al. Association between year of birth and 1-year survival among extremely preterm infants in Sweden during 2004-2007 and 2014-2016. JAMA. 2019;321:1188–99.
7. Nakanishi H, Suenaga H, Uchiyama A, Kono Y, Kusuda S, Neonatal Research Network, Japan. Trends in the neurodevelopmental outcomes among preterm infants from 2003–2012: a retrospective cohort study in Japan. J Perinatol. 2018;38:917–28.
8. Serenius F, Ewald U, Farooqi A, et al; Extremely Preterm Infants in Sweden Study Group. Neurodevelopmental outcomes among extremely preterm infants 6.5 years after active perinatal care in Sweden. JAMA Pediatr 170:954–963.
9. Doyle L, Roberts G, Anderson P; Victorian Infant Collaborative Study Group. Outcomes at age 2 years of infants <28 weeks' gestational age born in Victoria in 2005. J Pediatr. 2010;156:49–53.e1.
10. Adams-Chapman I, Heyne R, DeMauro S, et al.; Follow-Up Study of the Eunice Kennedy Shriver National Institute of Child Health and Human Development Neonatal Research Network. Neurodevelopmental impairment among extremely preterm infants in the Neonatal Research Network. Pediatrics. 2018;141:e20173091.
11. Myrhaug H, Brurberg K, Hov L, Markestad T. Survival and impairment of extremely premature infants: a meta-analysis. Pediatrics. 2019;143:e20180933.
12. Bonet M, Cuttini M, Piedvache A, et al.; MOSAIC and EPICE Research Groups. Changes in management policies for extremely preterm births and neonatal outcomes from 2003 to 2012: two population-based studies in ten European regions. BJOG Int J Obstet Gynaecol. 2017;124:1595–1604.

13. **DRAFT** perinatal management of extreme preterm birth before 27 weeks of gestation: a framework for practice. In: British Association of Perinatal Medicine; 2019. https://www.bapm.org/resources/extremepreterm. Accessed 17 Jun 2019.

14. Marlow N, Bennett C, Draper E, Hennessy E, Morgan A, Costeloe K. Perinatal outcomes for extremely preterm babies in relation to place of birth in England: the EPICure 2 study. Arch Dis Child Fetal Neonatal Ed. 2014;99:F181–8.

15. Smith LK, Draper ES, Manktelow BN, et al, on behalf of the MBRRACE-UK Collaboration. MBRRACE-UK report on survival up to one year of age of babies born before 27 weeks gestational age for births in Great Britain from January to December 2016. Leicester: The Infant Mortality and Morbidity Studies, Department of Health Sciences, University of Leicester; 2018.

16. Ding S, Lemyre B, Daboval T, Barrowman N, Moore G. A meta-analysis of neurodevelopmental outcomes at 4-10 years in children born at 22-25 weeks gestation. Acta Paediatr. 2019;108(7):1237–44. https://doi.org/10.1111/apa.14693.

17. Batton B, Li L, Newman N, et al; Eunice Kennedy Shriver National Institute of Child Health & Human Development Neonatal Research Network. Early blood pressure, antihypotensive therapy and outcomes at 18–22 months' corrected age in extremely preterm infants. Arch Dis Child Fetal Neonatal Ed. 2016;101:F201–F206.

18. Hess J. Experiences gained in a thirty year study of prematurely born infants. Pediatrics. 1953;11:425–34.

19. Backes C, Söderström F, Ågren J, et al. Outcomes following a comprehensive versus a selective approach for infants born at 22 weeks of gestation. J Perinatol. 2018;39:39–47.

20. Brumbaugh J, Hansen N, Bell E, et al. Outcomes of extremely preterm infants with birth weight less than 400 g. JAMA Pediatr. 2019;173:434–45.

21. Saigal S. Differences in preferences for neonatal outcomes among health care professionals, parents, and adolescents. JAMA. 1999;281:1991–7.

22. Tyson J, Parikh N, Langer J, Green C, Higgins R, for the National Institute of Child Health and Human Development Neonatal Research Network. Intensive care for extreme prematurity— moving beyond gestational age. N Engl J Med. 2008;358:1672–81.

23. Overview|Developmental follow-up of children and young people born preterm|Guidance|NICE. In: Nice.org.uk. 2019. https://www.nice.org.uk/guidance/NG72. Accessed 17 Jun 2019.

24. Farooqi A, Hagglof B, Sedin G, Serenius F. Impact at age 11 years of major neonatal morbidities in children born extremely preterm. Pediatrics. 2011;127:e1247–57.

25. Ting JY, Synnes A, Lee S, Shah P, Canadian Neonatal Network and Canadian Neonatal Follow Up Network. Association of admission temperature and death or adverse neurodevelopmental outcomes in extremely low-gestational age neonates. J Perinatol. 2018;38:844–9.

26. Synnes A, Luu T, Moddemann D, et al.; Canadian Neonatal Network and the Canadian Neonatal Follow-Up Network. Determinants of developmental outcomes in a very preterm Canadian cohort. Arch Dis Child Fetal Neonatal Ed. 2016;102:F235–F234.

27. Ambalavanan N, Carlo W, Tyson J, et al.; Generic Database: Subcommittees of the Eunice Kennedy Shriver National Institute of Child Health and Human Development Neonatal Research Network. Outcome trajectories in extremely preterm infants. Pediatrics. 2012;130:e115-e125.

28. Cheong J, Lee K, Boland R, et al.; for the Victorian Infant Collaborative Study Group. Changes in long-term prognosis with increasing postnatal survival and the occurrence of postnatal morbidities in extremely preterm infants offered intensive care: a prospective observational study. Lancet Child Adolesc Health. 2018;2:872–879.

29. Overview|Specialist neonatal respiratory care for babies born preterm|Guidance|NICE. In: Nice.org.uk. 2019. https://www.nice.org.uk/guidance/ng124. Accessed 17 Jun 2019.

30. Linsell L, Malouf R, Morris J, Kurinczuk J, Marlow N. Risk factor models for neurodevelopmental outcomes in children born very preterm or with very low birth weight: a systematic review of methodology and reporting. Am J Epidemiol. 2017;185:601–12.

31. Bax M, Goldstein M, Rosenbaum P, Leviton A, Paneth N, Dan B, Jacobsson B, Damiano D, Executive Committee for the Definition of Cerebral Palsy. Proposed definition and classification of cerebral palsy, April 2005. Dev Med Child Neurol. 2007;47:571–571.

32. Palisano R, Cameron D, Rosenbaum P, Walter S, Russell D. Stability of the gross motor function classification system. Dev Med Child Neurol. 2006;48(6):424–8. https://doi.org/10.1111/dmcn.13903.
33. Alliance C. Manual ability classification system (MACS)|cerebral palsy alliance. In: Cerebralpalsy.org.au. 2019. https://cerebralpalsy.org.au/our-research/about-cerebral-palsy/what-is-cerebral-palsy/severity-of-cerebral-palsy/manual-ability-classification-system/. Accessed 17 Jun 2019.
34. Larroque B, Ancel P, Marret S, et al.; EPIPAGE Study Group. Neurodevelopmental disabilities and special care of 5-year-old children born before 33 weeks of gestation (the EPIPAGE study): a longitudinal cohort study. Lancet. 2008;371:813–820.
35. De Groote I, Vanhaesebrouck P, Bruneel E, et al; Extremely Preterm Infants in Belgium (EPIBEL) Study Group. Outcome at 3 years of age in a population-based cohort of extremely preterm infants. Obstet Gynecol. 2007;110:855–864.
36. Hirvonen M, Ojala R, Korhonen P, Haataja P, Eriksson K, Gissler M, Luukkaala T, Tammela O. Cerebral palsy among children born moderately and late preterm. Pediatrics. 2014;134:X23.
37. Himmelmann K, Uvebrant P. The panorama of cerebral palsy in Sweden part XII shows that patterns changed in the birth years 2007-2010. Acta Paediatr. 2018;107:462–8.
38. Glinianaia S, Rankin J, Colver A, North of England Collaborative Cerebral Palsy Survey. Cerebral palsy rates by birth weight, gestation and severity in north of England, 1991-2000 singleton births. Arch Dis Child. 2010;96:180–5.
39. Pascal A, Govaert P, Oostra A, Naulaers G, Ortibus E, Van den Broeck C. Neurodevelopmental outcome in very preterm and very-low-birthweight infants born over the past decade: a meta-analytic review. Dev Med Child Neurol. 2018;60:342–55.
40. Wood N, Marlow N, Costeloe K, Gibson A, Wilkinson A. Neurologic and developmental disability after extremely preterm birth. EPICure Study Group. N Engl J Med. 2000;343:378–84.
41. Marlow N, Wolke D, Bracewell M, Samara M, EPICure Study Group. Neurologic and developmental disability at six years of age after extremely preterm birth. N Engl J Med. 2005;352:9–19.
42. Johnson S, Fawke J, Hennessy E, Rowell V, Thomas S, Wolke D, Marlow N. Neurodevelopmental disability through 11 years of age in children born before 26 weeks of gestation. Pediatrics. 2009;124:e249–57.
43. Serenius F, Källén K, Blennow M, et al.; EXPRESS Group. Neurodevelopmental outcome in extremely preterm infants at 2.5 years after active perinatal care in Sweden. JAMA. 2013;309:1810–1820.
44. Hutchinson E, De Luca C, Doyle L, Roberts G, Anderson P, Victorian Infant Collaborative Study Group. School-age outcomes of extremely preterm or extremely low birth weight children. Pediatrics. 2013;131:e1053–61.
45. Doyle L, Anderson P, the Victorian Infant Collaborative Study Group. Improved neurosensory outcome at 8 years of age of extremely low birthweight children born in Victoria over three distinct eras. Arch Dis Child Fetal Neonatal Ed. 2005;90:F484–8. https://doi.org/10.1136/adc.2004.063362.
46. Joseph R, O'Shea T, Allred E, Heeren T, Hirtz D, Jara H, Leviton A, Kuban K, for the ELGAN Study Investigators. Neurocognitive and academic outcomes at age 10 years of extremely preterm newborns. Pediatrics. 2016;137:e20154343.
47. Flynn J. What is intelligence? Cambridge: Cambridge University Press; 2009.
48. Moore T, Johnson S, Haider S, Hennessy E, Marlow N. Relationship between test scores using the second and third editions of the Bayley scales in extremely preterm children. J Pediatr. 2012;160:553–8.
49. Anderson P, Doyle L. Cognitive and educational deficits in children born extremely preterm. Semin Perinatol. 2008;32:51–8.
50. Linsell L, Johnson S, Wolke D, O'Reilly H, Morris J, Kurinczuk J, Marlow N. Cognitive trajectories from infancy to early adulthood following birth before 26 weeks of gestation: a prospective, population-based cohort study. Arch Dis Child. 2018;103:363–70.

51. Roberts G, Anderson P, Doyle L, Victorian Infant Collaborative Study Group. The stability of the diagnosis of developmental disability between ages 2 and 8 in a geographic cohort of very preterm children born in 1997. Arch Dis Child. 2009;95:786–90.

52. Cheong J, Anderson P, Burnett A, Roberts G, Davis N, Hickey L, Carse E, Doyle L, for the Victorian Infant Collaborative Study Group. Changing neurodevelopment at 8 years in children born extremely preterm since the 1990s. Pediatrics. 2017;139:e20164086.

53. Johnson S, Hennessy E, Smith R, Trikic R, Wolke D, Marlow N. Academic attainment and special educational needs in extremely preterm children at 11 years of age: the EPICure study. Arch Dis Child Fetal Neonatal Ed. 2009;94:F283–9.

54. Hack M, Taylor H, Drotar D, Schluchter M, Cartar L, Wilson-Costello D, Klein N, Friedman H, Mercuri-Minich N, Morrow M. Poor predictive validity of the Bayley scales of infant development for cognitive function of extremely low birth weight children at school age. Pediatrics. 2005;116:333–41.

55. Wong H, Santhakumaran S, Cowan F, Modi N. Developmental assessments in preterm children: a meta-analysis. Pediatrics. 2016;138:e20160251.

56. Preterm birth information for education professionals. In: Nottingham.ac.uk. 2019. https://www.nottingham.ac.uk/helm/dev/prism/index.html. Accessed 17 Jun 2019.

57. Blaggan S, Guy A, Boyle E, Spata E, Manktelow B, Wolke D, Johnson S. A parent questionnaire for developmental screening in infants born late and moderately preterm. Pediatrics. 2014;134:e55–62.

58. Saigal S, Stoskopf B, Boyle M, Paneth N, Pinelli J, Streiner D, Goddeeris J. Comparison of current health, functional limitations, and health care use of young adults who were born with extremely low birth weight and Normal birth weight. Pediatrics. 2007;119:e562–73.

59. Moster D, Lie R, Markestad T. Long-term medical and social consequences of preterm birth. N Engl J Med. 2008;359:262–73.

60. Lindstrom K, Winbladh B, Haglund B, Hjern A. Preterm infants as young adults: a Swedish National Cohort Study. Pediatrics. 2007;120:70–7.

61. Hack M. Young adult outcomes of very-low-birth-weight children. Semin Fetal Neonatal Med. 2006;11:127–37.

62. Stewart A, Reynolds E, Lipscomb A. Outcome for infants of very low birthweight: survey of world literature. Lancet. 1981;317:1038–41.

Chapter 20
Long Term Effects Following Extreme Prematurity: Respiratory Problems

John Lowe, Sarah J. Kotecha, and Sailesh Kotecha

Definitions

Preterm birth, defined as birth prior to 37 completed weeks of gestational age, accounts for 7–10% of all live births in the UK. This percentage is rising worldwide, especially in the late preterm gestations (34–36 weeks of gestation) [1]. There have been large-scale advances in the treatment of preterm birth in the last two decades and consequently many more of the most immature infants survive today with the limit of viability being around 22–23 weeks of gestation. Infants born at ≤28 weeks of gestation, often called 'extremely preterm', now represent the group who are likely to require significant neonatal care immediately following birth, requiring hospital stays of weeks or months. Infants born at the limit of viability require substantial multidisciplinary follow-up post-discharge, which places a significant burden on healthcare resources and on families.

Lung Development

To contextualise the reasons for longer term lung sequelae in children born extremely preterm, it is first useful to review the key stages of normal lung development: Embryonic (0–7 weeks of gestational age), pseudoglandular (7–17 weeks), canalicular (17–27 weeks), saccular (28–36) and alveolar (36 weeks until at least 2–3 years of age) [2]. Thus, the lungs of an extremely preterm born infant are in the late canalicular and early saccular growth stages, prior to the development of alveoli and type 2 pneumocytes, and provide only a nascent surface for facilitating gas

J. Lowe · S. J. Kotecha · S. Kotecha (✉)
Department of Child Health, Cardiff University School of Medicine, Cardiff, UK
e-mail: LoweJ3@cardiff.ac.uk; kotechasj@cardiff.ac.uk; kotechas@cardiff.ac.uk

© Springer Nature Switzerland AG 2020
E. M. Boyle, J. Cusack (eds.), *Emerging Topics and Controversies in Neonatology*, https://doi.org/10.1007/978-3-030-28829-7_20

exchange. Secondary to the neonatal interventions required to support life, and early exposure to the hyperoxic extrauterine environment, a period of dysregulated lung growth follows, coupled with abnormal vascular development [3]. Infants still receiving respiratory support at 36 weeks post-menstrual age may be diagnosed with bronchopulmonary dysplasia (BPD), also known as chronic lung disease of prematurity (CLD), which is a common occurrence at the extremes of gestation [4]. Due to advances in neonatal care including exogenous surfactant, antenatal cortico-steroids, and more gentle forms of ventilation, the pathology of BPD/CLD has changed to that reflecting the level of gestational immaturity, rather than the iatro-genic effects of neonatal care attributed to 'old BPD' [5], as described below.

Lung Pathology and Imaging

Debate on the relative importance of structural and functional aspects of lung dis-ease in extremely preterm born children has been ongoing [6]. Until recently, insights into the structural abnormalities of the extremely preterm lung have been limited to a handful of port-mortem examinations of children with fatal lung dis-ease, and to animal models. These show evidence of simplified alveoli (enlarged and reduced in number), poorly developed vasculature, and fibrosis. Cross-sectional studies of extremely preterm born children using CT scans have similarly noted opacities and hypo-attenuation which may reflect pre-emphysematous changes [7], as well as bronchial wall thickening [6]. These structural abnormalities decrease the surface area available for gas exchange, contribute to airway obstruction respec-tively, and are unsurprisingly more severe at lower gestation and in children with a history of BPD. Recent innovations in hyperpolarised ^{3}He MRI scanning have pro-vided novel insights into the lung structure of preterm born children, which indicate that the alveolar surface area continues to increase at least in to adolescence [8]. Moreover, the possibility also exists that the lungs of preterm born children may exhibit a degree of 'catch-up' alveolarisation by adolescence and beyond [9] with survivors of extreme prematurity having similar alveolar size as term born children. However evidence exists to the contrary, suggesting that school- age BPD survivors have fewer, larger, alveoli [10]. In the adolescent and young adult population, there are no studies of tissue samples [11] save from a case report of a 12 year-old with fatal asthma exacerbation [12]. The limited studies using CT imaging in this group have consistently reported abnormal lung structures which correlated with measures of lung function [13, 14].

Respiratory Infection and Morbidity

It is well-established that extremely preterm born infants have significantly more respiratory sequelae in the first years of life [15], and beyond [16–20]. Initially, this often manifests as increased hospital admissions for acute respiratory illness, primarily driven by respiratory syncytial virus (RSV) infection. While the majority of infants will contract RSV infection during the first 2 years of life, rates of admission are substantially higher in the extremely preterm population. A recent analysis from a large population based, data-linkage study reported a 12% increase in the frequency of infection-related hospitalisation during childhood per week reduction in gestational age [21]. The primary driver is likely to be an immature and dysregulated immune response to pathogens resulting from prenatal and postnatal exposures associated with extremely preterm birth, a topic which has been thoroughly reviewed [22]. Increased respiratory morbidity is often, but not always, associated with decrements in spirometry indices [23] with evidence of tracking throughout childhood [24, 25]. The systematic review of childhood wheezing disorders by Been and colleagues noted increased risk of wheeze in preterm-born children (OR1.17; 95% CI 1.57–1.87), reporting a sample size of over 1.5 million subjects and a strong dose-response effect of gestational age, with a 6% decrease in risk of wheezing disorder for every additional week up until the fortieth week of gestation at birth (Fig. 20.1) [26]. Similarly, reports from studies recruiting adult survivors of BPD note increased symptoms and inhaler use [27], when compared to terms controls, but not exclusively [28]. Although the available cross-sectional data support the notion of 'tracking' of poor respiratory health [29], we currently rely on studies of individuals whose neonatal course was vastly different to contemporary graduates of the neonatal unit who survive with 'new BPD' [30]. Thus, it is essential that longitudinal data are obtained to investigate if outcomes are improved for the 'post-surfactant' cohorts of children, how these change over time, and the mechanisms driving that change.

Lung Function

Unsurprisingly, lung function in extremely preterm born children is already suboptimal at birth and in the following months and early years [31–33]. These deficits are more pronounced in infants with a history of BPD/CLD.

The recent systematic review by Kotecha et al. noted decrements in lung function framed as reduction of approximately 7% in Forced Expiratory Volume in 1 second (FEV_1) for individuals born <37 weeks of gestation without a history of BPD/CLD when compared to term born controls up to the age of 23 years [34]. Individuals with BPD/CLD had increased deficits of between approximately 16–19% when compared to controls. Interestingly, most studies report normal Forced Vital Capacity (FVC), indicating obstructive disease, which affects peripheral and distal airways, but not lung volume. This concept of disproportionate growth between lung size and airway calibre has been termed 'dysanapsis' [35] and recently gained interest as a potential clinically important measure of lung function, especially in relation to obesity and asthma [36]. Extremely preterm born children, with their neonatal history of dysregulated lung growth, may be at an increased risk of this phenomenon. The aetiology is likely to be complex but is perhaps mediated by a chronic inflammatory response, and exacerbated by methods of nutrition and exposure to noxious substances including tobacco smoke [37].

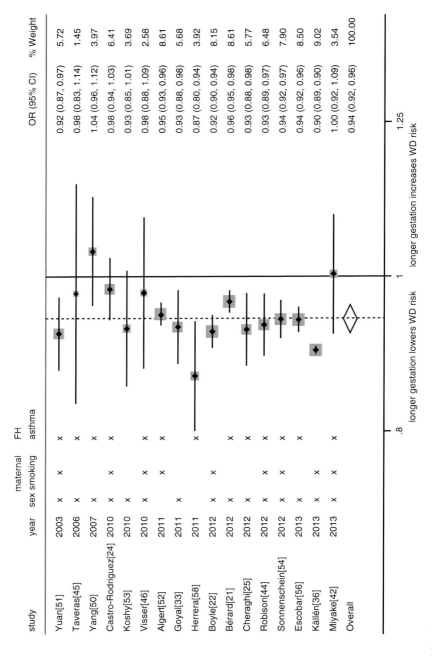

Fig. 20.1 Forest plot representing a per-week dose-response effect of increasing gestation on the odds of wheezing disorders. The effect estimate is OR 0.94. (Reproduced with permission from Been et al. [26])

The effect of extreme prematurity on the peripheral airways is now being characterised using the latest pulmonary function techniques providing evidence of modified airway and lung tissue mechanics in relation to reflecting increased airway obstruction (increased resistance) and altered elastic properties (decreased reactance), respectively [38, 39]. In contrast, evidence for the use of techniques for assessment of ventilation inhomogeneity (such as lung clearance index and the forced oscillation technique), or impaired gas exchange is more conflicting. That being said, interesting data from a cohort of preterm born children demonstrated evidence of ventilation inhomogeneity of the peripheral conducting airways, especially when the gestational age was <28 weeks of gestation, and lends further weight to the concept of dysanapsis between the airways and lung parenchyma [40].

There is strong evidence that decrements in lung function track or deteriorate, but do not improve through childhood in extremely preterm born children. The longitudinal studies available from the surfactant era of lung function note that, whilst some improvements may be observed in the more moderately preterm group by young adulthood [41], generally airway obstruction is observed to be consistently low in extremely preterm born individuals across the time period, and is more pronounced for the survivors of BPD/CLD (Fig. 20.2) [11, 24, 25]. Worryingly, this is exacerbated if there was also exposure to tobacco smoke [42]. Secondary effects

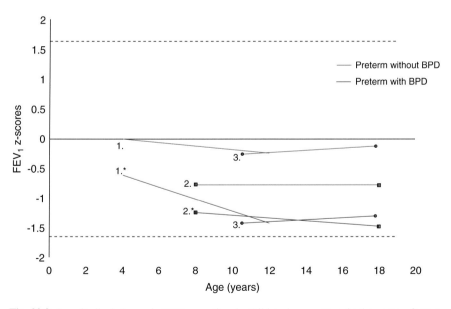

Fig. 20.2 Longitudinal change in FEV$_1$ over time in children born preterm in the post surfactant era with and without BPD. (1) Simpson et al. [25]; (2) Doyle et al. [42]; and (3) Vollsaeter et al. [11]. Upper and lower limits of normal are represented by dotted lines. ∗ Indicates significant lung function decline over time relative to a representative population of term-born controls. These studies have shown lung function tracks at z-scores of zero for healthy term-born children. (Reproduced with permission from Urs et al. [47])

may include reduced exercise capacity [43, 44] and reduced physical activity [45] at school age and in adulthood [46], which have the capacity to impact upon quality of life.

Taken together, these studies provide strong evidence that respiratory morbidity in adulthood has its origins early in life, and that these deficits track over time. The onset of age-related decline in lung function is not clinically relevant due to the large lung reserves available, However, preterm birth exacerbates these deficits, and imposes an additional burden, which may further prevent attainment of peak lung function.

The longer term impact of preterm birth on lung health is now starting to be realised as graduates of neonatal care from the 1970s onwards have entered adulthood. The recent systematic review by Gough and colleagues collated data from eight eligible studies and reported evidence of increased respiratory symptoms and airflow obstruction in adults born preterm, especially those with a history of BPD/CLD. This was accompanied by evidence of structural lung changes on radiological imaging, which likely reflect lung injury during the neonatal period [29].

Primary data collected by the same group also reported increased respiratory symptoms and medication use in BPD/CLD adults. FEV_1 and Forced Expiratory Flow at 25–75% of FVC (FEF_{25-75}) were also significantly lower than in non-BPD preterms and term controls. These decrements were also accompanied by a lower EQ-5D score, potentially reflecting a perceived lower quality of life [27]. Follow-up work by Caskey and colleagues noted that adult survivors of BPD/CLD had increased rates of fixed airway obstruction, greater impairment in gas transfer, and reduced exercise capacity when compared to the term-born group. Lung clearance index as measured by multiple breath washout was also higher in the BPD/CLD compared to term-born controls [14].

In the healthy population, peak lung function is attained approximately at 21–22 years of age, by which time there has been a 30-fold increase in lung volume and a 20-fold increase in gas exchange surface since birth [48]. From this plateau, both FEV_1 and FVC gradually decline as lung elasticity is lost [49]. However, it is of great concern that the structural and functional abnormalities noted above may predispose extremely preterm born adults to an early and accelerated decline in pulmonary function later in life and lead to early manifestation of chronic obstructive pulmonary disease (COPD) which impose restrictions on quality of life (Fig. 20.3) [50–53]. Encouragingly there is evidence that more contemporary cohorts of extremely preterm born individuals do fare better [54], but notwithstanding, interventions have been recommended to reduce the risk of chronic respiratory disease [55].

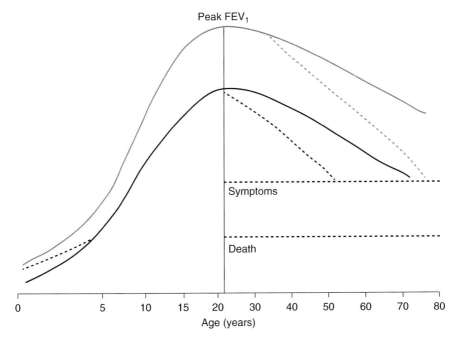

Fig. 20.3 Diagrammatic representation of the potential early respiratory decline in individuals born with sub-optimal lung function. After failure to achieve peak FEV_1 in early adulthood in comparison with a normal trajectory (blue line), symptoms of disease may occur at a younger age (red line). The effect is exacerbated in the presence of other risk factors, e.g. tobacco smoking (dotted red line). (Reproduced with permission from Stocks et al. [53])

Unanswered Questions, Future Research Directions

Phenotypes and Mechanisms of Disease

A combination of pathophysiology and symptomology have been used to define phenotypes of respiratory disease in children, namely asthma [56]. Often, extremely preterm born children are labelled as having higher rates of asthma [20]. However, there is growing consensus that the mechanisms and phenotypes of disease are different and that the term 'asthma' should be avoided when describing prematurity associated respiratory disease [57]. Recent evidence suggest that atopy does not play a role in the phenotype of wheezy disorder experienced by preterm born children. In the study by Edwards [16], rates of wheeze were noted to be similar in both preterm born children with a family history of atopy and those without a family history when compared to term controls (Fig. 20.4).

Moreover, airway inflammation in preterm born children may be mediated by neutrophils as opposed to eosinophils [58] and there are isolated reports of oxidative stress [59] and inflammation [60] in extremely preterm born children when compared to term born controls, but this is not consistent [61, 62]. Thus, it is unknown

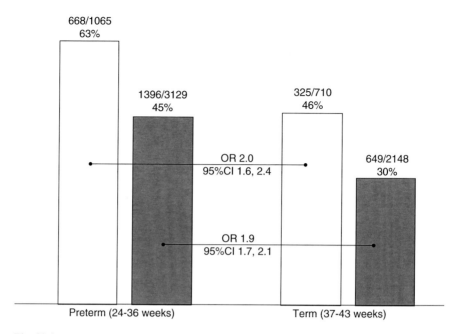

Fig. 20.4 The prevalence of wheeze-ever within the RANOPS cohort for preterm-born children and term-born controls. The white bars denote family history of atopy and the grey bars denote no family history. The odds ratio for wheeze-ever is similar when comparing preterm-born children with, or without family history to term controls. (Reproduced with permission from Edwards et al. [16])

if lung disease following preterm birth is a result of structural deficits acquired as result of developmental insults and necessary neonatal intervention, or an active process characterised by factors including inflammation and bronchial hyper-responsiveness. Until this question is resolved, continuing inflammation should be an important consideration alongside the long-held view that early airway remodelling and dysfunctional alveolar development are responsible for the long-term respiratory sequelae in extremely preterm born children.

New "systems biology" methods of biomarker profiling may offer one way to elucidate sub-phenotypes of respiratory disease. Metabolomics is one such approach that can be used for hypothesis-free biomarker profiling. With the aid of bioinformatics tools and multivariate statistical analysis, metabolic profiles are generated which are capable of discriminating between groups of individuals. Untargeted metabolomic analysis using urine sampling has recently shown promise in profiling children with recurrent respiratory infections against healthy peers, and following treatment with immuno-stimulant [63]. Moreover, another study was able to determine differences in metabolite profile from exhaled breath condensate between children with and without asthma using NMR-based methods [64]. A further opportunity exists within the development "breathomics": studying the molecular profile of breath through the analysis of gaseous volatile organic compounds in exhaled air, which differs from the metabolomics approach of analysing metabolites in exhaled breath condensate [65, 66]. Discrimination between asthmatic and non-asthmatic children is already possible, along with differing patterns between preschool asthma and transient wheeze [67], and between children with recent respiratory tract infection and those without [68]. With many believing that asthma should no longer be considered a single disease and that efforts should be made to identify the different biochemical-inflammatory profiles underlying asthma symptoms [69], it does not seem unreasonable to take a similar approaches in extremely preterm born children whose respiratory disease undoubtedly has a different aetiology.

Treatment: Infection

Extremely preterm born children are more susceptible to viral infections during the first years of life [70], potentially due to immune dysfunction acquired in utero and by alterations in microbial colonisation which occur by virtue of birth via caesarean section. This dysfunction may be further modulated as result of increased levels of pulmonary inflammation and oxidative stress in the neonatal period [71] and beyond, although the data are limited (as described above). Respiratory syncytial virus (RSV) lower respiratory tract infections and subsequent bronchiolitis is implicated in the pathogenesis of recurrent wheeze [72] and potentially atopic status [72], with increased hospitalisation and poorer lung function at school age [73], as shown in many observational studies [74].

The IMpact trial showed a 55% reduction in RSV related hospital admissions in high risk infants ($\leq$36 weeks' gestation or with BPD) in the first 2 years of life using monthly injections of palivizumab, a monoclonal antibody therapy [75], and supported licensing of the product in the United States. However, policy guidance on the use of palivizumab for RSV prophylaxis is cost-benefit driven. Current recommendations in the US are that infants born before 29 weeks of gestation who are younger than 12 months of age at the start of the RSV season are administered palivizumab prophylactically, although, infants born <32 weeks' gestation may qualify if they have a history of BPD/CLD. Treatment in the second year of life is considered only for infants with a history of BPD/CLD who continue to require medical support (defined as chronic corticosteroid therapy, diuretic therapy, or supplemental oxygen) during the 6-month period before the start of the second RSV season [76].

In comparison, guidance in the UK is more restrictive, with the recommendation for passive immunisation using palivizumab being for children born at <35 weeks' gestation, and less than 6 months old, to receive prophylactic 15 mg/kg doses on a monthly basis throughout the RSV season up to a maximum of five doses (Fig. 20.5) [77]. Pharmacokinetic data have demonstrated that serum levels of following five doses remain at or above protective levels for at least 3 months [78]. However, randomised placebo-controlled trials performed in the United States of infants born moderately preterm (33–35 weeks' gestation), aged 6 months or younger, noted a significant reduction in parent-reported wheezy days, and a reduction in

	Gestational age at birth (weeks+days)						
Age (months)	≤24+0	24+1to 26+0	26+1to 28+0	28+1to 30+0	30+1to 32+0	32+1to 34+0	≥34+1
<1.5							
1.5 to<3							
3 to <6							
6 to <9							
≥9							

Fig. 20.5 Cost-effective use of RSV prophylaxis as described in the UK guidelines. Green cells represent the appropriate combinations of gestational age and current age to receive treatment. (Reproduced from Public Health England: *The Green Book* chapter 27a [77])

bronchodilator usage, in the first year of life [79]. Follow-up of the same cohort at 6 years of age noted reduced rates of 'current asthma', defined as parent reported wheeze plus the use of asthma medication within the last 12 months. No differences were observed in physician diagnosed asthma or in lung function, leading the authors to conclude "that RSV prevention does not reduce clinically relevant asthma symptoms at age 6 years" [80].

Similar results were observed in the case-control study by Mochizuki. Palivizumab prophylaxis administered to preterm infants did not suppress the onset of atopic asthma but resulted in a significantly lower incidence of recurrent wheezing during the first 6 years of life [81]. A strength of this study was the capture of each wheeze episode, which may more accurately identify individuals with recurrent illness. This raises an interesting question as to whether recurrent preterm born wheezers may form part of a non-atopic phenotype which may benefit from sustained prophylactic treatment to avoid impairments in early childhood lung growth and development which manifest as flow limitation [31] and dysanapsis [37]. Indeed, the reported cost-effectiveness models do not include potential cost savings associated with readmissions for early childhood viral-induced wheeze in the vulnerable group of extremely preterm born children [82]. Thus, a low cost formulation of anti-RSV antibody would certainly extend the debate around the treatment of viral-induced wheeze.

Treatment: Inhaled Therapies

Worryingly, the lack of mechanistic understanding of respiratory disease in extremely preterm born individuals prevents the targeting of appropriate therapies, and it is of substantial concern that few practitioners, including paediatric specialists, do not know if their patients were born prematurely [83]. Indeed, a recent systematic review [84] identified only two small studies using serial doses of inhaled treatment in preterm born children: one of a single daily dose of beta-2 agonist for two weeks, and a second of a daily dose of budesonide for a four-month period [85, 86]. This lack of robust evidence is of concern, since use of inhaled medication has been reported to be significantly higher in the extremely preterm born population (especially ≤32 weeks of gestation) [16] but others report less than half with identified defects in lung function are receiving medication which is also of concern as is contrary to the evidence of reversible airway obstruction at rest [20] or following exercise [87] in preterm-born children when compared to term-born controls. Thus, the question arises as to whether children are being under-treated, or whether therapies such as inhaled corticosteroids (which can have significant side effects with long-term use), are being advocated with little prospect of effectiveness. Clearly, more robust evidence to optimise management of lung disease of preterm born children is needed. Small trials conducted in adults with 'non-eosinophilic' asthma revealed little response to a relatively short course of inhaled corticosteroid therapy [88, 89]. However, within these studies, and in the wider discussion [90], the role of extreme prematurity is not discussed, although other risk factors known to be affected by gestational age at birth such as viral infection, pollution and exposure to tobacco smoke are considered. The authors also note that many any of the features seen in non-eosinophilic asthma could occur in chronic obstructive pulmonary disease. In any case, the optimal management strategy will only be identified with modern mechanistic studies, and large-scale randomised controlled trials of commonly-used inhaled bronchodilators, corticosteroids, and perhaps leukotriene receptor antagonists. Moreover, the "omics" approaches described above, in time, may enable treatment with specifically targeted therapies.

Conclusion

It is increasingly evident that extremely preterm born individuals are bound for life-long respiratory disease. Thus, it is crucial that the most recent graduates of neonatal care are followed longitudinally, whilst at the same time novel methods of elucidating factors important in the mechanisms of the disease process are further developed. Identifying such characteristics which are amenable to therapy using systems biology methods may provide a more targeted approach to treatment.

References

1. Blencowe H, Cousens S, Oestergaard MZ, Chou D, Moller A-B, Narwal R, et al. National, regional, and worldwide estimates of preterm birth rates in the year 2010 with time trends since 1990 for selected countries: a systematic analysis and implications. Lancet. 2012;379(9832):2162–72.
2. Joshi S, Kotecha S. Lung growth and development. Early Hum Dev. 2007;83(12):789–94.

3. Chakraborty M, McGreal EP, Kotecha S. Acute lung injury in preterm newborn infants: mechanisms and management. Paediatr Respir Rev. 2010;11(3):162–70; quiz 70.
4. Costeloe K, Hennessy E, Gibson AT, Marlow N, Wilkinson AR. The EPICure study: outcomes to discharge from hospital for infants born at the threshold of viability. Pediatrics. 2000;106(4 I):659–71.
5. Jobe AH, Bancalari E. Bronchopulmonary dysplasia. Am J Respir Crit Care Med. 2001;163(7):1723–9.
6. Simpson SJ, Logie KM, O'Dea CA, Banton GL, Murray C, Wilson AC, et al. Altered lung structure and function in mid-childhood survivors of very preterm birth. Thorax. 2017;72(8):702–11.
7. Aukland SM, Rosendahl K, Owens CM, Fosse KR, Eide GE, Halvorsen T. Neonatal bronchopulmonary dysplasia predicts abnormal pulmonary HRCT scans in long-term survivors of extreme preterm birth. Thorax. 2009;64(5):405–10.
8. Narayanan M, Owers-Bradley J, Beardsmore CS, Mada M, Ball I, Garipov R, et al. Alveolarization continues during childhood and adolescence: new evidence from helium-3 magnetic resonance. Am J Respir Crit Care Med. 2012;185(2):186–91.
9. Narayanan M, Beardsmore CS, Owers-Bradley J, Dogaru CM, Mada M, Ball I, et al. Catch-up alveolarization in ex-preterm children: evidence from (3)He magnetic resonance. Am J Respir Crit Care Med. 2013;187(10):1104–9.
10. Flors L, Mugler JP III, Paget-Brown A, Froh DK, de Lange EE, Patrie JT, et al. Hyperpolarized Helium-3 diffusion-weighted magnetic resonance imaging detects abnormalities of lung structure in children with bronchopulmonary dysplasia. J Thorac Imaging. 2017;32(5):323–32.
11. Vollsaeter M, Roksund OD, Eide GE, Markestad T, Halvorsen T. Lung function after preterm birth: development from mid-childhood to adulthood. Thorax. 2013;68(8):767–76.
12. Cutz E, Chiasson D. Chronic lung disease after premature birth. N Engl J Med. 2008;358(7):743–6.
13. Wong PM, Lees AN, Louw J, Lee FY, French N, Gain K, et al. Emphysema in young adult survivors of moderate-to-severe bronchopulmonary dysplasia. Eur Respir J. 2008;32(2):321–8.
14. Caskey S, Gough A, Rowan S, Gillespie S, Clarke J, Riley M, et al. Structural and functional lung impairment in adult survivors of bronchopulmonary dysplasia. Ann Am Thorac Soc. 2016;13(8):1262–70.
15. Pramana IA, Latzin P, Schlapbach LJ, Hafen G, Kuehni CE, Nelle M, et al. Respiratory symptoms in preterm infants: burden of disease in the first year of life. Eur J Med Res. 2011;16(5):223–30.
16. Edwards MO, Kotecha SJ, Lowe J, Richards L, Watkins WJ, Kotecha S. Management of prematurity-associated wheeze and its association with atopy. PLoS One. 2016;11(5):e0155695.
17. Paranjothy S, Dunstan F, Watkins WJ, Hyatt M, Demmler JC, Lyons RA, et al. Gestational age, birth weight, and risk of respiratory hospital admission in childhood. Pediatrics. 2013;132(6):e1562–9.
18. Boyle EM, Poulsen G, Field DJ, Kurinczuk JJ, Wolke D, Alfirevic Z, et al. Effects of gestational age at birth on health outcomes at 3 and 5 years of age: population based cohort study. BMJ. 2012;344:e896.
19. Hennessy EM, Bracewell MA, Wood N, Wolke D, Costeloe K, Gibson A, et al. Respiratory health in pre-school and school age children following extremely preterm birth. Arch Dis Child. 2008;93(12):1037–43.
20. Fawke J, Lum S, Kirkby J, Hennessy E, Marlow N, Rowell V, et al. Lung function and respiratory symptoms at 11 years in children born extremely preterm: the EPICure study. Am J Respir Crit Care Med. 2010;182(2):237–45.
21. Miller JE, Hammond GC, Strunk T, Moore HC, Leonard H, Carter KW, et al. Association of gestational age and growth measures at birth with infection-related admissions to hospital throughout childhood: a population-based, data-linkage study from Western Australia. Lancet Infect Dis. 2016;16(8):952–61.
22. Townsi N, Laing IA, Hall GL, Simpson SJ. The impact of respiratory viruses on lung health after preterm birth. Eur Clin Respir J. 2018;5(1):1487214.

23. Narang I, Rosenthal M, Cremonesini D, Silverman M, Bush A. Longitudinal evaluation of airway function 21 years after preterm birth. Am J Respir Crit Care Med. 2008;178(1):74–80.

24. Filippone M, Bonetto G, Cherubin E, Carraro S, Baraldi E. Childhood course of lung function in survivors of bronchopulmonary dysplasia. JAMA. 2009;302(13):1418–20.

25. Simpson SJ, Turkovic L, Wilson AC, Verheggen M, Logie KM, Pillow JJ, et al. Lung function trajectories throughout childhood in survivors of very preterm birth: a longitudinal cohort study. Lancet Child Adolesc Health. 2018;2(5):350–9.

26. Been JV, Lugtenberg MJ, Smets E, van Schayck CP, Kramer BW, Mommers M, et al. Preterm birth and childhood wheezing disorders: a systematic review and meta-analysis. PLoS Med. 2014;11(1):e1001596.

27. Gough A, Linden M, Spence D, Patterson CC, Halliday HL, McGarvey LPA. Impaired lung function and health status in adult survivors of bronchopulmonary dysplasia. Eur Respir J. 2014;43(3):808.

28. Landry JS, Tremblay GM, Li PZ, Wong C, Benedetti A, Taivassalo T. Lung function and bronchial hyperresponsiveness in adults born prematurely. a cohort study. Ann Am Thorac Soc. 2016;13(1):17–24.

29. Gough A, Spence D, Linden M, Halliday HL, McGarvey LP. General and respiratory health outcomes in adult survivors of bronchopulmonary dysplasia: a systematic review. Chest. 2012;141(6):1554–67.

30. Jobe AJ. The new BPD: an arrest of lung development. Pediatr Res. 1999;46(6):641–3.

31. Friedrich L, Pitrez PM, Stein RT, Goldani M, Tepper R, Jones MH. Growth rate of lung function in healthy preterm infants. Am J Respir Crit Care Med. 2007;176(12):1269–73.

32. Fakhoury KF, Sellers C, Smith EO, Brian RJA, Fan LL. Serial measurements of lung function in a cohort of young children with bronchopulmonary dysplasia. Pediatrics. 2010;125(6):e1441.

33. Proietti E, Riedel T, Fuchs O, Pramana I, Singer F, Schmidt A, et al. Can infant lung function predict respiratory morbidity during the first year of life in preterm infants? Eur Respir J. 2014;43(6):1642–51.

34. Kotecha SJ, Edwards MO, Watkins WJ, Henderson AJ, Paranjothy S, Dunstan FD, et al. Effect of preterm birth on later FEV1: a systematic review and meta-analysis. Thorax. 2013;68(8):760–6.

35. Green M, Mead J, Turner JM. Variability of maximum expiratory flow-volume curves. J Appl Physiol. 1974;37(1):67–74.

36. Forno E, Weiner DJ, Mullen J, Sawicki G, Kurland G, Han YY, et al. Obesity and airway dysanapsis in children with and without asthma. Am J Respir Crit Care Med. 2017;195(3):314–23.

37. Lowe J, Kotecha SJ, Watkins WJ, Kotecha S. Effect of fetal and infant growth on respiratory symptoms in preterm-born children. Pediatr Pulmonol. 2018;53(2):189–96.

38. Udomittipong K, Sly PD, Patterson HJ, Gangell CL, Stick SM, Hall GL. Forced oscillations in the clinical setting in young children with neonatal lung disease. Eur Respir J. 2008;31(6):1292–9.

39. Vrijlandt EJLE, Boezen HM, Gerritsen J, Stremmelaar EF, Duiverman EJ. Respiratory health in prematurely born preschool children with and without bronchopulmonary dysplasia. J Pediatr. 2007;150(3):256–61.

40. Yammine S, Schmidt A, Sutter O, Fouzas S, Singer F, Frey U, et al. Functional evidence for continued alveolarisation in former preterms at school age. Eur Respir J. 2016;47(1):147–55.

41. Kotecha SJ, Watkins WJ, Paranjothy S, Dunstan FD, Henderson AJ, Kotecha S. Effect of late preterm birth on longitudinal lung spirometry in school age children and adolescents. Thorax. 2012;67(1):54–61.

42. Doyle LW, Adams AM, Robertson C, Ranganathan S, Davis NM, Lee KJ, et al. Increasing airway obstruction from 8 to 18 years in extremely preterm/low-birthweight survivors born in the surfactant era. Thorax. 2017;72(8):712–9.

43. Edwards MO, Kotecha SJ, Lowe J, Watkins WJ, Henderson AJ, Kotecha S. Effect of preterm birth on exercise capacity: a systematic review and meta-analysis. Pediatr Pulmonol. 2015;50(3):293–301.

44. Clemm HH, Vollsaeter M, Roksund OD, Eide GE, Markestad T, Halvorsen T. Exercise capacity after extremely preterm birth. Development from adolescence to adulthood. Ann Am Thorac Soc. 2014;11(4):537–45.
45. Lowe J, Watkins WJ, Kotecha SJ, Kotecha S. Physical activity and sedentary behavior in preterm-born 7-year old children. PLoS One. 2016;11(5):e0155229.
46. Kaseva N, Wehkalampi K, Strang-Karlsson S, Salonen M, Pesonen AK, Raikkonen K, et al. Lower conditioning leisure-time physical activity in young adults born preterm at very low birth weight. PLoS One. 2012;7(2):e32430.
47. Urs R, Kotecha S, Hall GL, Simpson SJ. Persistent and progressive long-term lung disease in survivors of preterm birth. Paediatr Respir Rev. 2018;28:87–94.
48. Stocks J, Sonnappa S. Early life influences on the development of chronic obstructive pulmonary disease. Ther Adv Respir Dis. 2013;7(3):161–73.
49. Quanjer PH, Stanojevic S, Cole TJ, Baur X, Hall GL, Culver BH, et al. Multi-ethnic reference values for spirometry for the 3-95-yr age range: the global lung function 2012 equations. Eur Respir J. 2012;40(6):1324–43.
50. Bush A. COPD: a pediatric disease. COPD. 2008;5:53–67.
51. Barker DJ, Osmond C, Forsen TJ, Thornburg KL, Kajantie E, Eriksson JG. Foetal and childhood growth and asthma in adult life. Acta Paediatr. 2013;102(7):732–8.
52. Narang I. Review series: What goes around, comes around: childhood influences on later lung health? Long-term follow-up of infants with lung disease of prematurity. Chron Respir Dis. 2010;7(4):259–69.
53. Stocks J, Hislop A, Sonnappa S. Early lung development: lifelong effect on respiratory health and disease. Lancet Respir Med. 2013;1(9):728–42.
54. Vollsaeter M, Skromme K, Satrell E, Clemm H, Roksund O, Oymar K, et al. Children born preterm at the turn of the millennium had better lung function than children born similarly preterm in the early 1990s. PLoS One. 2015;10(12):e0144243.
55. Bolton CE, Bush A, Hurst JR, Kotecha S, McGarvey L. Lung consequences in adults born prematurely. Thorax. 2015;70(6):574–80.
56. Henderson J, Granell R, Heron J, Sherriff A, Simpson A, Woodcock A, et al. Associations of wheezing phenotypes in the first 6 years of life with atopy, lung function and airway responsiveness in mid-childhood. Thorax. 2008;63(11):974–80.
57. Filippone M, Carraro S, Baraldi E. The term "asthma" should be avoided in describing the chronic pulmonary disease of prematurity. Eur Respir J. 2013;42(5):1430.
58. Teig N, Allali M, Rieger C, Hamelmann E. Inflammatory markers in induced sputum of school children born before 32 completed weeks of gestation. J Pediatr. 2012;161(6):1085–90.
59. Filippone M, Bonetto G, Corradi M, Frigo AC, Baraldi E. Evidence of unexpected oxidative stress in airways of adolescents born very pre-term. Eur Respir J. 2012;40(5):1253–9.
60. Halvorsen T, Skadberg BT, Eide GE, Roksund O, Aksnes L, Oymar K. Characteristics of asthma and airway hyper-responsiveness after premature birth. Pediatr Allergy Immunol. 2005;16(6):487–94.
61. Suursalmi P, Kopeli T, Korhonen P, Lehtimaki L, Nieminen R, Luukkaala T, et al. Very low birthweight bronchopulmonary dysplasia survivors show no substantial association between lung function and current inflammatory markers. Acta Paediatr. 2015;104(3):264–8.
62. Korhonen PH, Suursalmi PH, Kopeli T, Nieminen R, Lehtimaki L, Luukkaala T, et al. Inflammatory activity at school age in very low birth weight bronchopulmonary dysplasia survivors. Pediatr Pulmonol. 2015;50(7):683–90.
63. Bozzetto S, Pirillo P, Carraro S, Berardi M, Cesca L, Stocchero M, et al. Metabolomic profile of children with recurrent respiratory infections. Pharmacol Res. 2017;115:162–7.
64. Carraro S, Rezzi S, Reniero F, Heberger K, Giordano G, Zanconato S, et al. Metabolomics applied to exhaled breath condensate in childhood asthma. Am J Respir Crit Care Med. 2007;175(10):986–90.
65. Tenero L, Zaffanello M, Piazza M, Piacentini G. Measuring airway inflammation in asthmatic children. Front Pediatr. 2018;6:196.

66. Neerincx AH, Vijverberg SJH, Bos LDJ, Brinkman P, van der Schee MP, de Vries R, et al. Breathomics from exhaled volatile organic compounds in pediatric asthma. Pediatr Pulmonol. 2017;52(12):1616–27.
67. Smolinska A, Klaassen EMM, Dallinga JW, van de Kant KDG, Jobsis Q, Moonen EJC, et al. Profiling of volatile organic compounds in exhaled breath as a strategy to find early predictive signatures of asthma in children. PLoS One. 2014;9(4):e95668.
68. Robroeks CM, van Berkel JJ, Jobsis Q, van Schooten FJ, Dallinga JW, Wouters EF, et al. Exhaled volatile organic compounds predict exacerbations of childhood asthma in a 1-year prospective study. Eur Respir J. 2013;42(1):98–106.
69. Anderson GP. Endotyping asthma: new insights into key pathogenic mechanisms in a complex, heterogeneous disease. Lancet. 2008;372(9643):1107–19.
70. Greenough A, Alexander J, Burgess S, Bytham J, Chetcuti PAJ, Hagan J, et al. Health care utilisation of prematurely born, preschool children related to hospitalisation for RSV infection. Arch Dis Child. 2004;89(7):673–8.
71. Melville JM, Moss TJ. The immune consequences of preterm birth. Front Neurosci. 2013;7:79.
72. Roman M, Calhoun WJ, Hinton KL, Avendano LF, Simon V, Escobar AM, et al. Respiratory syncytial virus infection in infants is associated with predominant Th-2-like response. Am J Respir Crit Care Med. 1997;156(1):190–5.
73. Greenough A, Alexander J, Boit P, Boorman J, Burgess S, Burke A, et al. School age outcome of hospitalisation with respiratory syncytial virus infection of prematurely born infants. Thorax. 2009;64(6):490–5.
74. Régnier SA, Huels J. Association between respiratory syncytial virus hospitalizations in infants and respiratory sequelae: Systematic review and meta-analysis. Pediatr Infect Dis J. 2013;32(8):820–6.
75. The IMpact-RSV Study Group. Palivizumab, a humanized respiratory syncytial virus monoclonal antibody, reduces hospitalization from respiratory syncytial virus infection in high-risk infants. Pediatrics. 1998;102(3 Pt 1):531–7.
76. AAo P. Updated guidance for palivizumab prophylaxis among infants and young children at increased risk of hospitalization for respiratory syncytial virus infection. Pediatrics. 2014;134(2):e620.
77. Public Health England. Respiratory syncytial virus: the green book, Chapter 27a. 2015. https://www.gov.uk/government/publications/respiratory-syncytial-virus-the-green-book-chapter-27a. Accessed 30 Jun 2018.
78. Robbie GJ, Zhao L, Mondick J, Losonsky G, Roskos LK. Population pharmacokinetics of palivizumab, a humanized anti-respiratory syncytial virus monoclonal antibody, in adults and children. Antimicrob Agents Chemother. 2012;56(9):4927–36.
79. Blanken MO, Rovers MM, Molenaar JM, Winkler-Seinstra PL, Meijer A, Kimpen JLL, et al. Respiratory syncytial virus and recurrent wheeze in healthy preterm infants. N Engl J Med. 2013;368(19):1791–9.
80. Scheltema NM, Nibbelke EE, Pouw J, Blanken MO, Rovers MM, Naaktgeboren CA, et al. Respiratory syncytial virus prevention and asthma in healthy preterm infants: a randomised controlled trial. Lancet Respir Med. 2018;6(4):257–64.
81. Mochizuki H, Kusuda S, Okada K, Yoshihara S, Furuya H, Simões EAF, et al. Palivizumab prophylaxis in preterm infants and subsequent recurrent wheezing. Six-year follow-up study. Am J Respir Crit Care Med. 2017;196(1):29–38.
82. Fitzgerald DA. Preventing RSV bronchiolitis in vulnerable infants: the role of palivizumab. Paediatr Respir Rev. 2009;10(3):143–7.
83. Bolton CE, Bush A, Hurst JR, Kotecha S, McGarvey L, Stocks J, et al. Are early life factors considered when managing respiratory disease? A British Thoracic Society survey of current practice. Thorax. 2012;67(12):1110.
84. Kotecha SJ, Edwards MO, Watkins WJ, Lowe J, Henderson AJ, Kotecha S. Effect of bronchodilators on forced expiratory volume in 1 s in preterm-born participants aged 5 and over: a systematic review. Neonatology. 2015;107(3):231–40.

85. Pelkonen AS, Hakulinen AL, Turpeinen M. Bronchial lability and responsiveness in school children born very preterm. Am J Respir Crit Care Med. 1997;156(4 Pt 1):1178–84.

86. Pelkonen AS, Hakulinen AL, Hallman M, Turpeinen M. Effect of inhaled budesonide therapy on lung function in schoolchildren born preterm. Respir Med. 2001;95(7):565–70.

87. Joshi S, Powell T, Watkins WJ, Drayton M, Williams EM, Kotecha S. Exercise-induced bronchoconstriction in school-aged children who had chronic lung disease in infancy. J Pediatr. 2013;162(4):813–8.

88. Berry M, Morgan A, Shaw DE, Parker D, Green R, Brightling C, et al. Pathological features and inhaled corticosteroid response of eosinophilic and non-eosinophilic asthma. Thorax. 2007;62(12):1043–9.

89. Wenzel S, Schwartz L, Langmack E, Halliday J, Trudeau J, Gibbs R, et al. Evidence that severe asthma can be divided pathologically into two inflammatory subtypes with distinct physiologic and clinical characteristics. Am J Respir Crit Care Med. 1999;160(3):1001–8.

90. Haldar P, Pavord ID. Noneosinophilic asthma: a distinct clinical and pathologic phenotype. J Allergy Clin Immunol. 2007;119(5):1043–52.

Chapter 21
Behavioural and Educational Outcomes Following Extremely Preterm Birth: Current Controversies and Future Directions

Jayne Trickett, Samantha Johnson, and Dieter Wolke

Introduction

Extremely preterm (EP) births, before 28 weeks of gestation, continue to pose one of the greatest challenges to neonatal medicine, not just in terms of reducing mortality and short term morbidity, but in minimising the impact of immaturity at birth on lifelong health and development. Since the advent of contemporary neonatal care in the 1980s, and the continued improvement in survival rates, the long term consequences of EP birth have garnered increasing public, parent and professional concern. This has resulted in a growing body of research in which outcomes throughout childhood and adolescence have been well documented, particularly relating to the risk for neurodevelopmental impairments (see Chap. 20). As rates of severe sensory disabilities have fallen, and follow up has become increasingly interdisciplinary, greater attention has been paid to the impact of EP birth on behavioural and educational outcomes and quality of life. Here we present an overview of what is known about behavioural and educational outcomes following EP birth and outline current controversies in the field.

Where possible, we present data from EP birth cohort studies that have utilised gestational age defined inclusion criteria. However, given the continuity in outcomes across the full spectrum of preterm gestations, evidence from extremely low birthweight (ELBW; <1000 g) cohorts, very preterm/very low birthweight (VP/VLBW; <32 weeks of gestation/<1500 g) cohorts or whole population studies are included where these illustrate pertinent findings or where data from EP cohorts are lacking.

J. Trickett · S. Johnson (✉)
Department of Health Sciences, University of Leicester, George Davies Centre, Leicester, UK
e-mail: sjj19@le.ac.uk

D. Wolke
School of Psychology, University of Warwick, Coventry, UK

© Springer Nature Switzerland AG 2020
E. M. Boyle, J. Cusack (eds.), *Emerging Topics and Controversies in Neonatology*, https://doi.org/10.1007/978-3-030-28829-7_21

Attention, Social and Emotional Problems

Herein we adopt a broad definition of behavioural outcomes, encompassing research relating to behaviour, attention, social and emotional problems and mental disorders. The majority of extant data stem from VP/VLBW cohort studies, and from the use of parent, teacher or self completed rating scales given their utility on a large scale. The results of such studies are largely convergent, and have identified a greater risk for internalising than externalising problems among children born EP. For example, a recent meta-analysis of parent reported outcomes in EP/ELBW children compared with term born controls identified a moderate effect size for internalising problems (Standardised Mean Difference (SMD) 0.42; 95% CI 0.26, 0.58; 11 studies) and a small effect size for externalising problems (SMD 0.15; 95% CI 0.02, 0.28; 5 studies) (Fig. 21.1a) [1].

Results on such summary scales can mask differences in outcomes across functional domains. When the same authors analysed data for specific disorders, they found a large effect size for symptoms of combined Attention-Deficit/Hyperactivity Disorder (ADHD) and moderate effect sizes for inattention, hyperactivity, social problems and autism symptoms. In contrast, there was a small effect size for conduct problems and no significant difference in oppositional defiant disorder (ODD) problems between EP/ELBW children and controls (Fig. 21.1a) [1]. Although there are fewer studies in adolescence, their meta-analyses revealed similar findings. As shown in Fig. 21.1b, there were no significant differences between EP/ELBW adolescents and controls in parent reported externalising, conduct disorder or ODD problems; a small effect size for hyperactivity, but moderate effect sizes for social problems, combined ADHD symptoms, inattention and internalising problems (Fig. 21.1b) [1]. Indeed EP children identify poor peer relationships and mental wellbeing as salient characteristics [2].

These findings are reflective of the broader literature, including studies of VP/VLBW cohorts, which have led to the putative 'preterm behavioural phenotype'. This is a universal pattern of outcomes, characterised by an excess of problems and disorders associated with inattention, emotional symptoms, and social problems [3]; these are typically paralleled by a smaller or, in some cases, no increased risk for conduct disorder or ODD problems [3, 4]. This phenotype was evidenced in early reports by a strikingly similar pattern of outcomes in five European and North American EP/ELBW cohorts born in the 1970s–1990s [5, 6]. In each cohort, parents rated EP/ELBW children with a significant excess of attention, social and thought problems on the Child Behavior Checklist (CBCL) compared with term born controls; this was alongside no increased risk for aggressive or delinquent behaviour problems. These studies highlighted the cross-cultural and temporal consistency in outcomes despite improved neonatal care and the consequent increase in survival of EP babies over this period.

Whilst the majority of research has focused on middle childhood, problems are already evident in the early years [7–9]. Among children born at <29 weeks of gestation in the French EPIPAGE Study, 24% had clinically significant problems compared with 9% of full term controls at 3 years of age [10]. At 5 years of age,

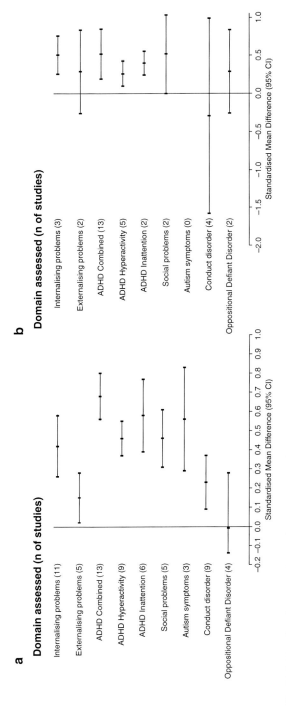

Fig. 21.1 Results of meta-analyses of parent reports of mental health outcomes for extremely low birth weight (<1000 g) survivors compared with term born (≥37 weeks' gestation) controls. Results are shown as standardised mean differences (SMD) and 95% Confidence Intervals (95% CI) for children aged 5 to 13 years (**a**) and adolescents aged 14 to 18 years (**b**). (Figures created using data published by Mathewson KJ, Chow CHT, Dobson KG, Pope EI, Schmidt LA, van Lieshout RJ. Mental health of extremely low birth weight survivors: a systematic review and meta-analysis. Psychol Bull. 2017;143(4):347–83)

38% of Norwegian children born <28 weeks of gestation had clinically significant problems compared with 11% of controls (OR 5.1; 95% CI 3.7, 7.1) [11]. An increased risk for regulatory problems, poor socio-emotional competence and withdrawn behaviour has also been observed in EP born infants [12–15] which has been associated with an increased risk for mental disorders later in life [16, 17].

A number of studies have also identified an increased risk of conduct problems among children born EP [8, 10, 11, 18], which may be inconsistent with the behavioural phenotype described above. However, externalising problems in early childhood may manifest as inattention, autistic traits or mental disorders later in life [16, 17]. In addition, the phenotype was observed from the co-occurrence of problems at a population level. Although there is greater comorbidity of psychological problems in EP children than controls [19], the extent to which ADHD, ASD and emotional disorders cluster within individuals is less well defined, particularly as many EP survivors will go on to have no long term morbidity. Using latent profile analysis, it was recently reported that 20% of EP survivors exhibit an outcome profile consistent with the preterm behavioural phenotype, with the remaining having only minimal difficulties (55%) or having elevated scores in multiple behavioural domains (25%) [20].

Mental Disorders

In a meta-analysis of five cohort studies of children born preterm (<37 weeks of gestation) or with low birthweight (LBW; <2500 g), prevalence estimates for mental disorders ranged from 21% to 28%, with a pooled Odds Ratio (OR) of 3.66 (95% CI 2.57, 5.21) relative to term born controls [21]. The authors also identified an increased risk for emotional disorders (anxiety or depression) in preterm/LBW survivors (OR 2.86; 95% CI 1.73, 4.73; 5 studies) [21]. Another recent meta-analysis reported a pooled OR of 4.05 (95% CI 2.38, 6.87; 4 studies) for ADHD in EP/ELBW children [22].

There is growing concern regarding the high risk for ASD in children born preterm, fuelled by reports that 13%–41% of EP children screen positive for autism in the first 2 years of life [23–26]. However, screening for ASD in EP populations is confounded by the high risk for other neurodevelopmental sequelae [25, 27]. Thus, the predictive validity of early screens is poor, with sensitivity and positive predictive values estimated to be 52% and 20%, respectively, for later ASD diagnoses [28]. A recent meta-analysis identified an ASD prevalence of 7% among children born VP [29], which is markedly increased relative to the prevalence of 62/10,000 reported in the general population [30].

Behavioural Outcomes: Current Controversies and Research Directions

One of the key current questions relates to the extent to which behavioural problems observed in childhood persist into adulthood; in particular, whether early sequelae represent a developmental delay, or whether EP birth limits developmental plasticity thus conferring deficits that persist across the lifespan. Data for EP adults remain sparse, but as the VP/VLBW/ELBW cohorts from the 1970s and 1980s transition to adulthood these questions are beginning to be answered.

In a recent narrative review of six studies, the authors reported that ELBW adults are at increased risk for internalising behaviours, anxiety problems, shyness, poor mental health and reduced social functioning. However, they found no excess of ADHD and externalising behaviour problems, and a decreased risk for substance use disorders [1]. This is similar to the results of a recent meta-analysis, which identified that VP/VLBW adults are more likely to have internalising problems and avoidant personality than term born adults, but are less likely to have externalising problems and anti-social behaviour [31]. These studies are also consistent with other reports in which VP/VLBW adults have been found to be more agreeable, socially withdrawn and introverted, and less likely to engage in substance use and risk taking behaviours [32, 33].

The most recent data available for EP survivors are from the UK and Irish EPICure Study in which trajectories of parent reported behaviour, attention, social and emotional problems have been explored (Fig. 21.2). Using the Strengths and Difficulties Questionnaire (SDQ) at 6, 11, 16 and 19 years of age, mean scores for ADHD and emotional problems were persistently higher in EP than term born individuals, but the risk for clinically significant problems declined from childhood to adulthood, with the group difference at 19 years no longer being significant. In contrast, the risk for clinically significant peer relationship problems was increased at all ages in EP survivors, peaking in adolescence. Notably, the risk for conduct problems was only increased at 6 years of age and progressively declined with age relative to controls [34].

However, these results were based on parent report. Most recently, the results of self-completed evaluations among this cohort at 19 years of age revealed higher scores for symptoms of anxiety, depression, withdrawn behaviour and avoidant personality. However, there was no increased risk for clinically significant problems in these areas, or for mood and anxiety disorders at 19 years of age [35], similar to reports of mood and anxiety disorders in VP/VLBW samples [36]. This is reassuring and suggests that, whilst sub-clinical problems may persist to adulthood, mental health outcomes for EP survivors may be better than once anticipated. The decreasing risk may be a result of reduced statistical power due to participant attrition, therefore these findings require confirmation in larger studies.

Another focus of current interest is the need to identify interventions to improve outcomes in this population, with a key question being whether these need to be population-specific, reflecting different mechanisms for psychiatric sequelae in preterm populations, or whether existing therapies are likely to be effective. Forging an understanding of the underlying risk pathways for mental health disorders is therefore a focus of current research, and is particularly evident in relation to ADHD.

In a recent meta-analysis of VP/VLBW cohort studies, the risk for symptoms of inattention (SMD 1.31; 95% CI 0.66, 1.96) was larger than for hyperactivity (SMD 0.74; 95% CI 0.35, 1.13), a finding that has been observed in other population based cohorts [37–40]. These findings are indicative of a different clinical presentation and, potentially, a different aetiology for ADHD in preterm born children. Recent

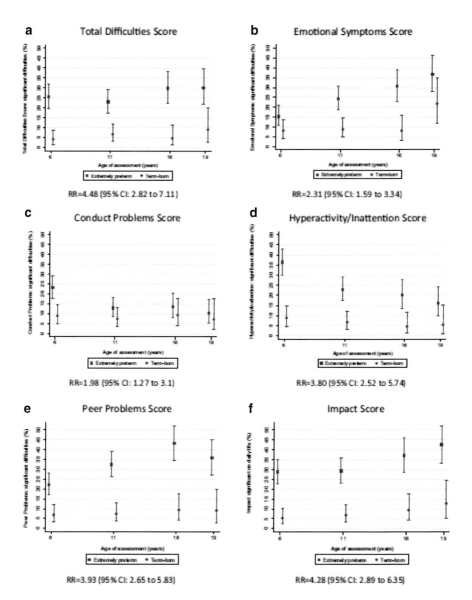

Fig. 21.2 Percentage in the abnormal range and 95% confidence intervals for Strengths and Difficulties Questionnaire (SDQ) Total difficulties and sub-scale scores in extremely preterm participants and term born controls at age 6, 11, 16 and 19 years. (Figure reprinted from Linsell L. Johnson S, Wolke D, Morris J, Kurinczuk J, Marlow N. Trajectories of behaviour, attention, social and emotional problems from childhood to early adulthood following extremely preterm birth: a prospective cohort study. Eur Child Adolesc Psychiatry. 2019;28(4):531–42)

studies have thus focused on elucidating the cognitive processes underlying ADHD in preterm populations and have suggested that, whilst some cognitive impairments are overlapping between VP children and term born children with ADHD, VP children show additional impairments reflecting more wide-ranging cognitive deficits [41–43]. Interruption to fetal brain development in the third trimester may result in trauma to the brain networks associated with ADHD [44], in addition to networks associated with other impairments, resulting not just in ADHD symptoms but in increased comorbidity in neurodevelopmental disorders observed in this population [41]. Similarly, there is growing evidence for an association between deficits in general cognitive functions, such as in executive function and/or working memory, and attention and social problems in children born preterm [45–49]. Improving these cognitive abilities may therefore be a potential target for intervention, the efficacy of which is discussed in the following sections.

Academic Attainment and Special Educational Needs

It is well documented that children born EP are at increased risk for intellectual impairments (see Chap. 20). Deficits in a range of general cognitive abilities are frequently reported, including poorer executive function, processing speed, working memory and visuospatial skills relative to term born controls [50–52]. It is therefore unsurprising that preterm birth has a marked impact on children's academic attainment and the need for special educational provision.

Deficits in the acquisition of early learning skills between EP children and their term born peers are already evident before the start of schooling. For example, significant deficits in school readiness have been observed in children born ELBW/VP [53–55], and these have been shown to predict later achievement in reading, spelling and mathematics [56]. Already at age five, VP children in the UK have poorer attainment at the end of the reception year, with 66% failing to have a good level of achievement compared with 51% of children born at term (RR 1.19; 95% CI 1.00, 1.42) [57]. By age seven, in the same cohort, 43% of VP children failed to have a good level of achievement in reading, writing and mathematics, compared with 18% of children born at full term (RR 1.78, 95% CI 1.24, 2.54) [58].

Outcomes for EP children are likely to be even poorer given the gestational age related gradient in outcomes. Indeed poorer mathematical and reading skills have been observed among EP/ELBW children compared with controls at age five in a representative sample of children in the US [59]. In middle childhood, by 8 years of age, EP/ELBW children continue to have significantly poorer attainment in reading, spelling and arithmetic compared to children born at term [60], and by 10–11 years of age, substantial deficits in mathematics and reading and poorer performance in national tests have been observed among EP/ELBW children [61, 62]. By the end of primary school, half of all EP children in the EPICure Study of births before 26 weeks of gestation had attainment below the national average compared with just 5% of their term born peers (OR 18.2, 95% CI 8.0, 41.4) [63].

Underachievement compared to term born peers continues to be evidenced at the end of formal schooling. At age 16, poorer scores on school leaving qualifications in mathematics, literacy and foreign language learning have been observed among adolescents born at <29 weeks of gestation, and poorer reading, spelling and mathematics skills have been reported at age 18 years in EP/ELBW young adults [64, 65]. Children born EP are also less likely to complete basic school than their term born peers, a risk that increases with decreasing gestational age at birth, particularly below 31 weeks of gestation [66].

Poor academic attainment has broader economic consequences, which are evidenced in the increased receipt of special educational needs (SEN) support among children born EP. School census data from Scotland show a clear gestational age related gradient in SEN, with the proportion of children requiring support increasing with decreasing gestational age at birth (Fig. 21.3). Among those born EP in this study, 29% had SEN compared with just 4% of children born at 40 weeks of gesta-

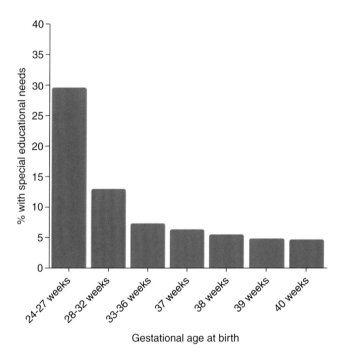

Gestational age at birth

Fig. 21.3 Prevalence of special educational needs in relation to gestational age at birth in a geographic population based cohort in Scotland. (Figure created using data published by Mackay D, Smith GCS, Dobbie R, Pell JP. Gestational age at delivery and special educational need: retrospective cohort study of 407,503 school children. PLoS Med. 2010;7(6):e10000289)

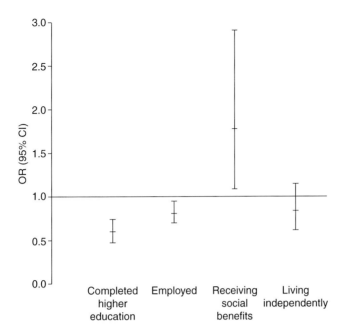

Fig. 21.4 Meta-analysis of 23 studies of the impact of very preterm birth/very low birthweight on educational, occupational and functional outcomes in adulthood. (Data shown are Odds Ratios with 95% Confidence Intervals. Figure created using data published by Bilgin A, Mendonca M, Wolke D. Preterm birth/low birth weight and markers reflective of wealth in adulthood: a meta-analysis. Pediatrics. 2018;142(1):e20173625)

tion (adjusted OR 6.92, 95% CI 5.58, 8.58) [67]. The proportion with SEN is even greater amongst the most immaturely born children, with 62% of children born below 26 weeks of gestation in the EPICure Study having SEN or attending special school compared with just 11% of term born controls (OR 13.1, 95% CI 7.4, 23.3) [62].

Ultimately, poorer educational outcomes result in poorer occupational status and wealth in adulthood [68]. A recent meta-analysis of 23 studies identified that VP/VLBW adults are less likely to complete education beyond high school and to be employed, and are more likely to be in receipt of benefits than adults born at term; however there was no significant difference in the proportion living independently (Fig. 21.4) [69].

Developmental Delay or Developmental Deficit?

Just as is the case for behavioural outcomes, a key controversy relates to whether poorer educational outcomes in childhood represent developmental deficits that persist across the lifespan, or whether, as EP children mature, they catch up with their peers. Similar to studies tracking IQ in EP/VP/VLBW cohorts [70, 71], recent longitudinal studies have failed to provide robust evidence of catch-up in academic outcomes. In a study of VP children and term born controls assessed through Grades 1–6 in the Netherlands, there was no significant difference in the trajectories of VP children and controls in either arithmetic, reading comprehension or spelling. This indicates that between-group differences remained stable over time and that VP children did not catch up with their peers by the end of primary education [72]. Most recently, an investigation of trajectories in results on national school attainment tests at ages 7, 11, 14 and 16 years in the UK found that children born preterm displayed some catch-up between 7 and 11 years, after which they had similar trajectories to their term born peers. As such, term born adolescents continued to outperform their preterm counterparts at the end of compulsory schooling [73]. It may be that EP birth places even greater limits on developmental plasticity and that trajectories may be more immutable in this population. To investigate this, the authors examined trajectories for those born VP and, whilst the overall trajectory was similar to the total preterm group, some of the catch-up observed between age 7 and 11 years was lost at secondary school [73]. The trajectory of attainment in EP children remains to be determined.

Current evidence is consistent with a developmental deficit rather than delay. However, the authors of the above studies argue that, despite the persistent deficits in academic attainment, the similarity in trajectories between preterm and term born children suggests that preterm children have intact learning abilities, thus affording opportunities for intervention [72, 73]. It is therefore important to elucidate the cognitive mechanisms underlying poor academic attainment in preterm populations in order to inform the development of intervention strategies, as discussed in the following sections.

Supporting the Learning of Children Born Preterm

Supporting the learning and academic attainment of EP children has never been more crucial since recent reports suggest that motor, cognitive and academic outcomes may be deteriorating despite ongoing advances in neonatal care [74–76]. Interest initially focused on preventive interventions delivered during the neonatal period or during the first few years of life. Whilst there was initial enthusiasm following reports that these might improve outcomes in the short term, meta-analyses have shown that the long term benefit of such programmes is limited; beneficial effects are rarely sustained beyond the period of intervention delivery and any impact on cognitive function is washed out by school age [77, 78]. Thus, if the aim is to improve academic outcomes, then intervention at school age may be most effective.

The aetiology of academic underachievement following EP birth is a focus of current research, especially in mathematics as EP children have greatest difficulties in this subject [62, 79, 80]. Such studies indicate that EP children's poor achievement in mathematics is not related to a specific deficit in numerical magnitude processing, but rather to deficits in general cognitive abilities such as working memory, executive function, visuospatial skills and processing speed [48, 52, 81–83]. Thus, converging evidence suggests that poor general cognitive abilities may underlie both behavioural and educational problems in EP children and that improving these may improve a range of outcomes. The notion that a single intervention may improve outcomes across multiple developmental domains is certainly enticing; however attempts so far have met with little success. For example, attention has focused on the use of computerised adaptive working memory training for improving cognitive and academic outcomes. Whilst some studies have reported short term positive effects in VP/VLBW samples, these have lacked an active control or have been underpowered [84, 85]. There remains no robust evidence of long term benefits of working memory training, particularly for enhancing academic attainment [86–88]. Given the evidence to date, it is perhaps time to focus efforts on identifying other strategies for improving outcomes in this population.

One approach gaining ground lies in improving educational support in the classroom. Knowledge and preparation about health conditions is crucial for the provision of appropriate educational management [89, 90], yet research has shown that teachers lack training about preterm birth and have poor knowledge of the impact it may have on children's learning [91]. As education professionals have a key role to play in supporting preterm children in the long term, this represents a significant public health concern. This was recognised in the recent European Standards of Care for Newborn Health in which it was recommended that education professionals receive training about preterm birth [92]. Improved communication of clinical research to teachers and better information sharing between healthcare and education services may serve to improve educational support for children born preterm. An evidence-based e-learning resource that has been shown to significantly improve teachers' knowledge of the consequences of preterm birth and their confidence in supporting children in the classroom [93] was released in 2019 (see: www.pretermbirth.info). The impact of this on improving educational support and learning outcomes for children born preterm remains to be seen.

Delayed School Entry

Perhaps one of the most controversial potential approaches to supporting the development of children born preterm is that of delayed school entry. The implicit underlying theoretical model for delayed school entry is that, given time, EP children will continue to develop and will reach the same level of cognitive and social maturity as term born children who enter compulsory education at the appropriate age. This is in stark contrast to the studies presented above, which consistently show that deficits in cognitive, attention and emotional function persist into adulthood [34, 70, 71].

The evidence for or against delayed school entry has been recently reviewed and existing studies are inconclusive [94, 95]. Using a natural experiment we recently investigated the effects of delayed versus age-appropriate school entry on children's academic attainment and attention using data from the Bavarian Longitudinal Study. The results indicated that delayed school entry had no beneficial effect on teacher ratings of academic performance at the end of the first year of schooling, but was associated with poorer performance in standardised tests of reading, writing, mathematics and attention at 8 years of age [95, 96]. Thus keeping children back for a whole year did not have a noticeable "maturation effect", but deprived these children from learning opportunities so that they did worse in achievement tests at the same age as those who had entered school at the compulsory entry age. Considering the adverse effects that low socio-economic status (SES) or poor parenting can have on the development of EP children, delaying school entry for EP infants from disadvantaged families may increase social disadvantage further.

Nonetheless, parents of preterm born children often believe that delayed school entry may be helpful. Indeed, preterm children should not be disadvantaged compared to term born children due to their preterm birth. For example, in the UK, children enter school in the September after their fourth birthday. However, EP born children who would have had their expected date of delivery in October may be born in July but are expected to enter school, considering post-conceptional age, younger than their term born peers. In these circumstances, delayed entry may be indicated to allow an EP child to enter school at the same time as children of the same post-conceptional age. However, delaying entry for all EP children due to the increased risk for developmental problems may not be beneficial according to the evidence to date.

To test whether delayed school entry may be a simple intervention that works, a randomised controlled trial is needed. Our recent feasibility study indicated that such a trial would not be feasible as parents expressed that the decision about whether or not to delay entry for their child was too important to be determined by randomisation [94]. Despite the controversial evidence, a report published in the UK in 2018 highlighted that the number of parents of summer born children that requested delayed entry doubled in 2016–2017 after legislation allowing this came into force [97]. The report also provided no evidence that delayed school entry improved children's scores in a phonics screening test in Year 1. Thus, evidence will have to rely on future observational studies tracking the impact of delayed school entry on academic achievement controlling carefully for social selection factors.

The Need for Theory Driven Research

Moving forwards, the elucidation of effective interventions requires a greater focus on theory driven research. Most EP cohort studies have used a simple main factor model investigating perinatal differences at birth, such as in gestational age or neonatal complications, and documenting whether these are associated with adverse developmental outcomes. This approach ignores that many other influences may operate between birth and outcomes in childhood and adulthood. One simple environmental factor to assess is the socioeconomic status (SES) of the family. For example, studies have shown that being born into a high versus low SES family has as much of an effect on long term outcomes as being born VP versus at term [98]. Similarly, having a mother whose highest educational attainment was at primary or secondary school compared to one who has received postgraduate education has the same adverse effect on the IQ of EP children as having suffered severe IVH or chronic lung disease [99]. It is thus no surprise that SES has been reported as one of the major influences on cognitive outcomes in VP children [100, 101]. It is, however, disconcerting that, by 2018, only 15 of 70 studies included in a meta-analysis of VP birth and IQ considered some marker of SES [102].

We recognise that measurement of SES is challenging since it can reflect a multitude of factors including social, family and parenting factors [103]. However, if we wish to unlock the black box of how these factors influence development, we need to measure them in as much detail as we have perinatal complications [103] which will require greater collaboration across disciplines in the design of follow-up studies. Let us consider two examples of such an approach. As described above, EP children are at higher risk for emotional problems in adolescence. Similarly, it is well documented that children who are exposed to trauma, such as being bullied by peers, are at higher risk of emotional problems [104, 105]. In a recent investigation, we noted that a major part of the effect of EP birth on emotional problems was explained by EP children being more than twice as likely to be bullied than their term born peers, which in turn explained the excess of emotional problems in adolescence. Thus bullying was a mediator of the effects of EP birth on emotional problems [106]. Furthermore, it has been shown that the academic achievement of healthy term born children is only minimally influenced by good or poor parenting. In contrast, VP children are strongly and adversely affected by low sensitive parenting while, on the other hand, very sensitive parenting has been found to lead to academic achievement on a par with children born at term [107].

These examples indicate that parenting and peer behaviour are important mediators or moderators of outcomes in the EP population. There is also increasing evidence that EP birth makes children more sensitive to adverse environmental risk factors [108]. This increased vulnerability leads to even worse outcomes if children are exposed to an average or poor environment, but EP survivors may attain outcomes similar to term born children when exposed to optimal environments. The effects are therefore best described using a diathesis-stress model [109]. Research that considers environmental influences from SES and parenting to peers and friendships and how these protect against, mediate or moderate the impact of EP birth on developmental outcomes is needed. Understanding such developmental mechanisms will be a major step change in current research as it may point to factors that are modifiable and thus are prime targets for intervention.

Summary

EP birth places infants at high risk for attention, social and emotional problems and disorders and for academic deficits later in life. Studies of VP/VLBW cohorts have shown that these deficits persist into adult life but a greater understanding of trajectories of educational and behavioural outcomes for EP survivors are needed. These will naturally ensue as the earliest EP cohorts born in the 1990s transition through adulthood. Attempts to improve long term outcomes for EP children have typically focused on the efficacy of early parenting interventions or on training children's cognitive abilities, but these have met with little success. Ongoing efforts to identify effective interventions to improve outcomes for EP children need to be intensified, for which a greater focus on theory driven research may hold the answer.

References

1. Mathewson KJ, Chow CH, Dobson KG, Pope EI, Schmidt LA, Van Lieshout RJ. Mental health of extremely low birth weight survivors: a systematic review and meta-analysis. Psychol Bull. 2017;143(4):347–83.
2. Gire C, Resseguier N, Brevaut-Malaty V, Marret S, Cambonie G, Souksi-Medioni I, et al. Quality of life of extremely preterm school-age children without major handicap: a cross-sectional observational study. Arch Dis Child. 2019;104(4):333–9.
3. Johnson S, Marlow N. Preterm birth and childhood psychiatric disorders. Pediatr Res. 2011;69(5):11r–8r.
4. Johnson S, Wolke D. Behavioural outcomes and psychopathology during adolescence. Early Hum Dev. 2013;89(4):199–207.
5. Hille ETM, den Ouden AL, Saigal S, Wolke D, Lambert M, Whitaker A, et al. Behavioural problems in children who weigh 1000g or less at birth in four countries. Lancet. 2001;357:1641–3.
6. Farooqi A, Hagglof B, Sedin G, Gothefors L, Serenius F. Mental health and social competencies of 10- to 12-year-old children born at 23 to 25 weeks of gestation in the 1990s: a Swedish national prospective follow-up study. Pediatrics. 2007;120(1):118–33.
7. Scott MN, Taylor HG, Fristad MA, Klein N, Espy KA, Minich N, et al. Behavior disorders in extremely preterm/extremely low birth weight children in kindergarten. J Dev Behav Pediatr. 2012;33(3):202–13.
8. Woodward LJ, Moor S, Hood KM, Champion PR, Foster-Cohen S, Inder TE, et al. Very preterm children show impairments across multiple neurodevelopmental domains by age 4 years. Arch Dis Child Fetal Neonatal Ed. 2009;94(5):F339–44.
9. Delobel-Ayoub M, Arnaud C, White-Koning M, Casper C, Pierrat V, Garel M, et al. Behavioral problems and cognitive performance at 5 years of age after very preterm birth: the EPIPAGE study. Pediatrics. 2009;123(6):1485–92.
10. Delobel-Ayoub M, Kaminski M, Marret S, Burguet A, Marchand L, N'Guyen S, et al. Behavioural outcome at 3 years of age in very preterm infants: the EPIPAGE study. Pediatrics. 2006;117(6):1996–2005.
11. Elgen SK, Leversen KT, Grundt JH, Hurum J, Sundby AB, Elgen IB, et al. Mental health at 5 years among children born extremely preterm: a national population-based study. Eur Child Adolesc Psychiatry. 2012;21(10):583–9.
12. Boyd LA, Msall ME, O'Shea TM, Allred EN, Hounshell G, Leviton A. Social-emotional delays at 2 years in extremely low gestational age survivors: correlates of impaired orientation/engagement and emotional regulation. Early Hum Dev. 2013;89(12):925–30.
13. Spittle AJ, Treyvaud K, Doyle LW, Roberts G, Lee KJ, Inder TE, et al. Early emergence of behavior and social-emotional problems in very preterm infants. J Am Acad Child Adolesc Psychiatry. 2009;48(9):909–18.
14. Ritchie K, Bora S, Woodward LJ. Social development of children born very preterm: a systematic review. Dev Med Child Neurol. 2015;57(10):899–918.

15. Clark CAC, Woodward LJ, Horwood LJ, Moor S. Development of emotional and behavioral regulation in children born extremely preterm and very preterm: biological and social influences. Child Dev. 2008;79(5):1444–62.
16. Treyvaud K, Ure A, Doyle LW, Lee KJ, Rogers CE, Kidokoro H, et al. Psychiatric outcomes at age seven for very preterm children: rates and predictors. J Child Psychol Psychiatry. 2013;54(7):772–9.
17. Johnson S, Hollis C, Kochhar P, Hennessy E, Wolke D, Marlow N. Psychiatric disorders in extremely preterm children: longitudinal finding at age 11 years in the EPICure study. J Am Acad Child Adolesc Psychiatry. 2010;49(5):453–63.e1.
18. Samara M, Marlow N, Wolke D, for the ESG. Pervasive behavior problems at 6 years of age in a total-population sample of children born at <=25 weeks of gestation. Pediatrics. 2008;122(3):562–73.
19. Johnson S, Marlow N. Growing up after extremely preterm birth: lifespan mental health outcomes. Semin Fetal Neonatal Med. 2014;19(2):97–104.
20. Burnett AC, Youssef G, Anderson PJ, Duff J, Doyle LW, Cheong JLY, et al. Exploring the "Preterm Behavioral Phenotype" in children born extremely preterm. J Dev Behav Pediatr. 2019;40(3):200–7.
21. Burnett AC, Anderson PJ, Cheong J, Doyle LW, Davey CG, Wood SJ. Prevalence of psychiatric diagnoses in preterm and full-term children, adolescents and young adults: a meta-analysis. Psychol Med. 2011;41(12):2463–74.
22. Franz AP, Bolat GU, Bolat H, Matijasevich A, Santos IS, Silveira RC, et al. Attention-deficit/hyperactivity disorder and very preterm/very low birth weight: a meta-analysis. Pediatrics. 2018;141(1):e20171645.
23. Limperopoulos C, Bassan H, Sullivan NR, Soul JS, Robertson RL, Moore M, et al. Positive screening for autism in ex-preterm infants: prevalence and risk factors. Pediatrics. 2008;121:758–65.
24. Kuban KCK, O'Shea TM, Allred EN, Tager-Flusberg H, Goldstein DJ, Leviton A. Positive screening on the modified checklist for autism in Toddlers (M-CHAT) in extremely low gestational age newborns. J Pediatr. 2009;154(4):535–40.
25. Moore T, Johnson S, Hennessy E, Marlow N. Screening for autism in extremely preterm infants: problems in interpretation. Dev Med Child Neurol. 2012;54(6):514–20.
26. Gray PH, Edwards DM, O'Callaghan MJ, Gibbons K. Screening for autism spectrum disorder in very preterm infants during early childhood. Early Hum Dev. 2015;91(4):271–6.
27. Luyster RJ, Kuban KCK, O'Shea TM, Paneth N, Allred EN, Leviton A, et al. The modified checklist for autism in Toddlers in extremely low gestational age newborns: individual items associated with motor, cognitive, vision and hearing limitations. Paediatr Perinat Epidemiol. 2011;25(4):366–76.
28. Kim SH, Joseph RM, Frazier JA, O'Shea TM, Chawarska K, Allred EN, et al. Predictive validity of the modified checklist for autism in Toddlers (M-CHAT) born very preterm. J Pediatr. 2016;178:101–7 e2.
29. Agrawal S, Rao SC, Bulsara MK, Patole SK. Prevalence of autism spectrum disorder in preterm infants: a meta-analysis. Pediatrics. 2018;142(3):e20180134.
30. Elsabbagh M, Divan G, Koh YJ, Kim YS, Kauchali S, Marcin C, et al. Global prevalence of autism and other pervasive developmental disorders. Autism Res. 2012;5(3):160–79.
31. Pyhala R, Wolford E, Kautiainen H, Andersson S, Bartmann P, Baumann N, et al. Self-reported mental health problems among adults born preterm: a meta-analysis. Pediatrics. 2017;139(4):e20162690.
32. Eryigit-Madzwamuse S, Strauss V, Baumann N, Bartmann P, Wolke D. Personality of adults who were born very preterm. Arch Dis Child Fetal Neonatal Ed. 2015;100(6):F524–9.
33. Hack M, Flannery D, Schluchter M, Cartar L, Borawski E, Klein N. Outcomes in young adulthood for very-low-birth-weight infants. N Engl J Med. 2002;346(3):149–57.
34. Linsell L, Johnson S, Wolke D, Morris J, Kurinczuk JJ, Marlow N. Trajectories of behavior, attention, social and emotional problems from childhood to early adulthood following extremely preterm birth: a prospective cohort study. Eur Child Adolesc Psychiatry. 2019;28(4):531–42.

35. Johnson S, O'Reilly H, Ni Y, Wolke D, Marlow N. Psychiatric symptoms and disorders in extremely preterm young adults at 19 years of age and longitudinal findings from middle childhood. J Am Acad Child Adolesc Psychiatry. 2019;S0890–8567(19):30260–6.

36. Jaekel J, Baumann N, Bartmann P, Wolke D. Mood and anxiety disorders in very pre-term/very low-birth weight individuals from 6 to 26 years. J Child Psychol Psychiatry. 2018;59(1):88–95.

37. Ask H, Gustavson K, Ystrom E, Havdahl KA, Tesli M, Askeland RB, et al. Association of gestational age at birth with symptoms of attention-deficit/hyperactivity disorder in children. JAMA Pediatr. 2018;172(8):749–56.

38. Johnson S, Kochhar P, Hennessy E, Marlow N, Wolke D, Hollis C. Antecedents of attention-deficit/hyperactivity disorder symptoms in children born extremely preterm. J Dev Behav Pediatr. 2016;37(4):285–97.

39. Jaekel J, Wolke D, Bartmann P. Poor attention rather than hyperactivity/impulsivity pre-dicts academic achievement in very preterm and full-term adolescents. Psychol Med. 2013;43(1):183–96.

40. Shum D, Neulinger K, O'Callaghan M, Mohay H. Attentional problems in children born with very preterm or with extremely low birth weight at 7–9 years. Arch Clin Neuropsychol. 2008;23:103–12.

41. Rommel AS, James SN, McLoughlin G, Brandeis D, Banaschewski T, Asherson P, et al. Association of preterm birth with attention-deficit/hyperactivity disorder-like and wider-ranging neurophysiological impairments of attention and inhibition. J Am Acad Child Adolesc Psychiatry. 2017;56(1):40–50.

42. James SN, Rommel AS, Cheung C, McLoughlin G, Brandeis D, Banaschewski T, et al. Association of preterm birth with ADHD-like cognitive impairments and additional subtle impairments in attention and arousal malleability. Psychol Med. 2018;48(9):1484–93.

43. Retzler J, Johnson S, Groom M, Hollis C, Budge H, Cragg L. Cognitive predictors of parent-rated inattention in very preterm children: the role of working memory and processing speed. Child Neuropsychol. 2019;25(5):617–35.

44. Finke K, Neitzel J, Bauml JG, Redel P, Muller HJ, Meng C, et al. Visual attention in preterm born adults: specifically impaired attentional sub-mechanisms that link with altered intrinsic brain networks in a compensation-like mode. Neuroimage. 2015;107:95–106.

45. Alduncin N, Huffman LC, Feldman HM, Loe IM. Executive function is associated with social competence in preschool-aged children born preterm or full term. Early Hum Dev. 2014;90(6):299–306.

46. Kroll J, Karolis V, Brittain PJ, Tseng CJ, Froudist-Walsh S, Murray RM, et al. Real-life impact of executive function impairments in adults who were born very preterm. J Int Neuropsychol Soc. 2017;23(5):381–9.

47. Mulder H, Pitchford NJ, Marlow N. Inattentive behaviour is associated with poor working memory and slow processing speed in very pre-term children in middle childhood. Br J Educ Psychol. 2011;81(Pt 1):147–60.

48. Aarnoudse-Moens CS, Weisglas-Kuperus N, Duivenvoorden HJ, van Goudoever JB, Oosterlaan J. Executive function and IQ predict mathematical and attention problems in very preterm children. PLoS One. 2013;8(2):e55994.

49. Loe IM, Feldman HM, Huffman LC. Executive function mediates effects of gestational age on functional outcomes and behavior in preschoolers. J Dev Behav Pediatr. 2014;35(5):323–33.

50. Brydges CR, Landes JK, Reid CL, Campbell C, French N, Anderson M. Cognitive outcomes in children and adolescents born very preterm: a meta-analysis. Dev Med Child Neurol. 2018;60(5):452–68.

51. Aarnoudse-Moens CS, Weisglas-Kuperus N, van Goudoever JB, Oosterlaan J. Meta-analysis of neurobehavioral outcomes in very preterm and/or very low birth weight children. Pediatrics. 2009;124(2):717–28.

52. Simms V, Gilmore C, Cragg L, Clayton S, Marlow N, Johnson S. Nature and origins of mathematics difficulties in very preterm children: a different etiology than developmental dyscalculia. Pediatr Res. 2015;77(2):389–95.

53. Reid LD, Strobino DM. A population-based study of school readiness determinants in a large urban public school district. Matern Child Health J. 2019;23(3):325–34.
54. Pritchard VE, Bora S, Austin NC, Levin KJ, Woodward LJ. Identifying very preterm children at educational risk using a school readiness framework. Pediatrics. 2014;134(3):e825–32.
55. Roberts G, Lim J, Doyle LW, Anderson PJ. High rates of school readiness difficulties at 5 years of age in very preterm infants compared with term controls. J Dev Behav Pediatr. 2011;32(2):117–24.
56. Taylor R, Pascoe L, Scratch S, Doyle LW, Anderson P, Roberts G. A simple screen performed at school entry can predict academic under-achievement at age seven in children born very preterm. J Paediatr Child Health. 2016;52(7):759–64.
57. Quigley MA, Poulsen G, Boyle E, Wolke D, Field D, Alfirevic Z, et al. Early term and late preterm birth are associated with poorer school performance at age 5 years: a cohort study. Arch Dis Child Fetal Neonatal Ed. 2012;97(3):F167–73.
58. Chan E, Quigley MA. School performance at age 7 years in late preterm and early term birth: a cohort study. Arch Dis Child Fetal Neonatal Ed. 2014;99(6):F451–7.
59. Lee M, Pascoe JM, McNicholas CI. Reading, mathematics and fine motor skills at 5 years of age in US children who were extremely premature at birth. Matern Child Health J. 2017;21(1):199–207.
60. Hutchinson EA, De Luca CR, Doyle LW, Roberts G, Anderson PJ, Group VICS. School-age outcomes of extremely preterm or extremely low birth weight children. Pediatrics. 2013;131(4):e1053–e61.
61. Joseph RM, O'Shea TM, Allred EN, Heeren T, Hirtz D, Jara H, et al. Neurocognitive and academic outcomes at age 10 years of extremely preterm newborns. Pediatrics. 2016;137(4):e20154343.
62. Johnson S, Hennessy E, Smith R, Trikic R, Wolke D, Marlow N. Academic attainment and special educational needs in extremely preterm children at 11 years. The EPICure Study. Arch Dis Child Fetal Neonatal Ed. 2009;94:F283–F9.
63. Johnson S, Wolke D, Hennessy E, Marlow N. Educational outcomes in extremely preterm children: neuropsychological correlates and predictors of attainment. Dev Neuropsychol. 2011;36(1):74–95.
64. Doyle LW, Cheong JL, Burnett A, Roberts G, Lee KJ, Anderson PJ. Biological and social influences on outcomes of extreme-preterm/low-birth weight adolescents. Pediatrics. 2015;136(6):e1513–20.
65. Hallin A-L, Hellström-Westas L, Stjernqvist K. Follow-up of adolescents born extremely preterm: cognitive function and health at 18 years of age. Acta Paediatr. 2010;99(9):1401–6.
66. Mathiasen R, Hansen BM, Andersen AM, Forman JL, Greisen G. Gestational age and basic school achievements: a national follow-up study in Denmark. Pediatrics. 2010;126(6):e1553–61.
67. MacKay DF, Smith GC, Dobbie R, Pell JP. Gestational age at delivery and special educational need: retrospective cohort study of 407,503 schoolchildren. PLoS Med. 2010;7(6):e1000289.
68. Basten M, Jaekel J, Johnson S, Gilmore C, Wolke D, et al. Psychol Sci. 2015;26(10):1608–19.
69. Bilgin A, Mendonca M, Wolke D. Preterm birth/low birth weight and markers reflective of wealth in adulthood: a meta-analysis. Pediatrics. 2018;142(1):e20173625.
70. Linsell L, Johnson S, Wolke D, O'Reilly H, Morris JK, Kurinczuk JJ, et al. Cognitive trajectories from infancy to early adulthood following birth before 26 weeks of gestation: a prospective, population-based cohort study. Arch Dis Child. 2018;103(4):363–70.
71. Breeman LD, Jaekel J, Baumann N, Bartmann P, Wolke D. Preterm cognitive function into adulthood. Pediatrics. 2015;136(3):415–23.
72. Twilhaar ES, de Kieviet JF, van Elburg RM, Oosterlaan J. Academic trajectories of very preterm born children at school age. Arch Dis Child Fetal Neonatal Ed. 2018;104(4):F419–23.
73. Odd D, Evans D, Emond AM. Prediction of school outcome after preterm birth: a cohort study. Arch Dis Child. 2019;104(4):348–53.

74. Spittle AJ, Cameron K, Doyle LW, Cheong JL, Victorian Infant Collaborative Study Group. Motor impairment trends in extremely preterm children: 1991–2005. Pediatrics. 2018;141(4):e20173410.
75. Cheong JLY, Anderson PJ, Burnett AC, Roberts G, Davis N, Hickey L, et al. Changing neurodevelopment at 8 years in children born extremely preterm since the 1990s. Pediatrics. 2017;139(6):e20164086.
76. Burnett AC, Anderson PJ, Lee KJ, Roberts G, Doyle LW, Cheong JLY, et al. Trends in executive functioning in extremely preterm children across 3 birth eras. Pediatrics. 2018;141(1):e20171958.
77. Spittle A, Orton J, Anderson PJ, Boyd R, Doyle LW. Early developmental intervention programmes provided post hospital discharge to prevent motor and cognitive impairment in preterm infants. Cochrane Database Syst Rev. 2015;11:CD005495.
78. Symington A, Pinelli J. Developmental care for promoting development and preventing morbidity in preterm infants. Cochrane Database Syst Rev. 2006;(2):CD001814.
79. Akshoomoff N, Joseph RM, Taylor HG, Allred EN, Heeren T, O'Shea TM, et al. Academic achievement deficits and their neuropsychological correlates in children born extremely preterm. J Dev Behav Pediatr. 2017;38(8):627–37.
80. Simms V, Cragg L, Gilmore C, Marlow N, Johnson S. Mathematics difficulties in children born very preterm: current research and future directions. Arch Dis Child Fetal Neonatal Ed. 2013;98(5):F457–63.
81. Jaekel J, Wolke D. Preterm birth and dyscalculia. J Pediatr. 2014;164(6):1327–32.
82. Tatsuoka C, McGowan B, Yamada T, Espy KA, Minich N, Taylor HG. Effects of extreme prematurity on numerical skills and executive function in kindergarten children: an application of partially ordered classification modeling. Learn Individ Differ. 2016;49:332–40.
83. Mulder H, Pitchford NJ, Marlow N. Processing speed and working memory underlie academic attainment in very preterm children. Arch Dis Child Fetal Neonatal Ed. 2010;95(4):F267–72.
84. Grunewaldt KH, Lohaugen GC, Austeng D, Brubakk AM, Skranes J. Working memory training improves cognitive function in VLBW preschoolers. Pediatrics. 2013;131(3):e747–54.
85. Aarnoudse-Moens CSH, Twilhaar ES, Oosterlaan J, van Veen HG, Prins PJM, van Kaam A, et al. Executive function computerized training in very preterm-born children: a pilot study. Games Health J. 2018;7(3):175–81.
86. Anderson PJ, Lee KJ, Roberts G, Spencer-Smith MM, Thompson DK, Seal ML, et al. Long-term academic functioning following cogmed working memory training for children born extremely preterm: a randomized controlled trial. J Pediatr. 2018;202:92–7 e4.
87. Roberts G, Quach J, Spencer-Smith M, Anderson PJ, Gathercole S, Gold L, et al. academic outcomes 2 years after working memory training for children with low working memory: a randomized clinical trial. JAMA Pediatr. 2016;170(5):e154568.
88. Melby-Lervag M, Hulme C. Is working memory training effective? A meta-analytic review. Dev Psychol. 2013;49(2):270–91.
89. Johnson MP, Lubker BB, Fowler MG. Teacher needs assessment for the educational management of children with chronic illnesses. J Sch Health. 1988;58(6):232–5.
90. Brook U, Galili A. Knowledge and attitudes of high school teachers towards pupils suffering from chronic diseases. Patient Educ Couns. 2001;43(1):37–42.
91. Johnson S, Gilmore C, Gallimore I, Jaekel J, Wolke D. The long-term consequences of preterm birth: what do teachers know? Dev Med Child Neurol. 2015;57(6):571–7.
92. Infants EFftCoN. European standards of care for newborn health. Munich, Germany; 2018.
93. Johnson S, Bamber D, Bountziouka V, Clayton S, Cragg L, Gilmore C, et al. Improving developmental and educational support for children born preterm: evaluation of an e-learning resource for education professionals. BMJ Open. 2019;9(6):e029720.
94. Wolke D, Dosanjh S, Johnson S, Jaekel J, Dantchev S. Delayed school entry for preterm children assessing the feasibility of a randomized controlled trial. 2018. https://www.nuffieldfoundation.org/sites/default/files/files/Wolke%2040442%20-%20Nuffield%20report_delayed%20school%20entry%20(Oct17).pdf. Accessed 20 Jun 2019.

95. Jaekel J, Strauss VY, Johnson S, Gilmore C, Wolke D. Delayed school entry and academic performance: a natural experiment. Dev Med Child Neurol. 2015;57:652–9.
96. Fastenau PS. Are the data on delayed school entry compelling enough to change policy ... or even pediatrician recommendations? Dev Med Child Neurol. 2015;57(7):596–7.
97. Cirin R, Lubwama J. Delayed School admissions for summer born pupils: Reserach report. Department of Education, her Majesty's Government; 2018.
98. Eryigit Madzwamuse S, Baumann N, Jaekel J, Bartmann P, Wolke D. Neuro-cognitive performance of very preterm or very low birth weight adults at 26 years. J Child Psychol Psychiatry. 2015;56(8):857–64.
99. Benavente-Fernandez I, Synnes A, Grunau RE, Chau V, Ramraj C, Galss T, et al. Association of socioeconomic status and brain injury with neurodevelopmental outcomes of very preterm children. JAMA Netw Open. 2019;2(5):e192914.
100. Linsell L, Malouf R, Morris J, Kurinczuk JJ, Marlow N. Prognostic factors for poor cognitive development in children born very preterm or with very low birth weight: a systematic review. JAMA Pediatr. 2015;169(12):1162–72.
101. Breeman LD, Jaekel J, Baumann N, Bartmann P, Wolke D. Neonatal predictors of cognitive ability in adults born very preterm: a prospective cohort study. Dev Med Child Neurol. 2017;59(5):477–83.
102. Twilhaar E, Wade RM, de Kieviet JF, van Goudoever JB, van Elburg RM, Oosterlaan J. Cognitive outcomes of children born extremely or very preterm since the 1990s and associated risk factors: a meta-analysis and meta-regression. JAMA Pediatr. 2018;172(4):361–7.
103. Editorial WD. Is social inequality in cognitive outcomes increased by preterm birth-related complications? JAMA Netw Open. 2019;2(5):e192902.
104. Zwierzynska K, Wolke D, Lereya TS. Peer victimization in childhood and internalizing problems in adolescence: a prospective longitudinal study. J Abnorm Child Psychol. 2013;41(2):309–23.
105. Wolke D, Lereya ST. Long-term effects of bullying. Arch Dis Child. 2015;100(9):879–85.
106. Wolke D, Baumann N, Strauss V, Johnson S, Marlow N. Bullying of preterm children and emotional problems at school age: cross-culturally invariant effects. J Pediatr. 2015;166(6):1417–22.
107. Wolke D, Jaekel J, Hall J, Baumann N. Effects of sensitive parenting on the academic resilience of very preterm and very low birth weight adolescents. J Adolesc Health. 2013;53(5):642–7.
108. Van Lieshout RJ, Boyle MH, Favotto L, Krzeczkowski JE, Savoy C, Saigal S, et al. Impact of extremely low-birth-weight status on risk and resilience for depression and anxiety in adulthood. Child Psychol Psychiatry. 2018;59(5):596–603.
109. Jaekel J, Pluess M, Belsky J, Wolke D. Effects of maternal sensitivity on low birth weight children's academic achievement: a test of differential susceptibility versus diathesis stress. Child Psychol Psychiatry. 2015;56(6):693–701.

Part V
The Infant Born Near Term

Chapter 22
Early Outcomes in Babies Born Close to Term

Elaine M. Boyle

Introduction

For the last few decades, neonatal research has focused on improving outcomes for babies born very preterm (28^{+0} to 31^{+6} weeks of gestation) [hereafter gestation will be expressed in complete weeks i.e.28–31 weeks and so on] or extremely preterm (23–27 weeks). The reasons for this are understandable, as these infants represent the smallest, sickest and most vulnerable group of all newborn babies [1]. Very preterm infants invariably need highly specialised care within a neonatal unit and are most likely to suffer adverse long term health problems because of their preterm birth [2, 3]. Advances in maternity care mean that many of these high risk babies are now being handed to neonatologists at birth in much better condition than previously. In turn, we, as neonatal intensive care practitioners, now have a myriad of different modalities of support at our disposal, and can offer more complex and superior care than previously. Neonatology has triumphed in the care of these tiny patients, and neonatal research has sought to build on this success further.

In contrast, babies born beyond 34 weeks of gestation have been considered mature, and therefore at low risk of complications. Many of these babies are cared for alongside their mothers in similar postnatal settings to those born at 37 or more weeks of gestation, though practice varies [4, 5]. For the most part, we do not expect them to darken the doors of the neonatal unit. Discharge from hospital often occurs within 48 h of birth, and only infrequently do we offer post-discharge follow-up. These babies have been "under the radar", and so it is, perhaps, no surprise that they have been described as the "forgotten" babies [6, 7].

Yet this has not always been so. In 1963, a sad, but important event occurred that was to spark a sharp increase in interest in neonatal intensive care. Patrick Bouvier Kennedy, the baby son of the President of the United States of America, John F

E. M. Boyle (✉)
Department of Health Sciences, University of Leicester, Leicester, UK
e-mail: eb124@leicester.ac.uk; eb124@le.ac.uk

© Springer Nature Switzerland AG 2020
E. M. Boyle, J. Cusack (eds.), *Emerging Topics and Controversies in Neonatology*, https://doi.org/10.1007/978-3-030-28829-7_22

Kennedy, was born just three weeks early, yet died at 39 h of age from surfactant deficient respiratory distress syndrome (RDS) [8]. Such a high profile neonatal death spurred on researchers to work to improve knowledge and management of respiratory disease in preterm infants. The babies whom we now view as "mature" and "straightforward" were indeed, the vulnerable infants of that period, with many succumbing to relatively minor complications of prematurity.

The last decade however, has seen renewed interest in more mature babies, not because of the severity of their illness in the neonatal period, but because new evidence has given us a better understanding of the difficulties experienced by these infants, and the potential effects of these problems. Around 35,000 babies are born at 34–36 weeks of gestation per year in England and Wales, and around 130,000 at 37–38 weeks of gestation [9]. Unlike the much smaller (approximately 2000 births per year), but extensively investigated extremely preterm group, these infants have been the subject of only limited research. Indeed, some have regarded the results of recent work in babies born at 34 or more weeks of gestation as a "wake-up call", highlighting the need to redress the balance [10].

Definitions

Definitions around gestational age at birth historically reflected a perceived dichotomy, with birth at 37 or more weeks of gestation classed as "term", and birth before 37 weeks as "preterm". North American data suggesting increased early mortality in babies born at 32–36 weeks of gestation [11] were some of the first to prompt researchers and clinicians to question the appropriateness of this. Terminology around gestational age was variable, confused, and definitions were lacking in consistency. Preterm infants born after 32 weeks of gestation have variously been referred to as "marginally preterm", "moderately preterm", "mildly preterm" and "minimally preterm", but perhaps the most commonly used expression was "near term". However, it was felt that this did not acknowledge the emerging knowledge about the effects of immaturity in this group. In order to reduce variability and better reflect the risks associated with birth at more mature preterm gestations, a new system of classification was proposed and births at 34–36 weeks of gestation were defined as "late preterm" [12, 13]. A little later, "moderately preterm" was coined to define birth at 32–33 week of gestation.

Further analysis of large population-based datasets has suggested that even within the "term" group, both neonatal problems and long term outcomes may differ [14–22]. This has led to the recognition of a gradient of risk associated with decreasing gestational age at birth that extends up to 39–41 weeks of gestation. In the light of this, those born at 37–38 weeks of gestation and those born at 39–41 weeks are now classified as "early term" and "full term" respectively. An increase in morbidity has long been recognised in infants born post term (after 42 weeks of gestation) when compared with those born at full term. Whilst the risk of severe disease for any individual late preterm or early term (LPET) infant is small when compared with extremely preterm counterparts, the effects of an increase in even minor morbidities in much larger numbers of these bigger, and more mature babies is significant at a population level, particularly if this risk persists across the whole lifespan (Fig. 22.1).

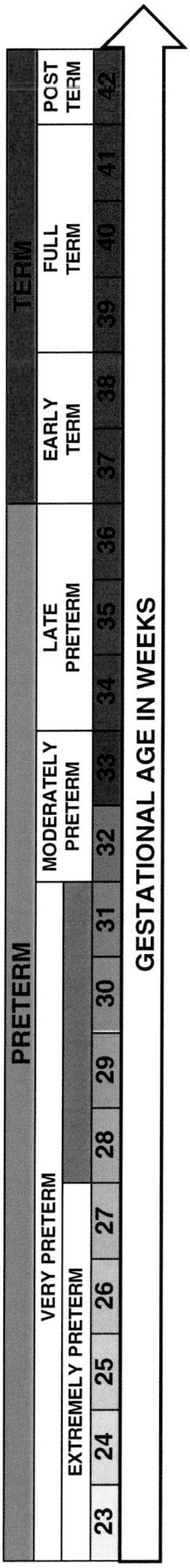

Fig. 22.1 The concept of gestational age as a continuum

Neonatal Morbidity

For the majority of LPET babies, neonatal care can be managed alongside their mother on a normal postnatal ward, but around 30–40% require admission to a neonatal unit [4]. In a small number of LPET babies, the need for continuing support can be clearly identified at the time of birth. For others, problems may take some time to develop or to be recognised, and in these cases, neonatal unit admission is delayed for up to several hours after birth [4]. The Late And Moderately preterm Birth Study (LAMBS), was a population-based study of birth at 32–36 weeks of gestation in the East Midlands region of the United Kingdom. It highlighted that, of all late preterm babies who were not admitted to a neonatal unit, more than 80% nevertheless required additional input from the specialist team for a variety of neonatal health problems related to their prematurity [4]. When such additional care is needed, it may be delivered in a number of different settings, including the postnatal ward, or dedicated transitional care area, and according to different models of care, depending on available facilities and staff. Skills of staff caring for these babies also vary. In the absence of evidence-based guidance, and with still limited awareness among clinicians about outcomes for these understudied babies, the approach to care may differ considerably between hospitals and even between clinicians in the same centre [4]. The effects of such variability in early care in LPET infants is unknown.

The commonest neonatal morbidities encountered by LPET neonates are hypoglycaemia, hypothermia and jaundice [23, 24]. These often occur together, and all are associated with immaturity of feeding and metabolic control [25]. Of these, arguably, hypoglycaemia is the most important, with potential long term adverse consequences. With respect to jaundice, kernicterus has been shown to be increased in late preterm babies managed as healthy full term infants, but the risk remains low [24].

Neonatal hypoglycaemia affects 5–15% of otherwise healthy term babies, but up to 50% of late preterm and 'at-risk' early term babies [4, 26–28]. Physiological immaturity is a risk factor for hypoglycaemia in late preterm babies [25]. Adaptation after birth is less good, the normal postnatal fall in blood glucose is greater, and compensatory mechanisms to protect the brain from effects of hypoglycaemia are not fully developed, increasing risk of adverse outcomes [23, 29]. Risk factors for hypoglycaemia in term infants include being small for gestational age, maternal diabetes and maternal beta blocker therapy [30]. Early term babies with these additional risk factors are especially vulnerable to adverse effects of hypoglycaemia. Symptoms of neonatal hypoglycaemia include irritability, jitteriness, increased heart and respiratory rates, poor feeding, change in consciousness, and seizures [29], but babies with very low blood glucose levels frequently appear asymptomatic, and hypoglycaemia may go undetected in 25% of at-risk babies [31, 32]. Early feeding, with breast feeding being the preferred method, reduces the risk of hypoglycaemia, yet feeding difficulties are common in these babies.

Recent UK guidance for the management of hypoglycaemia in babies born at or beyond 37 weeks of gestation recommends treatment for blood glucose levels of

2.0 mmol/L in asymptomatic babies [30]. The Children with Hypoglycemia and Their Later Development (CHYLD) study, of 528 babies above 35 weeks of gestation at risk of hypoglycaemia, found no association with adverse neurological outcomes at two year follow up [31]. However, in the same cohort at 4.5 years, an increased risk of poor executive and visual motor function was observed, not only in children exposed to severe or recurrent hypoglycaemia, but also in those where hypoglycaemia had not been detected by usual monitoring [33]. The threshold in this study, and all studies to date was 2.6 mmol/L. The threshold of 2.0 mmol/L for the treatment of hypoglycaemia in at-risk term babies is therefore untested. For late preterm babies, no UK recommendations currently exist for the prevention or management of hypoglycaemia. However, anecdotal reports suggest that the guidance intended for babies of more than 37 weeks of gestation has been adopted in some centres for less mature babies. Audit of this practice is needed to ensure that LPET infants with hypoglycaemia are managed safely.

Breast Feeding

Observational and qualitative data have highlighted low rates of successful breast feeding in LPET babies, compared with full term and even very preterm infants [34, 35]. The known benefits of breast feeding are well recognised; preterm and small for gestational age infants, with their increased vulnerability, likely stand to benefit particularly from receiving their mother's breast milk. LPET infants, by virtue of their larger size and perceived maturity, are often expected to behave like their more mature, full term counterparts and are managed in a similar way [36]. However, early breast feeding difficulties are much more common [35, 37]. They are more sleepy in the first few days of life and have relatively immature suck and swallow [38].

There is often a perception of inadequate breast milk supply among mothers, but also among clinical staff. This often results in medicalisation of their care to try to prevent or treat hypoglycaemia and other related morbidities [39]. The most common interventions are the introduction of infant formula or donated breast milk in some centres, nasogastric tube feeding and admission to a neonatal unit for intravenous fluids.

Feeding with infant formula is sometimes perceived as an effective way of hastening discharge from hospital. However, giving infant formula to LPET babies whose mothers plan to fully breast feed can adversely affect breast milk supply, undermine confidence, and decrease the likelihood of establishing successful long term breast feeding [40]. Of all mothers who initiate breast feeding, only 40–45% are exclusively breast feeding at discharge [4]. Reports suggest that 30–70% of term babies receive some formula during the hospital stay [40, 41]. Mothers whose babies receive infant formula in hospital are more likely to discontinue breast feeding than those who receive only mother's own breast milk[35].

Care on a neonatal unit is costly and necessitates separation of mother and baby, often for several days; this also interferes with mother-infant bonding and establishment of breast feeding [42]. Some mothers feel that they have failed their baby and many abandon their plans to breast feed [34, 40]. The psychological impact of challenges with feeding and the unanticipated separation of mother and baby is significant. Illness in the baby in the neonatal period, can make successful breast feeding even more challenging. These early problems, and increased risk of hospital readmission in the neonatal period [43, 44], together with evidence of poorer long term neurodevelopmental and health outcomes in these babies [4, 19, 20, 45–48], suggest that current management may be suboptimal.

Neonatal Respiratory Disease

Although RDS is most prominent in the most immature babies, it is also the most frequent respiratory diagnosis in LPET infants [49, 50], and a common reason for these babies to need admission to a neonatal unit [51–53]. Other respiratory conditions, often characterised by secondary inactivation of surfactant, such as respiratory infection, are also common in these babies [49, 54]. In contrast to the management of very preterm babies with significant RDS, who are routinely treated with exogenous surfactant [55], respiratory maturity is often assumed for LPET babies. It is expected that they will not need surfactant and not all babies with a diagnosis of RDS will receive this treatment [4]. In a proportion of these babies, respiratory distress worsens and non-invasive respiratory support or mechanical ventilation is required, with their associated potential complications. The upcoming SurfON (Surfactant Or Not) Trial, funded by the National Institute for Health Research, will randomise LPET babies with respiratory distress to receive early surfactant therapy or expectant management, and will examine the effects on length of hospital stay and severity of respiratory illness. Evidence is mounting for the persistence of respiratory morbidity into childhood, adolescence and adulthood in individuals born LPET [20, 56–60]. We do not know whether this ongoing respiratory deficit is due to immaturity *per se* or whether the presence of neonatal respiratory disease, and its management plays a part in long term adverse outcomes. Evidence considering whether exposure to neonatal intensive care, including mechanical ventilation, leads to poorer outcomes is sparse [61].

Obstetric Antecedents of Late Preterm and Early Term Birth

The only sure-fire way to avoid the effects of prematurity is to prevent preterm birth. Before information was available about outcomes of LPET birth, it was not uncommon, particularly in the US, for babies to be delivered because of maternal choice rather than for fetal or maternal morbidity. At this time, the preterm birth rate was increasing rapidly, fuelled mainly by these elective early births [62]. There have since been concerted efforts to reduce the number of LPET births that are not medically indicated. Guidance from the American College of Obstetricians and Gynecologists was produced and, in some states, there was withdrawal of funding for non-indicated births before 39 weeks of gestation [63]; these efforts have been largely successful, and the late preterm birth rate has plateaued in more recent years, indicating a better understanding of potential risks. However, obstetricians now have the unenviable task of balancing the uncertain risks of LPET birth with risks of stillbirth associated with continuing the pregnancy in the face of pregnancy-related problems. This is a challenging dilemma, and one which is difficult to study prospectively; given the choice between these two outcomes, it is probably reasonable to suppose that parents would wish to avoid the latter risk.

Two randomised controlled trials have looked at the management of preterm rupture of membranes at LPET gestation. The PPROM Expectant Management versus Induction of Labor (PPROMEXIL-2) trial compared induction of labour and a "watch and wait" approach in women with spontaneous rupture of membranes at 34–37 weeks of gestation. In this trial, pregnancy was prolonged by four days with expectant management, and the risk of neonatal infection was not increased [64]. The larger PPROMT (Immediate delivery compared with expectant management after preterm pre-labour rupture of the membranes close to term) trial randomised 1839 women to immediate delivery of expectant management, and also found no benefit with delivering immediately in spontaneous rupture of the membranes at 34–36 weeks of gestation [65]. Both recommend ongoing surveillance for development of overt signs of maternal sepsis that would necessitate delivery.

Intrauterine growth restriction (IUGR) is a common reason for LPET delivery, because of the association between IUGR and stillbirth. The optimal timing for delivery is, however, controversial and evidence is limited, resulting in variation in practice. The Disproportionate Intrauterine Growth Intervention Trial at Term (DIGITAT trial), an equivalence trial, showed that in women with suspected IUGR, outcomes following induction of expectant management did not differ in women delivered at 36 weeks gestation and beyond [66]. A recent large population-based observational study sought to compare outcomes in pregnancies affected by IUGR at 34–37 weeks of gestation [67]. Their analyses suggested that delivery at 37 weeks is advantageous in terms of reducing stillbirth, but this was a retrospective study, performed in a single centre and so results should be interpreted with some caution.

Antenatal Corticosteroids in Late Preterm and Early Term Labour

The use of antenatal steroids in threatened preterm labour from 24 to 33 + 6 weeks of gestation is common practice as it is known to accelerate lung development and reduce the risk of RDS in babies born preterm. Gyamfi-Bannerman et al. performed a large randomised controlled trial to study the use and potential benefits of antenatal corticosteroids before late preterm delivery and to evaluate neonatal respiratory outcomes [68]. They randomised women in late preterm labour to receive beta-methasone or placebo and measured the need for respiratory support in the babies at 72 h. Results showed that infants were less likely to need respiratory support, and that they were less likely to have severe respiratory morbidity. However, adverse long term effects of early postnatal corticosteroids have been observed in studies of extremely preterm infants [69], so some have urged caution in adopting this as routine treatment before long-term outcomes have been studied [70]. Also of note was the observation that babies whose mothers received betamethasone had a significantly higher incidence of hypoglycaemia [68] compared with those who did not, and this has been suggested as further reason to await follow-up [71]. Despite acknowledgement that more research is needed to confirm the safety of postnatal steroids in the late preterm population, the practice has been widely adopted [72].

The Impact of Late Preterm and Early Term Birth on Families

The impact on mothers and families of a baby's illness in the LPET population should not be underestimated. The need for specialised care for babies born extremely preterm is recognised and accepted by the public in general. Antenatal counselling by a senior clinician is usual for couples affected by threatened preterm labour or medically indicated delivery, and they are sensitively prepared for the events that will or might ensue, especially where delivery at the threshold of viability is anticipated. Most mothers delivering at 34–38 weeks of gestation, however, do not anticipate that their baby will have problems in the neonatal period. Indeed, the widely held perception of both the public and many clinicians about babies born "just a few weeks early", or "close to term" has been that they are not at increased risk. Prolonged neonatal hospitalisation of these more mature babies and unexpected separation of mothers and babies therefore causes significant psychological distress for families [73, 74].

Burden on Health Care Services

Large numbers of LPET babies contribute substantially to the workload of neonatal units and can generate high costs for the health care services. If the neonatal stay is significantly prolonged, this can lead to lack of availability of intensive care capacity for sicker or more preterm babies needing tertiary level care. In the United Kingdom, LPET births are spread across all levels of maternity units, including those with facilities for only low dependency neonatal care. Unlike an anticipated extremely preterm delivery, there is no mechanism to ensure delivery takes place in a centre offering neonatal intensive care. This is reasonable, as many LPET babies will need minimal, if any intervention; yet for an unexpectedly sick baby, postnatal transfer to a neonatal intensive care unit carries inherent risks of transport, disrupts the family unit and is costly. Health economic evaluations have highlighted high costs associated with LPET birth and perinatal care in comparison with costs of care for full term infants [75, 76].

Implications for Clinical Practice

In general, early morbidities in LPET infants are certainly fewer and milder than in babies born close to the limit of viability. Nevertheless, because of the very large numbers of babies affected by LPET birth, they represent a substantial burden of disease. In terms of disease severity, respiratory problems predominate in the newborn period, but other morbidities, often associated with poor establishment of feeding are common and are often the cause of post discharge hospital attendances [77–79]. In contrast to the number of studies performed in the extremely preterm population, there is a paucity of research in individuals born at LPET gestations, with a limited number of prospective studies and no focused randomised controlled trials. At present, it is not clear which antecedents are most important in terms of predicting adverse pregnancy, neonatal or long-term outcomes, although certain maternal morbidities, as well as socioeconomic factors may be important [80, 81]. Consequently, there is currently little to guide the clinicians in the management of women delivering at this gestation or their babies. The development of sound evidence based guidance will necessitate further research to identify groups at particular risk, and inform the development of targeted antenatal or postnatal interventions.

In the meantime, the optimisation of antenatal care and avoidance of unnecessary early birth should be of paramount importance. Effective communication between obstetric and neonatal teams should facilitate this. For babies unavoidably born at this gestation, early recognition and appropriate management of common neonatal problems is important, but undue over-medicalisation of care should be avoided. Breast feeding and early bonding are best supported when care for the baby is provided alongside the mother. Appropriate education of the mother and wider family will help in the establishment of feeding and healthy parent-infant interaction. Where severity of illness in either mother or baby means that they cannot be cared for in the same setting, it is important not to underestimate the adverse psychological effects mothers can experience when they are unexpectedly separated from their baby.

Some have called for routine neurodevelopmental follow-up in late preterm babies because of known long term adverse outcomes. Given the similar problems that are now being identified in the early term population, it might be expected that follow-up for this group might also be suggested before long. However, routine follow-up of such a large number of babies would not be feasible, in terms of costs and personnel, and nor would it be appropriate. While acknowledging the increased risk associated with LPET birth, we also know that this risk is not the same across the board. The majority of LPET babies will fall within normal parameters, do well over time, and go on to lead healthy and productive adult lives. The challenge lies in the prediction of those that will not.

Conclusions

We are on a steep learning curve with respect to the most appropriate management of LPET babies. We need now to turn our attention to what the data actually means. Should we be very anxious about outcomes for these babies? Has the initial surprise of seeing different outcomes by gestational age made us worry unnecessarily about small differences in babies and children that may not affect their future to a large extent? The answer is not yet known, but it is likely that both neonatal and ongoing management of this population can be more cost-effective, and may be improved such that greater numbers of children are likely to realise their full potential. The time is now right for long term follow-up studies, prospective studies and interventional trials of therapies in these understudied populations. Only when there is a much greater understanding of the influences at play in LP and ET birth will clinicians be able to direct care to those at greatest risk and to optimise ongoing health outcomes for this large and important population.

References

1. Costeloe KL, et al. Short term outcomes after extreme preterm birth in England: comparison of two birth cohorts in 1995 and 2006 (the EPICure studies). BMJ. 2012;345:e7976.
2. Vohr BR. Neurodevelopmental outcomes of extremely preterm infants. Clin Perinatol. 2014;41(1):241–55.
3. Wood NS, et al. Neurologic and developmental disability after extremely preterm birth. EPICure Study Group. N Engl J Med. 2000;343(6):378–84.
4. Boyle EM, et al. Neonatal outcomes and delivery of care for infants born late preterm or moderately preterm: a prospective population-based study. Arch Dis Child Fetal Neonatal Ed. 2015;100(6):F479–85.
5. Fleming PF, et al. A national survey of admission practices for late preterm infants in England. BMC Pediatr. 2014;14:150.
6. Demestre X. Late preterm, the forgotten infants: a personal perspective. Rev Chil Pediatr. 2017;88(3):315–7.
7. Paes B. Respiratory syncytial virus in otherwise healthy prematurely born infants: a forgotten majority. Am J Perinatol. 2018;35(6):541–4.
8. Patrick Bouvier Kennedy Biography. The Famous People. 2019. https://www.thefamouspeople.com/profiles/patrick-bouvier-kennedy-35151.php. Accessed 9 Jun 2019.
9. Office for National Statistics. Gestation specific infant mortality 2013. Office for National Statistics; 2015.
10. Escobar GJ, Clark RH, Greene JD. Short-term outcomes of infants born at 35 and 36 weeks gestation: we need to ask more questions. Semin Perinatol. 2006;30(1):28–33.
11. Kramer MS, et al. The contribution of mild and moderate preterm birth to infant mortality. Fetal and Infant Health Study Group of the Canadian Perinatal Surveillance System. JAMA. 2000;284(7):843–9.

12. Engle WA. A recommendation for the definition of "late preterm" (near-term) and the birth weight-gestational age classification system. Semin Perinatol. 2006;30(1):2–7.

13. Raju TN. The problem of late-preterm (near-term) births: a workshop summary. Pediatr Res. 2006;60(6):775–6.

14. Brown HK, et al. Neonatal morbidity associated with late preterm and early term birth: the roles of gestational age and biological determinants of preterm birth. Int J Epidemiol. 2014;43(3):802–14.

15. Chan E, Quigley MA. School performance at age 7 years in late preterm and early term birth: a cohort study. Arch Dis Child Fetal Neonatal Ed. 2014;99(6):F451–7.

16. Engle WA. Morbidity and mortality in late preterm and early term newborns: a continuum. Clin Perinatol. 2011;38(3):493–516.

17. Kajantie E, et al. Adult outcomes of being born late preterm or early term—what do we know? Semin Fetal Neonatal Med. 2019;24(1):66–83.

18. King JP, Gazmararian JA, Shapiro-Mendoza CK. Disparities in mortality rates among US infants born late preterm or early term, 2003-2005. Matern Child Health J. 2014;18(1):233–41.

19. Quigley MA, et al. Early term and late preterm birth are associated with poorer school performance at age 5 years: a cohort study. Arch Dis Child Fetal Neonatal Ed. 2012;97(3):F167–73.

20. Boyle EM, et al. Effects of gestational age at birth on health outcomes at 3 and 5 years of age: population based cohort study. BMJ. 2012;344:e896.

21. Crump C, et al. Gestational age at birth and mortality in young adulthood. JAMA. 2011;306(11):1233–40.

22. Crump C, et al. Early-term birth (37-38 weeks) and mortality in young adulthood. Epidemiology. 2013;24(2):270–6.

23. Laptook A, Jackson GL. Cold stress and hypoglycemia in the late preterm ("near-term") infant: impact on nursery of admission. Semin Perinatol. 2006;30(1):24–7.

24. Bhutani VK, Johnson L. Kernicterus in late preterm infants cared for as term healthy infants. Semin Perinatol. 2006;30(2):89–97.

25. Raju TN. Developmental physiology of late and moderate prematurity. Semin Fetal Neonatal Med. 2012;17(3):126–31.

26. Craighead DV, Elswick RK Jr. The influence of early-term birth on NICU admission, length of stay, and breastfeeding initiation and duration. J Obstet Gynecol Neonatal Nurs. 2014;43(4):409–21.

27. Harris DL, Weston PJ, Harding JE. Incidence of neonatal hypoglycemia in babies identified as at risk. J Pediatr. 2012;161(5):787–91.

28. Wang ML, et al. Clinical outcomes of near-term infants. Pediatrics. 2004;114(2):372–6.

29. Garg M, Devaskar SU. Glucose metabolism in the late preterm infant. Clin Perinatol. 2006;33(4):853–70; abstract ix-x.

30. BAPM. Identification and management of neonatal hypoglycaemia in the full term infant—a framework for practice. 2017.

31. McKinlay CJ, et al. Neonatal glycemia and neurodevelopmental outcomes at 2 years. N Engl J Med. 2015;373(16):1507–18.

32. Rozance PJ, Hay WW Jr. New approaches to management of neonatal hypoglycemia. Matern Health Neonatol Perinatal. 2016;2:3.

33. McKinlay CJD, et al. Association of neonatal glycemia with neurodevelopmental outcomes at 4.5 years. JAMA Pediatr. 2017;171(10):972–83.

34. Kair LR, et al. The experience of breastfeeding the late preterm infant: a qualitative study. Breastfeed Med. 2015;10(2):102–6.

35. Radtke JV. The paradox of breastfeeding-associated morbidity among late preterm infants. J Obstet Gynecol Neonatal Nurs. 2011;40(1):9–24.

36. Raju TN, et al. Optimizing care and outcome for late-preterm (near-term) infants: a summary of the workshop sponsored by the National Institute of Child Health and Human Development. Pediatrics. 2006;118(3):1207–14.

37. Goyal NK, Attanasio LB, Kozhimannil KB. Hospital care and early breastfeeding outcomes among late preterm, early-term, and term infants. Birth. 2014;41(4):330–8.

38. Adamkin DH. Feeding problems in the late preterm infant. Clin Perinatol. 2006;33(4):831–7; abstract ix.

39. Pierro J, et al. Factors associated with supplemental formula feeding of breastfeeding infants during postpartum hospital stay. Breastfeed Med. 2016;11:196–202.

40. Chantry CJ, et al. In-hospital formula use increases early breastfeeding cessation among first-time mothers intending to exclusively breastfeed. J Pediatr. 2014;164(6):1339–45 e5.

41. Boban M, Zakarija-Grkovic I. In-hospital formula supplementation of healthy newborns: practices, reasons, and their medical justification. Breastfeed Med. 2016;11:448–54.

42. Bystrova K, et al. Early contact versus separation: effects on mother-infant interaction one year later. Birth. 2009;36(2):97–109.

43. Jain S, Cheng J. Emergency department visits and rehospitalizations in late preterm infants. Clin Perinatol. 2006;33(4):935–45; abstract xi.

44. Oddie SJ, et al. Early discharge and readmission to hospital in the first month of life in the Northern Region of the UK during 1998: a case cohort study. Arch Dis Child. 2005;90(2):119–24.

45. Johnson S, et al. Neurodevelopmental outcomes following late and moderate prematurity: a population-based cohort study. Arch Dis Child Fetal Neonatal Ed. 2015;100(4):F301–8.

46. Kerstjens JM, et al. Neonatal morbidities and developmental delay in moderately preterm-born children. Pediatrics. 2012;130(2):e265–72.

47. Kerstjens JM, et al. Developmental delay in moderately preterm-born children at school entry. J Pediatr. 2011;159(1):92–8.

48. Talge NM, et al. Late-preterm birth and its association with cognitive and socioemotional outcomes at 6 years of age. Pediatrics. 2010;126(6):1124–31.

49. Consortium on Safe Labor. Respiratory morbidity in late preterm births. JAMA. 2010;304(4):419–25.

50. Mahoney AD, Jain L. Respiratory disorders in moderately preterm, late preterm, and early term infants. Clin Perinatol. 2013;40(4):665–78.

51. Natile M, et al. Short-term respiratory outcomes in late preterm infants. Ital J Pediatr. 2014;40:52.

52. Parikh LI, et al. Neonatal outcomes in early term birth. Am J Obstet Gynecol. 2014;211(3):265 e1–265 e11.

53. Robinson S, et al. Respiratory outcomes in late and moderately preterm infants: results from a population-based study. J Pediatr Neonatal Individ Med. 2015;4(2):19–20.

54. Deshpande S, et al. Surfactant therapy for early onset pneumonia in late preterm and term neonates needing mechanical ventilation. J Clin Diagn Res. 2017;11(8):SC09–12.

55. Suresh GK, Soll RF. Overview of surfactant replacement trials. J Perinatol. 2005;25(Suppl 2):S40–4.

56. Isayama T, et al. Health services use by late preterm and term infants from infancy to adulthood: a meta-analysis. Pediatrics. 2017;140(1):e20170266.

57. Kotecha SJ, Dunstan FD, Kotecha S. Long term respiratory outcomes of late preterm-born infants. Semin Fetal Neonatal Med. 2012;17(2):77–81.

58. Kotecha SJ, Gallacher DJ, Kotecha S. The respiratory consequences of early-term birth and delivery by caesarean sections. Paediatr Respir Rev. 2016;19:49–55.

59. Kotecha SJ, et al. Effect of early-term birth on respiratory symptoms and lung function in childhood and adolescence. Pediatr Pulmonol. 2016;51(11):1212–21.

60. Kotecha SJ, et al. Effect of late preterm birth on longitudinal lung spirometry in school age children and adolescents. Thorax. 2012;67(1):54–61.

61. McGowan JE, et al. Impact of neonatal intensive care on late preterm infants: developmental outcomes at 3 years. Pediatrics. 2012;130(5):e1105–12.

62. Engle WA, Kominiarek MA. Late preterm infants, early term infants, and timing of elective deliveries. Clin Perinatol. 2008;35(2):325–41, vi.

63. ACOG. ACOG committee opinion no. 561: nonmedically indicated early-term deliveries. Obstet Gynecol. 2013;121(4):911–5.

64. van der Ham DP, et al. Management of late-preterm premature rupture of membranes: the PPROMEXIL-2 trial. Am J Obstet Gynecol. 2012;207(4):276 e1–10.
65. Morris JM, et al. Immediate delivery compared with expectant management after preterm prelabour rupture of the membranes close to term (PPROMT trial): a randomised controlled trial. Lancet. 2016;387(10017):444–52.
66. Boers KE, et al. Induction versus expectant monitoring for intrauterine growth restriction at term: randomised equivalence trial (DIGITAT). BMJ. 2010;341:c7087.
67. Rabinovich A, et al. Late preterm and early term: when to induce a growth restricted fetus? A population-based study. J Matern Fetal Neonatal Med. 2018;31(7):926–32.
68. Gyamfi-Bannerman C, et al. Antenatal betamethasone for women at risk for late preterm delivery. N Engl J Med. 2016;374:1311–20.
69. Doyle LW, et al. Early (< 8 days) systemic postnatal corticosteroids for prevention of bronchopulmonary dysplasia in preterm infants. Cochrane Database Syst Rev. 2017;10:CD001146.
70. Kamath-Rayne BD, et al. Antenatal corticosteroids beyond 34 weeks gestation: what do we do now? Am J Obstet Gynecol. 2016;215(4):423–30.
71. Crowther CA, Harding JE. Antenatal glucocorticoids for late preterm birth? N Engl J Med. 2016;374(14):1376–7.
72. Battarbee AN, et al. Practice variation in antenatal steroid administration for anticipated late preterm birth: a physician survey. Am J Perinatol. 2019;36(2):200–4.
73. Rogers CE, Lenze SN, Luby JL. Late preterm birth, maternal depression, and risk of preschool psychiatric disorders. J Am Acad Child Adolesc Psychiatry. 2013;52(3):309–18.
74. Tully KP, et al. The relationship between infant feeding outcomes and maternal emotional well-being among mothers of late preterm and term infants: a secondary, exploratory analysis. Adv Neonatal Care. 2017;17(1):65–75.
75. Khan KA, et al. Economic costs associated with moderate and late preterm birth: a prospective population-based study. BJOG. 2015;122(11):1495–505.
76. Petrou S. Health economic aspects of late preterm and early term birth. Semin Fetal Neonatal Med. 2019;24(1):18–26.
77. Iacobelli S, et al. Gestational age and 1-year hospital admission or mortality: a nation-wide population-based study. BMC Pediatr. 2017;17(1):28.
78. Kuzniewicz MW, et al. Hospital readmissions and emergency department visits in moderate preterm, late preterm, and early term infants. Clin Perinatol. 2013;40(4):753–75.
79. Paranjothy S, et al. Gestational age, birth weight, and risk of respiratory hospital admission in childhood. Pediatrics. 2013;132(6):e1562–9.
80. Potijk MR, et al. Behavioural and emotional problems in moderately preterm children with low socioeconomic status: a population-based study. Eur Child Adolesc Psychiatry. 2015;24(7):787–95.
81. Potijk MR, et al. Developmental delay in moderately preterm-born children with low socioeconomic status: risks multiply. J Pediatr. 2013;163(5):1289–95.

Chapter 23
Long Term Outcomes in Moderate and Late Preterm Infants

Jeanie L. Y. Cheong and Lex W. Doyle

Introduction

Moderate and late preterm (MLP) births are increasing worldwide and comprise the largest proportion of all preterm births. In England and Wales, 6.5% of all births in 2016 were MLP (between 32 + 0–36 + 6 weeks of gestation), comprising over 80% of all preterm births [1]. In Australia, the rates of MLP births have risen from to 5.5% in 1994 [2] to 7.0% of all livebirths in 2015 [3]. In the USA, the overall rise in the rates of preterm birth (from 9.57% in 2014 to 9.85% in 2016) has mostly been attributed to a rise in late preterm (LP, 34 + 0–36 + 6 weeks of gestation) births, from 6.87% to 7.09% over the same period [4]. As they comprise a large group, any morbidity experienced by children born MLP has the potential to have a significant ongoing burden on health and educational resources.

Although previously thought to have similar health and developmental outcomes to children born at term, the last decade has seen increasing evidence that MLP birth is associated with increased health and neurodevelopmental morbidity, from the in-hospital period up to childhood and older, compared with birth at term.

J. L. Y. Cheong (✉)
Neonatal Services, Royal Women's Hospital, Melbourne, VIC, Australia

Department of Obstetrics and Gynaecology, University of Melbourne, Melbourne, VIC, Australia

Clinical Sciences, Murdoch Children's Research Institute, Melbourne, VIC, Australia
e-mail: jeanie.Cheong@thewomens.org.au

L. W. Doyle
Neonatal Services, Royal Women's Hospital, Melbourne, VIC, Australia

Department of Obstetrics and Gynaecology, University of Melbourne, Melbourne, VIC, Australia

Clinical Sciences, Murdoch Children's Research Institute, Melbourne, VIC, Australia

Department of Paediatrics, University of Melbourne, Melbourne, VIC, Australia

© Springer Nature Switzerland AG 2020
E. M. Boyle, J. Cusack (eds.), *Emerging Topics and Controversies in Neonatology*, https://doi.org/10.1007/978-3-030-28829-7_23

403

This review will focus on outcomes beyond the neonatal period, and on the domains of neurodevelopment, respiratory and functional outcomes where most data on long term outcomes have been reported. We have reviewed studies that include either MLP or LP births.

Neurodevelopment

Infancy

There is now robust evidence from several large studies that children born MLP are more likely to have developmental delay at 18–24 months compared with children born at term (Table 23.1). Most of the delay has been reported in the cognitive

Table 23.1 Developmental outcomes (up to 3 years of age) contrasted between moderate or late preterm children and term controls

Study	Participants	Age of assessment	Assessment tools	Outcomes in moderate and late preterm children compared with term
Romeo et al. [8]	33–36 weeks of gestation (n = 61), term infants (n = 60)	12 and 18 months corrected age	Bayley-2	MDI lower if uncorrected age used. No differences when comparing corrected ages
Woythaler et al. [6]	34–37 weeks ofgestation (n = 1200), term infants (n = 6300)	24 months (uncorrected age)	BSF-R	Higher odds of mental developmental delay (OR 1.52; 95% CI 1.26, 1.82), and physical developmental delay (OR 1.56; 95% CI 1.30, 1.89)
Voight et al. [7]	32–36 weeks ofgestation (n = 88), term controls (n = 86)	24 months corrected age	Bayley-2	Lower MDI: mean (SD) of 100.59 (11.30) vs 106.25 (8.94)
Johnson et al. [9]	32–36 weeks of gestation (n = 638), term controls (n = 765)	24 months corrected age	Questionnaire for neurosensory impairment, PARCA-R	Higher risk of neurosensory impairment 1.6% vs 0.3% (RR 4.89; 95% CI 1.07, 22.2), and cognitive impairment: 6.3% vs 2.4% (RR 2.09; 95% CI 1.19, 3.64)
Cheong et al. [5]	32–36 weeks of gestation (n = 198), term controls (n = 193)	24 months corrected age	Bayley-3	Higher odds of cognitive delay (aOR 1.8; 95% CI 1.1, 3.0), language delay (aOR 3.1; 95% CI 1.8, 5.2), motor delay (aOR 2.4; 95% CI 1.3, 4.5), problems with social-emotional competence (aOR 3.9; 95% CI 1.4, 10.9)

Bayley-2 Bayley Scales of Infant Development II, *BSF-R* Bayley Scales of Infant Development Short Form: Research Edition, *Bayley-3* Bayley Scales of Infant Development III, *MDI* Mental Developmental Index, *PARCA-R* Parent Report of Children's Abilities-Revised, *OR* odds ratio, *aOR* adjusted odds ratio, *RR* relative risk, *CI* confidence interval, *SD* standard deviation domain [5–9]; however, there are also reports of language and motor delay [5, 6] in MLP children compared with their term-born counterparts. More recently, two studies have reported delayed social competence in MLP children compared with term children at 2 years' corrected age [5, 10]. Johnson et al. [10] reported an adjusted relative risk (95% confidence interval (CI)) of 1.28 (1.03–1.58) for delayed social competence in a geographic population of MLP 2-year-olds (corrected) born in the UK compared with term-born children.

Cheong et al. [5], in a cohort study from a high-risk maternity hospital that contained a neonatal intensive care unit, also reported rates of delayed social competence in 13% (23/176) of children born MLP compared with only 3% (5/150) in controls born at term (adjusted odds ratio = 3.9; 95% CI 1.4, 10.9). Delayed social-emotional competence is associated with later psychiatric disorders in children born very preterm (less than 32 weeks of gestation) [11, 12]. Therefore, it is vital to follow up MLP cohorts into later childhood to determine the long term importance of delayed social competence in MLP children.

Pre-school and School Age

Cognitive Functioning and School Performance

At preschool age, a higher rate of poorer school readiness (adjusted odds ratio (aOR) 1.52; 95% CI 1.06, 2.18) was identified in LP children compared with term children in the Early Childhood Longitudinal Study, Birth Cohort at kindergarten age (around 65 months) [13]. In that study, school readiness was assessed using a composite measure derived from a battery of tests that assessed reading, mathematics, and expressive language.

A recent systematic review and meta-analysis summarised the long term cognitive and school outcomes following LP birth [14]. LP children had a 38% increased risk of lower general cognitive ability, defined as performing −1 standard deviation (SD) lower, relative to the test mean, compared with term children [14]. Although the two studies reporting outcomes in adolescence did not find differences between LP and term groups [15, 16], studies in adulthood identified differences in general cognitive ability in the order of −0.05 SD lower in men born LP compared with those born at term [17, 18]. General school performance at early school age in the UK Millennium cohort was poorer in MLP children compared with term children at age 5 years compared with full term children [19]. Note that this age was comparable to that of the Early Childhood Longitudinal Study, Birth Cohort in the USA, although the children in the latter cohort were still in preschool due to the different ages of school commencement between the countries.

The reports from individual categories of academic functioning, however, are less conclusive. Several studies have reported poorer language and mathematics achievement at school age [19, 20]. One study that assessed performance at intervals during primary school reported poorer reading and mathematics skills that persisted up to the fifth grade [21]. It will be interesting to see if the gap in academic achievement changes with age between MLP and term-born children.

In keeping with the concerns about poorer academic functioning in MLP children, there are several reports of higher rates of special educational needs and school retention in children born MLP compared with children born at term. The risk of attending special education was up to threefold higher in children born MLP compared with children born at term, and grade repetition was up to twofold higher in the 5–10 year age group [20–24].

Behaviour and Psychiatric Outcomes

Higher rates of emotional problems have been reported in MLP children from as early as age 3 years. A report from the Norwegian Mother and Child Cohort study of births from 1999 to 2008 assessed emotional and behavioural problems in LP children compared with term-born controls at 36 months [25]. They reported increased odds of emotional (aOR 1.26; 95% CI 1.04, 1.52) but not behavioural problems in the LP group compared with controls. Interestingly, the sex stratified analysis showed increased odds in girls only, but not in boys. In contrast, a Dutch study of MLP children at 4 years identified both internalising (emotional) and externalising (behavioural) problems in the MLP children compared with controls [26]. The difference in conclusions about externalising problems between the studies may have been partly explained by the inclusion of moderately preterm children in the latter study, which may reflect a group at higher risk of behavioural problems. Another study reported increased behavioural problems in LP infants who were admitted to a neonatal intensive care unit compared with those who were not, suggesting that "medical sickness" in the neonatal period conferred a higher risk for later behavioural problems [27].

Both emotional and behavioural problems have been identified at higher rates in MLP children at older ages compared with term controls. Talge et al. [28] found higher rates of teacher-reported behavioural problems, most likely involving the internalising and attention domains, in children born MLP compared with controls, but no effect of sex or social class. Higher rates of attention and hyperactivity problems at school age and into adolescence have also been reported in several other studies [24, 29, 30]. However, some studies were not able to demonstrate a difference in rates of attention deficit hyperactivity disorder between children born LP and children born at term [31].

Adulthood

The few studies of outcomes into adulthood suggest that LP birth is associated with increased neurocognitive and psychiatric problems. The Helsinki Birth Cohort study of adults born in the 1930s–1940s described lifelong disadvantages in neurocognitive performance and socio-economic attainment [32, 33]. In a study of Norwegian male army conscripts born between 1967–1979, 19% (2084/10836) of those born at 34–36 weeks of gestation had low IQ scores compared with 16% (34,382/209191) of those born at 39–41 weeks of gestation (aOR 1.14; 95% CI 1.08, 1/20) [17]. However, data from a Finnish cohort born in 1985–1986 suggests that LP birth is not associated with increased neurocognitive deficits in early adulthood, and the risk is only present for LP adults who were also growth restricted at birth [34]. Increased psychiatric morbidity in adulthood has been reported in some studies [35], but not others [36].

Respiratory Outcomes

Vulnerability of the MLP Lung

MLP infants are born in the third trimester of pregnancy, a period where lung maturation is at its greatest [37]. This is a period of transition between the saccular and alveolar periods of lung development, characterised by a rapid increase in lung volumes and surface area [37]. An interruption of this process by MLP birth may affect optimal alveolar development. There are additional challenges following MLP birth that may also add to lung vulnerability. In the *ex utero* environment, the lungs of MLP newborns are exposed to higher oxygen concentrations than they would have been *in utero* [38]. In addition, delayed lung fluid clearance [39], *in utero* growth restriction (a common risk factor for MLP birth) [40], *ex utero* suboptimal weight growth [41], and immature humoral immunity [42] are all potential contributory factors to the increased respiratory morbidities described in MLP children [43].

Infancy and Childhood Outcomes

Respiratory morbidity in infancy and early childhood is well described in MLP children. Hospitalisations with respiratory syncytial virus (RSV) are increased in MLP children. A recent systematic review reported an incidence of RSV hospitalisations up to 2 years of age ranged from 3.2% to 6.6% in those who did not receive RSV passive immunoglobulin prophylaxis [44]. However, it would be uncommon for MLP newborns to receive RSV prophylaxis. Another study of children under the age of 3 years enrolled in the Tennessee Medicaid program over a 4-year period reported higher rates of RSV admissions to hospital in infants born between 33 and 36 completed weeks (57 per 1000 child-years of RSV season), compared with 30 per 1000 in term infants [45]. The rates in the MLP children were approaching those of more immature preterm infants born at less than 33 weeks of gestation (66–70 per 1000) [45].

Preterm birth is associated with an increased risk of asthma and wheezing in childhood, and this includes those born MLP. A large meta-analysis of 147,000 European children from 31 cohorts reported that children born before 40 weeks of gestation had an increased risk of pre-school wheezing until four years of age and of school-age asthma at 5–10 years [41]. Although the risk was highest in children born at less than 28 weeks of gestation, those born in the MLP period were still at increased risk (mean odds ratios of up to 2.0) compared with term-born children [41]. Results from the regional Dutch Longitudinal Preterm Outcome Project (LOLLIPOP) of over 2000 children concurred with the meta-analysis. Compared with full term pre-school children, MLP children in the LOLLIPOP study had more cough and wheeze, both during (63% vs. 50%, respectively) and without a cold (23% vs. 15%, respectively) [46]. MLP children also reported more use of inhaled corticosteroids (9% vs. 6%, respectively) and antibiotics for respiratory illnesses (12% vs. 7%, respectively) than their term counterparts [46].

A similar trend was noted in the UK Millennium cohort. At both 3 and 5 years of age, the mean adjusted odds ratios for wheezing episodes in the 12 months prior to the assessment in children born MLP were in the range of 1.3–1.7, and the mean adjusted odds ratios for any prescribed asthma medication was between 2.2 and 2.8 compared with term-born controls [47]. Not all studies are in agreement with these findings. A large retrospective study of physician-diagnosed asthma in LP children aged up to 83 months of age did not show a significant association between prematurity and asthma [48]. The difference in results of the studies may be related to the different definitions of asthma, i.e. parent-reported symptoms compared with physician-diagnosed asthma.

Adolescence and Adulthood

There are few reports on long term respiratory outcomes in adolescence and adulthood in those born MLP. A retrospective Swedish registry study of births in the 1970s did not find a significant association between MLP birth and asthma medication use between the ages of 25 and 35 years [49]. This was in keeping with earlier studies where there was little evidence for associations between late prematurity and asthma [50].

Lung Function Studies

The studies that have reported lung function in MLP children have mostly described differences between MLP children and term controls. Todisco et al. reported lung function at age 8–15 years in 34 children born LP and 34 siblings born at term [51]. The LP children had "low respiratory risk" in that they did not have respiratory distress syndrome or mechanical ventilation in the neonatal period. Although mean values for residual volumes in both groups were in the upper limit of the normal range, the LP group had significantly higher residual volume and residual volume/total lung capacity than controls. Bronchial responsiveness was similar between the groups [51].

Using participants from the Avon Longitudinal Study of Parents and Children (ALSPAC), Kotecha et al. studied lung spirometry at 8–9 years and again, at

14–17 years [52]. At 8–9 years, children born at 33–34 weeks of gestation had lower forced expired volumes in 1 s (FEV_1) (adjusted mean difference in z-scores; −0.48; 95% CI −0.72, −0.25 SD) and forced vital capacity (FVC) (adjusted mean difference in z-scores; −0.35; 95% CI -0.59, −0.12 SD) than term controls, differences which were of similar magnitude when comparing term controls with those born at less than 32 weeks of gestation. By 14–17 years of age, the differences between those born 33–34 weeks and those born at term had attenuated. Children born at 35–36 weeks had similar values to those born at term at both ages [52].

Thus, an encouraging message from this study was that lung function may improve with age in moderately preterm adolescents; indeed those born at 33–34 weeks had improved values for $zFEV_1$ between 8–9 years and 14–17 years (adjusted mean difference in z-scores; 0.35; 95% CI 0.02, 0.68 SD), whereas there were no substantial changes between the two ages in other gestational age subgroups.

However, not all studies have reported improvements in expiratory flows with age in children born MLP. In a Swedish study of children born between 1994 and 1996 in Stockholm, Thunqvist et al. [53] reported that z-scores for FEV_1 were − 0.36 (95% CI -0.54, −0.08) lower for girls at 8 years compared with female controls, but there were no substantial differences between males at 8 years. However, by 16 years of age z-scores for FEV_1 were lower for both sexes compared with controls. Even fewer data are available in adolescence and adulthood. A study of 381 individuals aged 45–50 years showed a significant linear relationship between birth weight and FEV_1 and FVC [40].

Hospitalisation and Health Services Use

A recent systematic review and meta-analysis concluded that respiratory causes were an important contributor to health services use throughout the lifespan in those born LP compared with term controls [54]. Hospital admissions for bronchiolitis, asthma, and "non-infectious respiratory problems" were increased in LP children up to 6 years' of age [54]. For the one study in that systematic review that reported outcomes after 6 years of age, there was no significant increase in asthma rates in LP compared with term controls [55]. The differences however, were still present into adolescence with any admissions with non-infectious respiratory problems. A drawback of this systematic review is the heterogeneity of the studies included which precluded meta-analyses and firm conclusions to be drawn.

Functional and Other Outcomes

Several large population-based cohort studies from Scandinavian countries have reported functional and other outcomes for adults born MLP and those born at term. In a Swedish study of 522,310 births between 1973–1979, as 23–29 year-olds, those born at 33–36 weeks of gestation compared with term-born controls had higher rates of needing social welfare for more than 6 months (33–36 weeks, 2.9%, 39–41 weeks 1.8%) or receiving disability assistance (33–36 weeks, 2.7%, 39–41 weeks 1.5%) [56]. In a Norwegian study of over 900,000 births 2.4% of those born at 34–36 weeks were receiving a disability pension compared with 1.7% in those born at term [57].

Adults born MLP compared with controls in Sweden require higher rates of medications to treat hypertension [58] or diabetes [59]. In addition, MLP adults were less likely to attain a university degree, and they had a lower income compared with controls [56].

Research Gaps

There has been increasing awareness of the long term morbidities following MLP birth. Even though the frequency of various morbidities is lower than in their more immature counterparts, the potential public health impact is greater because they comprise more than 80% of all preterm births [1, 3, 4]. Neurodevelopmental and respiratory morbidities are well described into infancy and early childhood in survivors from more recent eras, and in large-scale epidemiological cohorts born more than 30 years ago, but more research is needed for longer term outcomes for more contemporaneous MLP survivors. Currently, MLP children receive little or no developmental or health surveillance as they are thought to have similar risks of morbidity compared with full term children. With increasing research, this approach may need to change as health professionals responsible for these children are made aware of the potential morbidities that MLP survivors face in childhood, adolescence and adulthood.

Conclusion

Mounting evidence suggests that MLP birth is associated with increased rates of long term health and neurodevelopmental problems compared with term birth. However, there is much to be learnt about the predictors for poorer outcomes, and about any protective factors. An understanding of the outcomes and the prognostic variables will be invaluable to develop risk stratification to target MLP at highest risk of poorer outcomes who might benefit from early intervention and ongoing surveillance.

References

1. Haines N. Births in England and Wales: 2017. Office for National Statistics; 2018.
2. Lancaster P, Huang J, Pedisich E. Australia's mothers and babies 1991. Perinatal statistics series no. 1. Sydney: AIHW National Perinatal Statistics Unit; 1994.

3. Australian Institute of Health and Welfare. Australia's mothers and babies 2015—in brief. Perinatal statistics series no. 33. Cat no. PER 91. Canberra: AIHW; 2017.
4. Martin JA, Hamilton BE, Osterman MJK, Driscoll AK, Drake P. Births: final data for 2016: National Vital Statistics Reports; 2018.
5. Cheong JL, Doyle LW, Burnett AC, Lee KJ, Walsh JM, Potter CR, et al. Association between moderate and late preterm birth and neurodevelopment and social-emotional development at age 2 years. JAMA Pediatr. 2017;171(4):e164805.
6. Woythaler MA, McCormick MC, Smith VC. Late preterm infants have worse 24-month neurodevelopmental outcomes than term infants. Pediatrics. 2011;127(3):e622–9.
7. Voigt B, Pietz J, Pauen S, Kliegel M, Reuner G. Cognitive development in very vs. moderately to late preterm and full-term children: can effortful control account for group differences in toddlerhood? Early Hum Dev. 2012;88(5):307–13.
8. Romeo DM, Di Stefano A, Conversano M, Ricci D, Mazzone D, Romeo MG, et al. Neurodevelopmental outcome at 12 and 18 months in late preterm infants. Eur J Paediatr Neurol. 2010;14(6):503–7.
9. Johnson S, Evans TA, Draper ES, Field DJ, Manktelow BN, Marlow N, et al. Neurodevelopmental outcomes following late and moderate prematurity: a population-based cohort study. Arch Dis Child Fetal Neonatal Ed. 2015;100(4):F301–8.
10. Johnson S, Matthews R, Draper ES, Field DJ, Manktelow BN, Marlow N, et al. Early emergence of delayed social competence in infants born late and moderately preterm. J Dev Behav Pediatr. 2015;36(9):690–9.
11. Treyvaud K, Doyle LW, Lee KJ, Roberts G, Lim J, Inder TE, et al. Social-emotional difficulties in very preterm and term 2 year olds predict specific social-emotional problems at the age of 5 years. J Pediatr Psychol. 2012;37(7):779–85.
12. Treyvaud K, Ure A, Doyle LW, Lee KJ, Rogers CE, Kidokoro H, et al. Psychiatric outcomes at age seven for very preterm children: rates and predictors. J Child Psychol Psychiatry. 2013;54(7):772–9.
13. Woythaler M, McCormick MC, Mao WY, Smith VC. Late preterm infants and neurodevelopmental outcomes at kindergarten. Pediatrics. 2015;136(3):424–31.
14. Chan E, Leong P, Malouf R, Quigley MA. Long-term cognitive and school outcomes of late-preterm and early-term births: a systematic review. Child Care Health Dev. 2016;42(3):297–312.
15. Gurka MJ, LoCasale-Crouch J, Blackman JA. Long-term cognition, achievement, socioemotional, and behavioral development of healthy late-preterm infants. Arch Pediatr Adolesc Med. 2010;164(6):525–32.
16. Narberhaus A, Segarra D, Caldu X, Gimenez M, Junque C, Pueyo R, et al. Gestational age at preterm birth in relation to corpus callosum and general cognitive outcome in adolescents. J Child Neurol. 2007;22(6):761–5.
17. Eide MG, Oyen N, Skjaerven R, Bjerkedal T. Associations of birth size, gestational age, and adult size with intellectual performance: evidence from a cohort of Norwegian men. Pediatr Res. 2007;62(5):636–42.
18. Ekeus C, Lindström K, Lindblad F, Rasmussen F, Hjern A. Preterm birth, social disadvantage, and cognitive competence in Swedish 18- to 19-year-old men. Pediatrics. 2010;125(1):e67–73.
19. Quigley MA, Poulsen G, Boyle E, Wolke D, Field D, Alfirevic Z, et al. Early term and late preterm birth are associated with poorer school performance at age 5 years: a cohort study. Arch Dis Child Fetal Neonatal Ed. 2012;97(3):F167–73.
20. Lipkind HS, Slopen ME, Pfeiffer MR, McVeigh KH. School-age outcomes of late preterm infants in New York City. Am J Obstet Gynecol. 2012;206(3):222.e221–6.
21. Chyi LJ, Lee HC, Hintz SR, Gould JB, Sutcliffe TL. School outcomes of late preterm infants: special needs and challenges for infants born at 32 to 36 weeks gestation. J Pediatr. 2008;153(1):25–31.
22. Odd DE, Emond A, Whitelaw A. Long-term cognitive outcomes of infants born moderately and late preterm. Dev Med Child Neurol. 2012;54(8):704–9.
23. Morse SB, Zheng H, Tang Y, Roth J. Early school-age outcomes of late preterm infants. Pediatrics. 2009;123(4):e622–9.
24. van Baar AL, Vermaas J, Knots E, de Kleine MJK, Soons P. Functioning at school age of moderately preterm children born at 32 to 36 weeks' gestational age. Pediatrics. 2009;124(1):251–7.

25. Stene-Larsen K, Lang AM, Landolt MA, Latal B, Vollrath ME. Emotional and behavioral problems in late preterm and early term births: outcomes at child age 36 months. BMC Pediatr. 2016;16(1):196.

26. Potijk MR, de Winter AF, Bos AF, Kerstjens JM, Reijneveld SA. Co-occurrence of developmental and behavioural problems in moderate to late preterm-born children. Arch Dis Child. 2016;101(3):217–22.

27. Boylan J, Alderdice FA, McGowan JE, Craig S, Perra O, Jenkins J. Behavioural outcomes at 3 years of age among late preterm infants admitted to neonatal intensive care: a cohort study. Arch Dis Child Fetal Neonatal Ed. 2014;99(5):F359–65.

28. Talge NM, Holzman C, Wang J, Lucia V, Gardiner J, Breslau N. Late-preterm birth and its association with cognitive and socioemotional outcomes at 6 years of age. Pediatrics. 2010;126(6):1124–31.

29. Lindstrom K, Lindblad F, Hjern A. Preterm birth and attention-deficit/hyperactivity disorder in schoolchildren. Pediatrics. 2011;127(5):858–65.

30. Huddy CLJ, Johnson A, Hope PL. Educational and behavioural problems in babies of 32–35 weeks gestation. Arch Dis Child Fetal Neonatal Ed. 2001;85(1):F23–8.

31. Harris MN, Voigt RG, Barbaresi WJ, Voge GA, Killian JM, Weaver AL, et al. ADHD and learning disabilities in former late preterm infants: a population-based birth cohort. Pediatrics. 2013;132(3):e630–6.

32. Heinonen K, Eriksson JG, Kajantie E, Pesonen A-K, Barker DJ, Osmond C, et al. Late-preterm birth and lifetime socioeconomic attainments: the Helsinki Birth Cohort Study. Pediatrics. 2013;132(4):647–55.

33. Heinonen K, Eriksson JG, Lahti J, Kajantie E, Pesonen AK, Tuovinen S, et al. Late preterm birth and neurocognitive performance in late adulthood: a birth cohort study. Pediatrics. 2015;135(4):e818–25.

34. Heinonen K, Lahti J, Sammallahti S, Wolke D, Lano A, Andersson S, et al. Neurocognitive outcome in young adults born late-preterm. Dev Med Child Neurol. 2018;60(3):267–74.

35. Lindstrom K, Lindblad F, Hjern A. Psychiatric morbidity in adolescents and young adults born preterm: a Swedish national cohort study. Pediatrics. 2009;123(1):e47–53.

36. Sammallahti S, Heinonen K, Andersson S, Lahti M, Pirkola S, Lahti J, et al. Growth after late-preterm birth and adult cognitive, academic, and mental health outcomes. Pediatr Res. 2017;81(5):767–74.

37. Langston C, Kida K, Reed M, Thurlbeck WM. Human lung growth in late gestation and in the neonate. Am Rev Respir Dis. 1984;129(4):607–13.

38. Jobe AH, Bancalari E. Bronchopulmonary dysplasia. Am J Respir Crit Care Med. 2001;163(7):1723–9.

39. Smith DE, Otulakowski G, Yeger H, Post M, Cutz E, O'Brodovich HM. Epithelial Na(+) channel (ENaC) expression in the developing normal and abnormal human perinatal lung. Am J Respir Crit Care Med. 2000;161(4 Pt 1):1322–31.

40. Edwards CA, Osman LM, Godden DJ, Campbell DM, Douglas JG. Relationship between birth weight and adult lung function: controlling for maternal factors. Thorax. 2003;58(12):1061–5.

41. Sonnenschein-van der Voort AM, Arends LR, de Jongste JC, Annesi-Maesano I, Arshad SH, Barros H, et al. Preterm birth, infant weight gain, and childhood asthma risk: a meta-analysis of 147,000 European children. J Allergy Clin Immunol. 2014;133(5):1317–29.

42. Collins A, Weitkamp JH, Wynn JL. Why are preterm newborns at increased risk of infection? Arch Dis Child Fetal Neonatal Ed. 2018;103(4):F391–f394.

43. Pike KC, Lucas JS. Respiratory consequences of late preterm birth. Paediatr Respir Rev. 2015;16(3):182–8.

44. Mauskopf J, Margulis AV, Samuel M, Lohr KN. Respiratory syncytial virus hospitalizations in healthy preterm infants: systematic review. Pediatr Infect Dis J. 2016;35(7):e229–38.

45. Boyce TG, Mellen BG, Mitchel EF Jr, Wright PF, Griffin MR. Rates of hospitalization for respiratory syncytial virus infection among children in medicaid. J Pediatr. 2000;137(6):865–70.

46. Vrijlandt EJ, Kerstjens JM, Duiverman EJ, Bos AF, Reijneveld SA. Moderately preterm children have more respiratory problems during their first 5 years of life than children born full term. Am J Respir Crit Care Med. 2013;187(11):1234–40.

47. Boyle EM, Poulsen G, Field DJ, Kurinczuk JJ, Wolke D, Alfirevic Z, et al. Effects of gestational age at birth on health outcomes at 3 and 5 years of age: population based cohort study. BMJ. 2012;344:e896.
48. Abe K, Shapiro-Mendoza CK, Hall LR, Satten GA. Late preterm birth and risk of developing asthma. J Pediatr. 2010;157(1):74–8.
49. Crump C, Winkleby MA, Sundquist J, Sundquist K. Risk of asthma in young adults who were born preterm: a Swedish national cohort study. Pediatrics. 2011;127(4):e913–20.
50. Braback L, Hedberg A. Perinatal risk factors for atopic disease in conscripts. Clin Exp Allergy. 1998;28(8):936–42.
51. Todisco T, de Benedictis FM, Iannacci L, Baglioni S, Eslami A, Todisco E, et al. Mild prematurity and respiratory functions. Eur J Pediatr. 1993;152(1):55–8.
52. Kotecha SJ, Watkins WJ, Paranjothy S, Dunstan FD, Henderson AJ, Kotecha S. Effect of late preterm birth on longitudinal lung spirometry in school age children and adolescents. Thorax. 2012;67(1):54–61.
53. Thunqvist P, Gustafsson PM, Schultz ES, Bellander T, Berggren-Brostrom E, Norman M, et al. Lung function at 8 and 16 years after moderate-to-late preterm birth: a prospective cohort study. Pediatrics. 2016;137(4):e20152056.
54. Isayama T, Lewis-Mikhael AM, O'Reilly D, Beyene J, McDonald SD. Health services use by late preterm and term infants from infancy to adulthood: a meta-analysis. Pediatrics. 2017;140(1):e20170266.
55. Leung JY, Lam HS, Leung GM, Schooling CM. Gestational age, birthweight for gestational age, and childhood hospitalisations for asthma and other wheezing disorders. Paediatr Perinat Epidemiol. 2016;30(2):149–59.
56. Lindstrom K, Winbladh B, Haglund B, Hjern A. Preterm infants as young adults: a Swedish national cohort study. Pediatrics. 2007;120(1):70–7.
57. Moster D, Lie RT, Markestad T. Long-term medical and social consequences of preterm birth. N Engl J Med. 2008;359(3):262–73.
58. Crump C, Winkleby MA, Sundquist K, Sundquist J. Risk of hypertension among young adults who were born preterm: a Swedish national study of 636,000 births. Am J Epidemiol. 2011;173(7):797–803.
59. Crump C, Winkleby MA, Sundquist K, Sundquist J. Risk of diabetes among young adults born preterm in Sweden. Diabetes Care. 2011;34(5):1109–13.

Part VI
General Principles in Neonatal Care

Chapter 24
Delivery Room Stabilisation

(… just when you thought you knew what you were doing)

Victoria J. Monnelly, Sean B. Ainsworth, and Jonathan P. Wyllie

Introduction

Every 5 years up to 2015 [1] the International Liaison Committee on Resuscitation (ILCOR) has published a Consensus on Science with Treatment Recommendations which has informed national and international guidelines. The process robustly assesses available evidence for the questions addressed and meets accepted standards for reviews and guidelines. ILCOR evidence evaluation is changing to a continuous process with position statements when appropriate and triggered by new research.

It is likely that formal collation of UK and European guidelines will remain five yearly. Whilst new research may not trigger ILCOR evaluation, it may cause controversy and uncertainty. This chapter aims to look at some of those areas, including relevant recent ILCOR statements and evidence available, to guide practitioners in their personal approach and future research.

V. J. Monnelly
Simpson Centre for Reproductive Health, Royal Infirmary of Edinburgh, Edinburgh, UK
e-mail: vix.monnelly@nhslothian.scot.nhs.uk

S. B. Ainsworth
Victoria Hospital, NHS Fife, Kirkcaldy, Scotland, UK
e-mail: sean.ainsworth@nhs.net

J. P. Wyllie (✉)
The James Cook University Hospital, Middlesbrough, UK

Paediatrics and Neonatology, University of Durham, Durham, UK
e-mail: jonathan.wyllie@nhs.net

© Springer Nature Switzerland AG 2020
E. M. Boyle, J. Cusack (eds.), *Emerging Topics and Controversies in Neonatology*, https://doi.org/10.1007/978-3-030-28829-7_24

Management of the Umbilical Cord After Birth

Re-introducing 'Normal' Cord Care

The concept that the umbilical cord should not be clamped immediately is termed "delayed" cord clamping (DCC). Unfortunately, this implies that "immediate" cord clamping (ICC) is the normal or natural timing for cord clamping; evidence and history suggest otherwise [2]. Successive recommendations have documented an increasing recognition of the benefits of DCC (Table 24.1) and that ICC is potentially injurious and implemented without clear evidence of benefit.

Whilst there is consensus that the cord should not be immediately clamped in babies not requiring resuscitation, there is no uniform definition of when this should happen. Definitions vary; including time limits (of 30 s–5 min), after the first breaths or ventilations ("physiological") and when the cord stops pulsating.

Alternatives to Immediate Cord Clamping

Babies requiring resuscitation or stabilisation are thought to be more likely to benefit from DCC; however few studies have included them. Alternatives to ICC and resuscitation include:

1. Umbilical cord milking with intact cord—where the cord is milked up to 3–5 times, resulting in a faster blood flow than occurs with passive return due to uterine contraction. During 3–5 milkings, a term infant receives 50 mL of blood [15]. The cord is clamped and cut after milking and the infant is taken to the resuscitaire [16].
2. Umbilical cord milking from a length of cord (~25 cm) after clamping and cutting. Blood volume from this is less than from an intact cord, but still gives the term infant about 25 mL more than would otherwise have been received [15]. The infant is taken to the resuscitaire immediately and milking occurs during resuscitation [17, 18].
3. A pause to delay cord clamping followed by stabilisation and resuscitation [16, 19].
4. Resuscitation/stabilisation with an intact cord [20].

Since the latest ILCOR recommendations, more studies [19, 21, 22] and a meta-analysis [23] have further informed the practice of cord management. Meta-analysis

Table 24.1 Successive ILCOR recommendations for the timing of umbilical cord clamping

1999/2000	*"The cord can usually be clamped about a minute after delivery"* [3–6]
2005	No recommendations about cord clamping [7, 8]
2010	*"Delay in umbilical cord clamping for at least 1 min is recommended for newborn infants **not** requiring resuscitation."* [9–12]
2015	*"For **uncompromised** babies, a delay in cord clamping of at least 1 min from the complete delivery of the infant, is now recommended for term and preterm babies."* [1, 13, 14]

showed that in preterm infants (<37 weeks) DCC reduced pre-discharge mortality (risk ratio [RR], 0.68; 95% confidence interval [CI], 0.52–0.90). Furthermore, subgroup analysis of very preterm infants (<28 weeks) showed this benefit is maintained in even the smallest infants (RR, 0.70; 95% CI 0.51–0.95). In addition to newer trial evidence, equipment allowing resuscitation at the mother's side has been developed and is commercially available [24].

Updating the Guidelines

ILCOR are re-examining umbilical cord care and outputs are expected in 2020. Data from trials will be re-examined; but assuming outputs reflect the meta-analysis, resuscitation with an intact cord and the alternatives of umbilical cord milking could become part of routine practice. Given the myriad causes of fetal compromise during labour and different methods of delivery, it may be that no single method will suit all circumstances and a flexible approach involving any of the methods described could be required.

Practicalities

There are concerns DCC may lead to more hypothermic infants unless additional steps are taken to address this, although this was not an issue in the largest DCC trial [19]. Implementing optimised cord care will, nonetheless, require unprecedented teamwork across all specialties involved in intra-partum care if the results from randomised trials are to be replicated in everyday practice [25].

Temperature Optimisation

Fetal tissues are metabolically active, producing large quantities of heat; this dissipates into maternal tissues leaving the fetal temperature ~0.5 °C higher than the mother's [26]. Newborn infants lose heat through conduction, convection, evaporation and radiation and, if these are not addressed, their temperature can drop by 2–4 °C within 10–20 min [27].

Uncompromised Babies

Since 2015, ILCOR has recommended that uncompromised newborn infants are maintained between 36.5 and 37.5 °C [13]. Sadly, newborn hypothermia remains a global issue [28]. Not so well recognised, is that hyperthermia (>37.5 °C) may also cause or exacerbate neonatal brain injury [29].

Besides drying and wrapping, various approaches, either singly or in combination, to maintain normothermia:

- Maintaining delivery room temperature of 23–25 °C for infants 28 or more weeks of gestation (>25 °C for more immature infants) [30]. This can be challenging; one trial of occlusive wraps in preterm infants reported room temperatures of 15–36 °C. Post-hoc analyses demonstrated warmer rooms resulted in higher neonatal unit (NNU) admission temperature [31].
- Skin-to-skin care is used in healthy term or near-term infants who do not require resuscitation [32]. Infants are dried, placed skin-to-skin and covered, including the head, with dry linen to maintain normothermia.
- Radiant warmers are integral to most resuscitaires and infants needing intervention are positioned under such devices. Unfortunately, there are no standards for these devices and exposure temperatures vary considerably resulting in both hypothermia and hyperthermia [33]. In prolonged resuscitation it seems prudent either to check the infant's temperature regularly or to use a servo-controlled device.
- The head represents more than 20% of the infant's body surface area, and heat loss from it can be considerable. Using a hat has long been known to reduce heat loss [34] but is frequently neglected. Polyethylene total body wraps (also covering the head) [35] and polyethylene caps [36] are effective in preterm infants.
- Polyethylene wrapping or bags minimise evaporative heat loss in preterm infants. Recent meta-analysis showed significantly fewer hypothermic infants below 28 weeks of gestation and at 28–34 weeks; others, however, became hyperthermic [37].
- Mattresses containing gel that crystallises exothermically within about 90 s reach 38–42 °C and maintain this temperature for up to 2 h. As with wrappings or bags, hyperthermia can be a problem; one trial was stopped because of this [38].
- Using humidified and heated gases is standard practice in the NNU yet in the delivery room cold dry gases, which can contribute to heat loss, are commonplace. Use of humidified and heated gases is feasible and effective [39].

Combining different interventions with quality improvement initiatives may be key to maintaining normothermia. Recording NNU admission temperature should allow benchmarking however the interventions used may vary depending on the individual situation.

Instituting Therapeutic Hypothermia at the Right Time

Therapeutic hypothermia is now standard care for moderate to severe hypoxic ischaemic encephalopathy in term infants. Whilst consideration is given to starting cooling sooner rather than later to maximise its effect, most delivery rooms are poorly equipped to monitor temperature and excessive cooling can occur. Early cooling may also divert attention from life-saving interventions and be harmful in unrecognised septicaemia. Because of these risks, normothermia should be maintained until a decision to cool is made by a senior clinician. Servo-controlled devices maintain the target temperature better than passive cooling [40] and, if available, can avoid uncontrolled hypothermia. A recent paper [41] using Bayesian analysis, has suggested that therapeutic hypothermia may be helpful up to 24 h after birth but, this is not as yet universally accepted.

Monitoring of Resuscitation

Although birth is a complex physiological process, the fetus is rarely monitored to the same degree as an infant in the NNU. The vigorous healthy infant needs little monitoring but in complex or prolonged resuscitations monitoring it may be highly informative.

Heart Rate

Heart rate, and its response, should guide resuscitation [1]. Intermittent palpation of central pulses (e.g. base of the umbilicus) or auscultation of the heart is easy to implement and requires only a stethoscope. These are, however, less accurate than pulse oximetry or electrocardiography (ECG), both of which also give a continuous measurement [42]. Accurate pulse oximetry of heart rate and oxygen saturation can take 1–2 min [43, 44]. Other limitations include motion artefact, data accuracy, signal quality, low perfusion states and costs of the oximeter and single-use sensors. ECG monitoring is more accurate and provides data quicker than pulse oximetry [45–47]. It cannot, however, give information about cardiac output and in low output states may be misleading [48, 49]. Getting traditional ECG gel electrodes to stick to a newborn infant can be problematic but newer technologies including dry-electrode ECG [50], digital stethoscopes [51], hand-held Doppler [52] are being investigated.

Increased accuracy from these devices allows re-evaluation of several widely-held beliefs about heart rate in the postpartum period; several studies now show that a heart rate of <100/min in the first minute is neither unusual, nor necessarily abnormal, but may vary according to the method of cord management (Fig. 24.1) [53–55]. Others challenge the view that it takes only 15 s for the heart rate respond to resuscitation [56, 57]. Evidence also suggests that below 30 weeks of gestation a heart rate of more than 100 beats per minute may not predict stability, but rather that above 120 or 150 beats per minute may be a better target [56].

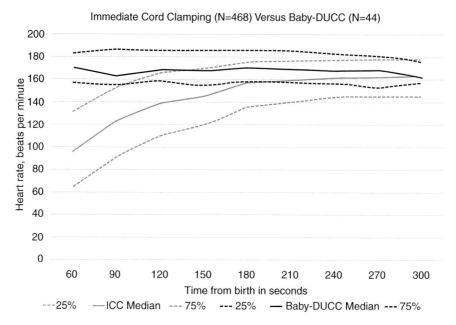

Fig. 24.1 Heart rate after birth showing historic reference ranges from Dawson et al. [43] compared to more recent data obtained during a study of delayed umbilical cord clamping (DUCC). (Reprinted from Blank DA, et al. Baby-directed umbilical cord clamping: a feasibility study. Resuscitation. 2018;131:1–7 [55]. Copyright 2018, with permission from Elsevier)

Respiratory Function Monitoring

Respiratory function monitoring (RFM) has revolutionised care of ventilated infants; it is virtually unheard of in the delivery room yet effective ventilation is the cornerstone of newborn resuscitation. Critical key respiratory parameters (such as pressure, volume, and duration) remain poorly defined. Potential methods to monitor delivery room ventilation include visual assessment of chest rise, oxygen saturation, exhaled CO_2 detection and RFM.

Most people now accept that assessment of colour is a poor substitute for oxygenation [58], so too is assessment of chest excursion for tidal volume [59]. Face-mask leak is common and frequently underestimated [60]. Measuring exhaled CO_2 may be problematic; partially fluid-filled lungs, reduced pulmonary blood flow, respiratory circuit dead space may affect measurement and to further confuse the issue, exhaled CO_2 values are typically lower in apnoeic than in spontaneously breathing infants [61], nonetheless, exhaled CO_2 can give information about improved ventilation before the heart rate improves [62].

RFM can provide instant and accurate feedback about peak pressures, positive end expiratory pressure (PEEP), expiratory tidal volumes, flow patterns and mask leak [63, 64]. Use improves performance in manikins [65] but little is yet known about benefits, or potential for harm, in clinical practice. Current understanding of lung aeration and maintenance of functional residual capacity is largely informed by intubated or tracheotomised animal models using phase-contrast x-rays [66], extrapolation to humans may not be entirely appropriate. RFM may allow refinement of tidal volumes required to displace fetal lung fluid and aerate the lung without causing damage.

Airway Management

Continuous Positive Airway Pressure With or Without Surfactant

For spontaneously breathing preterm infants, nasal continuous positive airway pressure (CPAP), if required, is the preferred method of respiratory support and can be instituted during stabilisation. Surfactant is not always necessary, but if it is required, this can be given in a controlled manner in the NNU using one of following:

- Intubation, surfactant administration and ventilation; the standard approach since early surfactant trials;
- INSURE (**I**ntubation, **SUR**factant and **E**xtubate) involves intubating, administration of surfactant and extubation after a brief period of ventilation [67]. This procedure requires analgesia and sedation, which may delay the return to CPAP;
- Surfactant administration in the spontaneously breathing infant via a fine catheter or feeding tube. Several techniques with a confusing array of acronyms—Less Invasive Surfactant Administration (LISA), Minimally Invasive Surfactant Therapy (MIST), Less Invasive Surfactant Therapy (LIST)—all involve use of a catheter to instil surfactant into the trachea of the spontaneously breathing infant on nasal CPAP or high flow oxygen [68]. This may be done without analgesia or sedation but requires skilled operators to pass the catheter through the vocal cords.
- Surfactant administration using a laryngeal mask airway (LMA) has the potential for wider use among individuals who intubate infrequently but is currently limited to larger infants due to sizes of available LMAs [69].
- Surfactant administration directly into the oropharynx is presently also under investigation in the POPART trial (https://ecrin.org/news/popart-trial-reducing-endotracheal-intubation-preterm-babies-respiratory-failure).

All of these techniques have their proponents but supporting evidence comes largely from tertiary centres with clear protocols and expert practitioners. Wider implementation has not been studied.

Sustained Lung Inflation

Residual fetal fluid must be cleared during transition. Higher peak inflation pressures may achieve this but can cause heterogeneous lung recruitment with overdistension and acute lung injury in areas already aerated. An alternative strategy is to apply a "sustained inflation" of lower pressure for longer (at least 10 s). Encouraging animal and early clinical data suggested improved short-term outcomes after sustained inflation.

The recent Sustained Aeration of Infant Lungs (SAIL) trial suggested that up to 2 sustained inflations (one at 20 cm H_2O for 15 s, followed, if needed, by a second of 25 cm H_2O for 15 s) offered no advantage over a standard approach in preterm infants of 23–26 weeks for the primary outcome of death or BPD (RR 1.10; 95% CI 0.9–1.3) [70]. An excess of early deaths (<48 h of age) in the sustained inflation arm (7.5% vs 1.4%, p = 0.002) led to premature study termination. Worryingly, in a blinded adjudication, 63% of early deaths were considered possibly attributable to resuscitation.

Laryngeal Mask Airways

In adults and children requiring resuscitation, LMAs have become increasingly common almost to the exclusion of tracheal intubation. A range of LMAs are available and there is growing experience of use in the newborn [71]. The LMA is inserted orally so that its lumen sits over the supraglottic airway. Not requiring laryngoscopy, it seems ideal for inexperienced providers who, after teaching, can successfully insert an LMA in <5 s [72]. Randomised controlled trials (RCTs) have shown initial respiratory management with an LMA is feasible, safe, and, in some cases, more effective than a face-mask [73, 74].

Current guidelines support LMA or supraglottic airway device use in rescue situations, particularly if face-mask ventilation is unsuccessful or tracheal intubation cannot be achieved, in newborns weighing 2000 g or more, or of 34 weeks of gestation or greater [14]. Complications of gastric distension [73] and trauma to the epiglottis and uvula [75] are reported and there are limited data supporting long-term ventilation via an LMA. Cost is another issue, an LMA being approximately 5 times more expensive than a facemask.

Oxygen: How Much and When?

Oxygen, usually 100%, was traditionally used to stabilise newborn infants. In the 1990s, air was shown to be as effective as pure oxygen for the respiratory support of asphyxiated term/near-term infants requiring ventilation [76]. When outcomes from this and four other trials were combined in a meta-analysis [77] that showed infants resuscitated with air were significantly less likely to die (RR 0.71; 95% CI 0.54–0.94) expert opinion began to change; the 2005 ILCOR guidelines suggested air could be used instead of pure oxygen to stabilise such infants [8].

Term and Near-Term Infants

In 2010 ILCOR strongly recommended starting to resuscitate term infants using air [12]. However, these early studies were undertaken before pulse oximetry and oxygen titration using blenders were widely utilised and studies of longer-term outcomes were of poor quality [78]. The question arises in current practice as to whether pulse oximetry with oxygen titration could individualise treatment so that the infant receives exactly the right amount.

In healthy spontaneously breathing term and late preterm newborns oxygen saturations rise gradually and it takes 7–8 min before preductal saturations exceed 90% [79]. It is not known whether target values derived from these infants are suitable for those who require resuscitation.

Preterm Babies (Below 37 Weeks of Gestation)

In 2015 ILCOR suggested starting with up to 30% oxygen, and that oxygen saturations should guide management [1]. Compared to term and near-term infants, there are more RCTs that compare low oxygen (FiO_2 less than 0.3) versus high oxygen (FiO_2 greater than 0.65) in the stabilisation or resuscitation of preterm infants. Meta-analysis of outcomes in 914 infants recruited to these trials, which include infants born below37 weeks gestation, supports starting in low concentration of oxygen [80].

In one individual patient analysis of 8 RCTs, infants (below 32 weeks) were less likely to have reached saturations of 80% by 5 min if resuscitation was started with up to 30% oxygen. Crucially, saturation below 80% was associated with lower heart rates, IVH and increased risk of death [81].

Very Preterm Babies (Below 28 Weeks of Gestation)

Fewer robust data exist for very preterm infants but one meta-analysis generated interesting data [82]. Overall, there was no difference between the two groups for mortality however when the studies were analysed according to whether they were masked or not; in masked studies there were fewer deaths in the low oxygen arms (RR 0.46; 95% CI 0.23–0.92) whereas in unmasked studies there were more (RR 1.97; 95% CI 1.02–3.68).

The largest unmasked study (To2rpido) [83] raised provocative questions. Only 5% of eligible infants in recruiting centres were enrolled and the study was terminated after reaching only 15% of its target sample size because of loss of equipoise when clinicians became concerned about use of high amounts of oxygen. It is ironic that post hoc and unprespecified analysis showed infants under 28 weeks of gestation initially receiving FiO_2 0.21 were almost 4 times likely to die (RR 3.9, 95% CI 1.1–13.4). Undoubtedly, early closure and extremely low rates of recruitment make it unwise to base any change in practice on this study. If anything, data highlight the need for further research and that some guidelines are based on low-quality evidence.

The Most Recent ILCOR Evidence Evaluation for Initial Oxygen Concentration in Babies Requiring Respiratory Support

The impact of the results of the To2rpido study in the clinical community was such that it led to the first review as part of ILCOR's continuous evidence evaluation and utilised GRADE methodology to rate the quality of evidence and the strength of recommendations [84]. For term and near-term (35 weeks or above) infants there were no new studies since those that informed 2010 guidelines, and the recommendation remains to start resuscitation in air. This recommendation was graded as a *weak recommendation*; however the group *strongly recommend* against starting with 100% oxygen. In both cases for reasons discussed previously these recommendation were graded as being based on evidence of *low certainty* [85].

For preterm infants (34 weeks or less) the review recommends starting with a lower oxygen concentration (21–30%) rather than higher oxygen concentration (60–100%) with subsequent titration of oxygen concentration using pulse oximetry (*weak recommendation, very low certainty of evidence*) [86]. The review also downgraded the importance of the To2rpido study due to its early cessation, lack of blinding, and overall risk of bias.

Both reviews acknowledge that we do not have the complete answer; what we do know is limited and large gaps in our knowledge still exist (Table 24.2).

When Should We Stop Resuscitation?

The 2015 recommendation that '*if the heart rate of a newly born baby is not detectable and remains undetectable for 10 min, it may be appropriate to **consider** stopping resuscitation*' [1] attracted criticism, in part, because it was misinterpreted as saying resuscitation should stop at 10 min [87]. The recommendation did, however, prompt the publication of several reports from institutions where infants could be offered therapeutic hypothermia after resuscitation [88–90]. These suggest that absence of heart rate at 10 min is not universally associated with a poor outcome and that return of spontaneous circulation (ROSC) at 11–17 min is seen in survivors. ROSC requires effective resuscitation and intact survival is more likely if therapeutic hypothermia is available. If there is no ROSC by 25 min survival does not occur.

Table 24.2 Knowledge gaps about the starting concentration of oxygen for term, late preterm and preterm babies identified by the recent ILCOR reviews [85, 86]

Term and late pre-term babies
• Are the requirements for late preterm babies the same as for term babies? Relatively few late preterm babies were included in studies.
• Does titration to oxygen saturation targets impact on outcomes?
• What are the effects of starting with an intermediate amount of oxygen (i.e. somewhere between air and 100%)?
• Does delayed cord clamping have any impact on oxygen exposure?
• What is the optimal oxygen concentration during prolonged bradycardia and when chest compressions are required?

Pre-term babies
• What are the long-term neurodevelopmental effects of different oxygen concentrations?
• Do different degrees of prematurity require different starting oxygen concentrations (i.e. is there a different requirement for the babies born at 24–26 weeks compared to those born at 28–30 weeks)?
• Are we sure that suggested oxygen saturation targets are the right ones for preterm babies?
• How do we titrate oxygen in the delivery room?
• Does delayed cord clamping have any impact on oxygen exposure?
• What is the optimal oxygen concentration during prolonged bradycardia and when chest compressions are required?

Gestation is important; there were no survivors among infants <32 weeks gestation admitted to a NNU after a late ROSC [90], and extremely preterm infants (<27 weeks) who have a heart rate of zero at 5 min do not survive even to NNU admission [91].

Deciding to stop resuscitation needs to be individualised and take into consideration gestation, duration of effective resuscitation and availability of intensive care and therapeutic hypothermia. Ten minutes is probably the time to begin to think about (i.e. *consider*) where things are heading, to examine these things, but nonetheless to continue effective resuscitation until the clinical situation or circumstances suggest that further resuscitation is futile.

Resuscitation and Stabilisation of Infants Born at the Margins of Viability

Threshold viability in many developed countries is currently around 22–23 weeks of gestation. Decision-making for these infants is complex and intricate. Whilst guidelines comment on whether to initiate or withhold resuscitation [92] their 'black and white' nature fails to reflect the 'greyness' of this situation. Population statistics cannot predict an individual's chances of survival and such statistics are highly variable, depending upon societal and practice norms [93]. The decision not to resuscitate at 22 weeks leads to the self-fulfilling prophecy that outcomes at that gestation are poor [94].

First trimester crown-rump length measurements gives the most accurate estimate of gestation but even this carries a margin for error of 5–7 days [95]. This can be of critical importance at peri-viable gestations. Additionally, decision-making using only gestation ignores many factors (e.g. gender, antenatal corticosteroids, birth weight, and single/multiple birth) that greatly impact survival and long-term outcomes [96].

The uncertain immediate and long-term outcomes must be acknowledged and sensitively communicated to parents who, for the majority, serve as the infant's best surrogate decision-makers [97]. Deciding not to resuscitate is a difficult decision, but for some families (and in some clinical situations) it may be the right one. Importantly, offering resuscitation does not mandate continuation of intensive care, especially if this results in survival with intolerable disability. Of paramount importance is establishing a good relationship with the family, Regular assessments of the dynamic, and often tumultuous, clinical course of peri-viable infants enable clinicians to respond to any changes and facilitates joint decision-making about appropriateness of on-going intensive care.

The immediate approach to peri-viable infants is similar to that at most other gestations, taking extra care to allow placental transfusion, maintain normothermia and limit lung injury. The need for chest compressions and medications, and a 5 min Apgar ≤ 2, are very clearly associated with adverse neurodevelopmental outcomes [98, 99]. Many clinicians might counsel parents that if the peri-viable infant does not respond to initial ventilation then it may not be in their infant's best interests to continue; and that a dignified death, without painful invasive procedures, may be appropriate. An immense number of complex decisions face families and clinicians shortly after the birth of a peri-viable infant. Clinicians should be responsive to the progress or deterioration of the infant and, in doing so, offer an appropriate level of care.

A Cautionary Note

(…What you read today was accurate when written, but may not be accurate when you read it, and what is used today may become obsolete in future)

Despite difficulties gaining consent [100] for studies of newborn resuscitation the numbers of published studies are increasing (Fig. 24.2).

Some generate thought-provoking (but potentially biased) results; in SAIL [70] and To2rpido [83] data conflict with preclinical and other clinical studies that support a potential short term advantage. Both studies were terminated before reaching their target sample size (72% and 15% respectively), in part, due to investigator concerns about safety or a lack of equipoise. It is important that large RCTs are not stopped prematurely; emerging trends may be due to chance, produce erroneous conclusions and threaten validity [101].

This is not the only problem; of published RCTs in newborns, 35% have discrepancies between proposed and actual sample sizes [102]. Furthermore, almost 40% of studies remain incomplete or unpublished [102]. Non-publication, discontinua-

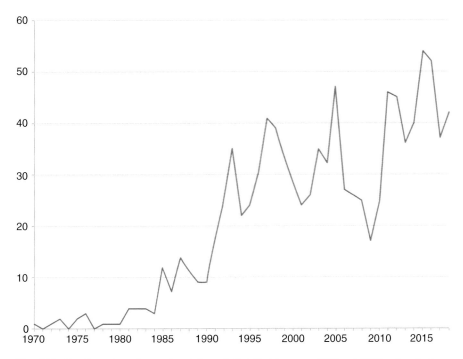

Fig. 24.2 Numbers of studies retrieved through PubMed between 1970 and 2018 using the keyword *"resuscitation"* with limits of *"clinical trial"* and *"age: newborn–1 month"*. It does not include laboratory or animal studies

tion and early termination raises ethical concerns, wastes resources and exposes participants to unknown risks without any potential benefit. In order to provide high quality guidelines, data from which any conclusions are drawn need to be comprehensive, robust and free from bias.

Outputs from ILCOR continue to reflect the uncertainty regarding the optimum management of resuscitation or stabilisation at birth. Technology and changing practice raise new questions which make it even more important to continue a constant cycle of reliable up-to-date evidence from well-planned and well-conducted RCTs, avoiding any bias.

References

1. Wyllie J, Perlman JM, Kattwinkel J, Wyckoff MH, Aziz K, Guinsburg R, Kim HS, Liley HG, Mildenhall L, Simon WM, Szyld E, Tamura M, Velaphi S, Neonatal Resuscitation Chapter Collaborators. Part 7: Neonatal resuscitation: 2015 International Consensus on Cardiopulmonary Resuscitation and Emergency Cardiovascular Care Science with Treatment Recommendations. Resuscitation. 2015;95:e169–201.
2. Downey CL, Bewley S. Historical perspectives on umbilical cord clamping and neonatal transition. J R Soc Med. 2012;105:325–9.

3. Phillips B, Zideman D, Wyllie J, Richmond S, van Reempts P, European Resuscitation Council. European Resuscitation Council Guidelines 2000 for Newly Born Life Support. A statement from the Paediatric Life Support Working Group and approved by the Executive Committee of the European Resuscitation Council. Resuscitation. 2001;48:235–9.
4. Kattwinkel J, Niermeyer S, Nadkarni V, Tibballs J, Phillips B, Zideman D, Van Reempts P, Osmond M. Resuscitation of the newly born infant: an advisory statement from the Pediatric Working Group of the International Liaison Committee on Resuscitation. Eur J Pediatr. 1999;158:345–58.
5. Kattwinkel J, Niermeyer S, Nadkarni V, Tibballs J, Phillips B, Zideman D, Van Reempts P, Osmond M. ILCOR advisory statement: resuscitation of the newly born infant. An advisory statement from the pediatric working group of the International Liaison Committee on Resuscitation. Circulation. 1999;99:1927–38.
6. Kattwinkel J, Niermeyer S, Nadkarni V, Tibballs J, Phillips B, Zideman D, Van Reempts P, Osmond M. An advisory statement from the Pediatric Working Group of the International Liaison Committee on Resuscitation. Pediatrics. 1999;103:e56.
7. International Liaison Committee on Resuscitation. The International Liaison Committee on Resuscitation (ILCOR) consensus on science with treatment recommendations for pediatric and neonatal patients: neonatal resuscitation. Pediatrics. 2006;117:e978–88.
8. International Liaison Committee on Resuscitation. The International Liaison Committee on Resuscitation (ILCOR) consensus on science with treatment recommendations for pediatric and neonatal patients: pediatric basic and advanced life support. Pediatrics. 2006;117:e955–77.
9. Perlman JM, Wyllie J, Kattwinkel J, Atkins DL, Chameides L, Goldsmith JP, Guinsburg R, Hazinski MF, Morley C, Richmond S, Simon WM, Singhal N, Szyld E, Tamura M, Velaphi S, Neonatal Resuscitation Chapter Collaborators. Part 11: Neonatal resuscitation: 2010 International Consensus on Cardiopulmonary Resuscitation and Emergency Cardiovascular Care Science with Treatment Recommendations. Circulation. 2010;122(16 Suppl 2):S516–38.
10. Perlman JM, Wyllie J, Kattwinkel J, Atkins DL, Chameides L, Goldsmith JP, Guinsburg R, Hazinski MF, Morley C, Richmond S, Simon WM, Singhal N, Szyld E, Tamura M, Velaphi S, Neonatal Resuscitation Chapter Collaborators. Neonatal resuscitation: 2010 International Consensus on Cardiopulmonary Resuscitation and Emergency Cardiovascular Care Science with Treatment Recommendations. Pediatrics. 2010;126:e1319–44.
11. Richmond S, Wyllie J. European Resuscitation Council Guidelines for Resuscitation. 2010 Section 7. Resuscitation of babies at birth. Resuscitation. 2010;81:1389–99.
12. Wyllie J, Perlman JM, Kattwinkel J, Atkins DL, Chameides L, Goldsmith JP, Guinsburg R, Hazinski MF, Morley C, Richmond S, Simon WM, Singhal N, Szyld E, Tamura M, Velaphi S, Neonatal Resuscitation Chapter Collaborators. Part 11: Neonatal resuscitation: 2010 International Consensus on Cardiopulmonary Resuscitation and Emergency Cardiovascular Care Science with Treatment Recommendations. Resuscitation. 2010;81(Suppl 1):e260–87.
13. Perlman JM, Wyllie J, Kattwinkel J, Wyckoff MH, Aziz K, Guinsburg R, Kim HS, Liley HG, Mildenhall L, Simon WM, Szyld E, Tamura M, Velaphi S, Neonatal Resuscitation Chapter Collaborators. Part 7: Neonatal Resuscitation: 2015 International Consensus on Cardiopulmonary Resuscitation and Emergency Cardiovascular Care Science With Treatment Recommendations. Circulation. 2015;132(16 Suppl 1):S204–41.
14. Wyllie J, Bruinenberg J, Roehr CC, Rüdiger M, Trevisanuto D, Urlesberger B. European Resuscitation Council Guidelines for Resuscitation. 2015: Section 7. Resuscitation and support of transition of babies at birth. Resuscitation. 2015;95:249–63.
15. McAdams RM, Fay E, Delaney S. Whole blood volumes associated with milking intact and cut umbilical cords in term newborns. J Perinatol. 2018;38:245–50.
16. Katheria AC, Truong G, Cousins L, Oshiro B, Finer NN. Umbilical cord milking versus delayed cord clamping in preterm infants. Pediatrics. 2015;136:61–9.
17. Upadhyay A, Gothwal S, Parihar R, Garg A, Gupta A, Chawla D, Gulati IK. Effect of umbilical cord milking in term and near term infants: randomized control trial. Am J Obstet Gynecol. 2013;208:120.e1–6.

18. Jaiswal P, Upadhyay A, Gothwal S, Chaudhary H, Tandon A. Comparison of umbilical cord milking and delayed cord clamping on cerebral blood flow in term neonates. Indian J Pediatr. 2015;82:890–5.

19. Tarnow-Mordi W, Morris J, Kirby A, Robledo K, Askie L, Brown R, Evans N, Finlayson S, Fogarty M, Gebski V, Ghadge A, Hague W, Isaacs D, Jeffery M, Keech A, Kluckow M, Popopat H, Sebastian L, Aagaard K, Belfort M, Pammi M, Abdel-Latif M, Reynolds G, Ariff S, Sheikh L, Chen Y, Colditz P, Liley H, Pritchard M, de Luca D, de Waal K, Forder P, Duley L, El-Naggar W, Gill A, Newnham J, Simmer K, Groom K, Weston P, Gullam J, Patel H, Koh G, Lui K, Marlow N, Morris S, Sehgal A, Wallace E, Soll R, Young L, Sweet D, Walker S, Watkins A, Wright I, Osborn D, Simes J, Australian Placental Transfusion Study Collaborative Group. Delayed versus immediate cord clamping in preterm infants. N Engl J Med. 2017;377:2445–55.

20. Katheria A, Poeltler D, Durham J, Steen J, Rich W, Arnell K, Maldonado M, Cousins L, Finer N. Neonatal Resuscitation with an intact cord: a randomized clinical trial. J Pediatr. 2016;178:75–80.e3.

21. Duley L, Dorling J, Pushpa-Rajah A, Oddie SJ, Yoxall CW, Schoonakker B, Bradshaw L, Mitchell EJ, Fawke JA, Cord Pilot Trial Collaborative Group. Randomised trial of cord clamping and initial stabilisation at very preterm birth. Arch Dis Child Fetal Neonatal Ed. 2018;103:F6–14.

22. Katheria AC, Brown MK, Faksh A, Hassen KO, Rich W, Lazarus D, Steen J, Daneshmand SS, Finer NN. Delayed cord clamping in newborns born at term at risk for resuscitation: a feasibility randomized clinical trial. J Pediatr. 2017;187:313–7.e1.

23. Fogarty M, Osborn DA, Askie L, Seidler AL, Hunter K, Lui K, Simes J, Tarnow-Mordi W. Delayed vs early umbilical cord clamping for preterm infants: a systematic review and meta-analysis. Am J Obstet Gynecol. 2018;218:1–18.

24. Weeks AD, Watt P, Yoxall CW, Gallagher A, Burleigh A, Bewley S, Heuchan AM, Duley L. Innovation in immediate neonatal care: development of the Bedside Assessment, Stabilisation and Initial Cardiorespiratory Support (BASICS) trolley. BMJ Innov. 2015;1:53–8.

25. Batey N, Yoxall CW, Fawke JA, Duley L, Dorling J. Fifteen-minute consultation: stabilisation of the high-risk newborn infant beside the mother. Arch Dis Child Educ Pract Ed. 2017;102:235–8.

26. Power GG, Blood AB. Perinatal thermal physiology. In: Polin R, Fox R, Abman SH, editors. Fetal and neonatal physiology. 4th ed. Philadelphia, PA: Saunders; 2011. p. 611–24.

27. Dahm LS, James LS. Newborn temperature and calculated heat loss in the delivery room. Pediatrics. 1972;49:504–13.

28. Lunze K, Bloom DE, Jamison DT, Hamer DH. The global burden of neonatal hypothermia: systematic review of a major challenge for newborn survival. BMC Med. 2013;11:24.

29. Kasdorf E, Perlman JM. Hyperthermia, inflammation, and perinatal brain injury. Pediatr Neurol. 2013;49:8–14.

30. Jia YS, Lin ZL, Lv H, Li YM, Green R, Lin J. Effect of delivery room temperature on the admission temperature of premature infants: a randomized controlled trial. J Perinatol. 2013;33:264–7.

31. Reilly MC, Vohra S, Rac VE, Dunn M, Ferrelli K, Kiss A, Vincer M, Wimmer J, Zayack D, Soll RF, Vermont Oxford Network Heat Loss Prevention (HeLP) Trial Study Group. Randomized trial of occlusive wrap for heat loss prevention in preterm infants. J Pediatr. 2015;166:262–8.e2.

32. Moore ER, Bergman N, Anderson GC, Medley N. Early skin-to-skin contact for mothers and their healthy newborn infants. Cochrane Database Syst Rev. 2016;11:CD003519.

33. Trevisanuto D, Coretti I, Doglioni N, Udilano A, Cavallin F, Zanardo V. Effective temperature under radiant infant warmer: does the device make a difference? Resuscitation. 2011;82:720–3.

34. Stothers JK. Head insulation and heat loss in the newborn. Arch Dis Child. 1981;56:530–4.

35. Doglioni N, Cavallin F, Mardegan V, Palatron S, Filippone M, Vecchiato L, Bellettato M, Chiandetti L, Trevisanuto D. Total body polyethylene wraps for preventing hypothermia in preterm infants: a randomized trial. J Pediatr. 2014;165:261–6.e1.

36. Trevisanuto D, Doglioni N, Cavallin F, Parotto M, Micaglio M, Zanardo V. Heat loss prevention in very preterm infants in delivery rooms: a prospective, randomized, controlled trial of polyethylene caps. J Pediatr. 2010;156:914–7e1.

37. Li S, Guo P, Zou Q, He F, Xu F, Tan L. Efficacy and safety of plastic wrap for prevention of hypothermia after birth and during nicu in preterm infants: a systematic review and meta-analysis. PLoS One. 2016;11:e0156960.

38. McCarthy LK, Molloy EJ, Twomey AR, Murphy JF, O'Donnell CP. A randomized trial of exo-thermic mattresses for preterm newborns in polyethylene bags. Pediatrics. 2013;132:e135–41.

39. te Pas AB, Lopriore E, Dito I, Morley CJ, Walther FJ. Humidified and heated air during stabilization at birth improves temperature in preterm infants. Pediatrics. 2010;125:e1427–32.

40. Akula VP, Joe P, Thusu K, Davis AS, Tamaresis JS, Kim S, Shimotake TK, Butler S, Honold J, Kuzniewicz M, DeSandre G, Bennett M, Gould J, Wallenstein MB, Van Meurs K. A ran-domized clinical trial of therapeutic hypothermia mode during transport for neonatal enceph-alopathy. J Pediatr. 2015;166:856–61.e1–2.

41. Laptook AR, Shankaran S, Tyson JE, Munoz B, Bell EF, Goldberg RN, Parikh NA, Ambalavanan N, Pedroza C, Pappas A, Das A, Chaudhary AS, Ehrenkranz RA, Hensman AM, Van Meurs KP, Chalak LF, Khan AM, Hamrick SEG, Sokol GM, Walsh MC, Poindexter BB, Faix RG, Watterberg KL, Frantz ID 3rd, Guillet R, Devaskar U, Truog WE, Chock VY, Wyckoff MH, McGowan EC, Carlton DP, Harmon HM, Brumbaugh JE, Cotten CM, Sánchez PJ, Hibbs AM, Higgins RD, Eunice Kennedy Shriver National Institute of Child Health and Human Development Neonatal Research Network. Effect of therapeutic hypothermia ini-tiated after 6 hours of age on death or disability among newborns with hypoxic-ischemic encephalopathy: a randomized clinical trial. JAMA. 2017;318:1550–60.

42. Murphy MC, De Angelis L, McCarthy LK, O'Donnell CPF. Comparison of infant heart rate assessment by auscultation, ECG and oximetry in the delivery room. Arch Dis Child Fetal Neonatal Ed. 2018;103:F490–2.

43. Dawson JA, Kamlin CO, Wong C, te Pas AB, Vento M, Cole TJ, Donath SM, Hooper SB, Davis PG, Morley CJ. Changes in heart rate in the first minutes after birth. Arch Dis Child Fetal Neonatal Ed. 2010;95:F177–81.

44. Gandhi B, Rich W, Finer N. Time to achieve stable pulse oximetry values in VLBW infants in the delivery room. Resuscitation. 2013;84:970–3.

45. van Vonderen JJ, Hooper SB, Kroese JK, Roest AA, Narayen IC, van Zwet EW, te Pas AB. Pulse oximetry measures a lower heart rate at birth compared with electrocardiography. J Pediatr. 2015;166:49–53.

46. Iglesias B, Rodrí Guez MAJ, Aleo E, Criado E, Martí Nez-Orgado J, Arruza L. 3-lead elec-trocardiogram is more reliable than pulse oximetry to detect bradycardia during stabilisation at birth of very preterm infants. Arch Dis Child Fetal Neonatal Ed. 2018;103:F233–7.

47. Katheria A, Rich W, Finer N. Electrocardiogram provides a continuous heart rate faster than oximetry during neonatal resuscitation. Pediatrics. 2012;130:e1177–81.

48. Dyson A, Jeffrey M, Kluckow M. Measurement of neonatal heart rate using handheld Doppler ultrasound. Arch Dis Child Fetal Neonatal Ed. 2017;102:F116–9.

49. Luong DH, Cheung P-Y, O'Reilly M, Lee TF, Schmolzer GM. Electrocardiography vs aus-cultation to assess heart rate during cardiac arrest with pulseless electrical activity in newborn infants. Front Pediatr. 2018;6:366.

50. Linde JE, Schulz J, Perlman JM, Øymar K, Francis F, Eilevstjønn J, Ersdal HL. Normal new-born heart rate in the first five minutes of life assessed by dry-electrode electrocardiography. Neonatology. 2016;110:231–7.

51. Gaertner VD, Kevat AC, Davis PG, Kamlin COF. Evaluation of a digital stethoscope in tran-sitioning term infants after birth. Arch Dis Child Fetal Neonatal Ed. 2017;102:F370–1.

52. Shimabukuro R, Takase K, Ohde S, Kusakawa I. Handheld fetal Doppler device for assessing heart rate in neonatal resuscitation. Pediatr Int. 2017;59:1069–73.
53. Smit M, Dawson JA, Ganzeboom A, Hooper SB, van Roosmalen J, te Pas AB. Pulse oximetry in newborns with delayed cord clamping and immediate skin-to-skin contact. Arch Dis Child Fetal Neonatal Ed. 2014;99:F309–14.
54. Pichler G, Baik N, Urlesberger B, Cheung PY, Aziz K, Avian A, Schmölzer GM. Cord clamping time in spontaneously breathing preterm neonates in the first minutes after birth: impact on cerebral oxygenation—a prospective observational study. J Matern Fetal Neonatal Med. 2016;29:1570–2.
55. Blank DA, Badurdeen S, Omar F, Kamlin C, Jacobs SE, Thio M, Dawson JA, Kane SC, Dennis AT, Polglase GR, Hooper SB, Davis PG. Baby-directed umbilical cord clamping: a feasibility study. Resuscitation. 2018;131:1–7.
56. Yam CH, Dawson JA, Schmölzer GM, Morley CJ, Davis PG. Heart rate changes during resuscitation of newly born infants <30 weeks gestation: an observational study. Arch Dis Child Fetal Neonatal Ed. 2011;96:F102–7.
57. Hooper SB, Fouras A, Siew ML, Wallace MJ, Kitchen MJ, te Pas AB, Klingenberg C, Lewis RA, Davis PG, Morley CG, Schmölzer GM. Expired CO2 levels indicate degree of lung aeration at birth. PLoS One. 2013;8:e70895.
58. O'Donnell CP, Kamlin CO, Davis PG, Carlin JB, Morley CJ. Clinical assessment of infant colour at delivery. Arch Dis Child Fetal Neonatal Ed. 2007;92:F465–7.
59. Poulton DA, Schmölzer GM, Morley CJ, Davis PG. Assessment of chest rise during mask ventilation of preterm infants in the delivery room. Resuscitation. 2011;82:175–9.
60. Schmölzer GM, Kamlin OC, O'Donnell CP, Dawson JA, Morley CJ, Davis PG. Assessment of tidal volume and gas leak during mask ventilation of preterm infants in the delivery room. Arch Dis Child Fetal Neonatal Ed. 2010;95:F393–7.
61. van Vonderen JJ, Lista G, Cavigioli F, Hooper SB, te Pas AB. Effectivity of ventilation by measuring expired CO2 and RIP during stabilisation of preterm infants at birth. Arch Dis Child Fetal Neonatal Ed. 2015;100:F514–8.
62. Blank D, Rich W, Leone T, Garey D, Finer N. Pedi-cap color change precedes a significant increase in heart rate during neonatal resuscitation. Resuscitation. 2014;85:1568–72.
63. Schmölzer GM, Morley CJ, Wong C, Dawson JA, Kamlin CO, Donath SM, Hooper SB, Davis PG. Respiratory function monitor guidance of mask ventilation in the delivery room: a feasibility study. J Pediatr. 2012;160:377–81.e2.
64. Verbeek C, van Zanten HA, van Vonderen JJ, Kitchen MJ, Hooper SB, te Pas AB. Accuracy of currently available neonatal respiratory function monitors for neonatal resuscitation. Eur J Pediatr. 2016;175:1065–70.
65. Wood FE, Morley CJ, Dawson JA, Davis PG. A respiratory function monitor improves mask ventilation. Arch Dis Child Fetal Neonatal Ed. 2008;93:F380–1.
66. Hooper SB, Te Pas AB, Kitchen MJ. Respiratory transition in the newborn: a three-phase process. Arch Dis Child Fetal Neonatal Ed. 2016;101:F266–71.
67. Pfister RH, Soll RF. Initial respiratory support of preterm infants: the role of CPAP, the INSURE method, and noninvasive ventilation. Clin Perinatol. 2012;39:459–81.
68. Aldana-Aguirre JC, Pinto M, Featherstone RM, Kumar M. Less invasive surfactant administration versus intubation for surfactant delivery in preterm infants with respiratory distress syndrome: a systematic review and meta-analysis. Arch Dis Child Fetal Neonatal Ed. 2017;102:F17–3.
69. Pinheiro JM, Santana-Rivas Q, Pezzano C. Randomized trial of laryngeal mask airway versus endotracheal intubation for surfactant delivery. J Perinatol. 2016;36:196–201.
70. Kirpalani H, Ratcliffe SJ, Keszler M, Davis PG, Foglia EE, Te Pas A, Fernando M, Chaudhary A, Localio R, van Kaam AH, Onland W, Owen LS, Schmölzer GM, Katheria A, Hummler H, Lista G, Abbasi S, Klotz D, Simma B, Nadkarni V, Poulain FR, Donn SM, Kim HS, Park WS, Cadet C, Kong JY, Smith A, Guillen U, Liley HG, Hopper AO, Tamura M, SAIL Site Investigators. Effect of sustained inflations vs intermittent positive pressure ventilation on

bronchopulmonary dysplasia or death among extremely preterm infants: the SAIL randomized clinical trial. JAMA. 2019;321:1165–75.

71. Bansal SC, Caoci S, Dempsey E, Trevisanuto D, Roehr CC. The Laryngeal Mask Airway and its use in neonatal resuscitation: a critical review of where we are in 2017/2018. Neonatology. 2018;113:152–61.

72. Gandini D, Brimacombe J. Manikin training for neonatal resuscitation with the laryngeal mask airway. Pediatr Anaesth. 2004;14:493–4.

73. Zhu XY, Lin BC, Zhang QS, Ye HM, Yu RJ. A prospective evaluation of the efficacy of the laryngeal mask airway during neonatal resuscitation. Resuscitation. 2011;82:1405–9.

74. Trevisanuto D, Cavallin F, Nguyen LN, Nguyen TV, Tran LD, Tran CD, Doglioni N, Micaglio M, Moccia L. Supreme laryngeal mask airway versus face mask during neonatal resuscitation: a randomized controlled trial. J Pediatr. 2015;167:286–91.

75. Esmail N, Saleh M, Ali A. Laryngeal mask airway versus endotracheal intubation for Apgar score improvement in neonatal resuscitation. Egypt J Anaesth. 2002;18:115–21.

76. Ramji S, Ahuja S, Thirupuram S, Rootwelt T, Rooth G, Saugstad OD. Resuscitation of asphyxic newborn infants with room air or 100% oxygen. Pediatr Res. 1993;34:809–12.

77. Davis PG, Tan A, O'Donnell CP, Schulze A. Resuscitation of newborn infants with 100% oxygen or air: a systematic review and meta-analysis. Lancet. 2004;364:1329–33.

78. Saugstad OD, Vento M, Ramji S, Howard D, Soll RF. Neurodevelopmental outcome of infants resuscitated with air or 100% oxygen: a systematic review and meta-analysis. Neonatology. 2012;102:98–103.

79. Dawson JA, Kamlin CO, Vento M, Wong C, Cole TJ, Donath SM, Davis PG, Morley CJ. Defining the reference range for oxygen saturation for infants after birth. Pediatrics. 2010;125:e1340–7.

80. Lui K, Jones LJ, Foster JP, Davis PG, Ching SK, Oei JL, Osborn DA. Lower versus higher oxygen concentrations titrated to target oxygen saturations during resuscitation of preterm infants at birth. Cochrane Database Syst Rev. 2018;5:CD010239.

81. Oei JL, Finer NN, Saugstad OD, Wright IM, Rabi Y, Tarnow-Mordi W, Rich W, Kapadia V, Rook D, Smyth JP, Lui K, Vento M. Outcomes of oxygen saturation targeting during delivery room stabilisation of preterm infants. Arch Dis Child Fetal Neonatal Ed. 2018;103:F446–54.

82. Oei JL, Vento M, Rabi Y, Wright I, Finer N, Rich W, Kapadia V, Aune D, Rook D, Tarnow-Mordi W, Saugstad OD. Higher or lower oxygen for delivery room resuscitation of preterm infants below 28 completed weeks gestation: a meta-analysis. Arch Dis Child Fetal Neonatal Ed. 2017;102:F24–30.

83. Oei JL, Saugstad OD, Lui K, Wright IM, Smyth JP, Craven P, Wang YA, McMullan R, Coates E, Ward M, Mishra P, De Waal K, Travadi J, See KC, Cheah IG, Lim CT, Choo YM, Kamar AA, Cheah FC, Masoud A, Tarnow-Mordi W. Targeted oxygen in the resuscitation of preterm infants, a randomized clinical trial. Pediatrics. 2017;139:e20161452.

84. Guyatt GH, Oxman AD, Vist GE, Kunz R, Falck-Ytter Y, Alonso-Coello P, Schünemann HJ, GRADE Working Group. GRADE: an emerging consensus on rating quality of evidence and strength of recommendations. BMJ. 2008;336:924–6.

85. Welsford M, Nishiyama C, Shortt C, Isayama T, Dawson JA, Weiner G, Roehr CC, Wyckoff MH, Rabi Y, on behalf of the International Liaison Committee on Resuscitation Neonatal Life Support Task Force. Room air for initiating term newborn resuscitation: a systematic review with meta-analysis. Pediatrics. 2019;143:e20181825.

86. Welsford M, Nishiyama C, Shortt C, Weiner G, Roehr CC, Isayama T, Dawson J, Wykoff M, Rabi Y, on behalf of the International Liaison Committee on Resuscitation Neonatal Life Support Task Force. Initial oxygen use for preterm newborn resuscitation: a systematic review with meta-analysis. Pediatrics. 2019;143:e20181828.

87. Wilkinson DJ, Stenson B. Don't stop now? How long should resuscitation continue at birth in the absence of a detectable heartbeat? Arch Dis Child Fetal Neonatal Ed. 2015;100:F476–8.

88. Shah P, Anvekar A, McMichael J, Rao S. Outcomes of infants with Apgar score of zero at 10 min: the West Australian experience. Arch Dis Child Fetal Neonatal Ed. 2015;100:F492–4.

89. Kasdorf E, Laptook A, Azzopardi D, Jacobs S, Perlman JM. Improving infant outcome with a 10 min Apgar of 0. Arch Dis Child Fetal Neonatal Ed. 2015;100:F102–5.

90. Sproat T, Hearn R, Harigopal S. Outcome of babies with no detectable heart rate before 10 minutes of age, and the effect of gestation. Arch Dis Child Fetal Neonatal Ed. 2017;102:F262–5.

91. Haines M, Wright IM, Bajuk B, Abdel-Latif ME, Hilder L, Challis D, Guaran R, Oei JL. Population-based study shows that resuscitating apparently stillborn extremely preterm babies is associated with poor outcomes. Acta Paediatr. 2016;105:1305–11.

92. Nuffield Council on Bioethics. Critical care decisions in fetal and neonatal medicine: ethical issues. England 2006. http://nuffieldbioethics.org/wp-content/uploads/2014/07/CCD-web-version-22-June-07-updated.pdf. Accessed 12 September 2019.

93. Draper ES, Zeitlin J, Fenton AC, Weber T, Gerrits J, Martens G, Misselwitz B, Breart G, MOSAIC Research Group. Investigating the variations in survival rates for very preterm infants in 10 European regions: the MOSAIC birth cohort. Arch Dis Child Fetal Neonatal Ed. 2009;94:F158–63.

94. Costeloe KL, Hennessy EM, Haider S, Stacey F, Marlow N, Draper ES. Short term outcomes after extreme preterm birth in England: comparison of two birth cohorts in 1995 and 2006 (the EPICure studies). BMJ. 2012;345:e7976.

95. Napolitano R, Dhami J, Ohuma EO, Ioannou C, Conde-Agudelo A, Kennedy SH, Villar J, Papageorghiou AT. Pregnancy dating by fetal crown-rump length: a systematic review of charts. BJOG. 2014;121:556–65.

96. Tyson JE, Parikh NA, Langer J, Green C, Higgins RD. Intensive care for extreme prematurity—moving beyond gestational age. N Engl J Med. 2008;358:1672–81.

97. Dupont-Thibodeau A, Barrington KJ, Farlow B, Janvier A. End-of-life decisions for extremely low-gestational-age infants: why simple rules for complicated decisions should be avoided. Semin Perinatol. 2014;38:31–7.

98. Shah PS. Extensive cardiopulmonary resuscitation for VLBW and ELBW infants: a systematic review and meta-analyses. J Perinatol. 2009;29:655–61.

99. Wyckoff MH, Salhab WA, Heyne RJ, Kendrick DE, Stoll BJ, Laptook AR, National Institute of Child Health and Human Development Neonatal Research Network. Outcome of extremely low birth weight infants who received delivery room cardiopulmonary resuscitation. J Pediatr. 2012;160:239–44.e2.

100. Foglia EE, Owen LS, Keszler M, Davis PG, Kirpalani H. Obtaining informed consent for delivery room research: the investigators' perspective. Arch Dis Child Fetal Neonatal Ed. 2017;102:F90–1.

101. Tarnow-Mordi W, Cruz M, Morris J. Design and conduct of a large obstetric or neonatal randomized controlled trial. Semin Fetal Neonatal Med. 2015;20:389–402.

102. Rüegger CM, Dawson JA, Donath SM, Owen LS, Davis PG. Nonpublication and discontinuation of randomised controlled trials in newborns. Acta Paediatr. 2017;106:1940–4.

Chapter 25
Principles of Family-Oriented and Family-Integrated Care

Liz McKechnie and Kathy Dewhurst

Introduction

Since incubators for preterm babies were invented around the turn of the twentieth century, the technology and understanding of newborn care has developed exponentially. However, consideration for parental and family involvement in care has not kept up this pace. Preterm, sick and vulnerable babies have been separated from their mothers and health professionals have assumed total care of the baby. Parents have become passive, often feeling like onlookers, or voyeurs in their baby's care [1].

However, times are changing. The importance of the whole family in long and short-term outcomes is becoming better understood and reflected in new ways to care for neonatal patients by actively encouraging prolonged parental presence and participation in care [2–4]. The UNICEF Baby Friendly Initiative has highlighted the positive contribution a mother can make in her baby's physiological, emotional and neurological development [5], and their neonatal standards [6] have emphasised the importance of "valuing parents as partners in care". There is good evidence to show that babies whose parents that get to know them well and become responsive to their needs have a better outcome [7].

The UK neonatal charity Bliss also champions parental presence and participation with their Baby Charter [8] and the Family Friendly Accreditation Scheme [9] that complements their seven standards.

L. McKechnie (✉)
Leeds Teaching Hospitals Trust, University of Leeds, Leeds, UK
e-mail: l.mckechnie@nhs.net

K. Dewhurst
University of Leeds, Leeds, UK
e-mail: K.Dewhurst@leeds.ac.uk

© Springer Nature Switzerland AG 2020
E. M. Boyle, J. Cusack (eds.), *Emerging Topics and Controversies in Neonatology*, https://doi.org/10.1007/978-3-030-28829-7_25

With support and education, parents can be ideal partners in care. They are perfectly suited to reduce their infant's stress by providing individualised, developmentally responsive care, regular and prolonged periods of skin to skin contact and provision of breast milk. These interventions have been shown to make significant improvements on outcomes [10–13] and parents want to be educated and involved [14].

Parents of preterm infants suffer significant distress during their baby's neonatal journey [15]. They experience a void in their parental role [16] as a result of the physical, psychological and emotional separation from their infant. They experience feelings of fear, blame, anxiety and anger [17, 18]. These negative feelings may last many years and have a detrimental effect on neurodevelopmental and behavioural outcome of the infant [19, 20]. Strategies that engage parents in the care of babies on the neonatal unit (NNU) enable them to reclaim their parental role. By promoting these models of care clinical staff can help to improve neonatal and parental outcomes.

However, the provision of truly family centred care (FCC) / integrated care (FIC) is sporadic at best. Often 'lip service' only is paid to it, particularly by medical professionals who may see FCC/FIC as a nursing role, in which they do not feel they play a part. True FCC/FIC comes from the whole team and nursing staff can find the challenge of implementing FCC/FIC insurmountable due to barriers that physicians sometimes erect.

We will discuss some of these challenges and controversies that we have found with our experience in family integrated care.

Parental Presence On Ward Rounds

One of the key tenets of FCC is open, honest communication and collaboration with parents [21]. FIC principles state that parents are essential to the baby's care and as such they should be involved in discussion and shared decision making around this [22].

As long ago as 1903 it was advocated that engaging the patient in bedside rounds were beneficial for learning, diagnosis and planning care [22, 23]. Subsequently, patient and family engagement on the ward round has been advocated in many different settings [24–29] and been found to improve communication and care planning.

However, the Picker Survey 2014 [30] demonstrated that at least a third of parents felt doctors on NNU were not available for discussion as much as they wanted. More recently still, parents highlight the lack of availability of doctors to discuss their babies' care, and the variation in quality of the information given [31]. For parents of sick children this is clearly unacceptable.

With this knowledge, many neonatal services now encourage parents to be present during the ward round for their own baby. Abdel-Latif [32] conducted a randomised controlled trial of parental presence at neonatal ward rounds and 95% of parents supported it, citing improved information, communication and collaboration with the care team that was also recognised by the health professionals. Families want to be present at ward rounds as it reduces stress, and they feel supported and informed [33]. They are more satisfied with the care their child receives [34] and believe that participation in rounds improves transparency in decision making, thereby fostering trust between parents and health professionals and enabling them to feel part of the team [35]. Parents are intimate with their infant and aware of subtle changes in their condition not evident to staff, that may change on a shift by shift basis [36].

Negatives

The evidence for parental presence on the ward round is compelling, but there are those that argue against it. Parents participating in ward round discussions may lengthen the ward round causing issues for the medical team. However, there is evidence that shows increase in time is negligible and has no negative impact on patient care. Parents see this as time well spent. Doctors recognised it can save time as they did not have to go back later to talk to the families [37].

Concern that parental presence will compromise teaching opportunities also has little evidence to support it. Phipps' study on paediatric intensive care units suggests it has no impact, with Muething et al. reporting that junior medical staff and other healthcare professionals found it improved quality of teaching [38].

Not all parents welcome the opportunity to participate in medical ward rounds. Some find it overwhelming or too intimidating to be present. Others find listening to the discussion increases anxiety and the conversation can be difficult to understand. Where units "allow" parents to be present at ward rounds, participation in the discussion is variable but, when staff have the relevant skills to convey information in a structured and meaningful way, parents feel less intimidated. FIC takes parental participation further by encouraging them to present information about their babies on the round. Early reports suggest that this helps parents build confidence to discuss their baby with the clinical team [39].

Why Should Parents Have 24/7 Access to Their Baby?

Whilst many neonatal units encourage parental presence on rounds for their own baby, they are then asked to leave the nursery until the round is over. With the variations in unit geography and capacity, parents and baby may experience long periods of separation. Some units may also ask parents to leave during nurse handover which may be up to 4-6 h a day [38] in total. Full participation in care to enable parents to get to know their baby means the need for unrestricted visiting and parents only being asked to leave their baby in exceptional circumstances.

Concerns Over 24 H Access

The most commonly voiced concern over 24 h parental access is that of confidentiality. There is conflicting evidence regarding this. Parents in one study admitted overhearing information about other babies and how they dealt with this was variable. Indeed, Dellogrammaticas also cites anecdotal evidence of parents hearing news about their baby through another parent [40]!

The opportunity for breaches in confidentiality at any time on the NNU must not be under-estimated. Both the Nursing and Midwifery Council (NMC) and General Medical Council (GMC) are clear on the ethical and legal implications of protecting a patient's personal information from "improper disclosure". The Royal College of Physicians and Royal College of Nursing pay some attention to this in their publication "Ward Rounds in Medicine" [41]. However, the advice is scant at best, stating "all members of the ward-round team should be aware of the immediate environment when discussing patient information".

Some units have tried innovative methods to change their ways of working in order to accommodate unrestricted parental access whilst protecting confidentiality. The use of 'board rounds' and 'huddles' away from the clinical area, are used on some NNUs to avoid open discussion of sensitive issues [42]. Some provide the ability for parents to "opt out" if they do not wish their baby to be discussed in the presence of other parents, whereas other neonatal units have adopted the use of noise cancelling headphones [43] which have been more successful in some units than others.

Siblings on the Neonatal Unit

The natural progression from unlimited parental access to their baby on the neonatal unit is to include the wider family. Practice across western healthcare varies widely in this respect. Within Europe there appears a north south divide with parental, sibling and family access being far more restrictive in Italy and Spain compared to northern European countries such as Denmark and Sweden [44].

Parents of babies requiring neonatal care frequently have other young children and find continuing the routine and normality of life for them very challenging to balance with care for their newborn baby. Parents are stressed and tired and, as health professionals caring for the family, we should be supportive, bearing this in mind.

However, there is considerable unease amongst many health professionals about having siblings on the neonatal unit. The main reason for concern is that of infection. Young children socialise with their peers in nursery or school which are both known "viral culture pots". They are frequent sufferers of infections and as such can pose a risk to the fragile preterm infant. However, a common sense approach to sibling visiting is backed up by evidence. A recent study in a large Tokyo neonatal unit used a simple health screening tool and found no increase in infection when siblings visited [45]. The authors comment that an earlier study in Boston showed a decrease in RSV infection when siblings less than 13 years old were banned during the RSV season. However, this study screened babies for RSV and the number of symptomatic infections did not increase [46].

A review of published neonatal intensive care unit (NICU) infectious outbreaks over a 2 year period from 2015 to 2017 revealed 39 outbreaks in total [47]. Over 50% of these were bacterial and only five viral. This shows that we would perhaps do better to improve our own infection prevention practices before banning healthy siblings from visiting their new brother or sister.

The parental stress that having a sick or premature baby uncovers is often communicated to siblings, whose routine and life is wholly upset. This may lead to negative emotions in the sibling who may not understand what has happened. Allowing siblings to visit the newborn baby may have benefits. Several studies have concluded that there is no negative impact on young children visiting their new sibling [48, 49], with one showing an improvement in some behaviours. This study randomised siblings to visit or not in the first 3 weeks after their sibling's birth. At the end of this period over a third of the non-visiting group could not even name their new baby, whereas the visitors were well-informed and participated in care [50].

To many health professionals, the benefits of a healthy sibling visiting the new baby are clear. It helps the family adjust, allows the parents not to worry about child care and decreases anxiety in the sibling who may not understand why the upset to his routine has occurred. The prolonged hospitalisation of a sibling may lead to separation anxiety, sibling rivalry, attention seeking and sleep disturbance [51].

However, like many things, understanding the problem and doing something about it are two different things. Young children have a limited attention span, with boundless energy and curiosity. Support for siblings should be provided a part of a family centred approach to neonatal care.

In the USA, programmes that support siblings and educate parents on how to support their other children are prevalent [52, 53]. Wainwright reports several different initiatives that aim to support children and parents alike adjusting to life with a sick newborn [54]. Initiatives such as these should be supported in the UK. Play specialists are not commonplace in the British neonatal nursery. Their inclusion to the neonatal team may well support the older neonate as well as their siblings. This will allow parents less stress and more time with their new baby, learning the essential skills to care for the baby and establish breastfeeding. This may lead to decreased hospital stays that offset the expense of the play specialist.

Accountability and Delegation

Supporting and educating the family are one of the pillars of FIC [55], but another is that of educating the professional care team. These two pillars of FIC, along with peer support and environmental adaptions to NNUs should allow an improvement in quality of care.

High quality neonatal care should treat parents as partners in care and enable them to be fully involved in their baby's care. Many studies and care programs report significant improvements in outcome when parental involvement is promoted consistently from the beginning of the baby's stay on the NNU. Starting as early as possible in their baby's journey, parents can provide simple interventions such as oral cares, comfort holds, and kangaroo care. Lester noted that the earlier parents start to participate in their baby's care, the more they do over their baby's stay and this increased contact promotes significant neurodevelopmental benefits for the baby. The FIC model also demonstrates the value of gradually integrating the parent into all aspects of their baby's care by improving breast feeding rates at discharge, increasing infant weight gain and reducing parental anxiety at discharge. As a consequence, the nursing role changes from primary carer to coach, mentor and educator. They provide the parents of a medically stable infant with sufficient education and skills to become a confident primary caregiver, under the supervision of the NNU team. Within O'Brien's study, FIC parents carry out tasks formerly considered within the nurse's remit including weighing, nasogastric feeding, and taking temperatures.

Models such as FIC shift the paradigm of care and roles of the nurse and parent. They are highly dependent on the enabling behaviour of staff in the creation of opportunities that empower parents to participate. However, the change in culture that this requires by healthcare professionals is challenging.

Staff voice concerns about the reduced control they have over the care of the infant [41] and that parents may cross professional boundaries [56]. They highlight the risks of allowing parents to participate in their baby's care as well as the effect this could have on their professional accountability. Indeed, the NMC mandates that, as registered professionals, we must preserve safety and reduce, as far as possible, the potential for harm. Thus, protecting a child against mistaken or accidental acts of over confident or unaware parents would seem appropriate and justified although others may argue that the least likely to cause harm to the infant would be the fully informed parent. O'Brien notes that there were no increases in incident reporting when FIC was introduced. We have seen the same in our own unit, alongside a significant decrease in complaints due, we believe, to much improved communication and relationships.

Concerns regarding health professionals' accountability can be allayed by considering the NMC guidance on delegation of care [56]. The NMC code [57] says, "registrants must be accountable for their decisions to delegate tasks and duties to other people." In this instance, the nurse would be accountable for the delegation of tasks to the parent within the same context as a student or non-registered practitioner. In translating guidance on delegation to the parental role it makes sense that only tasks that are within the parent's competence should be delegated and that they are adequately supervised and supported. The outcome of any task they perform should meet a required standard. The success of the FIC model comes with clearly documented competencies, matched with approved guidelines, standards and protocols, and clear boundaries that are communicated to staff and parents. Indeed, healthcare legal teams are more confident in parental care that is provided with clearly documented evidence of education and competency, than the more traditional way of parents providing care in an unmeasured, random manner.

The law imposes a duty of care on a healthcare practitioner in situations where it is "reasonably foreseeable" that they may cause harm to patients through their actions or omissions, with the NMC stating the need to be aware and reduce, as far as possible, the potential for harm. The poor neurodevelopmental outcomes of preterm and low birthweight survivors are starting to be connected to the stressful environment they are subjected to on a NNU, particularly when they do not have a parent to provide support during stressful experiences [58]. As accountable practitioners, we must reflect on the known benefits from promoting parental participation in care and address what it means if we fail to enable this.

Where FIC has been successfully embedded, it has been with the support of a robust staff education programme. These provide practical updates on clinical skills to ensure that staff are able to provide consistent and accurate advice to parents. They can build confidence in staff so that their concerns are addressed, and they can consider the benefits of the shift in their role and the impact it can have [59].

Conclusion

The essential role the family has to play in the healthcare outcomes of a family member is well recognised. To enable parents to become fully integrated into their baby's care requires a paradigm shift by healthcare professionals. New ways of working are necessary and old habits must be broken. It is no longer acceptable to create barriers between a parent and their infant. Allowing 24 h uninterrupted access for parents, participation in ward rounds and employing a sensible approach to sibling visiting are part of developing true Family Integrated Care. Although the culture change may initially be challenging, staff will recognise the benefits and embrace the opportunities it provides.

Ultimately, all neonatal health professionals are there for the same purpose—to ensure the best possible outcomes for a baby. We must work innovatively and collaboratively to provide the optimal environment for the baby and family to thrive [60].

References

1. Gooding JS, Cooper LG, Blaine AI, Franck LS, Howse JL, Berns SD. Family support and family-centered care in the neonatal intensive care unit: origins, advances, impact. Semin Perinatol. 2011;35:20–8.
2. Charpak N, Ruiz-Pelaez JG, Figueroa de CZ, Charpak Y. A randomised, controlled trial of kangaroo mother care: results of follow-up at 1 year of corrected age. Pediatrics. 2001;108(5):1072–9.

3. Melnyk BM, Feinstein NF, Alpert-Gillis L, Fairbanks E, Crean HF, et al. Reducing premature infants' length of stay and improving parents' mental health outcomes with the creating opportunities for parent empowerment (COPE) neonatal intensive care unit program: a randomized, controlled trial. Pediatrics. 2006;118(5):e1414–27.
4. O'Brien K, Bracht M, Macdonell K, McBride T, Robson T, O'Leary L, Christie K, Galarza M, Dicky T, Levin A, Lee SK. A pilot cohort analytic study of family integrated care ina Canadian Neonatal Intensive Care Unit. BMC Pregnancy Childbirth. 2013;13(suppl 1):S12.
5. UNICEF. The evidence and rationale for the UNICEF UK Baby Friendly Initiative Standards. London: UNICEF; 2013.
6. UNICEF. Guide to the Baby Friendly Initiative standards. London: UNICEF; 2012.
7. Neel MLM, Stark AR, Maitre NL. Parenting style impacts cognitive and behavioural outcomes of former preterm infants: a systematic review. Child Care Health Dev. 2018;44:507–15.
8. The Bliss Baby Charter Standards (Bliss 2009). https://www.bliss.org.uk/health-professionals/bliss-baby-charter. Accessed 9 Sept 2018.
9. Bliss Family friendly Accreditation Scheme. https://www.bliss.org.uk/health-professionals/bliss-baby-charter/whats-involved-in-the-bliss-baby-charter. Accessed 10 Sept 2018.
10. Landry SH, Smith KE, Swank PS. Responsive parenting: establishing early foundations for social, communication, and independent problem-solving skills. Dev Psychol. 2006;42(4):627–42.
11. Lester BM, et al. 18-month follow up of infants cared for in a single-family room Neonatal Intensive Care Unit. J Paediatr. 2016;177:84–9.
12. Warren I. FINE Family and Infant neurodevelopmental Education Level 1. Foundation Toolkit for family centred developmental care. London: FINE Partnership; 2015.
13. World Health Organization. Born too soon: the global action report on preterm birth. 2012. http://www.who.int/pmnch/media/news/2012/201204_borntoosoon-report.pdf Accessed 10 Sept 2018.
14. POPPY Steering Group. Family-centred care in neonatal units. A summary of research results and recommendations from the POPPY project. London: NCT; 2009.
15. Singer LT, Salvator A, Guo S, et al. Maternal psychological distress and parenting stress after the birth of a very low-birth-weight infant. JAMA. 1999;281:799–805.
16. Gibbs DP, Boshoff K, Stanley MJ. The acquisition of parenting occupations in neonatal intensive care: a prelimary perspective. Can J Occup Ther. 2016;83(2):91–102.
17. Flacking R, et al. Closeness and separation in neonatal intensive care. Acta Paediatr. 2012;101(10):1032–7.
18. Woodward LJ, Bora S, Clark CA, et al. Very preterm birth: maternal experiences of the neonatal intensive care environment. J Perinatol. 2014;34(7):555–61.
19. Gray RF, Indurkhya A, McCormick MC. Prevalence, stability, and predictors of clinically significant behavior problems in low birth weight children at 3, 5, and 8 years of age. Pediatrics. 2004;114:736.
20. Carter JD, Mulder RT, Bartram AF, Darlow BA. Infants in a neonatal intensive care unit: parental response. Arch Dis Child Fetal Neonatal Ed. 2005;90:F109–13.
21. Harrison H. Principles of neonatal family centred care. Pediatrics. 1993;92(5):643.
22. Lee SK, O'Brien K. Family integrated care: changing the NICU culture to improve whole-family health. J Neonatal Nurs. 2018;24(1):1–3.
23. The William Osler Papers. https://profiles.nlm.nih.gov/ps/retrieve/Narrative/GF/p-nid/363. Accessed 12 Sept 2018.
24. Davidson JE, Falk NL, Kleba P, Bull J. Summary of evidence: family participation in rounds. Nursing Alliance for Quality Care.
25. Bains J, Vassilas CA. Carers of people with dementia: their experience of ward rounds. Aging Ment Health. 1999;3(2):184–7.
26. Jacobowski N, Girard T, Mulder J, Ely W. Communication in critical care: family rounds in the intensive care unit. Am J Crit Care. 2010;19(5):421–30.
27. Aronson P, Yau J, Helfaer M, et al. Impact of family presence during pediatric intensive care unit rounds on the family and medical team. Pediatrics. 2009;124(4):1119–25.

28. Birtwistle L, Houghton JM, Rostill H. A review of surgical ward round in a large paediatric hospital. Does it acheive its aims? Med Educ. 2000;34(5):398–403.
29. Phipps LM, Bartke C. Spear assessment of parental presence during paediatric intensive care rounds: effect on duration, teaching and privacy. Pediatr Crit Care Med. 2007;8(3):220–4.
30. Burger SA. Parents' experiences of neonatal care: findings from a Neonatal Survey 2014. Oxford: The Picker Institute.
31. Deierl A, Platonos K, Aloysius A, Banerjee J. Evaluation of parental experience post-discharge and development of a parent focus group. J Neonatal Nurs. 2018;24:21–8.
32. Abdel Latif ME, Boswell D, Broom M, Smith J, Davis D. 2015 parental presence on neonatal intensive care unit clinical bedside rounds: randomised trial and focus group discussion. Arch Dis Fetal Neonatal Ed. 2015;100:F203–9.
33. Cameron MA, Schleien CL, Morris MA. Parental presence on pediatric Intensive care Rounds. J Pediatr. 2009;155(4):522–9.
34. Bramwell R, Weindling M. Families' views on ward rounds in neonatal units. Arch Dis Child Fetal Neonatal. 2005;90:F429–31.
35. Platonos K, Aloysius A, Banerjee J, Deierl. Integrated family delivered care project: parent education programme. J Neonatal Nurs. 2018;24:24–34.
36. Klieiber C, Davenport T, Freyenberger B. Open bedside rounds for families with children in pediatric intensive care units. Am J Crit Care. 2006;15(5):492–6.
37. Meuthing SE, Kotagal UR, Schoettker MS, Gonzalez del Rey J, DeWitt TG. Family centred bedside rounds: a new approach to patient care and teaching. Pediatrics. 2007;119(4):829–32.
38. Banerjee J, Aloysius A, Platonos K, Deierl. Family centred care and family delivered care—what are we talking about? J Neonatal Nurs. 2018;24:8–12.
39. Dellogrammaticas HD, Lacovidou N. Presence of parents during ward rounds: experience from a Greek NICU. Arch Dis Child Fetal Neonatal. 2006;91(6):F466–7.
40. Royal College of Physicians/Royal College of Nursing. Ward rounds in medicine principles for best practice. London: Royal College of Physicians/Royal College of Nursing; 2012.
41. Read K, Rattenbury L. Parents as partners in care: lessons from the baby friendly Initiative. J Neonatal Nurs. 2018;24:17–20.
42. Deierl A, Wright J, Hicks B, Armstrong B, Palmer SJ, Godambe S. Using sound blocking headphones on the neonatal unit to enable parents to stay with their baby during ward rounds and handovers. Poster Presentation JENS. 2015. p. 2015.
43. Greisen G, Mirante N, et al. Parents, siblings and grandparents in the Neonatal Intensive Care Unit. A survey of policies in eight European countries. Acta Paediatr. 2009;98(11):1744–50.
44. Horikoshi Y, et al. Sibling visits and viral infection in the neonatal intensive care unit. Pediatr Int. 2018;60(2):153–6.
45. Peluso AM, Harnish BA, Miller NS, Cooper ER, Fujii AM. Effect of young sibling visitation on respiratory syncytial virus activity in a NICU. J Perinatol. 2015;35(8):627–30.
46. Johnson J, Quach C. Outbreaks in the neonatal ICU: a review of the literature. Curr Opin Infect Dis. 2017;30:395–403.
47. Schwab F, Tolbert B, Bagnato S, Maisels MJ. Sibling visiting in a neonatal intensive care unit. Pediatrics. 1983;71(5):835–8.
48. Maloney JM, Ballard JL, Hollister L, Shank M. A prospective, controlled study of scheduled sibling visits to a newborn intensive care unit. J Am Acad Child Psychaitry. 1983;22(6):565–70.
49. Oehler JM, Vileisis RA. Effect of early sibling visitation in an Intensive Care Nursery. J Dev Behav Pediatr. 1990;11(1):6–12.
50. Beavis A. What about brothers and sisters? Helping siblings cope with a new baby brother or sister in the NICU. Infant. 2007;3(6):239.
51. Munch S, Levick J. I'm special too: promoting sibling adjustment on the neonatal Intensive Care Unit. Health Soc Care. 2001;26(1):58–64.
52. Levick J, Quinn M, Holder A, Nyberg A, Beaumont E, Munch S. Support for siblings of NICU patients: an interdisciplinary approach. Soc Work Health Care. 2010;49(10):919–33.
53. Wainwright L. Children with newborn siblings in a neonatal unit: learning from support programmes in the USA. J Health Visiting. 2013;1(8):468–73.

54. O'Brien K, Robson K, Bracht M, Cruz M, Lui K, Alvaro R, et al. Effectiveness of family integrated care in neonatal intensive care units on infant and parent outcomes: a multicentre, multinational, cluster-randomised, controlled trial. Lancet Child Adolesc Health. 2018;2(4):245–54.

55. Aloysius A, Platonos K, Theakstone-Owen A, Deierl A, Banarjee J. Integrated family delivered care: development of a staff education programme. J Neonatal Nurs. 2018;24:35–8.

56. NMC. Delegation and accountability. Supplementary information to the NMC Code. London: NMC; 2018.

57. NMC. Professional standards of practice and behaviour for nurses and midwives. London: NMC; 2015.

58. Lester BM, et al. Single-family room care and neurobehavioural and medical outcomes in preterm infants. Pediatrics. 2014;134(4):754.

59. Lim S. Neonatal nurses' perceptions of supportive factors and barriers to the implementation of skin-to-skin care in the extremely low birth weight (ELBW) infants—A qualitative study. J Neonatal Nurs. 2018;24:39–43.

60. Redshaw ME. Family centred care? facilities, information and support for parents in UK neonatal units. Arch Dis Child Fetal Neonatal Ed. 2010;95(5):F365–8.

Chapter 26
Quality and Patient Safety in Neonatal Care

K. Suresh Gautham

Quality and Safety: Terminology and Frameworks

The quality of healthcare is defined as 'the degree to which health services for individuals and populations increase the likelihood of desired health outcomes and are consistent with current professional knowledge' [1, 2] Many publications and expert reports [1, 3–5] have emphasized that, in addition to widespread deficiencies of quality in healthcare, preventable harm to hospitalised patients from medical errors is frequent. A medical error is defined as failure of a planned action to be completed as intended, or the use of a wrong plan to achieve an aim [5]. An adverse event is defined as an injury resulting from a medical intervention [5].

Institutions providing care for neonates should ideally monitor and continually improve the quality and safety of care provide to ensure that their patients receive the best care possible, avoid medical errors and preventable adverse events, and that they attain the best clinical outcomes possible. To ensure this, each neonatal intensive care unit should have a framework and approach for assessing, monitoring and improving the quality of care. Two frameworks in particular are useful—Donabedian's triad, and the six domains of quality described by the Institute of Medicine.

Donabedian's triad: An important framework for quality of care was proposed in the 1960s by Donabedian who proposed that the domains of quality are structure, process, and outcomes [6–8]. **Structure** denotes the facilities, equipment, services and manpower available for care, the environment in which care is provided, the qualifications, skills and experience of the health care professionals in that institution, and other characteristics of the hospital or system providing care. Therefore, for a neonatal unit it encompasses aspects of quality such as space per patient, the

K. S. Gautham (✉)
Baylor College of Medicine, Texas Children's Hospital, Houston, TX, USA
e-mail: gksuresh@texaschildrens.org

© Springer Nature Switzerland AG 2020   447
E. M. Boyle, J. Cusack (eds.), *Emerging Topics and Controversies in Neonatology*, https://doi.org/10.1007/978-3-030-28829-7_26

layout of the unit, the nurse-patient ratio, the availability of radiology facilities around the clock, the types of respiratory equipment used and the neonatology training and skills of the personnel. **Process** is defined as a "set of activities that go on between practitioners and patients". It refers to the content of care, i.e., how the patient was moved into, through and out of the health care system and the services that were provided during the care episode. Process is what physicians and other health care professionals do to and for patients. For a neonatal unit, process can include aspects of quality such as the percentage of personnel washing their hands prior to patient contact, the duration of time between birth and the first dose of surfactant, the percentage of infants in whom the examination for retinopathy of prematurity is performed on time, the efficiency with which a neonate is transported from a referring hospital, the frequency of medical errors and so on. Finally, outcomes are the end results of care. They are consequences to the health and welfare of individuals and society or alternatively, the measured health status of the individual or community. **Outcomes** of care have also been defined as 'the results of care…(which) can encompass biologic changes in disease, comfort, ability for self-care, physical function and mobility, emotional and intellectual performance, patient satisfaction and self-perception of health, health knowledge and compliance with medical care, and viability of family, job and social role functioning [9]. For NICU patients and their parents, examples of outcome measures are mortality rate, the frequency of chronic lung disease, the number of nosocomial blood stream infections per 1000 patient days, the percentage of NICU survivors that are developmentally normal, and parental satisfaction with the care of their baby. Table 26.1 demonstrates common quality measures in the field of neonatal respiratory care.

The Institute of Medicine's Domains of Quality: Six domains of quality were described by the Institute of Medicine in its 2001 report *Crossing the Quality Chasm*

Table 26.1 Errors and adverse events in neonatal intensive care

- Intra-tracheal administration of enteral feeds
- Intravenous lipid given through orogastric/nasogastric tube
- Hundred-fold overdose of insulin
- Administration of fosphenytoin instead of hepatitis B vaccine
- Sub-therapeutic dose of penicillin for Group B Streptococcal infection given for 3 days before discovery
- Infusion of total daily intravenous fluids over 1–2 h
- Intravenous administration of lidocaine instead of saline flush
- 'Stat' blood transfusion took 2.5 h
- Antibiotic given 4 h after ordering
- Delay of greater than an hour in obtaining intravenous dextrose to treat hypoglycaemia
- Medications given to the wrong patient
- Infant fed breast milk of wrong mother

Other errors

- Consent for a blood transfusion obtained from wrong infant's parent
- Infant falls from weighing scale, incubator and from swing
- Failure of supply of compressed air throughout neonatal intensive care unit
- Incubator drawn towards Magnetic Resonance Imaging machine requiring four security guards to pull it away

[1]—safety, timeliness, effectiveness, efficiency, equity and patient-centeredness (these can be remembered by the acronym STEEEP). A neonatal unit should try to provide respiratory care optimally in all these domains. **Safety** in particular is a high-priority domain that deserves separate emphasis and is defined as freedom from accidental injury (avoiding harm to patients from the care that is intended to help them). **Timeliness** is the reduction of delays and unnecessary waits for patients, their families and health professionals. **Effectiveness** is the provision of healthcare interventions supported by high-quality evidence to all eligible patients, and avoiding those that are unlikely to be beneficial. **Efficiency** is avoiding waste, including waste of equipment, supplies, ideas and energy. **Equity** is provision of care that does not vary based on a patient's personal characteristics such as gender, ethnicity, geographic location, and socioeconomic status. **Patient-centered care** is the provision of care that is respectful of, and responsive to an individual neonate's family preferences, needs, and values, and ensuring that the family's values guide all clinical decisions.

Clinical Microsystems

A clinical microsystem can be defined as the combination of a small group of people who work together on a regular basis to provide care and the subpopulation of patients who receive that care [9]. Each neonatal unit is a functioning clinical microsystem with the patient at the center and the physicians, nurses, respiratory therapists, and other professionals working with the patient and the family. It is the place where quality, safety, outcomes, satisfaction and staff morale are created. Multiple microsystems are nested within a mesosystem (departments such as the pediatric department, or service lines such as women and children's services), and multiple mesosystems are in turn components of a larger entity—the macrosystem or the larger organization. This macrosystem is embedded in the environment- the community, healthcare market, health policy and the regulatory milieu. Assessment and monitoring of the quality of care provided in a neonatal unit will ultimately be shaped by the culture and the environment of the organisation within which it is embedded.

Assessing and Monitoring the Quality of Neonatal Care

The quality of neonatal care can be assessed and monitored using a set of quality indicators that measure different domains of quality. Individual units should choose the exact indicators to monitor based on local priorities, local patterns of practice, ease of access to data and resources required to collect, analyse and display data. Quality indicators should be collected both for (1) Comparison and (2) Improvement.

Quality Indicators for Comparative Performance Measures

Such indicators are typically used to compare a unit's clinical performance (and not process measures) against comparators. Comparators can be the quality indicators of other similar units, national benchmarks, or targets. Ideally these data should be risk-adjusted in order to make the comparisons valid. Risk adjustment applies statistical methods to differentiate intrinsic heterogeneity among patients (e.g. comorbid conditions) and institutions (e.g. available hospital personnel and resources). With risk adjustment, an outcome can be better ascribed to the quality of clinical care provided by health professionals and institutions. Several models of risk adjustment have been developed for the NICU setting and used to evaluate inter-institutional variation.

When quality indicators are monitored, although there is often a long time lag between the events being measured and the analysis, display and comparison of the data, the discrepancy between an individual unit's performance and the comparators can be used to motivate change and launch improvement projects around specific topics. Quality indicators for such judgment may also be used by regulators and payors to rank neonatal units (sometimes publicly) according to the quality of care they provide (their performance), withhold payments, and provide incentive payments. They may also be used by families of patients, when choice is feasible (for example in an antenatally diagnosed fetal anomaly), to choose the hospital where the mother will deliver and their infant will receive care. Many neonatal networks such as the Vermont Oxford Network, the Mednax neonatal database, and the Canadian Neonatal Network, collect predefined data items from member neonatal units and provide reports to these units that include quality indicators. For example, the Vermont Oxford Network provides member units each quarter and each year a report that includes their rate of ventilation, use of postnatal steroids, use of surfactant, use of inhaled nitric oxide, pulmonary air leak, bronchopulmonary dysplasia and mortality.

Published data from several neonatal networks reveal the existence of wide variation in neonatal process measures and neonatal outcomes (including respiratory outcomes) that persists after risk-adjustment [10–14]. This suggests that the observed differences in outcomes are the result of the quality of care provided to the patients, and that the units with the poorer clinical outcomes have room to improve their quality of care.

A particularly important subset of quality indicators is that of patient safety events. Each neonatal unit should monitor medical errors and adverse events (patient safety events) related to respiratory care. These events are most commonly identified through reporting by health professionals involved in or witnessing the event, a method that is convenient and requires few resources [14] Other methods to identify patient safety events [15] are the use of trigger tools, chart review, random safety audits, mortality and morbidity meetings, autopsies and review of patient family complaints or medical-legal cases. These methods do not yield a true rate of these events and therefore cannot be used to evaluate a unit's performance against comparators. The ideal method to identify these events is prospective surveillance [16]. This system yields accurate rates and can be used for comparison, but is not widely used because it is laborious and requires many resources. A variety of medical errors and adverse events related to neonatal respiratory care have been described in the literature (Table 26.1) [17, 18]. In one study of ten Dutch neonatal intensive care units, 9% of patient safety incidents were related to mechanical ventilation. Of all recorded incidents, those related to mechanical ventilation and to blood products had the highest risk scores (an indicator of the likelihood of recurrence and likelihood of severe consequences) [19].

Quality Indicators for Improvement

These indicators are used to monitor the progress of a specific quality improvement project. These usually are a combination of outcome measures and process measures. They are collected in real-time and used by quality improvement teams (see below) to monitor the progress of the project, identify unintended consequences and draw inferences about the effects of their attempts to make change. Ideally these data are disaggregated as much as possible (not lumped together) and displayed over time (with time on the X axis and the indicator on the Y axis) in the form of either run charts or statistical process control charts as displayed in Fig. 26.1.

Improving the Quality of Care

Over the past two decades Quality Improvement (QI) has emerged as a strong movement in health care systems of developed countries. It reflects the effort to import into health care principles, tools, and techniques from other industries about improving product quality in order to meet their customers' needs and expectations. The basic premise of QI in health care is that improvements in patient care can be achieved by making a focused, conscious effort, using a defined set of scientific methods and by constant reflection on the results of our attempts to improve care. It is based heavily on systems thinking and therefore emphasizes the organization and systems of care. Many approaches to QI have been described (IMPROVE, Model for improvement, Lean or Lean-Six-sigma (DMAIC) or Toyota Production System, Rapid cycle improvement, Four key habits (VON), Advanced Training Program of Intermountain Healthcare, Microsystems approach) and all are broadly similar in their approaches. Of these, one simple and effective approach that can be used to improve the quality of care is the Model for Improvement (Fig. 26.1) that was formalized by Langley, Nolan and colleagues [20]. The use of this model and the use of Plan-Do-Study-Act cycles to achieve improvement is discussed below.

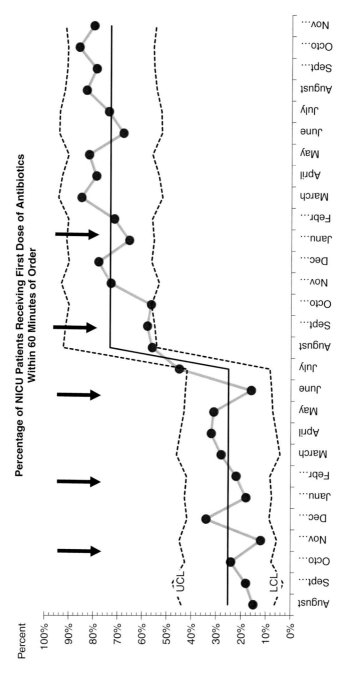

Fig. 26.1 Example of a statistical process control chart (P chart). Arrows represent sequential interventions implemented in Plan-Do-Study-Act cycles to achieve and sustain improvement. *UCL* upper control limit, *LCL* lower control limit

The Improvement Team

To successfully carry out Quality Improvement projects, it is important to have a core team of people in each unit. This is usually a multidisciplinary team composed of physicians, nurses and others who are directly or indirectly involved in aspects of the topic that is targeted for improvement. The more disciplines represented, the better the quality improvement efforts will be. The members of this team have to become skilled in several techniques, such as how to have productive meetings, how to work together as a team, how to bring about change in a unit, how to deal with barriers to improvement and how to collect, analyse and display data. The involvement of the entire NICU team in QI efforts increase buy in and heightens awareness of a problem thereby possibly creating a Hawthorne effect which is beneficial.

Collaboration

Improvement in patient care is impossible without cooperation—working together to produce mutual benefit or attain a common purpose. Collaboration and cooperation have to occur within each unit. Collaboration is a powerful force in motivating people toward improvement and in sustaining the momentum for change in each unit. The improvement team has to get 'buy-in' from other members in their unit and get them to participate in the improvement effort. Collaboration and cooperation among different units is also helpful. Different units can work together, share ideas and help each other to improve care. Clemmer and colleagues [21] suggest five methods to foster cooperation: (1) develop a shared purpose (2) create an open, safe, environment (3) include all those who share the common purpose and encourage diverse viewpoints (4) learn how to negotiate agreement and (5) insist on fairness and equity in applying rules.

Aim: What Are We Trying to Accomplish?

The first step in any improvement project is to set a clear aim. This can be done in three stages. First, a list of problems faced by the unit or opportunities for change is made. The existence of Quality Indicators as described above will assist the compilation of such a list. Second, the problems or opportunities for change that are listed are then prioritised using criteria such as the resources available, the probability of achieving change, emotional appeal, the importance to stakeholders (including patients and their families), and practicality. Third, one item is finally selected from this list as the aim for improvement. For those unfamiliar with Quality Improvement, it is best to choose for the initial project a small and well-focused topic on which data are easy to obtain that will generate interest among clinicians and nurses. Very low birth weight (VLBW) neonates have been the obvious target for quality improvement in many quality improvement initiatives. VLBW neonates contribute significantly to the mortality and morbidity burden in the neonatal units, consume largest proportion of resources, are easily identified and develop potentially preventable outcomes like nosocomial infections, intraventricular haemorrhage, bronchopulmonary dysplasia and retinopathy of prematurity. When an aim is selected, it should be specified as a SMART aim, i.e., it should be Specific, Measurable, Achievable, Realistic, and Time-bound. A good example of a SMART aim is—*"We aim to increase the percentage of NICU patients each month who receive the first dose of antibiotic within 60 minutes of the physician's order being placed, from the current level of 20% to 70% or greater by December 2020"*.

Measurement: How Will We Know That a Change Is an Improvement?

Measurement is key to QI. Measuring the quality of care serves three purposes: (1) It indicates the current status of the unit or practice. This is called assessing 'current reality'. Without objective measurement, clinicians will be left guessing or relying on subjective impressions. Objective measurement of structures, processes and outcomes provides strong motivation for a unit to embark on an improvement project. (2) Measurement of quality will inform QI teams whether or not they are actually making an improvement, without having to rely on subjective impressions or opinions, with the attendant risk of being misguided. (3) Measuring quality helps teams learn from attempts to make improvements and also learn from their successes as well as failures.

What Changes Can We Make That Will Result in an Improvement?

The answers to this question come from many sources. Some of these include

1. A detailed analysis and mapping of the process by which care is provided (process mapping). For medical errors and adverse events a detailed systems analysis [22] is recommended. Such an analysis (the most extensive form of which is a root cause analysis [23] attempts to identify work-place related, human-related, and organizational factors [24] that contributed to the occurrence and propagation of the event. Table 26.2 details the steps involved in the RCA process. It is critical for the leader of the RCA process to be well versed in RCA methodology and also be focused on identifying system related challenges rather than assignment of individual blame.

Table 26.2 Steps of a root cause analysis

Step 1: Identify a sentinel event
Step 2: Assemble a multidisciplinary team including executive and operational leadership, QI coaches and providers who come in contact with the system
Step 3: Verify facts surrounding the event and collect associated data
Step 4: Chart causal factors using process maps, brainstorming, pareto charts, fishbone diagrams etc
Step 5: Identify root causes by asking why five times for each issue, to get to the bottom of the cause
Step 6: Develop strategies and make recommendations for process change
Step 7: Present results to all stake holders
Step 8: Perform "Tests of change"

2. A review of published literature and using the principles of Evidence-based Medicine
3. Benchmarking, i.e., learning from superior performers in the area chosen for improvement
4. Advice from experts or others who have attempted improvement in similar topics
5. Brainstorming, critical thinking and hunches about the current system of care
6. Use of 'change concepts', a set of principles of redesign of process or work flow (such as 'change the sequence of steps' or 'eliminate unnecessary steps') [20]
7. Particularly for patients safety projects, use of knowledge of human psychology, the science of human factors engineering

Using one or a combination of these approaches, one or more interventions are identified that, if implemented, have the potential to result in improvements in patient care and outcomes. These interventions are variously known as 'change concepts' or 'potentially better practices' [25] or 'key clinical activities' [26] or, for patient safety events, 'safety practices.' They are sometimes grouped into a set of synergistic or complementary interventions that are known as 'bundles'.

The well-known Swiss Cheese model [27] (Fig. 26.2) depicts how an error reaches a patient in spite of a series of existing safety mechanisms because the 'holes in the Swiss Cheese line up' (multiple safety mechanisms fail concurrently or serially and allow propagation of the error). A key principle of improving patient safety and reducing medical errors is to focus not on individual healthcare providers as the cause of errors (the 'person approach'), but more broadly on the system of care (in which the provider is embedded) as the desired locus of prevention (the 'system approach'). Ensuring patient safety involves the establishment of operational systems and processes that minimise the likelihood of errors and maximises the likelihood of intercepting them when they occur [5]. Optimal design of equipment, tasks and the work environment can enhance error-free human performance and the use of principles of human factors engineering can successfully guide such optimal design.

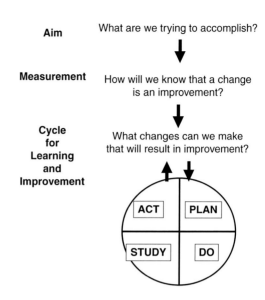

Fig. 26.2 The model for improvement. (Source: Langley GJ, Moen RD, Nolan KM, Nolan, TW, Normal CL, Provost LP. The improvement guide: a practical approach to enhancing organizational performance, 2nd edn.)

After the changes or potentially better practices or safety practices are selected it is not sufficient to implement them and assume that patient outcomes will improve. The next step in the improvement process is to carry out a series of Plan-Do-Study-Act cycles.

Plan-Do-Study-Act Cycles

No matter what the sources of our ideas for improvement are, there is no guarantee that these changes tried will make things better. The results of the implementation of these changes have to be studied, using the measures that have previously been set up when answering the question 'How will we know that a change is an improvement?' In other words, the change has to be tested. This process also allows process related obstacles to be identified and resolved. This process of testing a change is called a Plan-Do-Study-Act (PDSA) cycle. This is a critical step in the process of QI, since it allows trouble-shooting prior to wide spread implementation. The PDSA cycles include planning an intervention (e.g. steps to enhance adherence to hand-washing), carrying out the intervention, studying its effect (e.g. handwashing compliance rate, hospital-acquired infection rate) and finally implementing the intervention in day-to-day practice. Common questions the QI team should ask itself are—Why did we succeed? Why did we fail? What further changes do we now need to make in order to succeed? By doing a series of PDSA cycles and thus learning from each effort at improvement, the team can achieve lasting improvements in the way they provide patient care and in patient outcomes. The apparent simplicity of the PDSA cycle is deceptive. The cycle is a sophisticated, demanding way to achieve learning and change in complex systems [28].

Ensuring Success and Sustainability of QI Projects

Quality improvement projects often are not completed as intended, unsuccessful in achieving the desired results, or unable to achieve sustained results. The following ten tips can contribute to successful completion and sustained results:

1. Gain a deep understanding of the problem first using systems thinking [29] ('formulate the mess') before trying to implement solutions and resist quick 'off-the-shelf' solutions.
2. Avoid solely using a research mentality, especially with measurement. Successful QI requires a combination of rigorous scientific thinking as well as pragmatism. Particularly with measurement, seek usefulness, not perfection [30].
3. Focus on sustainability from the beginning, and not just on short-term wins.
4. Develop a consensus-based approach to decision-making when the evidence for interventions is sparse, incomplete or flawed.
5. Manage change carefully using published expert recommendations [31, 32]
6. Learn from 'failure' through multiple Plan-Do-Study-Act cycles. Understanding the reasons for failure can guide future refinements of the changes implemented, with eventual success.
7. Use the principles and methods of project management [33], including good meeting skills.
8. Go beyond just using jargon such as 'silo', 'low-hanging' fruit, and 'checklist'.
9. Use a QI coach if possible. Coaching can enhance the success of QI teams [34].
10. Do not get feel compelled to adhere rigidly to any one approach to quality improvement.

Leadership and Unit Culture

Finally, the involvement, support and encouragement of the leaders of the organization or the clinical unit, as well as a favorable organizational culture are crucial elements for the success of quality and safety improvement efforts. Without such support many improvement efforts will be doomed to failure and frustration. Leaders of neonatal units must focus on the quality of care as an important part of the mission of their units and must actively work to create an organisational culture in the unit that will encourage efforts to improve the quality of care. For patient safety in particular this involves fostering a culture where staff feel safe (i.e., not intimidated) in pointing out safety hazards, challenging authority, and stopping a work process or procedure if they feel it is unsafe ('stopping the line' [35]). One useful method to promote safety culture is 'executive walk rounds' [36], where senior organizational leaders periodically walk through the neonatal unit and talk to front-line staff about their perceptions of patient safety problems, hazards and requirements.

Why Is Quality Improvement Important in Neonatal Care?

Published literature on wide variation in neonatal process measures and neonatal morbidity that persists after risk-adjustment [10–14] suggests that the observed differences in outcomes are the result of the quality of care provided to the patients, that a significant proportion of neonates managed in NICUs suffer from preventable morbidity, and that the units with the poorer clinical outcomes have room to improve their quality of care. For example, one particular concern is the high incidence in very low birth weight infants of chronic lung disease (CLD), a condition that has major impact on long term pulmonary function, is associated with high healthcare and societal costs and neurodevelopmental morbidity. Despite significant advances in neonatal pulmonary care over the last three decades, the rates of CLD in infants <1500 g has remained relatively unchanged over the past decade, and also vary significantly across centers in the United States (despite adjustment for confounding factors). Neonatal health outcomes are influenced by a variety of endogenous and exogenous factors like birthweight, gestation, obstetric management during delivery, resuscitation practices, initial respiratory support, nutritional management and prevention of infections. Application of systematic QI efforts has the potential to reduce CLD and other forms of neonatal morbidity through reliable and consistent application of existing high-level evidence, without depending on new medications, technology or innovations to be developed. Such efforts are described below.

Examples of Quality and Safety Improvement in Neonatal Care

QI Projects in Individual Units

Birenbaum et al. reported significant reduction in rate of chronic lung disease (CLD) as a result of a QI project in their unit [37]. The rate of BPD in VLBW neonates was reduced by more than half by avoidance of intubation, adoption of new pulse oximeter limits, and early use of nasal continuous positive airway pressure therapy.

Nowadzky et al. [38] used QI methods to reduce CLD by implementing nasal bubble CPAP to reduce mechanical ventilation. Although the group was successful in implementing the use of bubble CPAP, the rate of CLD was unchanged and a concomitant increase in ROP rate was noted.

Merkel et al. [39] reduced unplanned extubations from 2.38 to 0.41 per 100 patient-intubated days by having at least two staff members participate in procedures such as retaping and securing endotracheal tubes, weighing, and transferring the patient out of the bed; placement of alert cards at the bedside indicating the risk level for an unplanned extubation, the security of the endotracheal tube, and the depth of placement at the gums along with documentation of proper care of the endotracheal tube; use of a commercial product to secure the endotracheal tube, education of staff by staff experts ("champions"), use of a real-time analysis form to identify causes of unplanned extubations, use of a centrally located display of the days since last unplanned extubation, and placing mittens or socks on infants' hands for intubated patients greater than 34 weeks' postmenstrual age. They suggest that the benchmark for unplanned extubation should be a rate less than 1 per 100 patient-intubated days.

Collaborative QI Projects

One successful approach that has been used in neonatology by the Vermont Oxford Network (VON) is that of collaborative quality improvement in which a group of neonatal units collaborate for the purpose of improving the quality of neonatal care [11, 40]. With this approach, a team of personnel from each hospital (from multiple disciplines involved in neonatal care, such as neonatologists, nurses, respiratory therapists and others) meet periodically, with ongoing collaboration in between meetings carried on by the use of email and telephone calls among these team members. The Network acts as a coordinator, facilitator and motivator of this collaborative effort and provides expert faculty members who work with individual sets of teams to facilitate their improvement efforts.

VON has implemented a number of such collaborative projects called the Neonatal Intensive Care Quality (NICQ) projects. The major components of NICQ projects included multidisciplinary collaboration within and among hospitals, feedback of information from the network database regarding clinical practice and patient outcome, training and quality improvement methods, site visits to project NICUs, benchmarking visits to superior performers within the network, identification and implementation of potentially better practices and evaluation of the results. In the first NICQ project, teams from the 10 hospitals worked together in cross-institutional improvement groups [11]. Six NICUs focused on reducing nosocomial infection and 4 units focused on reducing chronic lung disease. The potentially best practices that were proposed were based on an evidence review and careful analysis of other practices at best-performing centers. During the period of project from 1994 to 1996, the rate of infection with coagulase-negative Staphylococcus decreased from 22.0 to 16.6% at the 6 project NICUs in the infection group; the rate of supplemental oxygen at 36 weeks' adjusted gestational age decreased from 43.5 to 31.5% at the 4 NICUs in the chronic lung disease group. Another NIC/Q project was implemented in 16 centers of VON during 2001–2003 to reduce the incidence of BPD among VLBW neonates [41]. BPD rates dropped significantly in 2003 compared with the baseline year. In addition, severe retinopathy of prematurity, severe intraventricular hemorrhage, and supplemental oxygen at discharge dropped significantly. VON reported anther quality improvement project with an objective of promoting evidence-based surfactant treatment of preterm neonates [42]. Participating centers were randomized to control or intervention arm. Hospitals in intervention arm received quality improvement advice including audit and feedback, evidence reviews, an interactive training workshop, and ongoing faculty support via conference calls and email. Although there was no significant difference in incidence of pneumothorax or mortality, neonates born in intervention hospitals were more likely to receive surfactant in delivery room or within 2 h of birth.

Payne et al. [43] reported the results over nine years from eight NICUs that participated in a VON collaborative to reduce lung injury (the ReLI group). This group successfully decreased delivery room intubation, conventional ventilation and the use of postnatal steroids for BPD. They increased the use of nasal continuous positive airway pressure, and survival to discharge increased. Nosocomial infections decreased. However, BPD-free survival remained unchanged, and the BPD rate increased.

In a cluster randomised trial done by the Canadian Neonatal Network [44] six neonatal intensive care units were assigned to reduce nosocomial infection (infection group) and 6 units to reduce BPD (pulmonary group). Practice change interventions were implemented using rapid-change cycles for 2 years. The incidence of BPD decreased in the pulmonary group, and the incidence of nosocomial infections decreased significantly in both the infection and pulmonary groups.

In a cluster randomised QI trial, 14 centers of the National Institute of Child Health and Human Development Neonatal Research Network were randomised to intervention or control clusters [45]. Intervention centres implemented practices of 3 best performing centres of the network to reduce rate of BPD. Although intervention centres successfully implemented practices of best performing centres, the rate of BPD was not reduced in intervention or control centres. Explanations given for failure to reduce the rate of BPD were choosing interventions which were not evidence-based and targeting a multifactorial disease with single-prong strategy of reducing oxygen exposure.

More recently, state-wide collaboratives have been developed in multiple US states where some or all NICUs in the state work collaboratively on the same clinical topics using QI methods, share data, and learn from each other to make improvements in clinical outcomes and processes. Such state-wide collaboratives [46–49] have reported significant decreases in central line associated blood stream infections (CLABSIs), and are targeting other clinical outcomes as well.

Conclusions

Leaders of every neonatal unit should monitor the quality of care provided and continuously try to improve the process measures and outcomes of infants in their unit. It is important to recognize that QI methods do not replace formal randomised controlled trials (RCTs) as a research method, rather they complement RCTs in ensuring the implementation of evidence based practices to improve outcome. The complex multifactorial nature of neonatal outcomes such as CLD often raises challenges in implementation of potentially better practices that have been successful elsewhere. It is thus imperative that changes be based on review of evidence when possible, to mitigate the possibility of perceived improvement ideas. Using evidence-based practices adapted to local context within structured quality improvement projects neonatal units can reduce unplanned extubations, prevent BPD and improve other neonatal outcomes. Participation in a multicentre collaborative project may enhance such improvements.

References

1. Institute of Medicine (U.S.). Committee on Quality of Health Care in America. Crossing the quality chasm : a new health system for the 21st century. Washington, DC: National Academy Press; 2001.
2. Lohr K. Committee to design a strategy for quality review and assurance in medicare. In: Medicare: a strategy for quality assurance, vol. 1. Washington, DC: The National Academies Press; 1990.
3. McGlynn EA, Asch SM, Adams J, Keesey J, Hicks J, DeCristofaro A, Kerr EA. The quality of health care delivered to adults in the United States. N Engl J Med. 2003;348(26):2635–45. PubMed PMID: 12826639.
4. Mangione-Smith R, DeCristofaro AH, Setodji CM, Keesey J, Klein DJ, Adams JL, Schuster MA, McGlynn EA. The quality of ambulatory care delivered to children in the United States. N Engl J Med. 2007;357(15):1515–23. PubMed PMID: 17928599.
5. Kohn LT, Corrigan JM, Donaldson MS, editors. To err is human. In: Building a safer health system. Washington, DC: National Academy Press; 2000. pp. 28–29; 87, 101; 210–211.
6. Donabedian A. Evaluating the quality of medical care. Milbank Q. 1966;44:S166–206.
7. Donabedian A. The quality of care. How can it be assessed? JAMA. 1988;260:1743–8.
8. Donabedian A. Explorations in quality assessment and monitoring. In: The definition of quality and approaches to its assessment, vol. 1. Ann Arbor: Health Administration Press; 1980.
9. Council on Medical Service. Quality of care. JAMA. 1986;256:1032–4.
10. Lee SK, Lee DS, Andrews WL, Baboolal R, Pendray M, Stewart S. Higher mortality rates among inborn infants admitted to neonatal intensive care units at night. J Pediatr. 2003;143:592–7.
11. Horbar JD, Rogowski J, Plsek PE, Delmore P, Edwards WH, Hocker J, et al. Collaborative quality improvement for neonatal intensive care. NIC/Q Project Investigators of the Vermont Oxford Network. Pediatrics. 2001;107:14–22.
12. Lee SK, McMillan DD, Ohlsson A, Pendray M, Synnes A, Whyte R, et al. Variations in practice and outcomes in the Canadian NICU network: 1996–1997. Pediatrics. 2000;106:1070–9.
13. Murphy BP, Armstrong K, Ryan CA, Jenkins JG. Benchmarking care for very low birthweight infants in Ireland and Northern Ireland. Arch Dis Child Fetal Neonatal Ed. 2010;95:F30–5.
14. Leape LL. Reporting of adverse events. N Engl J Med. 2002;347(20):1633–8.
15. Thomas EJ, Petersen LA. Measuring errors and adverse events in health care. J Gen Intern Med. 2003;18(1):61–7.
16. Thomas EJ. The future of measuring patient safety: prospective clinical surveillance. BMJ Qual Saf. 2015;24(4):244–5.
17. Suresh G, Horbar JD, Plsek P, Gray J, Edwards WH, Shiono PH, Ursprung R, Nickerson J, Lucey JF, Goldmann D. Voluntary anonymous reporting of medical errors for neonatal intensive care. Pediatrics. 2004;113(6):1609–18. PubMed PMID: 15173481.
18. Snijders C, van Lingen RA, van der Schaaf TW, Fetter WP, Molendijk HA, NEOSAFE Study Group. Incidents associated with mechanical ventilation and intravascular catheters in neonatal intensive care: exploration of the causes, severity and methods for prevention. Arch Dis Child Fetal Neonatal Ed. 2011;96(2):F121–6.
19. Snijders C, van Lingen RA, Klip H, Fetter WP, van der Schaaf TW, Molendijk HA, NEOSAFE Study Group. Specialty-based, voluntary incident reporting in neonatal intensive care: description of 4846 incident reports. Arch Dis Child Fetal Neonatal Ed. 2009;94(3):F210–5.
20. Langley GJ, Nolan KM, Nolan TW, Normal CL, Provost LP. The improvement guide. In: A practical approach to enhancing organizational performance. San Fransisco: Jossey-Bass; 1996.
21. Clemmer TP, Spuhler VJ, Berwick DM, Nolan TW. Cooperation: the foundation of improvement. Ann Intern Med. 1998;128:1004–9.
22. Vincent C. Understanding and responding to adverse events. N Engl J Med. 2003;348(11):1051–6. PubMed PMID: 12637617.

23. Shaqdan K, Aran S, Daftari Besheli L, Abujudeh H. Root-cause analysis and health failure mode and effect analysis: two leading techniques in health care quality assessment. J Am Coll Radiol. 2014;11(6):572–9.
24. Suresh GK, Godfrey MM, Nelson EC, Batalden PB. Improving safety and anticipating hazards in clinical microsystems. Chapter 3, in: Value by design, eds. Nelson EC, Batalden PB, Godfrey MM, Lazar J. Jossey-Bass, 2011.
25. Payne NR, LaCorte M, Sun S, Karna P, Lewis-Hunstiger M, Goldsmith JP, Breathsavers Group. Evaluation and development of potentially better practices to reduce bronchopulmonary dysplasia in very low birth weight infants. Pediatrics. 2006;118(Suppl 2):S65–72. PubMed PMID: 17079625.
26. Bundy DG, Morawski LF, Lazorick S, Bradbury S, Kamachi K, Suresh GK. Education in quality improvement for pediatric practice: an online program to teach clinicians QI. Acad Pediatr. 2014;14(5):517–25.
27. Reason Reason J. Human error: models and management. BMJ. 2000;320(7237):768–70.
28. Berwick DM. Developing and testing changes in delivery of care. Ann Intern Med. 1998;128:651–6.
29. Plsek PE, Greenhalgh T. Complexity science: the challenge of complexity in health care. BMJ. 2001;323(7313):625–8.
30. Nelson EC, Splaine ME, Batalden PB, Plume SK. Building measurement and data collection into medical practice. Ann Intern Med. 1998;128(6):460–6.
31. Kotter JP, Schlesinger LA. Choosing strategies for change. Harv Bus Rev. 2008; 130–9.
32. Katzenbach JR, Steffen I, Kronley C. Cultural change that sticks. Harv Bus Rev. 2012; 110–7.
33. Sa Couto J. Project management can help to reduce costs and improve quality in health care services. J Eval Clin Pract. 2008;14(1):48–52.
34. Godfrey MM, Andersson-Gare B, Nelson EC, Nilsson M, Ahlstrom G. Coaching interprofessional health care improvement teams: the coachee, the coach and the leader perspectives. J Nurs Manag. 2014;22(4):452–64.
35. Furman C, Caplan R. Applying the toyota production system: using a patient safety alert system to reduce error. Jt Comm J Qual Patient Saf. 2007;33(7):376–86.
36. Weaver SJ, Lubomksi LH, Wilson RF, Pfoh ER, Martinez KA, Dy SM. Promoting a culture of safety as a patient safety strategy: a systematic review. Ann Intern Med. 2013;158(5 Pt 2):369–74.
37. Birenbaum HJ, Dentry A, Cirelli J, Helou S, Pane MA, Starr K, et al. Reduction in the incidence of chronic lung disease in very low birth weight infants: results of a quality improvement process in a tertiary level neonatal intensive care unit. Pediatrics. 2009;123:44–50.
38. Nowadzky T, Pantoja A, Britton JR. Bubble continuous positive airway pressure, a potentially better practice, reduces the use of mechanical ventilation among very low birth weight infants with respiratory distress syndrome. Pediatrics. 2009;123(6):1534–40.
39. Merkel L, Beers K, Lewis MM, Stauffer J, Mujsce DJ, Kresch MJ. Reducing unplanned extubations in the NICU. Pediatrics. 2014;133(5):e1367–72.
40. Horbar JD. The vermont oxford network: evidence-based quality improvement for neonatology. Pediatrics. 1999;103:350–9.
41. Payne NR, LaCorte M, Karna P, Chen S, Finkelstein M, Goldsmith JP, et al. Reduction of bronchopulmonary dysplasia after participation in the Breathsavers Group of the Vermont Oxford Network Neonatal Intensive Care Quality Improvement Collaborative. Pediatrics. 2006;118(Suppl 2):S73–7.
42. Horbar JD, Carpenter JH, Buzas J, Soll RF, Suresh G, Bracken MB, et al. Collaborative quality improvement to promote evidence based surfactant for preterm infants: a cluster randomised trial. BMJ. 2004;329:1004.
43. Payne NR, Finkelstein MJ, Liu M, Kaempf JW, Sharek PJ, Olsen S. NICU practices and outcomes associated with 9 years of quality improvement collaboratives. Pediatrics. 2010;125(3):437–46.
44. Lee SK, Aziz K, Singhal N, Cronin CM, James A, Lee DS, et al. Improving the quality of care for infants: a cluster randomized controlled trial. CMAJ. 2009;181:469–76.

45. Walsh M, Laptook A, Kazzi SN, Engle WA, Yao Q, Rasmussen M, Buchter S, Heldt G, Rhine W, Higgins R, Poole K, National Institute of Child Health and Human Development Neonatal Research Network. A cluster-randomized trial of benchmarking and multimodal quality improvement to improve rates of survival free of bronchopulmonary dysplasia for infants with birth weights of less than 1250 grams. Pediatrics. 2007;119(5):876–90.
46. Fisher D, Cochran KM, Provost LP, et al. Reducing central line-associated blood stream infections in North Carolina NICUs. Pediatrics. 2013;132(6):e1664–71.
47. Kaplan HC, Lannon C, Walsh MC, Donovan EF. Ohio statewide quality-improvement collaborative to reduce late-onset sepsis in preterm infants. Pediatrics. 2011;127:427–35.
48. Wirtschafter DD, Powers RJ, Pettit JS, Lee HC, Boscardin WJ, Ahmad Subeh M, et al. Nosocomial infection reduction in VLBW infants with a statewide quality-improvement model. Pediatrics. 2011;127:419–26.
49. Schulman J, Stricof R, Stevens TP, Horgan M, Gase K, Holzman IR, et al. Statewide NICU central-line-associated bloodstream infection rates decline after bundles and checklists. Pediatrics. 2011;127:436–44.

Chapter 27
Transport of the Sick Infant

Joanna Behrsin and Andrew Leslie

Introduction

Neonatal care models have evolved over time to ensure that the sickest and smallest babies are managed in specialised units, leading to a reduction in mortality and serious morbidity [1]. Development of neonatal transport provision is inherent to this model. In the early days of neonatal transport teams, they consisted of a neonatal doctor/nurse being deployed from a neonatal unit utilising a local transport platform e.g. emergency ambulance. The current norm in many countries, including the United Kingdom, Australia, Canada and the USA, is for transport to be delivered by stand-alone transport services. These may be services that only undertake neonatal transfers or may be combined with paediatric intensive care transport services. The delivery of transport by specialised, trained, designated teams working in services with a robust clinical governance structure has been demonstrated to improve outcomes [2].

There is a wealth of literature that reports an increased rate of mortality and morbidity following ex-utero transfer. There has been debate over many years regarding whether these apparent adverse effects of transfer are real or simply artefacts of selection bias [3–6]. Evidence is beginning to emerge that there are adverse effects of transport; if so, these are likely to be multifactorial, relating to pre-transport stabilisation as well as the risk of exposure to vibration and acceleration forces during transport [3, 7].

J. Behrsin (✉)
Leicester Neonatal Service, Leicester Royal Infirmary and CenTre Neonatal Transport, Leicester, UK
e-mail: Joanna.Behrsin@uhl-tr.nhs.uk

A. Leslie
CenTre Neonatal Transport, Leicester, UK
e-mail: Andrew.leslie@uhl-tr.nhs.uk

© Springer Nature Switzerland AG 2020
E. M. Boyle, J. Cusack (eds.), *Emerging Topics and Controversies in Neonatology*, https://doi.org/10.1007/978-3-030-28829-7_27

The risks of neonatal transport may be divided into several areas, each of which is covered in more detail below:

- Physiological effects of transport on the newborn;
- Working in the transport environment;
- Limitations of transport equipment to deliver optimal mobile intensive care;
- Communication between referring unit, receiving unit, and transport team;
- Skill-mix of staff undertaking transport and stabilising the infant in the referring centre.

Physiological Effects of Transport on the Newborn

This section reviews the additional physiological challenges for transported infants compared to those that are inborn in a tertiary centre. These are:

- Thermoregulation;
- Exposure to vibration and acceleration forces;
- Exposure to sound;
- Effect of altitude.

Thermoregulation in Neonatal Transport

Thermoregulation for the baby during neonatal transport can pose a challenge. The baby is exposed to a variety of temperatures within the transport episode when moving from the neonatal unit into the vehicle and vice-versa. Preterm babies are particularly susceptible to issues with thermoregulation due to their lack of both white fat (source of insulation) and brown fat (thermogenically active). It is well established that maintaining normothermia in preterm babies on the NICU improves survival [8] and poor temperature control in transported infants is associated with increased risk of death [9] Moreover hypothermia increases the risk of other morbidity, including worsening respiratory distress syndrome due to inactivation of surfactant, pulmonary hypertension and hypoglycaemia [10].

There are various strategies that can be implemented both in the transport setting and in the neonatal intensive care unit (NICU) to optimise thermoregulation. Heat loss may occur via conduction, convection, evaporation and radiation. There are strategies that can be put in place to minimise each of these modes. The use of incubator covers and heated humidified incubators reduces heat loss. Insulators such as "bubble-wrap" and chemical gel packs (Transwarmer ®) also have a role to play. Heat loss not only occurs through the skin but also via the airway. This can be reduced by the use of humidified gases [11]. Deploying staff for transport who are specifically trained and experienced in minimising these temperature challenges improves the rate of temperature stability for infants [12].

Exposure to Vibration and Acceleration Forces

During neonatal transport infants are exposed to rapid acceleration and deceleration forces. This can lead to a sudden shift in arterial or venous cerebral perfusion which is a risk factor for intraventricular haemorrhage in preterm babies. It is reported in the literature that there is an increased incidence of intraventricular haemorrhage in extremely preterm infants undergoing transport [6].

The infant is also exposed to significant vibration force during neonatal transport. This is dependent on both speed and road conditions. The effects of vibration from the road may be attenuated by the locking mechanisms used to secure the trolley in the ambulance safely [13]. Studies have shown that vibration exposure in the ambulance can exceed 0.5 m/s^2 (this is the "action value" threshold for adults in the workplace according to EU regulations) [14]. The effects of vibration do not improve with the addition of gel or sponge mattresses. In addition to the vibrational forces that vary with speed, road traffic accidents are more prevalent and lead to higher injury rates when lights and sirens are used. Emergency driving should be restricted to conditions where the reduction in journey time is likely to lead to demonstrable clinical benefit [15–17].

Exposure to Sound

There is international guidance regarding noise exposure in a NICU. It is recommended that noise levels do not exceed 50 db [18, 19]. The transport environment (both road and air) has been shown to be noisier than the intensive care setting. During the acceleration phase of aircraft take-off sound levels may almost double this limit [20].

There are measures that can be utilised to reduce noise. These include: incubator covers and ear muffs although these may only have a limited effect (Fig. 27.1).

More collaborative research between transport services, vehicle providers and medical equipment companies is needed in the future to develop transport systems that use technologies in the design that dampens exposure to noise and vibration as well as developing adjuncts such as effective ear protection and infant harnesses to address this issue.

Effect of Altitude

There are also particular risks of air transport for the newborn [21]:

- Risk of hypoxia—the barometric pressure decreases with altitude leading to a reduction in the partial pressure of oxygen and hence risk of hypoxia (Dalton's law). During stabilisation of the infant requiring air transport, it is important to be aware of this and ensure that oxygen delivery is optimised by maintaining an appropriate haemoglobin concentration and systemic blood pressure.

Fig. 27.1 Incubator covers and ear protectors are strategies to reduce noise during neonatal transport

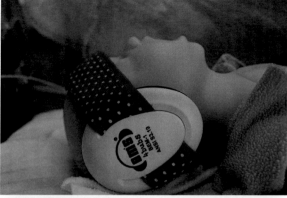

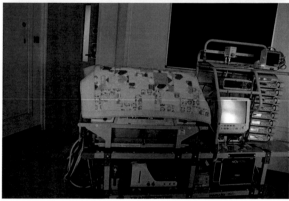

- Risk of air leak—air expands at increasing altitudes due to a reduction in baro-metric pressure (Boyle's law).This means that small air leaks at sea level may expand and have potential to cause significant clinical symptoms, for example, due to a tension pneumothorax. Any trapped air liable to cause a pneumothorax must be drained.
- Thermoregulation—temperature decreases with altitude and it is well documented that cold stress leads to worse outcomes [8, 9]. As in ground transport, the use of incubator covers, Transwarmers®, bubble-wrap and hats may improve the ability to maintain a normal body temperature during air transport.

These risks need to be balanced against potential benefits of air transport where the ride may be faster and smoother than a ground transfer.

Working in the Transport Environment

Working in the transport environment is challenging. Space is cramped, especially in a fixed wing aircraft or helicopter, making interventions and procedures difficult. The environment is noisy, which can have an impact on team work and communication.

The motion of the vehicle can lead to travel sickness which may manifest as vomiting or lethargy affecting physical abilities and decision making.

There is limited access to diagnostic equipment in the vehicle and the availability of resources in the referring centre can be varied. Some transport teams have developed innovative processes involving telemedicine and portable diagnostic equipment to perform investigations, for example echocardiography and cranial ultrasound [22]. In addition to these quantifiable challenges, there are also human factors issues that are increasingly well-understood and which require strategies to minimise their impact. For transport service staff key challenges include working in isolation apart from the usual sources of help, support and advice available on the NICU, and assuming responsibility for complex, unstable patients where the quality of the handover of information is critical [23].

The goal of the transport team is to ensure that neonates are transported when they are stable. There are rare situations, for example, transposition of the great arteries with an intact septum, where rapid transport to a specialist centre for life-saving intervention outweighs the risk of transporting an unstable infant.

Limitations of Transport Equipment to Deliver Mobile Intensive Care

The objective of transport equipment is to provide a mobile intensive care unit offering care that is as similar as possible to that on the neonatal unit. There are significant challenges to achieving this in practice. The statutory framework that regulates medical equipment in the European Union has evolved over time so that there is now an expectation that equipment should be demonstrably fit-for-purpose. For neonatal critical care transport this means equipment should be tested and approved for both neonatal intensive care use and for use in the transport environment. The market for transport equipment is small, so this, plus the additional regulatory complexities are tending to mitigate against innovation in this area. It is often some years after a new technology becomes available for NICU use that a transport-approved iteration arrives on the market.

The transport trolley needs to support an incubator and have space to carry gas cylinders. There needs to be equipment for respiratory support as well as monitoring equipment, and portable suction and infusion pumps. Devices for administering inhaled nitric oxide and providing servo-controlled therapeutic hypothermia in transit are also necessary (Fig. 27.2).

It is not possible to simply bolt the same equipment used on the neonatal intensive care onto a transport trolley as it is paramount that these are shown to be safe for use in a transport environment and risk assessed. Many pieces of equipment now have a specialist CE mark to demonstrate that they are safe to use in the transport setting. There are British/European standards detailing the requirements [24, 25].

These standards offer guidance on both mechanical and electrical safety and are an important framework to protect patients and staff. The weight of the equipment is critical and designs should strive to be as light as possible and securely attached

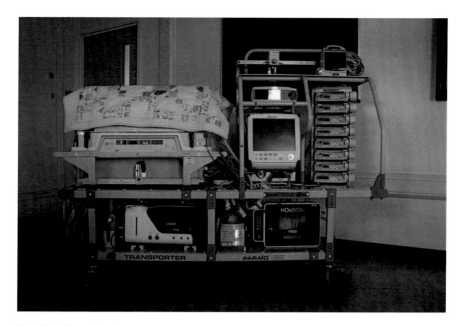

Fig. 27.2 Example of neonatal transport equipment permission from CenTre neonatal transport service, UK

to the trolley so that it will not move in transit and cause injury to staff or the baby. The increasing use of electrical equipment in transport that has high power requirements, such as oscillatory ventilators, active humidifiers and servo-controlled cooling machines, means that the power available in transit needs careful planning.

Respiratory Support During Neonatal Transport

There are a range of respiratory support modalities available on the NICU including low flow nasal cannula oxygen, high flow nasal cannula oxygen, continuous positive airway pressure (CPAP) and other modes of non-invasive respiratory support, various synchronised and non-synchronised modes of mechanical ventilation including volume targeted techniques and high frequency oscillatory ventilation (HFOV). More recently, high-flow nasal cannula oxygen has been shown to be used safely in the transport environment [26]. The use of transcutaneous CO_2 as well as saturation monitoring can be used to guide ventilation weaning during transport. End-tidal CO_2 has utility as a breath-by-breath indicator of tracheal intubation but has repeatedly been shown not to be a useful guide to ventilation status or trends in neonatal patients [27, 28].

Traditionally transport teams used gas driven ventilators such as the Babypac® (Smiths Medical), these had advantages in that they were robust, light and did not

Table 27.1 How to calculate the number of cylinders required for transport

Gas requirements for transfer [32]
The oxygen requirements (in L) of a baby can be estimated from the formula: Flow delivered (L/min) × FiO$_2$ × journey time (min) × 2
How long a cylinder supply will last may be estimated from the formula: Cylinder contents (L)/gas consumption (L/min)
Oxygen cylinder capacity (L)
E = 680   G = 3400 F = 1360   J = 6800

require a battery and so were unlikely to fail. However, because these ventilators are only able to deliver asynchronous, non-triggered, pressure limited, time cycled ventilation there has been a trend over the last 10 years to use more sophisticated modes of ventilation in transit. There is emerging evidence that volume-targeted ventilation, which is commonly used on the NICU can reduce the incidence of hypocarbia, air-leaks and bronchopulmonary dysplasia [29]. Modern transport ventilators enable transport teams to monitor the minute ventilation and other ventilatory parameters during transport enabling clinicians to assess variation in pulmonary mechanics and adjust the ventilation accordingly [30]. This may improve problems that can occur in transport such as hypocarbia, which has an impact on cerebral perfusion and has been shown to be a risk factor for intraventricular haemorrhage and periventricular leukomalacia. Whilst this technology has been available for several years, it is not yet the routine practice. A survey by Bhat et al. in 2015 reported that only 40% of UK transport teams have equipment available on transport systems to monitor parameters such as tidal volume during transport [31].

Consideration needs to be undertaken around gas and power consumption when using more modern ventilators as, at times, these can be so large as to make their use in transport impractical. Transport teams need to be able to titrate FiO$_2$ according to need from air to 100% FiO$_2$ and must carry enough gas for the duration of the journey, but also allowing extra in case of unpredictable delays in journeys. Table 27.1 shows cylinder capacity and gas requirement calculations for transfer to facilitate this.

Managing the Baby with Difficult Oxygenation/Ventilation During Transport

It is possible to use high frequency oscillation ventilation(HFOV) for babies during transport. The use of this modality, together with the availability of inhaled nitric oxide (iNO) for oxygenation difficulties associated with persistent pulmonary hypotension, means that it is possible to transport sicker babies safely for ongoing intensive care. In the first 6 months of 2018 in the UK there were 154 infants transferred on nitric oxide by neonatal transport teams and 48 infants transferred while receiving HFOV. Some of these transfers were for babies requiring Extracorporeal Membrane Oxygenation (ECMO).

Table 27.2 ECMO referral criteria

Criteria for an ECMO referral [32, 36]
1. A neonate with an OI of >30–35 on optimal treatment for 4 h, or >25 on iNO
2. An infant or child with a pneumonia/air leak/ARDS and an OI of >25 (assuming no right to left shunt)
3. An arterial CO_2 tension of >12 KPa for more than 3 h despite optimal treatment

The UK collaborative ECMO trial group publications have provided key evidence of the benefit of neonatal ECMO in reducing mortality and severe disability in neonates compared to conventional therapy [32, 33, 35]. The commonest respiratory ECMO indications in neonates are congenital diaphragmatic hernia (30%), meconium aspiration syndrome (25%) and persistent pulmonary hypertension (20%) [36].

An oxygenation index (OI) of 40 or greater has traditionally been considered the threshold for instituting neonatal ECMO support, but recent evidence suggests that earlier initiation of ECMO when the OI is between 25 and 40 may lead to a shorter hospital stay and a trend to improved outcomes. More recently it has been possible to initiate ECMO treatment by a specialised mobile ECMO team in the referring centre. This affords advantages in terms of earlier respiratory and cardiovascular support and seems to outweigh the risks of cannulation in an unfamiliar environment and transport of a patient on an ECMO circuit [34] (Table 27.2).

Transporting the Infant with Hypoxic Ischaemic Encephalopathy Requiring Therapeutic Hypothermia

There have been numerous randomised controlled trials demonstrating the benefits of therapeutic hypothermia on survival and neurodevelopmental outcome for treating babies who have sustained an hypoxic ischaemic insult at birth and meeting specific criteria [37, 38]. This involves reduction in body temperature to 33–34 °C. There is a critical window of 6 h when this treatment is most effective and may be of even greater benefit if the baby achieves this target temperature sooner [39]. Therapeutic hypothermia is usually delivered in specialised 'cooling' centres, necessitating postnatal transfer of babies that require this treatment. Options for achieving cooling in transport are passive cooling [40], active cooling using adjuncts such as refrigerated gel packs [41] or servo-controlled active cooling using devices such as Techotherm® (inspiration healthcare) or Criticool mini® (Charter Kontron). Recent evidence suggests that target temperature may be achieved sooner when servo-controlled hypothermia is used during transport [42–44] (Fig. 27.3).

Achieving target temperature within 6 h is challenging for referring units and transport teams and is affected by multiple factors:

- Timing of recognition of babies that meet cooling criteria by the referring centre;

Fig. 27.3 Example of active cooling in transport (Criticool mini® Charter Kontron)

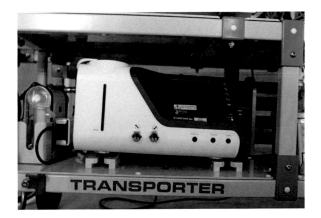

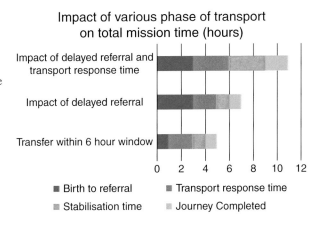

Fig. 27.4 Model of phases of transport to illustrate the various phases where delay may occur which may impede the possibility of achieving target temperature by 6 h of life

Impact of various phase of transport on total mission time (hours)

- Impact of delayed referral and transport response time
- Impact of delayed referral
- Transfer within 6 hour window

0 2 4 6 8 10 12

■ Birth to referral   ■ Transport response time
■ Stabilisation time   ■ Journey Completed

- Lack of availability of servo-controlled active cooling in smaller centres that primarily deliver low dependency neonatal care;
- Age at referral to the transport service;
- Speedy mobilisation of the transport team (dispatch time);
- Choice of mode of transport to reach the referring unit in a timely manner.
- Availability of servo-controlled cooling devices with the transport team.

In order to ensure appropriate infants are in target temperature within a 6 h window there must be prompt recognition by the cooling centre that the infant requires transport and timely referral to the transport service. The transport service needs to have adequate resource to promptly dispatch a team and choose a mode of transport that enables them to mount a timely response. Efficient stabilisation and packaging of the patient is then necessary to ensure the team can travel safely to the cooling centre [44]. Data modelling to demonstrate this concept is shown in (Fig. 27.4). Should the referral be delayed it is extremely challenging for a transport service to achieve cooling within a 6 h window this effect is further potentiated if there are delays in mobilising a transport team.

Active cooling in transit is commonplace in the UK with the referral time, transport response times and time taken to set up cooling equipment on the baby are now the only logistical factors in play to achieve target temperature in this group of babies. There is debate about whether it is appropriate to equip centres with low dependency facilities only with cooling equipment. Whilst this might ensure achievement of target temperature before arrival of the transport team, there are issues of maintaining training, familiarization and skills to be considered in centres that would rarely require this facility.

In the UK the majority of transport teams move infants using servo-controlled active cooling. Of 229 babies transferred using active cooling and in 154 (81%) of these, target temperature was achieved by 6 h [45].

Transferring such babies can be complex. Many will have difficulties in ventilation due to co-morbidities such as meconium aspiration, some of whom will have persistent pulmonary hypertension also requiring inhaled nitric oxide. These babies often have multi-organ failure requiring careful fluid management and inotropes. Disseminated intravascular coagulation is also not uncommon, posing the need for administration of blood products to correct clotting and platelet abnormalities.

Communication Between Referring Unit, Receiving Unit and Transport Teams

The transport process is complex and requires interaction between the referring clinicians, transport team, receiving clinicians and sometimes other specialists such as cardiologists or paediatric surgeons (Fig. 27.5). It is imperative that, from the first contact with the transport service, there are clear lines of communication and there is a streamlined process in place to enable an informed decision around securing a cot in an appropriate centre and any stabilisation that will be required from the referring team before arrival of the transport team.

Utilising a call conference facility makes this process more efficient and reduces risks of miscommunication. It also enables multidisciplinary discussion, which is helpful when discussing complex transfers and sensitive issues such as whether it is in a baby's best interests to continue intensive care due to a life-limiting diagnosis. If there is ability to record calls then this is valuable to feed into the clinical governance processes to review management of cases at a later stage.

The transport team is the intermediary between the referring team and the receiving team. Handover is a key part of the transport process ensuring that the transport team are familiar with the baby's care pathway to date and are able to plan stabilisation interventions prior to departure and to pass on the appropriate relevant information that will influence the baby's care in the receiving unit. Handover tools such as 'SBAR' (Situation, Background, Assessment, Recommendations) may be helpful here to facilitate effective handover.

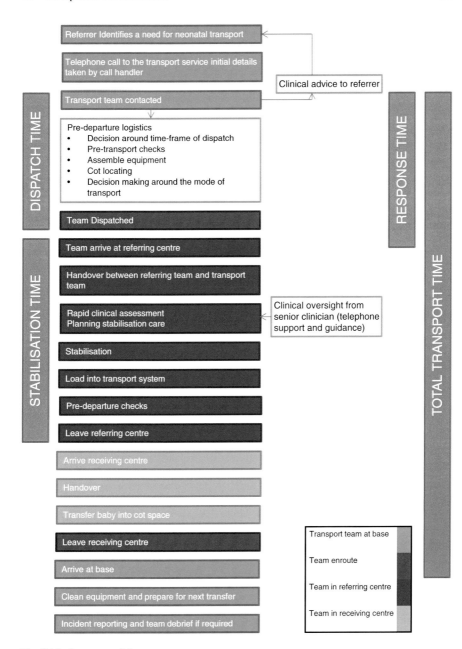

Fig. 27.5 Summary of the transport process

Decision Making Around Inutero and Exutero Transfers Is Complex

In Utero *Transfers*

Where possible, transfer of the mother before birth is preferable to transfer of the baby after birth. Organising an *in-utero* transfer (IUT) requires close working between obstetric, midwifery and neonatal teams to ensure that the woman is medically fit for transfer and that there is appropriate capacity and resources at the receiving hospital to manage obstetric care, delivery and neonatal care. The availability of transport resources (e.g. midwifery staff, vehicles and ambulance personnel) is also key.

There are several potential barriers to suboptimal rates of IUTregionally [46]:

- Birth before arrival at hospital or acute presentation in established labour meaning delivery is imminent;
- Suboptimal triage around the risks of preterm birth in transit;
- Lack of maternity or neonatal intensive care beds in tertiary services;
- Lack of availability of maternal transport capacity (both emergency vehicles and midwifery staff);
- Over-reliance on neonatal retrieval services as a substitute for IUT

Data from Victoria, Australia, demonstrate that births before arrival at hospital account for 4–5% of all out-born births below 32 weeks of gestation and being born extremely preterm (below 28 weeks) is associated with 4.8 times the risk of neonatal death compared to being born in hospital [47]. Threatened preterm labour is the commonest reason for IUT and this generates anxiety about the consequences for the infant of delivering en-route. Reviewing the literature the rate of this occurrence is low. Stewart [46] reports three births during IUT in Victoria, Australia in a 17 year period (2000-2017), which included more than 10,000 high risk transfers. Capacity of neonatal and maternity services is an important factor governing the ability to undertake IUT. This is compounded by the fact that in many cases a women will be transferred and may not deliver until much later. In some studies figures of 30% of women not delivering within 7 days after IUT have been reported [48, 49].

In the UK, IUT is poorly understood. Data on numbers of IUT and the outcomes of those transfers are scarce and often incomplete. There appears to have been little interest from policy-makers on how to increase the appropriate use of IUT to ensure infants are born in the right place while also aiming to decrease the inappropriate use of IUT to manage lack of capacity on neonatal units. The interests and concerns of the obstetric and neonatal specialities are at times not well-aligned [50].

Role of a "Flying-Squad" to Attend Births in Neonatal Transport

There is some evidence to suggest that dispatch of a specialised transport team to attend preterm deliveries and stabilise the infant may improve the outcomes of out-born babies [51, 52]. However there is still significant risk for the infant associated with neonatal transport compared to IUT.

Australian data demonstrates that the presence of a highly-skilled transport team present at the time of birth improves the quality of neonatal resuscitation by increasing intubation success rate, improving thermoregulation and achieving earlier vascular access [51]. The benefits of such an approach will vary depending on the infrastructure of neonatal care within that healthcare system and the relative distances between units providing care.

Transport Team Skill-Mix

Transport services need to be organised to ensure that the frontline staff transferring a baby have the appropriate competence to safely and effectively carry out the transport. There is a diverse multifaceted range of competencies that are required which can be divided up into a number of domains (Fig. 27.6). These are not mutually exclusive but are inherently interlinked. It is essential that the team provides a skill-mix to perform transport safely and efficiently [53].

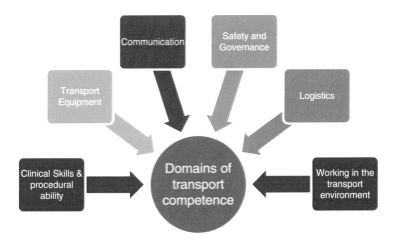

Fig. 27.6 Domains of competence for transport teams

An argument could be made for all staff to possess all the competencies required to do safe transport (cross-over training), particularly when reviewing equipment competencies to facilitate team performance [53]. however it may not be practical for all team members to develop the full range of competencies prior to undertaking transport, particularly if there are rotational staff members that have a fixed term contract of employment with the transport service e.g. a 6 months medical placement. A more sustainable model is to identify which are the essential core competencies for all staff and those which are dependent on the staff members' role.

Core competencies should include familiarity with equipment and knowledge of policies and procedures relating to the transport service. However there may be variances in the level of competence to be achieved depending on the role of the staff member. For example, doctor/ANNP must be able to perform endotracheal intubation, whereas a nurse may not need this skill.

The following are the essential prerequisites for a member of a transport team

- Procedural competence appropriate to role e.g.– chest drain insertion, endotracheal intubation, umbilical arterial and venous catheter placement, peripheral venous and arterial access, intra-osseous needle insertion;
- Familiarity with transport equipment;
- Ability to complete appropriate documentation;
- Generic skills of multidisciplinary team working, leadership and communication;
- Newborn resuscitation skills;
- Knowledge based competencies relevant to neonatal care within a transport setting and practitioner role (i.e. previous appropriate nursing, medical or advanced nurse practitioner experience of neonatal intensive care).

These competences are very much "entry-level" i.e. should be completed by all staff prior to embarking on a transport. Hence it is essential that all staff have appropriate orientation to the transport service before embarking on transport. There is a role for supervised transport experience by more senior members of the team during this process. It cannot be assumed that, because individuals have an appropriate skill-set to work in the NICU environment, this is directly transferrable to the transport setting. A survey of paediatric trainees in the United Kingdom in the 1990s demonstrated that many training-grade paediatricians lacked both the experience and training in transporting critically ill neonates. This was a factor that was found to affect their confidence in transferring sick neonates [53, 54].

The preparation of staff attending transfers has improved as transport has emerged as a sub-speciality. In the UK and elsewhere the role of the transport nurse is well-established and their attendance on neonatal transfers is near-universal. There is diversity in how medical skills are provided. There is a trend away from doctors-in-training being the sole providers of medical skills. They have been replaced by advanced neonatal nurse practitioners in some places and also by more senior doctors—in 2018 in the UK more than half (8/15) of transport services reported they had Consultants Neonatologists available at all times to attend transfers, an increase from 24% in 2013 [45].

The Challenges of Pre-transport Stabilisation by Referring Units

One of the challenges of managing a healthcare system where neonatal intensive care for the smallest infants is centralised is ensuring that there is a team available skilled in providing basic neonatal stabilisation for the smallest and sickest babies requiring intensive care.

This risk can be mitigated to some degree if there is a robust IUT policy [46, 47, 50]. However despite this, there will still be occasions when an unexpected preterm baby delivers in a non-NICU setting.

The development of managed clinical networks as in the UK, may facilitate good care by ensuring that there are standardised guidelines in place. Close working between transport services, clinical networks and centres to provide outreach education and training around stabilisation can aid in local clinicians maintaining skills. Teaching resources such as simulation training and procedural workshops can be useful to deliver this.

In the United Kingdom the Resuscitation Council has developed courses to deliver standardised training in basic newborn life support (NLS) and Advanced Resuscitation of the Newborn Infant (ARNI) which address not only delivery room management but stabilisation in the NICU for critically sick infants [55].

Importance of a Robust Clinical Governance Programme to Reduce Risk in Neonatal Transport

The safe transport of neonatal and paediatric patients requires monitoring of the quality of care delivered during transport and its impact on patient outcomes. The US Institute of Medicine [56] has outlined the elements of a quality health care system, suggesting that care must be safe, timely, equitable, efficient and patient-centred.

A typical clinical governance programme within a transport service will involve critical analysis of transport cases to identify learning to share with the team, regional hospitals and other transport services. Recognition and reporting of risk via an incident reporting processes is also essential as is local audit to drive service development and quality improvement. There should be collection and analysis of feedback from service users (hospitals served by the transport service and parents that have used the service). Development of targeted training programmes to ensure that all staff have appropriate induction and retention of skills as well as delivery of outreach education to hospital staff in the wider region (Fig. 27.7).

Data benchmarking enables transport services to compare workload and transport quality.

The **G**round **A**ir **M**edical q**U**ality **T**ransport (GAMUT) Quality Improvement Collaborative has established definitions for quality metrics in transport and has

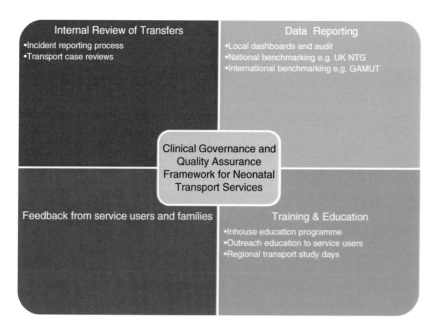

Fig. 27.7 Clinical governance in transport

devolved a database and infrastructure for transport services to track, report and analyse their performance compared to other programmes [57]. In the UK there is a robust system of data collection and benchmarking around neonatal transports performed by the Neonatal Transport Group [45]. There were 7594 transfers carried out by neonatal transport services in the UK between January and June 2018. Transports are categorised into standardised clinical and operational reasons for comparison (Table 27.3).

The dispatch time (time from start of referral call to team mobilisation) and response time (time from referral to arriving at the referring unit) will vary according to the nature of the transfer. For intensive care transfers (BAPM 2011 [58]) the response time standard for the UK is 3.5 h. For time critical transfers in the UK there is a dispatch time standard of 1 h. There are UK standardised definitions of time-critical transfers (Table 27.4). The purpose of the standardised list of time-critical conditions was so that transport services could perform meaningful benchmarking of their response to time-critical referrals in the knowledge that they are comparing like with like. The list includes situations that all UK teams agree should be treated as time-critical. Each service may in addition, have local criteria, but these are not included in the benchmarking data. In 2018 in the UK between January and June there were 315 timecritical transfers and the target of 1 h dispatch was met in 79% of them [45].

In addition to data benchmarking there are international accreditation standards. The Commission on Accreditation of Medical Transport Systems (CAMTS) [59] offers transport services the opportunity to be assessed for compliance against

Table 27.3 Neonatal transport group classifications

Primary clinical reason	Medical	Surgical	Cardiac	Neurological
	e.g. prematurity, sepsis, meconium aspiration	Any surgical specialty other than cardiac or neurological. Includes transfers for surgical review, even if surgery is not scheduled	Known or suspected cardiac abnormality Rhythm disorder PDA	HIE Therapeutic hypothermia Seizures Neuromuscular Intra-cranial haemorrhage
Primary operational reason	**Uplift**	**Resources/capacity**	**Repatriation**	**Outpatients**
	Transfer for care that the referring centre does not normally offer Day care surgery	Capacity (cot spaces) Staffing	Transfer to a centre closer to home "step-down" care	Includes cardiac Echocardiogram Investigations such as EEG or MRI

Table 27.4 Time critical transfer definitions, UK Neonatal Transfer Group 2017

Clinical Criteria for time critical transfers (BAPM and NTG dataset 2017)
1. Gastroschisis
2. Ventilated infant with trachea-oesophageal fistula ± atresia
3. Intestinal perforation
4. Suspected duct-dependent cardiac lesion not responding to prostin
5. Unstable respiratory of cardiovascular failure not responding to appropriate management: This is defined as when despite giving appropriate ventilation via endotracheal tube the infant's respiratory status remains unstable or severely compromised. This includes when: • There is a persistent unstable pneumothorax despite a chest drain insitu   • The infant requires 100% FiO_2 • Arterial oxygen <5 KPa on two consecutive blood gas measurements and pH <7.1 and pCO_2 > 9 KPa   • Persistent mean blood pressure below corrected gestational age (measured on an arterial line) or below corrected gestational age (cuff blood pressure) and metabolic acidosis with a pH <7.1

Note that this list refers only to situations where all transport services agree a time-critical response is necessary, so that like-with-like benchmarking may be undertaken. Operationally, any transfer may be treated as time-critical as decided by the clinical team responding

accreditation standards that demonstrate their service is of a certain quality. The standards address issues of patient care and safety both for air transport (fixed wing and rotary) and ground transport. Each standard has measurable criteria so that a transport service can demonstrate the level of quality delivered against each domain.

Summary

Developments in neonatal transport are leading to the emergence of a distinctive subspecialty. With many healthcare professionals now working in this area, more attention than ever before is being given to how to optimise the services that provide care for infants in transit. A broader understanding is emerging that the effectiveness of every single infant transfer is a result of the development of reliable patient-centred systems of care. In this chapter we have outlined the clinical, engineering, human and organisational factors that have to be accounted-for in the design and delivery of services for this vulnerable group of patients. We have also described the risks of ex-utero transport. Wherever possible process should be implemented to facilitate optimal *in-utero* transport, ensuring that the infant is born in an appropriate centre rather than moving critically ill neonates after delivery [3, 7, 46, 50].

References

1. Gale C, Santhakumaran N, Statnikov M. Impact of manages clinical networks on NHS specialist neonatal services in England: a population based study. BMJ. 2012;344:e2105.
2. Orr RA, Felmet KA, Han Y, et al. Pediatric specialized transport teams are associated with improved outcomes. Pediatrics. 2009;124:40–8.
3. Bowman E, Doyle LW, Murton LJ. Increased mortality of preterm infants transferred between tertiary perinatal centres. BMJ. 1988;297(6656):1098–100.
4. Harding JE, Morton SM. Adverse effects of neonatal transport between level 3 centres. J Pediatr Child Health. 1993;29:146–9.
5. Harding JE, Morton SM. Outcome of neonates transported between level 3 centres depends upon centre of care. J Pediatr Child Health. 1994;30:389–92.
6. Mohamed MA, Aly H. Transport of premature infants is associated with increased risk for intraventricular haemorrhage. Arch Dis Child Fetal Neonatal Ed. 2010;95(6):F403–7.
7. Marlow N, Bennett C, Draper E. Perinatal outcomes for extremely preterm babies in relation to place of birth in England: the EPICure 2 study. Arch Dis Child Fetal Neonatal Ed. 2014;99:F181–8.
8. Silverman WA, Fertig JW, Berger AP. The influence of the thermal environment upon the survival of the newly born premature infant. Pediatrics. 1958;22:876–86. 13600915.
9. Leslie A, Stephenson TJ. Audit of neonatal intensive care transport. Arch Dis Child. 1994;71:F61–6.
10. Bartels DB, Kreienbrock L, Dammann O, et al. Population based study on the outcome of small for gestational age newborns. Arch Dis Child Fetal Neonatal Ed. 2005;90:F53–9. 15613577.
11. Fassassi M, Michel F, Thomachot L, et al. Airway humidification with heat and moisture exchanger in mechanically ventilated neonates. Intensive Care Med. 2007;33:336–43. 17165022.
12. Leslie A, Stephenson TJ. Audit of neonatal intensive care transport—closing the loop. Acta Paediatr. 1997;86:1253–6.
13. Blaxter L, Yeo M, McNally D, Crowe J, Henry C, Hill S, Mansfield N, Leslie A, Sharkey D. Neonatal head and torso vibration exposure during inter-hospital transfer. Proc Inst Mech Eng H. 2017;231(2):99–113.
14. EU Directive 2002/44/EC-vibration. www.osha.europa.eu/en/legislation/directives/19.
15. Auerbach PS, Morris JA Jr, Phillips JB, et al. An analysis of ambulance accidents in Tennessee. JAMA. 1987;258:487–90.
16. Fenton AC, Leslie A, Skeoch CH. Optimising neonatal transfer. Arch Dis Child Fetal Neonatal Ed. 2004;89:F215–9.
17. Hunt RC, Brown LH, et al. Is ambulance transport time with lights and siren faster than that without? Ann Emerg Med. 1995;25(4):507–11.
18. Magnavita V, Arslan E, Benini F. Noise exposure in the neonatal intensive care units. Acta Otorhinolarygol Ital. 1994;14:489–51.

19. Statement AP. Noise: a hazard for the fetus and newborn. Pediatrics. 1997;100:724–7.
20. Buckland L, Austin N, Jackson A, et al. Excessive exposure of sick neonates to sound during transport. Arch Dis Child Fetal Neonatal Ed. 2003;88:F513–6.
21. Skeoch CH, Jackson L, Wilson AM, Booth P. Fit to fly: practical challenges in neonatal transfers by air. Arch Dis Child Fetal Neonatal Ed. 2005;90:F456–60.
22. Carmo K. The history of ultrasound and its use at point of care: neonatal ultrasound in transport. Curr Treat Options Pediatr. 2017;3(4):305–12. https://doi.org/10.1007/s40746-017-0101-0.
23. Senthilkumar R, Corpuz N, Ratnavel N, Sinha A, Mohinuddin S. Adverse events during emergency transfer of neonates performed by a regionalised dedicated transfer service. Arch Dis Child. 2011;96:A91. https://doi.org/10.1136/adc.2011.212562.211.
24. EN 13976-1:2018. Rescue systems—transportation of incubators—part 1: interface requirements.
25. EN 13976-2:2018. Rescue systems—transportation of incubators—part 2: system requirements.
26. Boyle MA, Dhar A, Chaudhary R, Kent S, O'Hare S, Dassios T, Broster S. Introducing high-flow nasal cannula to the transport environment. Acta Paediatr. 2017;106(3):509–12.
27. O'Connor TA, Grueber R. transcutaneous measurement of carbon dioxide tension during long distance transport of neonates receiving mechanical ventilation. J Perinatol. 1998;18(3):189–92.
28. Lilley CD, Stewart M, Morley CJ. Respiratory function monitoring during neonatal emergency transport. Arch Dis Child Fetal Neonatal Ed. 2005;90:F82–3.
29. Klingenberg C, Wheeler KI, MaCallion N, Morley CJ, Davis PG. Volume-targeted versus pressure limited ventilation in neonates. Cochrane Database Syst Rev. 2017;10:CD003666. https://doi.org/10.1002/14651858.
30. Goldsmith J, Karotkin E. Assisted ventilation of the neonate. 5th ed. New York: Elsevier Saunders; 2011.
31. Bhat P, Dhar A, Chaudhary R, O'Hare S, Kent S, Broster S, Curley A. Monitoring respiratory function parameters in ventilated infants during inter-hospital emergency neonatal transport. Arch Dis Child. 2015;100.
32. Barry P, Leslie A, editor. Paediatric and neonatal critical care transport.
33. Extracorporeal Life Support Organization. http://www.elso.org.
34. UK collaborative randomised trial of neonatal extracorporeal membrane oxygenation. UK Collaborative ECMO Trial Group. Lancet. 1996;348(9020):75–82.
35. Bennet CC, Johnson A, Field DJ, Elbourne D. UK collaborative ECMO trial group. UK collaborative randomised controlled trial of neonatal extracorporeal membrane oxygenation: follow-up to age 4 years. Lancet. 2001;357(9262):1094–6.
36. Robinson S, Peek G. The role of ECMO in neonatal and paediatric patients. Paediatr Child Health. 2015;25(5):222–7.
37. Azzopardi D, Brocklehurst P, Edwards D, Halliday H, Levene M, Thorensen M, et al. The TOBY Study. Whole body hypothermia for the treatment of perinatal asphyxial encephalopathy: a randomised controlled trial. BMC Pediatr. 2008;8:17.
38. Gluckman PD, Wyatt JS, Azzopardi D, et al. Selective head cooling with mild systemic hypothermia after neonatal encephalopathy: multicentre randomised trial. Lancet. 2005;365(9460):663–70.
39. Thorensen M, tooley J, Liu X, jary S, Fleming P, Luyt K, et al. Time is brain: starting therapeutic hypothermia within three hours after birth improves motor outcome in asphyxiated newborns. Neonatology. 2013;104(3):228–33.
40. UK TOBY cooling register clinicians handbook. Version 4. 2010. https://www.npeu.ox.ac.uk/downloads/files/tobyregister/Regis-Clinicians-Handbook1-v4-07-06-10.pdf
41. Jacobs S, Morley CJ, Inder TE, et al. Whole-body hypothermia for term and near-term newborns with hypoxic ischaemic encephalopathy. A randomized controlled trial. Arch Pediatr Adolesc Med. 2011;165(8):692–700.
42. Akula VP, Joe P, Thrusu K, Davis AS, Tamaresis JS, Kim S, et al. A randomized clinical trial of therapeutic hypothermia mode during transport for neonatal encephalopathy. J Pediatr. 2015;166(4):856–861.e2.

43. Goel N, Mohinuddin SM, Ratnavel N, Kempley S, Sinha A. Comparison of passive and servo-controlled active cooling for infants with hypoxic-ischaemic encephalopathy during neonatal transfers. Am J Perinatol. 2017;34(1):19–25.
44. Torre Monmany N, Behrsin J, Leslie A. Servo-controlled cooling during neonatal transport for babies with hypoxic-ischaemic encephalopathy is practical and beneficial: experience from a large UK neonatal transport service. J Paediatr Child Health. May 2019;55(5):518–22.
45. United Kingdom Neonatal Transport Group. https://ukntg.net/.
46. Stewart MJ, Smith J, Boland RA. Optimizing outcomes in regionalized perinatal care: integrating maternal and neonatal emergency referral, triage and transport. Curr Treat Options Pediatr. 2017;3:313–26.
47. Boland RA, Davis PG, Dawson JA, Stewart MJ, Smith J, Doyle LW. Very preterm birth before arrival at hospital. Aust N Z J Obstet Gynaecol. 2018;58:197–203.
48. Goh A, Browning Carmo K, Morris J, Berry A, Wall M, Abdel-Latif M. Outcomes of high-risk obstetric transfers in New South Wales and the Australian Capital Territory: the high-risk obstetric transfer study. Aust N Z J Obstet Gynaecol. 2015;55(5):434–9.
49. Hutchinson FH, Davies MW. Time to delivery after maternal transfer to a tertiary perinatal centre. Biomed Res Int. 2014;2014:325919.
50. Gale C, Hay A, Phillip C, Khan R, Santhakamaran S, Ratnavel N. Inutero transfer is too difficult: results from a prospective study. Early Hum Dev. 2012;88(3):147–50.
51. McNamara PJ, Mak W, Whyte HE. Dedicated neonatal retrieval teams improve delivery room resuscitation of outborn premature infants. J Perinatol. 2005;25(5):309–14.
52. Truffert P, Goujard J, Dehan M, Vodovar M, Breart G. Outborn status with a medical neonatal transport service and survival without disability at two years: a population based cohort survey of newborns of less than 33 weeks of gestation. Eur J Obstet Gynaecol Reprod Biol. 1998;79(1):13–8.
53. Ratnaval N. Safety and Governance issues for neonatal transport services. Early Hum Dev. 2009;85:483–6.
54. Davis P, Manktelow B, Bohin S, Field D. Paediatric trainees and the transportation of critically ill neonates: experience, training and confidence. Actapaediatrics. 2001;90:1068–72.
55. Resuscitation Council UK. www.resus.org.uk.
56. US Institute of Medicine. Committee on quality of health care in America; crossing the quality chasm: a new health system for the 21st century. Washington, DC: National Academy Press; 2001.
57. Ground Air Medical Quality Transport Quality Improvement Collaborative. http://gamutqi.org/.
58. https://www.bapm.org/resources/categories-care; 2011.
59. Commission on Accreditation of Medical Transport Systems. http://www.camts.org.

Chapter 28
Neonatal Pain

Ricardo Carbajal

Introduction

Before the 1980s, the reality of neonatal pain was widely unrecognised [1]. A survey published in 1986 on physicians' attitudes toward pain in children found that 40% of responders thought that newborn infants did not experience pain [2]. It was very common before the 1990s for neonates to undergo surgery with minimal anaesthesia, to receive little or no postoperative analgesia, or to undergo numerous painful procedures without consideration of their discomfort or potential long term consequences [1]. In the late 1980s, the seminal work of Anand et al. marked the dawn of a new era in the acknowledgment and management of neonatal pain [3–5].

Anand et al. found, in a randomised controlled trial (RCT), that preterm babies undergoing surgery with minimal anaesthesia mounted major hormonal responses to surgery compared to babies receiving anaesthesia with fentanyl [3]. Compared with the fentanyl group, the non-fentanyl group had increased circulatory and metabolic complications postoperatively.

During the last 25 years, the exponential growth of pain research has led to significant advances in many areas. These include: acknowledgment of the reality of neonatal pain; understanding of pain mechanisms, anatomical and functional development of pain structures; recognition of short and long term consequences of pain; assessment of neonatal responses to pain; and assessment of the efficacy and safety of numerous pharmacological and non-pharmacological interventions to relieve pain. Despite these impressive gains, many of the previously identified and newer

R. Carbajal (✉)
Pediatric Emergency Department, Armand Trousseau Hospital, Paris, France

INSERM UMR 1153, Obstetrical, Perinatal and Pediatric Epidemiology Research Team (EPOPé), Médecine Sorbonne Université, Paris, France
e-mail: ricardo.carbajal@trs.aphp.fr

© Springer Nature Switzerland AG 2020
E. M. Boyle, J. Cusack (eds.), *Emerging Topics and Controversies in Neonatology*, https://doi.org/10.1007/978-3-030-28829-7_28

challenges remain. One of the main reasons for the persistence of suboptimal neo-natal pain management is the large gap that exists between published research results and routine clinical practice [6].

Proven and safe therapies are currently under-used for routine minor, yet painful procedures as well as for continuous or prolonged pain. The prevention and treat-ment of neonatal pain using adequate anaesthetics and analgesics is an essential component of humane and optimal neonatal practice.

Hereafter, the author describes the recent advances in the understanding of the development on neonatal pain, the burden of neonatal pain, the controversial issue of pain assessment, recent data on the long term consequences of neonatal pain, and the current pharmacological and non-pharmacological interventions to treat pain.

Development of the Nociceptive Brain

Pain is a complex experience, has many dimensions and is processed at multiple different levels of the nervous system. It is accepted that a painful experience needs brain encoding of the sensory discriminative, cognitive-evaluative, and motivational-affective components of noxious stimulation. There is no specific area of the cortex for pain perception; rather, noxious stimulation elicits a diffuse pattern of activation in a network of many brain areas, including primary and secondary somatosensory cortices, anterior and mid cingulate cortex, insular cortex, the amygdala, and regions of the prefrontal cortex [7].

The development of this network and its processes in the newborn is currently incompletely understood [7]. It is worth noting that neonatal brain structures do not necessarily need to attain an adult structure to be functional; many temporary struc-tures develop and disappear during development. Thalamocortical connections are considered a requirement for cortical processing of external input. Thalamocortical afferents begin to reach the superficial subplate of the sensory and associative corti-ces by 20–22 weeks of gestation and the cortical plate by 23–26 weeks [8]. Although the anatomical development of limbic structures occurs earlier, the development of their function seems to parallel that of the cortical sensory area [7]. The develop-ment of nociceptive processing in the infant brain has recently been studied using neurophysiological and haemodynamic measures.

Cortical and Behavioural Measures of Pain

Neurophysiological evidence of nociceptive-related brain activity can be obtained non-invasively in human neonates using scalp electroencephalography (EEG).

Slater et al. time-locked an EEG recording to a clinically required heel lance in newborn infants aged 35–39 weeks postmenstrual age and found two consecutive event related potentials (ERP) maximal at the vertex [9]. The first ERP ('tactile') occurs between 100 and 400 ms post stimulation and can be evoked simply by tapping the heel, and therefore it likely represents a sensory response generated by the non-noxious aspects of the lance; the second ERP ('nociceptive') occurs at between 300 and 750 ms and is only present following skin-breaking stimulation [7].

This nociceptive ERP (nERP) does not seem to be related to activity in the somatic motor and autonomic circuits underlying the behavioural and physiological response to procedural pain in neonates, as sucrose administration reduces this activity, but not the nERP [10]. However, little is known about the underlying source of neural activity underlying the nERP, and it is not known whether the nERP magnitude is related to the level of pain experienced [11]. The nERP magnitude cannot therefore be simply interpreted as a measure of pain intensity. In adults, Moureau and Iannetti reported that nERP induced by laser stimulation does not directly reflect nociceptive specific neural activity [12].

Haemodynamic evidence of the development of the nociceptive cortical activity can be obtained non-invasively using near infrared spectroscopy (NIRS) [13, 14] and functional magnetic resonance imagery (fMRI) [15]. These techniques provide an indirect measure of neuronal activation by monitoring changes in blood flow within the brain in response to a stimulus [7]. As with EEG, haemodynamic responses to noxious and non-noxious stimuli are distinguishable with NIRS. Verriotis et al. have recorded NIRS and EEG responses simultaneously in the human infant following noxious heel lances and innocuous tactile cutaneous stimulation in 30 newborn infants. Noxious stimulation elicited a peak haemodynamic response that was ten-fold larger than that elicited by an innocuous stimulus and a distinct nociceptive-specific waveform in electrophysiological recordings [16]. Haemodynamic and electrophysiological responses co-occurred, at an individual level, in only 64% of noxious test occasions [16]. Cortical responses to noxious heel lance recorded with NIRS correlate well with pain behaviours measured using the Premature Infant Pain Profile (PIPP) scale, in particular with the facial component of the scale (correlation coefficient 0.74) [17].

However, cortical pain responses were still recorded in some infants who did not display a change in facial expression. The partial dissociation between cortical and behavioural responses suggests, as with the ERP recorded in EEG studies, that cortical activity is not directly related to the motor circuits underlying behavioural changes [7]. Jones et al. have simultaneously measured nociceptive behaviour (facial expression and PIPP score), brain activity (EEG), and levels of physiological stress (salivary cortisol and high frequency heart rate variability [HF HRV]) in newborn infants of 36–42 weeks of gestation during a heel lance [11].

The time-locked heel lance evoked a nERP with a characteristic N3P3 waveform in 67% of infants; the heel lance also produced characteristic nociceptive facial behaviour in 51% of infants. Numerous studies indicate that behavioural responses to a noxious stimulus are a good reflection of individual pain perception; the correlation found between behavioural responses and cortical activity further support this view. However, as mentioned above, a reduction in pain behaviour is not always accompanied by a reduction in pain-related cortical activity [17]. This had led to the questioning of using behavioural responses alone to assess infant pain [18].

Assessment of Neonatal Pain

The definitions used for pain assessment and management in the adult or older children obviously do not apply to neonates [19]. Thus, clear definitions for descriptors such as acute, persistent, prolonged or chronic pain in the neonate are necessary. Anand has suggested a starting point to better define these terms in neonates [20].

Accurate pain assessment in preterm and term neonates is essential in order to adequately manage pain. The use of analgesics should be guided by the assessment of its necessity and efficacy. Although extensive research has resulted in the availability of an important number of validated tools for assessing neonatal pain, this assessment is challenging in this nonverbal and vulnerable population who do not always display reliable indicators of pain; for example, discrepancies between behavioural and physiological pain indicators have been reported [21]. Based on behavioural and physiological responses to nociception, more than 40 tools have been developed to assess pain in neonates. It is not the purpose of this article to describe these tools and the reader is referred to excellent reviews on the subject [22, 23].

Neonatal intensive care units (NICUs) should choose a limited number of pain assessment tools based on the context of acute, procedural or prolonged pain. The difficulties in neonatal pain assessment is reflected in a recent multicentre study including 243 European NICUs that found that assessment of continuous pain occurred in less than one third of NICU admissions and daily in only 10% of neonates [24]. NICU staff should consider including routine assessments of continuous pain in newborns.

Since behavioural responses do not always correlate with nociception, some authors have suggested the use of multi-modal integrated methods to measure neural and behavioural responses to nociception [25]. This method includes synchronous recording of muscle and central nervous system activity with surface electromyography, scalp electroencephalography and NIRS coupled with behavioural and autonomic responses. Although this approach may be useful for procedural pain, its applicability for continuous pain has not been validated. In the future, "brain-oriented" approaches may provide a more objective measurement of pain in neonates, but in the meantime, validated neonatal pain assessment tools based on behavioural and physiological responses should be implemented in all NICUs, and their ongoing use optimised to form a consistent, reproducible basis for the safe and effective treatment of neonatal pain [26].

Long-Term Consequences of Neonatal Pain

Preterm neonates are particularly vulnerable to procedural stress and pain exposure during neonatal intensive care, at a time of rapid and complex brain development [27]. Given the number of invasive and painful procedures that are performed in these neonates, concerns have been raised regarding the long term effects of neonatal pain on brain development. Painful stimuli can affect the normal development of the CNS in a developing organism [28]. Studies using skin-breaking procedures as a proxy of nociception have shown that repeated neonatal pain leads to poorer cognition [29] and motor function [30], impaired brain development [31, 32] and altered pain responses [33]. As a result of this worrisome association between neonatal pain and adverse neurodevelopmental outcomes, the American Academy of Pediatrics recommends pre-emptive analgesia for moderate to severe pain and invasive procedures [34].

The Burden of Neonatal Pain

Newborn infants routinely undergo painful invasive procedures, even after an uncomplicated birth. The EPIPPAIN study conducted in all NICUs of the Paris region in France showed that neonates experienced a median of 75 (range, 3–364) painful procedures during the first 14 days of admission and 10 (range, 0–51) painful procedures per day of hospitalisation [6]. Regarding the use of analgesia, of all painful procedures, 2.1% were performed with only pharmacological therapy; 18.2% with only non-pharmacological interventions, 20.8% with pharmacological, non-pharmacological, or both types of therapy; and 79.2% without specific analgesia. 34.2% were performed while the neonate was receiving concurrent analgesic or anaesthetic infusions for other reasons [6].

An international systematic review of 18 studies on procedural pain in neonates found an average of 7.5–17.3 painful procedures per neonate per day [35]. The most frequent procedures were heel lance, suctioning, venepuncture and insertion of peripheral venous catheter. Pharmacological and non-pharmacological approaches were inconsistently applied [35].

Premature, or very sick neonates often need tracheal intubation and mechanical ventilation, which are major sources of neonatal pain and distress. A study conducted in 2012–2013 in 243 NICUs from 18 European countries and including 6680 neonates showed that 2142 (32%) neonates were given tracheal ventilation (TV), 1496 (22%) non-invasive ventilation (NIV), and 3042 (46%) were spontaneously breathing (SB) [36]. In the TV, NIV, and SB groups, respectively, 1746 (82%), 266 (18%), and 282 (9%) neonates were given sedation or analgesia as a continuous infusion, as intermittent doses, or both.

Analgesic Treatment

Both non-pharmacological approaches and pharmacological treatments are available for pain management in the neonate. Non-pharmacological interventions have a wide applicability, alone or in combination with pharmacological treatments.

Non-pharmacological interventions and sweet solutions are not necessarily substitutes or alternatives for pharmacological interventions, but rather are complementary [37]. These interventions can reduce pain in neonates indirectly, by reducing the total amount of noxious stimuli to which they are exposed, and directly, by blocking nociceptive transduction or transmission, or by activation of descending inhibitory pathways, or by activating attention and arousal systems that modulate pain [37].

Nonpharmacological Interventions

Prevention

One of the most effective methods for reducing pain in neonates is to prevent it. The least painful procedure is the one that is never performed. "Routine" procedures should be avoided and invasive procedures must only be performed if they are absolutely necessary for the diagnostic and/or therapeutic management of the baby.

In the French Epippain study, a neonate of 26 weeks of gestation underwent 95 heel sticks during the first 14 days after admission to the NICU and several others underwent more than 300 painful procedures during the first 2 weeks of NICU admission [6]. Given the burden that these procedures impose on the neonate, one may ask if all these heel sticks were absolutely necessary. Procedural pain can be minimised by efficient training of staff using indwelling lines for sampling, or by planning procedures so that an analgesic approach can be considered [38]. In some occasions, venepunctures may be preferred to heel lance as the former has also been reported to be less painful than the latter [39–41].

Sweet Solutions

Oral sucrose has been widely studied for relief of procedural pain in neonates. A Cochrane systematic review published in 2016 found that sucrose was effective for reducing procedural pain from single events such as heel lance, venipuncture and intramuscular injection in both preterm and term infants at the doses of 0.5–2.0 mL [42]. However, an optimal dose was not identified due to inconsistencies in effective sucrose dosage among studies. Sucrose was not effective in reducing pain from circumcision. The effectiveness of sucrose for reducing pain/stress from other interventions such as arterial puncture, subcutaneous injection, insertion of nasogastric or orogastric tubes, bladder catheterisation, eye examinations and echocardiography examinations were inconclusive [42]. There is some moderate quality evidence that sucrose, in combination with other non-pharmacological interventions such as nonnutritive sucking, is more effective than sucrose alone. No serious side effects or harms have been documented with this intervention.

The peak effect appears to occur at 2 min and lasts approximately 4 min [43]. Therefore, if the procedure exceeds this duration, another oral administration should be given [44]. Age parameters for efficacy are not very clear. Although sucrose continues to have an effect beyond the newborn period, some data show that this analgesic effect decreases with age and it is very modest at 2 months [45, 46].

Sucrose induced analgesia is triggered by stimulation of taste receptors in the oral cavity and is not due to post-ingestional mechanisms as direct stomach loading of sucrose is ineffective [47]. In animal studies, analgesia induced by sucrose in rats is blocked by systemic injection of opioid receptor antagonists [48, 49]. Regarding the neural circuit involved in sucrose analgesia, Anseloni et al. have found that intra-oral sucrose activates neurons in the periaqueductal gray and nucleus raphe magnus, two key brainstem sites critically involved in descending pain modulation [49].

Oral glucose has also been shown to be effective in reducing procedural pain in neonates during minor procedures; 30% glucose has been shown to be effective both in term neonates during heel stick [50] and during venepunctures [51], and in preterm neonates during subcutaneous injections [52]. A systematic review and meta-analysis found that glucose reduces pain scores and crying during single heel lances and venipuncture [53]. Results indicated that 20–30% glucose solutions have analgesic effects and can be recommended as an alternative to sucrose for procedural pain reduction in healthy term and preterm neonates.

In 2016, the American of Pediatrics issued an updated recommendation stating that oral sucrose and/or glucose solutions can be effective in neonates undergoing mild to moderately painful procedures, either alone or in combination with other pain relief strategies [34]. These recommendations underlined that fact that when sucrose or glucose is used as a pain management strategy, it should be prescribed and tracked as a medication.

Swaddling, "Facilitated Tucking", Touch, and Positioning

Swaddling is defined as an infant securely wrapped in a blanket to prevent the child's limbs from moving around excessively [54]. Facilitated tucking involves firmly containing the infant using a caregiver's hands on both head and lower limbs to maintain a 'folded-in' position. Infants may or may not be wearing clothes [54]. Swaddling has been shown to reduce pain-elicited distress during and after heel stick in neonates [55]. However, A Cochrane review found a very modest analgesic effect [54]. A RCT published in 2018 in preterm infants of 28–32 weeks of gestation concluded that the combined use of facilitated tucking and non-nutritive sucking did not significantly alleviate pain during the heel-stick procedure compared to non-nutritive sucking alone [56].

Nonnutritive Sucking

The pacifying effect of non-nutritive sucking (NNS) has been clearly shown in humans [57]. Recently, a Cochrane review concluded that for preterm infants, sucking is not efficacious in reducing pain reactivity but is effective for immediate pain regulation [54]. An analysis of significant studies suggests that pain relief is maximised if sucking begins at least three minutes prior to the painful stimuli. For term neonates, the results suggest that sucking is effective for pain reactivity and immediate pain regulation [54].

Skin-to-Skin Contact (Kangaroo Care)

Gray et al. found that 10–15 min skin-to-skin contact (SSC) between mothers and their newborns reduces crying, grimacing, and heart rate during heel lance procedures in full-term neonates [58].

A Cochrane review published in 2017 found 25 studies including 2001 infants and concluded that SSC appears to be effective as measured by composite pain indicators with both physiological and behavioural indicators and, independently, using heart rate and crying time. It was also shown to be safe for a single painful procedure in neonates [59].

Breast Feeding Analgesia

Breast feeding maintained throughout a procedure has been shown to be a potent analgesic to relieve procedural pain in term neonates [60–64]. In one study, neonates who were held and breast fed by their mothers during heel lance and blood collection had a reduction in crying of 91% and grimacing of 84%, as compared to infants who had the same blood test while being swaddled in their bassinets [60]. In another study, Carbajal et al. randomised 180 term infants undergoing venepuncture to receive four different analgesic interventions [61]: breast feeding, being held in their mothers' arms without breast feeding, 1 mL of oral placebo (sterile water) prior to venipuncture, and 1 mL of oral 30% glucose plus a pacifier prior to venipuncture. Significant reductions in pain scores were noted for the breast feeding and glucose plus pacifier groups compared to the other two groups. A 2012 Cochrane review, evaluating 10 studies confirmed the analgesic effects of breast feeding for procedural pain [64].

Pharmacological Treatment

Opioids

Opioids are the most common pharmacologic agents used for pain relief in hospitalised infants, with morphine and fentanyl most often used, especially for persistent pain [34]. In a study conducted in 243 European NICUs, opioids were given to invasively ventilated neonates [36]. Morphine and fentanyl were given to 43% and

29%, respectively, of ventilated neonates. Opioids bind to three major groups of membrane receptors in the spinal cord and brain: mu, kappa and delta. Binding to these receptors leads to a decrease in neuronal firing and nociceptive input to the brain [65]. Opioids also interact with local receptors in peripheral tissues. Analgesia is believed to occur after a minimum concentration of opioid is achieved in the serum; however, this minimal concentration may differ within the same patient from day to day [65, 66]. Furthermore, even if current knowledge allows an accurate prediction of serum morphine concentrations [67], we do not know yet the target concentrations at receptors that is needed [68].

The use of opioids for mechanically ventilated neonates has been the subject of considerable debate [34, 69]. Since pain, stress, agitation, irritability, and ventilator asynchrony commonly occur during mechanical ventilation of preterm and full term neonates, systemic analgesia and sedation have been extensively used in ventilated neonates [70]. Neonatal pain relief may, in itself, be a sufficient reason for treatment in the absence of other clinical benefits or adverse effects. However, effective management strategies for pain and sedation during mechanical ventilation remain elusive [34].

A recent systematic review reported that here is insufficient evidence to recommend the routine use of opioids in mechanically ventilated newborns [69]. Opioids should be used selectively, when indicated by clinical judgment and evaluation of pain indicators. Clinicians should be aware that if opioids are used for long periods of time, hyperalgesia may occur. Opioid-induced hyperalgesia has been reported as an explanation for diminished opioid analgesic efficacy in a neonate receiving morphine [71].

Morphine

Morphine is a naturally occurring opioid. It is metabolised primarily to two active compounds, morphine-3-glucuronide (M3G) and morphine-6-glucoronide (M6G) that are renally excreted with the parent compound [65]. M3G is an opioid antagonist whereas M6G is a potent opioid agonist. The relatively inactive M3G is produced as early as day 1 of life in preterm and term neonates, whereas the highly active M6G only appears on day 2; there is no obvious correlation of dose with analgesic/sedative effect during the first days of life, especially in preterm neonates [72]. Thus, the evaluation of pain control must be the primary guide for dosing. Following major neonatal surgery, continuous morphine at the dose of 10 µg/kg per hour or intermittent morphine at 30 µg/kg every 3 h were equally effective [73]. Neonates below 7 days of age had significantly higher morphine plasma concentrations and a lower ratio of M6G/morphine. Neonates who were mechanically ventilated for longer than 24 h had significantly higher morphine plasma concentrations than the spontaneously breathing neonates at 12 h and 24 h after surgery (29.1 vs. 13.1 ng/mL and 26.9 vs. 12.0 ng/mL, respectively).

Fentanyl

Fentanyl is a synthetic opioid that acts as an agonist binding to mu and kappa opioid receptors and has the properties of an analgesic, sedative and anaesthetic [74]. It has an onset of action of 2–3 min, a duration of action of 60 min with bolus doses and minimal haemodynamic effects [75].

Chest wall rigidity may occur with rapid fentanyl IV administration. Fentanyl has a high hepatic extraction ratio, and thus clearance is primarily dependent on hepatic perfusion [76]. Transient rebound in fentanyl plasma levels may occur in some patients, especially with prolonged infusions, reflecting sequestering and subsequent release of fentanyl [76]. Whereas the potency ratio of fentanyl compared to morphine in adults is 80–100 times, in infants it has been reported to be 13–20 times [77]. Tolerance to fentanyl develops rapidly, especially with infusions compared to boluses [75]. Furthermore, the risk of dependence and withdrawal is greater when compared to morphine [78].

Ancora et al. reported in 2013, a multicentre, double-blind, randomised controlled trial in 131 mechanically ventilated infants below 32 weeks of gestation designed to evaluate the analgesic efficacy and safety of continuous fentanyl infusions as compared to fentanyl boluses [79]. They found that continuous infusion of fentanyl does not reduce, in a clinically significant way, the level of prolonged pain as measured by the Échelle de Douleur et d'Inconfort du Nouveau-né (EDIN) scale during mechanical ventilation compared with placebo, when open-label boluses of fentanyl are allowed. However, the incidence of severe prolonged pain, as indicated by an EDIN score of greater than six, was significantly higher in the placebo group compared with the fentanyl group (10.6% vs. 6.8%; p = .003). The incidence of severe procedural pain, indicated by a PIPP score above 12, was higher in the placebo group (19.9% vs. 4.6%; p < .001).

Fentanyl analgesia is associated with fewer sedative or hypotensive effects, reduced effects on gastrointestinal motility or urinary retention, but greater opioid tolerance and withdrawal as compared with morphine [80]. A study compared infusions of fentanyl (1.5 µg/kg/h) versus morphine (20 µg/kg/h) in 163 ventilated neonates and reported similar pain scores, catecholamine responses, and vital signs in both groups [77]. There were no adverse respiratory effects or difficulties in weaning from ventilation in either group, but decreased beta-endorphin levels and gastrointestinal dysmotility occurred more frequently in the fentanyl group [77].

Fentanyl should be used, in a controlled setting, when a rapidly acting opioid is required for analgesia. Other indications include fentanyl analgesia for postoperative pain (following cardiac surgery), or for patients with pulmonary hypertension [80].

Remifentanil

Remifentanil is a synthetic opioid that has a chemical structure similar to that of fentanyl with twice its analgesic potency and an ultra-short duration of action (3–15 min) [80]. It is metabolised by plasma esterases in erythrocytes and tissue fluids; and its excretion is independent of liver and renal function [81].

Remifentanil is mainly used for short procedures such as endotracheal intubation [82, 83], laser surgery for retinopathy of prematurity [84] or for insertion of a percutaneous intravenous central catheter [85].

The analgesic and sedative effects of remifentanil disappear very soon after the infusion is discontinued [68]. Therefore, when used for major surgery, anticipation and replacement by another longer acting opioid or non-opioid analgesic is needed [68].

Long continuous infusions may lead to opioid-induced tolerance or hyperalgesia since these are more frequent with short elimination half-life opioids [68, 86]. Doses used for endotracheal intubation have ranged from 1 to 3 µg/kg [83, 87–89]. For percutaneous intravenous central catheter placement a dose of 0.25 µg/kg/min was more effective than 0.1 µg/kg/min [85]. Remifentanil has also been used for sedation and analgesia in mechanically ventilated neonates with doses around 0.15 µg/kg/min [90].

Paracetamol

Paracetamol (acetaminophen) has analgesic and antipyretic properties, but only very limited peripheral anti-inflammatory activity [91]. It inhibits the COX-2 enzymes in the brain [80]. Based on paracetamol pharmacokinetics in neonates, an oral dose of 25 mg/kg/day in premature neonates at 30 weeks of gestation, 45 mg/kg/day at 34 weeks and 60 mg/kg/day in term neonates has been suggested [91]. It has been suggested that the dosing regimen of intravenous paracetamol in neonates and infants of 32–44 postmenstrual age should consist of a loading dose of 20 mg/kg followed by a maintenance dose of 10 mg/kg every 6 h [92]. The interval between two maintenance doses should be increased up to 12 h if the PMA is below 31 weeks [92].

Paracetamol is not effective in reducing procedural pain (heel lances, retinopathy of prematurity screening) [91], but it is effective for continuous pain. A morphine sparing (66% less) effect of intravenous, but not rectal, paracetamol co-administration after neonatal surgery has been reported [93, 94]. Similarly, intravenous paracetamol was effective for traumatic pain after delivery, while rectal administration failed [95].

Topical Anesthetics

Hospitalised neonates undergo numerous painful skin-breaking procedures [6]. Topical anesthetics that are available for use in the neonate are lidocaine 2.5%-prilocaine 2.5% (Eutectic Mixture of Local Anesthetics—EMLA), tetracaine 4% gel (Ametop™, Pontocaine™), and liposomal lidocaine 4% cream (LMX4™). In the neonate, most research has been conducted with EMLA.

A 2017 Cochrane review evaluated the efficacy and safety of amethocaine and EMLA in preterm and term infants [96]. Only eight small randomised controlled trials met the inclusion criteria. For EMLA, two individual studies reported a statistically significant reduction in pain compared to placebo during lumbar puncture and venepuncture. Three studies found no statistical difference between the groups during heel lancing. For amethocaine, three studies reported a statistically significant reduction in pain compared to placebo during venepuncture and one study reported a statistically significant reduction in pain compared to placebo during cannulation. One study reported no statistical difference between the two groups during intramuscular injection. Two studies reported no methaemoglobinaemia with single application of EMLA. Overall, all the trials were small, and the effects of uncertain clinical significance. Thus, the evidence regarding the effectiveness or safety of these interventions is inadequate to support clinical recommendations. Furthermore, another 2019 review concluded that EMLA reveals minimal benefits in terms of reduction of pain due to venepuncture procedure in comparison with placebo and no benefit in comparison with sucrose and/or breast feeding when used in infants less than 3 months old [97].

Conclusions

The alleviation of pain is a basic need and human right regardless of age. Procedural pain is the principal source of pain in sick or preterm neonates. These neonates experience numerous heel sticks, tracheal aspirations, venous and arterial punctures, gastric tube placements, and tracheal intubations. Epidemiological studies show the need to improve procedural pain management in neonates. Several non-pharmacological and pharmacological interventions are effective in reducing procedural and continuous pain in neonates. Non-pharmacological interventions are simple, feasible, accessible, and can be easily given by those caring for neonates. Using these interventions may also be cost effective because they involve minimal effort and time and may reduce or, in some instances, obviate the need for pharmacological analgesics. Nonetheless, non-pharmacological interventions alone should be used for only minor invasive procedures. For more invasive procedures, potent pharmacological analgesics must be used; this is also true for post-operative or prolonged severe pain.

Although pain assessment is crucial to adequate pain management, studies still show that they are not systematically used, even in very sick neonates receiving potent analgesics. Even if pain assessment is challenging in preterm and term neonates, and controversies exist regarding discrepancies among behavioural, physiological or cortical neurophysiological and haemodynamic measures of pain, validated neonatal pain assessment tools based on behavioural and physiological responses should be implemented in all NICUs.

Excessive nociception and untreated pain have deleterious long term effects in neonates. Thus, the prevention and treatment of neonatal pain is essential.

References

1. Schechter NL, Berde CB, Yaster M. Pain in infants, children, and adolescents: an overview. In: Schechter NL, Berde CB, Yaster M, editors. Pain in infants, children, and adolescents. Philadelphia: Lippincott Williams & Wilkins; 2003. p. 3–18.
2. Schechter NL, Allen D. Physicians' attitudes toward pain in children. J Dev Behav Pediatr. 1986;7(6):350–4.
3. Anand KJ, Sippell WG, Aynsley-Green A. Randomised trial of fentanyl anaesthesia in preterm babies undergoing surgery: effects on the stress response. Lancet. 1987;1(8524):62–6. %U http://www.ncbi.nlm.nih.gov/pubmed/2879174.
4. Anand KJ, Sippell WG, Schofield NM, Aynsley-Green A. Does halothane anaesthesia decrease the metabolic and endocrine stress responses of newborn infants undergoing operation? Br Med J (Clin Res Ed). 1988;296(6623):668–72.
5. Anand KJ, Brown MJ, Causon RC, Christofides ND, Bloom SR, Aynsley-Green A. Can the human neonate mount an endocrine and metabolic response to surgery? J Pediatr Surg. 1985;20(1):41–8.
6. Carbajal R, Rousset A, Danan C, Coquery S, Nolent P, Ducrocq S, et al. Epidemiology and treatment of painful procedures in neonates in intensive care units. JAMA. 2008;300(1):60–70.
7. Verriotis M, Chang P, Fitzgerald M, Fabrizi L. The development of the nociceptive brain. Neuroscience. 2016;338:207–19. Epub 2016/10/27.
8. Kostovic I, Judas M. The development of the subplate and thalamocortical connections in the human foetal brain. Acta Paediatr. 2010;99(8):1119–27. Epub 2010/04/07.
9. Slater R, Worley A, Fabrizi L, Roberts S, Meek J, Boyd S, et al. Evoked potentials generated by noxious stimulation in the human infant brain. Eur J Pain. 2009;14(3):321–6.
10. Slater R, Cornelissen L, Fabrizi L, Patten D, Yoxen J, Worley A, et al. Oral sucrose as an analgesic drug for procedural pain in newborn infants: a randomised controlled trial. Lancet. 2010;376(9748):1225–32. Epub 2010/09/08.
11. Jones L, Fabrizi L, Laudiano-Dray M, Whitehead K, Meek J, Verriotis M, et al. Nociceptive cortical activity is dissociated from nociceptive behavior in newborn human infants under stress. Curr Biol. 2017;27(24):3846–51 e3. Epub 2017/12/05.
12. Mouraux A, Iannetti GD. Nociceptive laser-evoked brain potentials do not reflect nociceptive-specific neural activity. J Neurophysiol. 2009;101(6):3258–69. Epub 2009/04/03.
13. Slater R, Cantarella A, Gallella S, Worley A, Boyd S, Meek J, et al. Cortical pain responses in human infants. J Neurosci. 2006;26(14):3662–6.
14. Bartocci M, Bergqvist LL, Lagercrantz H, Anand KJ. Pain activates cortical areas in the pre-term newborn brain. Pain. 2006;122(1–2):109–17.
15. Goksan S, Hartley C, Emery F, Cockrill N, Poorun R, Moultrie F, et al. fMRI reveals neural activity overlap between adult and infant pain. Elife. 2015;4:e06356. Epub 2015/04/22.
16. Verriotis M, Fabrizi L, Lee A, Cooper RJ, Fitzgerald M, Meek J. Mapping cortical responses to somatosensory stimuli in human infants with simultaneous near-infrared spectroscopy and event-related potential recording. eNeuro. 2016;3(2). Epub 2016/05/21.
17. Slater R, Cantarella A, Franck L, Meek J, Fitzgerald M. How well do clinical pain assessment tools reflect pain in infants? PLoS Med. 2008;5(6):e129.
18. Pillai Riddell R, Fitzgerald M, Slater R, Stevens B, Johnston C, Campbell-Yeo M. Using only behaviours to assess infant pain: a painful compromise? Pain. 2016;157(8):1579–80. Epub 2016/06/10.
19. Anand KJ, Craig KD. New perspectives on the definition of pain. Pain. 1996;67(1):3–6. discussion 209-11.
20. Anand KJS. Defining pain in newborns: need for a uniform taxonomy? Acta Paediatr. 2017;106(9):1438–44. Epub 2017/05/31.
21. Ranger M, Johnston CC, Anand KJ. Current controversies regarding pain assessment in neonates. Semin Perinatol. 2007;31(5):283–8. Epub 2007/10/02.

22. Duhn LJ, Medves JM. A systematic integrative review of infant pain assessment tools. Adv Neonatal Care. 2004;4(3):126–40.

23. de Melo GM, Lelis AL, de Moura AF, Cardoso MV, da Silva VM. Pain assessment scales in newborns: integrative review. Revista paulista de pediatria. 2014;32(4):395–402. Epub 2014/12/17. Escalas de avaliacao de dor em recem-nascidos: revisao integrativa.

24. Anand KJS, Eriksson M, Boyle EM, Avila-Alvarez A, Andersen RD, Sarafidis K, et al. Assessment of continuous pain in newborns admitted to NICUs in 18 European countries. Acta Paediatr. 2017;106(8):1248–59. Epub 2017/03/04.

25. Worley A, Fabrizi L, Boyd S, Slater R. Multi-modal pain measurements in infants. J Neurosci Methods. 2012;205(2):252–7. Epub 2012/01/31.

26. Maxwell LG, Malavolta CP, Fraga MV. Assessment of pain in the neonate. Clin Perinatol. 2013;40(3):457–69. Epub 2013/08/27.

27. Ranger M, Grunau RE. Early repetitive pain in preterm infants in relation to the developing brain. Pain Manage. 2014;4(1):57–67. Epub 2014/03/20.

28. Kesavan K. Neurodevelopmental implications of neonatal pain and morphine exposure. Pediatr Ann. 2015;44(11):e260–4. Epub 2015/11/21.

29. Vinall J, Miller SP, Bjornson BH, Fitzpatrick KP, Poskitt KJ, Brant R, et al. Invasive procedures in preterm children: brain and cognitive development at school age. Pediatrics. 2014;133(3):412–21. Epub 2014/02/19.

30. Grunau RE, Whitfield MF, Petrie-Thomas J, Synnes AR, Cepeda IL, Keidar A, et al. Neonatal pain, parenting stress and interaction, in relation to cognitive and motor development at 8 and 18 months in preterm infants. Pain. 2009;143(1–2):138–46.

31. Anand KJ, Palmer FB, Papanicolaou AC. Repetitive neonatal pain and neurocognitive abilities in ex-preterm children. Pain. 2013;154(10):1899–901. Epub 2013/06/25.

32. Zwicker JG, Grunau RE, Adams E, Chau V, Brant R, Poskitt KJ, et al. Score for neonatal acute physiology-II and neonatal pain predict corticospinal tract development in premature newborns. Pediatr Neurol. 2013;48(2):123–9 e1. Epub 2013/01/23.

33. Taddio A, Katz J, Ilersich AL, Koren G. Effect of neonatal circumcision on pain response during subsequent routine vaccination. Lancet. 1997;349(9052):599–603.

34. American Academy of Pediatrics. Prevention and management of procedural pain in the neonate: an update. Pediatrics. 2016;137(2):1–13. Epub 2016/01/27.

35. Cruz MD, Fernandes AM, Oliveira CR. Epidemiology of painful procedures performed in neonates: a systematic review of observational studies. Eur J Pain. 2016;20(4):489–98. Epub 2015/08/01.

36. Carbajal R, Eriksson M, Courtois E, Boyle E, Avila-Alvarez A, Andersen RD, et al. Sedation and analgesia practices in neonatal intensive care units (EUROPAIN): results from a prospective cohort study. Lancet Respir Med. 2015;3(10):796–812. Epub 2015/10/01.

37. Stevens B, Gibbins S, Franck LS. Treatment of pain in the neonatal intensive care unit. Pediatr Clin North Am. 2000;47(3):633–50.

38. Menon G, Anand KJ, McIntosh N. Practical approach to analgesia and sedation in the neonatal intensive care unit. Semin Perinatol. 1998;22(5):417–24. Epub 1998/11/20.

39. Larsson BA, Tannfeldt G, Lagercrantz H, Olsson GL. Venipuncture is more effective and less painful than heel lancing for blood tests in neonates. Pediatrics. 1998;101(5):882–6.

40. Shah VS, Taddio A, Bennett S, Speidel BD. Neonatal pain response to heel stick vs. venepuncture for routine blood sampling. Arch Dis Child Fetal Neonatal Ed. 1997;77(2):F143–4.

41. Shah VS, Ohlsson A. Venepuncture versus heel lance for blood sampling in term neonates. Cochrane Database Syst Rev. 2011;10:CD001452. Epub 2011/10/07.

42. Stevens B, Yamada J, Ohlsson A, Haliburton S, Shorkey A. Sucrose for analgesia in newborn infants undergoing painful procedures. Cochrane Database Syst Rev. 2016;7:CD001069. Epub 2016/07/16.

43. Barr RG, Quek VS, Cousineau D, Oberlander TF, Brian JA, Young SN. Effects of intra-oral sucrose on crying, mouthing and hand-mouth contact in newborn and six-week-old infants. Dev Med Child Neurol. 1994;36(7):608–18.

44. Stevens B, Yamada J, Lee GY, Ohlsson A. Sucrose for analgesia in newborn infants undergoing painful procedures. Cochrane Database Syst Rev. 2013;(1):CD001069. Epub 2013/02/27.

45. Allen KD, White DD, Walburn JN. Sucrose as an analgesic agent for infants during immunization injections. Arch Pediatr Adolesc Med. 1996;150(3):270–4.

46. Barr RG, Young SN, Wright JH, Cassidy KL, Hendricks L, Bedard Y, et al. "Sucrose analgesia" and diphtheria-tetanus-pertussis immunizations at 2 and 4 months. J Dev Behav Pediatr. 1995;16(4):220–5.

47. Ramenghi LA, Evans DJ, Levene MI. "Sucrose analgesia": absorptive mechanism or taste perception? Arch Dis Child Fetal Neonatal Ed. 1999;80(2):F146–7.

48. Blass E, Fitzgerald E, Kehoe P. Interactions between sucrose, pain and isolation distress. Pharmacol Biochem Behav. 1987;26(3):483–9.

49. Anseloni VC, Weng HR, Terayama R, Letizia D, Davis BJ, Ren K, et al. Age-dependency of analgesia elicited by intraoral sucrose in acute and persistent pain models. Pain. 2002;97(1–2):93–103. Epub 2002/05/29.

50. Skogsdal Y, Eriksson M, Schollin J. Analgesia in newborns given oral glucose. Acta Paediatr. 1997;86(2):217–20.

51. Carbajal R, Chauvet X, Couderc S, Olivier-Martin M. Randomised trial of analgesic effects of sucrose, glucose, and pacifiers in term neonates. BMJ. 1999;319(7222):1393–7.

52. Carbajal R, Lenclen R, Gajdos V, Jugie M, Paupe A. Crossover trial of analgesic efficacy of glucose and pacifier in very preterm neonates during subcutaneous injections. Pediatrics. 2002;110(2 Pt 1):389–93.

53. Bueno M, Yamada J, Harrison D, Khan S, Ohlsson A, Adams-Webber T, et al. A systematic review and meta-analyses of nonsucrose sweet solutions for pain relief in neonates. Pain Res Manag. 2013;18(3):153–61. Epub 2013/06/12.

54. Pillai Riddell RR, Racine NM, Gennis HG, Turcotte K, Uman LS, Horton RE, et al. Non-pharmacological management of infant and young child procedural pain. Cochrane Database Syst Rev. 2015;12:CD006275. Epub 2015/12/03.

55. Campos RG. Soothing pain-elicited distress in infants with swaddling and pacifiers. Child Dev. 1989;60(4):781–92.

56. Perroteau A, Nanquette MC, Rousseau A, Renolleau S, Berard L, Mitanchez D, et al. Efficacy of facilitated tucking combined with non-nutritive sucking on very preterm infants' pain during the heel-stick procedure: a randomized controlled trial. Int J Nurs Stud. 2018;86:29–35. Epub 2018/07/01.

57. Field T, Goldson E. Pacifying effects of nonnutritive sucking on term and preterm neonates during heelstick procedures. Pediatrics. 1984;74(6):1012–5.

58. Gray L, Watt L, Blass EM. Skin-to-skin contact is analgesic in healthy newborns. Pediatrics. 2000;105(1):e14.

59. Johnston C, Campbell-Yeo M, Disher T, Benoit B, Fernandes A, Streiner D, et al. Skin-to-skin care for procedural pain in neonates. Cochrane Database Syst Rev. 2017;2:CD008435. Epub 2017/02/17.

60. Gray L, Miller LW, Philipp BL, Blass EM. Breastfeeding is analgesic in healthy newborns. Pediatrics. 2002;109(4):590–3.

61. Carbajal R, Veerapen S, Couderc S, Jugie M, Ville Y. Analgesic effect of breast feeding in term neonates: randomised controlled trial. Br Med J. 2003;326(7379):13–5.

62. Shendurnikar N, Gandhi K. Analgesic effects of breastfeeding on heel lancing. Indian Pediatr. 2005;42(7):730–2.

63. Phillips RM, Chantry CJ, Gallagher MP. Analgesic effects of breast-feeding or pacifier use with maternal holding in term infants. Ambul Pediatr. 2005;5(6):359–64.

64. Shah PS, Herbozo C, Aliwalas LL, Shah VS. Breastfeeding or breast milk for procedural pain in neonates. Cochrane Database Syst Rev. 2012;12:CD004950. Epub 2012/12/14.

65. Taddio A. Evidence for systemic morphine and fentanyl analgesia. In: Anand KJS, Stevens B, McGrath P, editors. Pain in neonates and infants. 3rd ed. Philadelphia: Elsevier; 2007. p. 141–54.

66. Chay PC, Duffy BJ, Walker JS. Pharmacokinetic-pharmacodynamic relationships of morphine in neonates. Clin Pharmacol Ther. 1992;51(3):334–42.
67. Krekels EH, DeJongh J, van Lingen RA, van der Marel CD, Choonara I, Lynn AM, et al. Predictive performance of a recently developed population pharmacokinetic model for morphine and its metabolites in new datasets of (preterm) neonates, infants and children. Clin Pharmacokinet. 2011;50(1):51–63. Epub 2011/01/01.
68. Allegaert K, Tibboel D, van den Anker J. Pharmacological treatment of neonatal pain: in search of a new equipoise. Semin Fetal Neonatal Med. 2013;18(1):42–7. Epub 2012/10/31.
69. Bellu R, de Waal K, Zanini R. Opioids for neonates receiving mechanical ventilation: a systematic review and meta-analysis. Arch Dis Child Fetal Neonatal Ed. 2010;95(4):F241–51. Epub 2009/06/18.
70. Aranda JV, Carlo W, Hummel P, Thomas R, Lehr VT, Anand KJ. Analgesia and sedation during mechanical ventilation in neonates. Clin Ther. 2005;27(6):877–99. Epub 2005/08/25.
71. Hallett BR, Chalkiadis GA. Suspected opioid-induced hyperalgesia in an infant. Br J Anaesth. 2012;108(1):116–8. Epub 2011/10/25.
72. Pacifici GM. Metabolism and pharmacokinetics of morphine in neonates: a review. Clinics (Sao Paulo). 2016;71(8):474–80. Epub 2016/09/15.
73. Bouwmeester NJ, Hop WC, van Dijk M, Anand KJ, van den Anker JN, Tibboel D. Postoperative pain in the neonate: age-related differences in morphine requirements and metabolism. Intensive Care Med. 2003;29(11):2009–15.
74. Pacifici GM. Clinical pharmacology of fentanyl in preterm infants. A review. Pediatr Neonatol. 2015;56(3):143–8. Epub 2014/09/02.
75. Anand KJ. Pharmacological approaches to the management of pain in the neonatal intensive care unit. J Perinatol. 2007;27(Suppl 1):S4–S11. Epub 2007/04/25.
76. Koehntop DE, Rodman JH, Brundage DM, Hegland MG, Buckley JJ. Pharmacokinetics of fentanyl in neonates. Anesth Analg. 1986;65(3):227–32.
77. Saarenmaa E, Huttunen P, Leppaluoto J, Meretoja O, Fellman V. Advantages of fentanyl over morphine in analgesia for ventilated newborn infants after birth: a randomized trial. J Pediatr. 1999;134(2):144–50.
78. Franck LS, Vilardi J, Durand D, Powers R. Opioid withdrawal in neonates after continuous infusions of morphine or fentanyl during extracorporeal membrane oxygenation. Am J Crit Care. 1998;7(5):364–9. Epub 1998/09/19.
79. Ancora G, Lago P, Garetti E, Pirelli A, Merazzi D, Mastrocola M, et al. Efficacy and safety of continuous infusion of fentanyl for pain control in preterm newborns on mechanical ventilation. J Pediatr. 2013;163(3):645–51 e1. Epub 2013/04/16.
80. Hall RW, Anand KJ. Pain management in newborns. Clin Perinatol. 2014;41(4):895–924. Epub 2014/12/03.
81. Welzing L, Roth B. Experience with remifentanil in neonates and infants. Drugs. 2006;66(10):1339–50. Epub 2006/08/15.
82. Audil HY, Tse S, Pezzano C, Mitchell-van Steele A, Pinheiro JMB. Efficacy, safety, and usability of remifentanil as premedication for INSURE in preterm neonates. Children (Basel). 2018;5(5):63. Epub 2018/05/24.
83. Choong K, AlFaleh K, Doucette J, Gray S, Rich B, Verhey L, et al. Remifentanil for endotracheal intubation in neonates: a randomised controlled trial. Arch Dis Child Fetal Neonatal Ed. 2010;95(2):F80–4. Epub 2010/03/17.
84. Sammartino M, Bocci MG, Ferro G, Mercurio G, Papacci P, Conti G, et al. Efficacy and safety of continuous intravenous infusion of remifentanil in preterm infants undergoing laser therapy in retinopathy of prematurity: clinical experience. Paediatr Anaesth. 2003;13(7):596–602. Epub 2003/09/03.
85. Shin SH, Kim HS, Lee J, Choi KY, Lee JH, Kim EK, et al. A comparative study of two remifentanil doses for procedural pain in ventilated preterm infants: a randomized, controlled study. Pediatr Crit Care Med. 2014;15(5):451–5. Epub 2014/04/11.
86. Allegaert K, Thewissen L, van den Anker JN. Remifentanil in neonates: a promising compound in search of its indications? Pediatr Neonatol. 2012;53(6):387–8. Epub 2013/01/02.

87. Avino D, Zhang WH, De Ville A, Johansson AB. Remifentanil versus morphine-midazolam premedication on the quality of endotracheal intubation in neonates: a noninferiority randomized trial. J Pediatr. 2014;164(5):1032–7. Epub 2014/03/04.
88. Badiee Z, Vakiliamini M, Mohammadizadeh M. Remifentanil for endotracheal intubation in premature infants: a randomized controlled trial. J Res Pharm Pract. 2013;2(2):75–82. Epub 2013/04/01.
89. Crawford MW, Hayes J, Tan JM. Dose-response of remifentanil for tracheal intubation in infants. Anesth Analg. 2005;100(6):1599–604. Epub 2005/05/28.
90. Kamata M, Tobias JD. Remifentanil: applications in neonates. J Anesth. 2016;30(3):449–60. Epub 2016/01/14.
91. Allegaert K, van den Anker JN. Perinatal and neonatal use of paracetamol for pain relief. Semin Fetal Neonatal Med. 2017;22(5):308–13. Epub 2017/07/20.
92. Veyckemans F, Anderson BJ, Wolf AR, Allegaert K. Intravenous paracetamol dosage in the neonate and small infant. Br J Anaesth. 2014;112(2):380–1. Epub 2014/01/17.
93. Ceelie I, de Wildt SN, van Dijk M, van den Berg MM, van den Bosch GE, Duivenvoorden HJ, et al. Effect of intravenous paracetamol on postoperative morphine requirements in neonates and infants undergoing major noncardiac surgery: a randomized controlled trial. JAMA. 2013;309(2):149–54. Epub 2013/01/10.
94. van der Marel CD, Peters JW, Bouwmeester NJ, Jacqz-Aigrain E, van den Anker JN, Tibboel D. Rectal acetaminophen does not reduce morphine consumption after major surgery in young infants. Br J Anaesth. 2007;98(3):372–9. Epub 2007/02/08.
95. Allegaert K, Naulaers G, Vanhaesebrouck S, Anderson BJ. The paracetamol concentration-effect relation in neonates. Paediatr Anaesth. 2013;23(1):45–50. Epub 2012/11/23.
96. Foster JP, Taylor C, Spence K. Topical anaesthesia for needle-related pain in newborn infants. Cochrane Database Syst Rev. 2017;2:CD010331. Epub 2017/02/06.
97. Shahid S, Florez ID, Mbuagbaw L. Efficacy and safety of EMLA cream for pain control due to venipuncture in infants: a meta-analysis. Pediatrics. 2019;143(1):e20181173. Epub 2018/12/28.

Chapter 29
Neonatal Infection

Janet Elizabeth Berrington and Eleri Jayne Williams

Neonatal Infection: Post Millennium But Still Not a Thing of the Past

'Neonatal infection' (occurring in the first 28 days of life) remains a leading cause of neonatal death worldwide [1] and reducing it by two thirds by 2015 was the United Nations Millennium Development Goal number 4, a target that the neonatal community failed to achieve [2]. The historical division into early onset sepsis (EOS) (up to 48–72 h) or late onset sepsis (LOS) (beyond this) remains helpful since aetiology, and thus prevention strategies, differ. Post millennium infection related deaths remain disappointingly high, vary widely country to country and between neonatal intensive care units (NICUs) [3], and vary with gestation and postnatal age [4].

Recent rates of EOS are between one and seven cases per 1000 live births in high income countries [5]. Late onset rates (within NICUs at all gestations) range from 0.61% (Japan [6]) to 13.9% in the Netherlands [7] and for preterm or very low birth weight (<1500 g; VLBW)) infants are up to 25% in the USA [8]. In lower income countries, the overall burden of EOS and LOS is significantly more difficult to ascertain with certainty, but importantly higher [9].

J. E. Berrington (✉)
Department of Neonatology, Newcastle upon Tyne Hospitals Foundation Trust, Newcastle upon Tyne, UK

Institute of Cellular Medicine, University of Newcastle, Newcastle upon Tyne, UK
e-mail: janet.berrington@nuth.nhs.uk; j.e.berrington@newcastle.ac.uk

E. J. Williams
Department of Paediatric Infectious Diseases, Newcastle upon Tyne Hospitals Foundation Trust, Newcastle upon Tyne, UK
e-mail: eleri.williams@nuth.nhs.uk

© Springer Nature Switzerland AG 2020
E. M. Boyle, J. Cusack (eds.), *Emerging Topics and Controversies in Neonatology*, https://doi.org/10.1007/978-3-030-28829-7_29

Infection related mortality in high income countries has a changing aetiology in preterm infants [10] but remains higher than desired and proportional to the degree of prematurity [11], disappointingly contributing increasingly to UK deaths in preterm infants [12]: 1 in 10 UK preterm deaths results from infection. Although understanding of mechanisms of adverse neurodevelopmental outcome after infection is better, our ability to prevent lifelong harm to survivors is not [13]. UK data (2013–2015) from a large randomised feeding trial of infants <32 weeks gestation, showed 31% of infants in the trial developed LOS [14]. This is despite many obstetric and neonatal interventions designed to reduce infection (maternal antibiotics, antenatal steroids, central line bundles, promoting breast milk use, hand washing and alcohol gels).

To change the incidence of neonatal infection we must accurately understand rates, variations, associated features, causative organisms and antibiotic use. Currently we lack standardised approaches: information is gathered through observational studies and surveillance mechanisms, and interventional studies, but each is challenging and non-standardised. The complexities involved were highlighted by the need for and development of the STROBE-NI statement (Strengthening The Reporting of Observational studies in Epidemiology for Newborn Infection) [15] designed to increase data utility, facilitate meta-analyses and enable pathogen specific burden estimates as a basis for new interventions. We await its effect. Surveillance mechanisms, an alternate or complimentary approach to observational data also operate in several countries and networks [16], but also lack standardisation, making comparisons difficult, using different mechanisms and definitions. In the UK, Public Health England offers laboratory-based surveillance systems with extremely good capture where an organism is isolated, but little clinical context, and no handle on 'culture negative' infection. Clinically oriented systems are less comprehensive (cases may be completely missed), depending on clinicians to remember and record cases, and determine context, but benefit from this context. Worldwide, at least nine significant surveillance programmes offer a web-based system and publicise rates, organisms, associated risk factors and other key features [16] offering rapid shared exploration of changing aetiology, causative organisms, sensitivity and resistance patterns, and the possibility of shared global learning.

Central line associated blood stream infection (CLABSI) rates are the focus of some of these surveillance reports, and rightly receive considerable attention, with these perhaps most easily prevented as 'matching Michigan' based approaches have shown [17]. Sustaining low rates is challenging though, [18] as is ensuring uniformity of reporting [19]. A question for all NICUs is whether 'zero CLABSI rates' are possible as proposed in adult settings [20]. This challenges our 'acceptance' that infection is inevitable for some, usually the most preterm, sick, or surgically treated infants, who have least reserve for the additional burden of infection, but the highest rates. Risk reviewing individual cases could promote zero tolerance, as would easy open access to individual unit rates through well-moderated systems with clear denominator and case descriptions, which could now be achieved through national electronic data collection systems, available in real time. A step towards this has been undertaken in the UK [21]. Most datasets confirm the increasing importance of coagulase negative *staphylococcal* species (CONS) that now numerically dominate LOS cases in in-patients in neonatal units in industrialised countries (proportional rates of 53–78%) and significant proportions in developing regions (up to 47%) [22]. Historically CONS infection was considered less detrimental developmentally, but increasingly data indicate adverse neurodevelopmental sequelae after neonatal CONS infection. The old perspective that CONS could be considered a contaminant, or if it were genuinely infecting a baby was probably minimally harmful, is being challenged.

Diagnostic Techniques and Biomarkers: Improvements and Future Promise

Molecular Tests

Ideally a rapid, accurate, sensitive and specific test that definitively confirmed or excluded bacterial infection in a neonate, and ideally identified the precise organism and sensitivity pattern would exist. The deficiencies of blood culture held to these standards have been recognised and explored, and attempts made to discern 'true infections' from 'contaminants' [23], but these important deficiencies have also driven the exploration of other diagnostic tests in the neonatal setting. Molecular based methods offer the possibility of detecting microbial DNA directly from body fluids without culture, and theoretically more rapid and accurate diagnosis [24, 25]. PCR (polymerase chain reaction) based techniques have previously been limited by contamination, but closed systems appear to have improved this [26] and a recent study targeting the eight most common LOS pathogens using PCR performed with 77% sensitivity and 81% specificity in a preterm population [27]. Slide based microarray systems allowing simultaneous detection of pathogen, virulence proteins and host response are also being developed, but being specific to key pathogens and not offering sensitivity information, do not currently look able to replace the blood culture. However, meta-analysis of the use of molecular approaches in adults with blood stream infections shows an associated reduction in mortality where these approaches are employed, and neonatal medicine may need to look further into appropriate more clinically relevant outcome measures for these techniques than simply 'sensitivity and specificity' [28].

Biomarkers

In the absence of a rapid sensitive and specific diagnostic test that identifies the organism of interest (or rules out bacteraemia) in neonates, there has been extensive effort to identify high quality laboratory biomarkers. Despite these efforts, no single biomarker currently appears adequate with combinations performing better. Until recently the combination of C-reactive protein (CRP) and immature neutrophil combination appeared most promising [29, 30]. However, the recently published 'Neopins' study [31] examined procalcitonin to aid decision making around antibiotic treatment and duration in term and near-term infants with suspected EOS. It demonstrated that an algorithm, with procalcitonin levels measured daily, reduced overall antibiotic exposure (from 65 to 55 h) at no apparent safety cost (reinfection or death) in comparison to standard clinical decision making. Overall antibiotic use was still high in relation to units that cover for the first 36–48 h only (stopping where cultures are negative) and the population studied was only infants of above 33 weeks gestation, preventing extrapolation to more preterm infants. Procalcitonin in preterm infants has been less well studied, but normal values exist based on 283 preterm Japanese infants, and in this cohort at least, infected preterm neonates had values above the 95th centile [32]. Procalcitonin may help to differentiate between LOS and NEC, as NEC does not appear to mount a procalcitonin response [33], although this study was small (NEC n = 8) differentiating NEC from LOS early remains a key aim. Circulating levels of cell free DNA in pilot work differ in infected mice, pigs and preterm humans compared to healthy controls, but to date no prospective trial of their utility as a biomarker has been undertaken [34]. Similarly cytokine profiles show promise in research settings, but cost and time preclude clinical use currently [35]. At present, biomarker studies have tended to focus on blood measures, but non-invasive samples (urine/stool/saliva) are attractive targets for the future [29].

Stool microbiome patterns have been shown to differ ahead of LOS development in comparison to healthy gestation and postnatally age matched controls [36]; bedside 16SrRNA techniques are emerging but have yet to be tested clinically. The large variability seen between infants and within infants even when well makes detecting relevant changes challenging even if technology were to improve [37]. Volatile organic compounds, a reflection of stool microbial and host metabolism, that can be sensed with a bedside monitor, are potentially more suitable for daily stool analysis looking for changes that precede LOS, and have been shown to discriminate certain types of LOS [38].

For similar practical reasons, using software to interpret changes in biological variations in physical parameters such as heart rate variability has been explored as a potential early warning marker of LOS, with an apparent reduction in mortality seen in association with such profiling [39, 40]. Subsequent clinical use of the technique does not however appear widespread.

Preventing Maternal to Infant Transmissions

Preventing mother to infant (vertical) transmission of infections has been the target of significant global effort in the run up to the millennium and beyond, with some successes, but important outstanding needs remain. Similarities in approach to reducing vertical transmission apply to HIV, syphilis, cytomegalovirus (CMV), and to some extent to hepatitis B, but success varies for these diseases.

A multi-pronged approach of increasing antenatal detection, maternal treatment where available to reduce infective load (e.g. antiretrovirals), choice of delivery mode and postnatal care of the baby with early treatment or vaccines is required. Employing all these has led to vertical transmission of HIV in the UK declining year-on-year to 0.27% in 2012–2014 [41]. However, this 'energy and resource rich' approach is not possible in many resource poor countries. Despite the improved access to antiretroviral drugs over the last two decades, over a million pregnant women living with HIV cannot access antiretroviral agents, with political and financial challenges remaining significant barriers to implementing what can clearly be a successful strategy [42].

Congenital syphilis should, in theory, be entirely preventable through antenatal screening and treatment of mothers in pregnancy. Since the 2007 World Health Organisation initiative to eliminate congenital syphilis there has been estimated global reduction in cases by 39% from 2009 to 2012 [43]. However, recent data from the UK with a robust antenatal healthcare service identifies ongoing congenital syphilis infections, with common themes of failure of early detection and early treatment as contributing to six cases of congenital syphilis in 2010–2011 [44].

Congenital Cytomegalovirus (cCMV) infection is becoming increasingly important on the public health stage: estimated to affect 3/1000 live-born babies in the UK, with 90% asymptomatic at birth but causing 25% childhood hearing loss [45] with significant cost related to long term neurodevelopmental impairment [46]. Randomised controlled trial evidence exists to support treatment of 'symptomatic' infants with cCMV starting in the first month of life with ganciclovir (or the oral prodrug valganciclovir) to improve hearing and neurodevelopmental outcome [47].

A number of questions remain however; what is the benefit of treatment if the only sign at birth is hearing loss detected through screening, is there benefit of treating if hearing loss is later identified and is there any benefit of universal newborn cCMV screening? Antenatal screening has been considered by the UK screening committee, but has not been adopted due to current difficulties in identifying at risk pregnancies (as both primary CMV and reactivation can cause congenital infection) and lack of evidence for in-utero treatment. There is, however, good evidence that education packages on CMV infection and behavioural interventions to reduce primary infection (such as simple handwashing) during pregnancy work, [48] but despite this, targeted public health initiatives related to cCMV prevention are lacking, and the impact of cCMV continues.

Vaccinations to Prevent Vertical Transmission

One potentially potent weapon in the armoury against vertically transmitted neonatal infection is maternal vaccination, and this is being used to effectively eliminate congenital rubella in many countries globally [49]. Other congenital infections that may be reducible with maternal vaccination are early onset Group B *streptococcal* disease (GBS) and cCMV. It is estimated that a maternal GBS vaccine with 80% efficacy and 90% coverage would prevent 229,000 infant and maternal GBS cases, and 108,000 stillbirths and infant deaths annually [50]. There are a number of candidate vaccines in development but not fully subjected to safety and efficacy studies [50]. There are also a number of CMV vaccines in development, including two phase 2 studies of glycoprotein B vaccines showing a 45–50% efficacy in reducing primary infection [47]. Since at least half of the women of childbearing age are CMV seropositive before pregnancy, it is unclear how a vaccine reducing primary infection would impact the rates of cCMV or indeed if another strategy (vaccinating young infants) would have better impact [51]. For all these diseases though, significant hope exists that the next years will see further reduction in vertical transmission.

Managing the Infant 'At Risk' of Early Onset Bacterial Infection

Correctly and quickly identifying the rare infant with genuine bacterial EOS is important in minimising adverse outcomes resulting from EOS, but it is also important in antibiotic governance terms to avoid over treatment of non-infected infants given the increased threat of antimicrobial resistance (AMR). This desire to balance risk and harm in the absence of fast, reliable diagnosis or accurate biomarkers has meant decision making around various 'risk factors' for EOS has become increasingly protocolised.

Whilst 'expert groups' previously advocated certain approaches to tolerance (or lack of) to risk factors, ranging from 'treat any risk factor' to 'only treat specific combinations' in 2012 the UK National Institute for Health and Care Excellence (NICE) produced guidelines [52] designed to 'reduce delays in recognising and treating sick babies and prevent unnecessary use of antibiotics'. Estimates are that such protocolisation currently leads to around 8% (~400,000) of European neonates being 'unnecessarily' treated for possible EOS to 'safeguard' the 0.1% with proven EOS [53]. Controversy has occurred in part due to the encouragement to use CRP as part of the decision to treat or stop treating (although recent data on normal variation in CRP may help stop this [54]) and partly because data after the introduction of the NICE guidance showed higher resource use, more investigation and greater antibiotic exposure [55], although smaller audit reports suggest this may not be universal [56].

Decisions on antibiotic treatment of infants >35 weeks of gestation at risk of EOS based on clinical assessment alone or with additional laboratory measurement, showed that clinical assessment alone resulted in less antibiotic use, shorter stay, and no adverse outcomes [57]. Despite this, it feels challenging to write guidance that relies solely on clinical acumen, although this view is now appearing in the literature [58], and attempts to refine our capacity using alternative strategies to predict EOS continue unabated.

A significant difference between the UK and AAP/CDC guidance [59, 60] is the lack of routine GBS screening in the UK, which remains controversial and at odds with European consensus guidance [61], although globally, fewer countries screen than do not screen [62]. This important difference needs to be accounted for when assessing how innovations like on-line sepsis calculators might perform in different settings. One such example is that developed by the Kaiser Permanente North California Hospital. Based on adding knowledge about GBS status, background rates of EOS, maternal temperatures, receipt of antibiotics and an assessment of health, the calculator reduced laboratory testing and antibiotic exposure without apparent risk [63], although it could be argued that experience, local knowledge and good history taking do the same! This calculator is now available on line (https://neonatalsepsiscalculator.kaiserpermanente.org/?kp_shortcut_referrer=kp.org/eoscalc), but caution is needed when applying it outside the population in which it has been tested. A retrospective application of the calculator to 896 infants screened for possible infection in Philadelphia showed that it only identified three of five culture positive infants as requiring treatment [64].

Alternative strategies include genome wide association studies seeking to identify which infants are at risk of infection. Although promising in theory, genome wide association studies in neonates have not so far identified candidate single nucleotide polymorphisms (SNPs) that met genome wide significance, but it is possible, in the future, that whole genome analysis may in the future identify infants at specific increased risk [65].

Antibiotic Choice, Duration and Governance

Surprisingly in this age of evidence based medicine, significant gaps in knowledge remain around important aspects of antibiotic choice and duration for treating either clinically suspected or culture proven neonatal infection, and for managing the interim period from clinical suspicion to culture result.

Most guidance still suggests relatively narrow spectrum agents as first line for late onset infection with flucloxacillin (or ampicillin) and gentamicin and data from the UK suggesting that this was still optimal for the vast majority of neonatal bacteraemias [66, 67]. However it was recently estimated that more than 200,000 of the deaths attributable to neonatal sepsis were due to resistant pathogens, mostly in developing countries [68]. This is increasingly reflected in first choice antibiotics no longer being narrow spectrum, with the resultant drive in further antimicrobial resistance becoming cyclical and self-fulfilling. Stopping this vicious cycle has to be one of the key goals for neonatal medicine in the near future [69]. Units should have rapid access to their own causative organisms with sensitivity data, in order to understand their own pathologies and make the narrowest spectrum choices possible. In conjunction with rapid stopping of antibiotics where infants are well and cultures are negative there are key local steps that can help break this ever increasing use of broad spectrum antibiotics driven by fear. Data from a single Australian centre reassures that stopping after

2–3 days with negative cultures is safe (no relapses identified in infants with negative cultures stopping antibiotics at this point over a 25 years series), but also suggested that even short exposure on its own may not be enough to limit risks of antimicrobial resistance development in this setting [70]. A recent systematic review of the risk of necrotising enterocolitis (NEC) by type of antibiotics suggests that we should also make our choices with this devastating complication of prematurity in mind [71].

Where blood cultures are positive, there is still remarkably little controlled trial data to guide us regarding duration of antibiotics. Chowdhary [72] compared 7 days treatment to 14 days treatment in infants who had reached clinical remission by day 5, showing that only for *Stapylococcus aureus* was there benefit (reduced relapse) from 14 days rather than 7.Gathwala [73] randomised at day seven (if clinically in remission) to either 10 or 14 days, showing no benefit to 14 days under these circumstances. Despite the lack of evidence, most current guidance recommends at least 7 days, and some 10 days for culture positive sepsis, depending on the organism isolated, and the clarity with which meningitis has been excluded [74]. Similarly the trial data on which to base decisions around duration for meningitis is minimal but newer technologies examining transcriptomic proteomic and metabolic data may be of assistance in the future for individualised decision making [75].

Neonatal medicine as a community, particularly in the age of increasing shared national data collection systems, potentially has the capacity to begin to address some of these outstanding questions. Cluster randomised controlled clinical trials comparing durations of antibiotics for sepsis with and without meningitis might easily answer these questions, and we might be surprised by the results. Data from developing countries shows that many infants are successfully treated with shorter duration of antibiotics and intramuscular or combination intramuscular or oral treatment is successful in resource poor settings [76].

Treatment Adjuncts

If we cannot prevent all infection, we should aim to treat optimally, and whilst antibiotics and supportive treatment are the mainstay of treatment, effective adjunct treatments would also be of benefit, but none is routinely used.

Is it possible that there are successful treatment adjuncts available to neonatal clinicians that are not being utilised currently? Are there small scale trials that point to what our next large scale trial(s) should be?

The neonatal community has devoted significant effort to testing several potential 'obvious' immune adjunct treatments: pooled IVIG given to neonates with suspected or proven infection failed in a large well powered study to reduce mortality [77]. In theory specific (e.g. anti-staphylococcal) immunoglobulins may be more effective—trials are under way in infants with infection or suspected infection, but these products have not shown prophylactic value [78]. Granulocyte colony-stimulating factor (GCSF) as adjunct treatment has been studied in small trials: Bilgin [79] demonstrated superior white cell counts and survival in neutropaenic neonates with clinical sepsis treated with recombinant granulocyte-macrophage colony-stimulating factor

(GM-CSF) in comparison to conventional treatment, but this finding was not confirmed in the more recent, but still small, study in Turkey [80] where higher neutrophil counts were not associated with an improvement in mortality.

Pentoxifylline also shows promise as a treatment adjunct. The Cochrane meta-analysis identified six studies of just over 400 neonates suggesting a reduction in all-cause mortality (RR 0.57 95% CI 0.35–0.93) when used in addition to antibiotics for LOS or NEC [81] with a number needed to treat for beneficial outcome of 13. A recent small neonatal trial focused on short term measures, showing lowering of CRP and heart rate responses in pentoxifylline treated, infected VLBW infants compared to those receiving immunoglobulin [82]. An Australian study is underway to examine this further (the PROTECT trial: NHMRC ACTRN12616000405415).

There has also been recent interest in the potential role of the gut microbiome and its dysregulation in contributing to LOS [36], with therapeutic manipulation of the microbiome a clinical goal with, for example probiotics and prebiotics as well as other enteral treatments (oral antibiotics or bioactive breast milk constituents such as lactoferrin). To date these have been trialled as prophylaxis rather than treatment adjuncts in neonates [83, 84].

Despite meta-analyses of prophylactic probiotic use in preterm infants showing important reductions in LOS they have not been widely adopted for reasons including fear of giving a live organism with subsequent probiotic septicaemia and questions around optimal dose and species. It is possible that targeted adjunct use in association with antibiotics, rather than broad prophylactic use may be more acceptable, and may have a role in gut mediated adverse events related to LOS or it's treatments [85]. Lactoferrin, an iron binding glycosylated whey protein has poly-antimicrobial activity in vitro and in animal studies [86], apparent success in reducing LOS in the first preterm human supplementation trial [84] and has recently been tested in two large trials of LOS prevention in preterm infants (n = 2200 (ELFIN enteral lactoferrin in neonates (UK)) and n = 1540 (LIFT lactoferrin infant feeding trial)). The results of the ELFIN study [87] do not support the use of lactoferrin to prevent late onset infection in this group. The embedded mechanistic work on the gut microbiome and metabolome (the MAGPIE trial ISRCTN12554594) may help understand the complex interactions between the microbiome, lactoferrin and health. Rates of LOS in Peruvian infants of <2500 g were reduced by lactoferrin, but only in a secondary analysis taking into account the time from commencing lactoferrin not in a primary intention to treat analysis [88], which may be relevant to the interpretation of the ELFIN data.

References

1. Lawn JE, Blencowe H, Kinney MV, Bianchi F, Graham WJ. Evidence to inform the future for maternal and newborn health. Best Pract Res Clin Obstet Gynaecol. 2016;36:169–83.
2. The Millennium Development Goals Report. New York: United Nations; 2015.
3. Oza S, Lawn JE, Hogan DR, Mathers C, Cousens SN. Neonatal cause-of-death estimates for the early and late neonatal periods for 194 countries: 2000–2013. Bull World Health Organ. 2015;93(1):19–28.

4. Shane AL, Sánchez PJ, Stoll BJ. Neonatal sepsis. Lancet. 2017;390(10104):1770–80.
5. Lukacs SL, Schrag SJ. Clinical sepsis in neonates and young infants, United States, 1988-2006. J Pediatr. 2012;160(6):960–5.e1. https://doi.org/10.1016/j.peds.2011.12.023.
6. Morioka I, Morikawa S, Miwa A, Minami H, Yoshii K, Kugo M, et al. Culture-proven neonatal sepsis in Japanese neonatal care units in 2006-2008. Neonatology. 2012;102(1):75–80.
7. Van Den Hoogen A, Gerards LJ, Verboon-Maciolek MA, Fleer A, Krediet TG. Long-term trends in the epidemiology of neonatal sepsis and antibiotic susceptibility of causative agents. Neonatology. 2009;97(1):22–8.
8. Boghossian NS, Page GP, Bell EF, Stoll BJ, Murray JC, Cotten CM, et al. Late-onset sepsis in very low birth weight infants from singleton and multiple-gestation births. J Pediatr. 2013;162(6):1120–4.
9. Seale AC, Blencowe H, Manu AA, Nair H, Bahl R, Qazi SA, et al. Estimates of possible severe bacterial infection in neonates in sub-Saharan Africa, south Asia, and Latin America for 2012: a systematic review and meta-analysis. Lancet Infect Dis. 2014;14(8):731–41.
10. Williams EJ, Embleton ND, Bythell M, Ward Platt MP, Berrington JE. The changing profile of infant mortality from bacterial, viral and fungal infection over two decades. Acta Paediatr. 2013;102(10):999–1004.
11. Vergnano S, Menson E, Kennea N, Embleton N, Russell AB, Watts T, et al. Neonatal infections in England: the neonIN surveillance network. Arch Dis Child Fetal Neonatal Ed. 2011;96(1):F9–F14.
12. Berrington JE, Hearn RI, Bythell M, Wright C, Embleton ND. Deaths in preterm infants: changing pathology over 2 decades. J Pediatr. 2012;160(1):49–53.
13. Jin C, Londono I, Mallard C, Lodygensky GA. New means to assess neonatal inflammatory brain injury. J Neuroinflammation. 2015;12:180. https://doi.org/10.1186/s12974-015-0397-2.
14. Oddie SJ, Young L, Mcguire W. Slow advancement of enteral feed volumes to prevent necrotising enterocolitis in very low birth weight infants. Cochrane Database Syst Rev. 2017;8:CD001241.
15. Fitchett EJA, Seale AC, Vergnano S, Sharland M, Heath PT, Saha SK, et al. Strengthening the reporting of observational studies in epidemiology for newborn infection (STROBE-NI): an extension of the STROBE statement for neonatal infection research. Lancet Infect Dis. 2016;16:e202–13.
16. Cailes B, Vergnano S, Kortsalioudaki C, Heath P, Sharland M. The current and future roles of neonatal infection surveillance programmes in combating antimicrobial resistance. Early Hum Dev. 2015;91(11):613–8.
17. Schulman J, Stricof R, Stevens TP, Horgan M, Gase K, Holzman IR, et al. Statewide NICU central-line-associated bloodstream infection rates decline after bundles and checklists. Pediatrics. 2011;127(3):436–44.
18. Bion J, Richardson A, Hibbert P, Beer J, Abrusci T, McCutcheon M, et al. Matching michigan: a 2-year stepped interventional programme to minimise central venous catheterblood stream infections in intensive care units in England. BMJ Qual Saf. 2013;22(2):110–23.
19. Ponnusamy V, Clarke P. "Matching michigan" in neonatal intensive care units: a plea for uniform data presentation. Pediatr Infect Dis J. 2013;32(8):927.
20. Palomar M, Álvarez-Lerma F, Riera A, Díaz MT, Torres F, Agra Y, et al. Impact of a national multimodal intervention to prevent catheter-related bloodstream infection in the ICU: the Spanish experience. Crit Care Med. 2013;41(10):2364–72.
21. Johnson AP, Muller-Pebody B, Budd E, Ashiru-Oredope D, Ladenheim D, Hain D, et al. Improving feedback of surveillance data on antimicrobial consumption, resistance and stewardship in England: putting the data at your fingertips. J Antimicrob Chemother. 2017;72(4):953–6.
22. Dong Y, Speer CP. Late-onset neonatal sepsis: recent developments. Arch Dis Child Fetal Neonatal Ed. 2015;100:F257–63.
23. Hossain B, Weber MW, Hamer DH, Hibberd PL, Ahmed ASMNU, Marzan M, et al. Classification of blood culture isolates into contaminants and pathogens on the basis of clinical and laboratory data. Pediatr Infect Dis J. 2016;35(5):S52–4.

24. Kasper DC, Altiok I, Mechtler TP, Böhm J, Straub J, Langgartner M, et al. Molecular detection of late-onset neonatal sepsis in premature infants using small blood volumes: proof-of-concept. Neonatology. 2013;103(4):268–73.
25. Pammi M, Flores A, Leeflang M, Versalovic J. Molecular assays in the diagnosis of neonatal sepsis: a systematic review and meta-analysis. Pediatrics. 2011;128(4):e973–85.
26. Altun O, Almuhayawi M, Ullberg M, Ozenci V. Clinical evaluation of the filmarray blood culture identification panel in identification of bacteria and yeasts from positive blood culture bottles. J Clin Microbiol. 2013;51(12):4130–6.
27. Van Den Brand M, Van Den Dungen FAM, Bos MP, Van Weissenbruch MM, Marceline Van Furth A, De Lange A, et al. Evaluation of a real-time PCR assay for detection and quantification of bacterial DNA directly in blood of preterm neonates with suspected late-onset sepsis. Crit Care. 2018;22:105. https://doi.org/10.1186/s13054-018-2010-4.
28. Timbrook TT, Morton JB, Mcconeghy KW, Caffrey AR, Mylonakis E, LaPlante KL. The effect of molecular rapid diagnostic testing on clinical outcomes in bloodstream infections: a systematic review and meta-analysis. Clin Infect Dis. 2017;64(1):15–23.
29. Ng PC, Ma TPY, Lam HS. The use of laboratory biomarkers for surveillance, diagnosis and prediction of clinical outcomes in neonatal sepsis and necrotising enterocolitis. Arch Dis Child Fetal Neonatal Ed. 2015;100:F448–52.
30. Gilfillan M, Bhandari V. Biomarkers for the diagnosis of neonatal sepsis and necrotizing enterocolitis: clinical practice guidelines. Early Hum Dev. 2017;105:25–33.
31. Stocker M, van Herk W, el Helou S, Dutta S, Fontana MS, Schuerman FABA, et al. Procalcitonin-guided decision making for duration of antibiotic therapy in neonates with suspected early-onset sepsis: a multicentre, randomised controlled trial (NeoPIns). Lancet. 2017;390(10097):871–81.
32. Fukuzumi N, Osawa K, Sato I, Iwatani S, Ishino R, Hayashi N, et al. Age-specific percentile-based reference curve of serum procalcitonin concentrations in Japanese preterm infants. Sci Rep. 2016;6:23871. https://doi.org/10.1038/srep23871.
33. Turner D, Hammerman C, Rudensky B, Schlesinger Y, Wine E, Muise A, et al. Low levels of procalcitonin during episodes of necrotizing enterocolitis. Dig Dis Sci. 2007;52(11):2972–6.
34. Nguyen DN, Stensballe A, Lai JCY, Jiang P, Brunse A, Li Y, et al. Elevated levels of circulating cell-free DNA and neutrophil proteins are associated with neonatal sepsis and necrotizing enterocolitis in immature mice, pigs and infants. Innate Immun. 2017;23(6):524–36.
35. Delanghe JR, Speeckaert MM. Translational research and biomarkers in neonatal sepsis. Clin Chim Acta. 2015;451(Pt A):46–64.
36. Mai V, Torrazza RM, Ukhanova M, Wang X, Sun Y, Li N, et al. Distortions in development of intestinal microbiota associated with late onset sepsis in preterm infants. PLoS One. 2013;8(1):e52876. https://doi.org/10.1371/journal.pone.0052876.
37. Wandro S, Osborne S, Enriquez C, Bixby C, Arrieta A, Whiteson K, et al. The microbiome and metabolome of preterm infant stool are personalized and not driven by health outcomes, including necrotizing enterocolitis and late-onset sepsis. mSphere. 2018;3(3):e00104–18. https://doi.org/10.1128/mSphere.00104-18.
38. Berkhout DJC, Van Keulen BJ, Niemarkt HJ, Bessem JR, De Boode WP, Cossey V, et al. Clinical infectious diseases late-onset sepsis in preterm infants can be detected preclinically by fecal volatile organic compound analysis: a prospective, multicenter cohort study. Clin Infect Dis. 2019;68(1):70–7. https://doi.org/10.1093/cid/ciy383.
39. Moorman JR, Carlo WA, Kattwinkel J, Schelonka RL, Porcelli PJ, Navarrete CT, et al. Mortality reduction by heart rate characteristic monitoring in very low birth weight neonates: A randomized trial. J Pediatr. 2011;159(6):900–6.
40. Fairchild KD, Schelonka RL, Kaufman DA, Carlo WA, Kattwinkel J, Porcelli PJ, et al. Septicemia mortality reduction in neonates in a heart rate characteristics monitoring trial. Pediatr Res. 2013;74(5):570–5.
41. Peters H, Francis K, Sconza R, Horn A, Peckham CS, Tookey PA, et al. UK mother-to-child HIV transmission rates continue to decline: 2012-2014. Clin Infect Dis. 2017;64(4):527–8.

42. Idele P, Hayashi C, Porth T, Mamahit A, Mahy M. Prevention of mother-to-child transmission of HIV and paediatric HIV care and treatment monitoring: from measuring process to impact and elimination of mother-to-child transmission of HIV. AIDS Behav. 2017;21:23–33.

43. Wijesooriya NS, Rochat RW, Kamb ML, Turlapati P, Temmerman M, Broutet N, et al. Global burden of maternal and congenital syphilis in 2008 and 2012: a health systems modelling study. Lancet Glob Health. 2016;4(8):e525–33.

44. Townsend CL, Francis K, Peckham CS, Tookey PA. Syphilis screening in pregnancy in the United Kingdom, 2010–2011: a national surveillance study. BJOG. 2017;124(1):79–86.

45. Williams EJ, Kadambari S, Berrington JE, Luck S, Atkinson C, Walter S, et al. Feasibility and acceptability of targeted screening for congenital CMV-related hearing loss. Arch Dis Child Fetal Neonatal Ed. 2014;99(3):F230–6.

46. Korndewal MJ, Weltevrede M, van den Akker-van Marle ME, et al. Healthcare costs attributable to congenital cytomegalovirus infection. Arch Dis Child. 2018;103:452–7.

47. Rawlinson WD, Boppana SB, Fowler KB, Kimberlin DW, Lazzarotto T, Alain S, et al. Congenital cytomegalovirus infection in pregnancy and the neonate: consensus recommendations for prevention, diagnosis, and therapy. Lancet Infect Dis. 2017;17(6):e177–88.

48. Revello MG, Tibaldi C, Masuelli G, Frisina V, Sacchi A, Furione M, et al. Prevention of primary cytomegalovirus infection in pregnancy. EBioMedicine. 2015;2(9):1205–10.

49. Grant GB, Reef SE, Patel M, Knapp JK, Dabbagh A. Progress in rubella and congenital rubella syndrome control and elimination—worldwide, 2000–2016. Morb Mortal Wkly Rep. 2017;66(45):1256–60.

50. Seale AC, Bianchi-Jassir F, Russell NJ, Kohli-Lynch M, Tann CJ, Hall J, et al. Estimates of the Burden of Group B Streptococcal Disease Worldwide for Pregnant Women, Stillbirths, and Children. Clin Infect Dis. 2017;65:S200–19.

51. Plotkin SA, Boppana SB. Vaccination against the human cytomegalovirus. Vaccine. 2018. https://doi.org/10.1016/j.vaccine.2018.02.089

52. Neonatal infection (early onset): antibiotics for prevention and treatment. 2012. nice.org.uk/guidance/cg149.

53. Van Herk W, El Helou S, Janota J, Hagmann C, Klingenberg C, Staub E, et al. Variation in current management of term and late-preterm neonates at risk for early-onset sepsis: an international survey and review of guidelines. Pediatr Infect Dis J. 2016;35(5):494–500.

54. Macallister K, Smith-Collins A, Gillet H, Hamilton L, davis J. Serial C-reactive protein measurements in newborn infants without evidence of early onset infection. Neonatology. 2019;116:85–91.

55. Mukherjee A, Davidson L, Anguvaa L, Duffy DA, Kennea N. NICE neonatal early onset sepsis guidance:Greater consistency, but more investigations, and greater length of stay. Arch Dis Child Fetal Neonatal Ed. 2015;100:F248–9.

56. Mitchell J, Kirolos S, Jackson L, Powls A. Implementation of the NICE prevention and treatment of early onset neonatal infection guideline: the Glasgow experience. Arch Dis Child Fetal Neonatal Ed. 2017;102(1):F91–2.

57. Berardi A, Fornaciari S, Rossi C, Patianna V, Bacchi Reggiani ML, Ferrari F, et al. Safety of physical examination alone for managing well-appearing neonates ≥35 weeks gestation at risk for early-onset sepsis. J Matern Neonatal Med. 2015;28(10):1123–7.

58. Benitz WE, Wynn JL, Polin RA. Reappraisal of guidelines for management of neonates with suspected early-onset sepsis. J Pediatr. 2015;166(4):1070–4.

59. Verani JR, McGee L, Schrag SJ. Prevention of perinatal group B streptococcal disease revised guidelines from CDC, 2010. Morb Mortal Wkly Rep. 2010;59(10RR):1–31.

60. Randis TM, Polin RA. Early-onset group B Streptococcal sepsis: new recommendations from the centres for disease control and prevention. Arch Dis Child Fetal Neonatal Ed. 2012;97(4):F291–4.

61. Di Renzo GC, Melin P, Berardi A, Blennow M, Carbonell-Estrany X, Donzelli GP, et al. Intrapartum GBS screening and antibiotic prophylaxis: a European consensus conference. J Matern Neonatal Med. 2015;28(7):766–82.

62. Le Doare K, O'Driscoll M, Turner K, Seedat F, Russell NJ, Seale AC, et al. Intrapartum antibiotic chemoprophylaxis policies for the prevention of group B streptococcal disease worldwide: systematic review. Clin Infect Dis. 2017;65:S143–51.
63. Kuzniewicz MW, Puopolo KM, Fischer A, Walsh EM, Li S, Newman TB, et al. A quantitative, risk-based approach to the management of neonatal early-onset sepsis. JAMA Pediatr. 2017;171(4):365–71. https://doi.org/10.1001/jamapediatrics.2016.4678.
64. Carola D, Vasconcellos M, Sloane A, McElwee D, Edwards C, Greenspan J, et al. Utility of early-onset sepsis risk calculator for neonates born to mothers with chorioamnionitis. J Pediatr. 2018;195:48–52.e1.
65. Srinivasan L, Page G, Kirpalani H, Murray JC, Das A, Higgins RD, et al. Genome-wide association study of sepsis in extremely premature infants. Arch Dis Child Fetal Neonatal Ed. 2017;102:F439–45.
66. Muller-Pebody B, Johnson AP, Heath PT, Gilbert RE, Henderson KL, Sharland M. Empirical treatment of neonatal sepsis: are the current guidelines adequate? Arch Dis Child Fetal Neonatal Ed. 2011;96(1):F4–8.
67. Blackburn RM, Verlander NQ, Heath PT, Muller-Pebody B. The changing antibiotic susceptibility of bloodstream infections in the first month of life: Informing antibiotic policies for early- and late-onset neonatal sepsis. Epidemiol Infect. 2014;142(4):803–11.
68. Laxminarayan R, Matsoso P, Pant S, Brower C, Røttingen J-A, Klugman K, et al. Access to effective antimicrobials: a worldwide challenge. Lancet. 2016;387(10014):168–75.
69. Holmes AH, Moore LSP, Sundsfjord A, Steinbakk M, Regmi S, Karkey A, et al. Understanding the mechanisms and drivers of antimicrobial resistance. Lancet. 2016;387(10014):176–87.
70. Carr D, Barnes EH, Gordon A, Isaacs D. Effect of antibiotic use on antimicrobial antibiotic resistance and late-onset neonatal infections over 25 years in an Australian tertiary neonatal unit. Arch Dis Child Fetal Neonatal Ed. 2017;102:F244–50.
71. Seale JV, Hutchinson RA, Fleming PF, Sinha A, Kempley ST, Husain SM, et al. Does antibiotic choice for the treatment of suspected late-onset sepsis in premature infants determine the risk of developing necrotising enterocolitis? A systematic review. Early Hum Dev. 2018;123:6–10.
72. Chowdhary G, Dutta S, Narang A. Randomized controlled trial of 7-day vs. 14-day antibiotics for neonatal sepsis. J Trop Pediatr. 2006;52(6):427–32.
73. Gathwala G, Sindwani A, Singh J, Choudhry O, Chaudhary U. Ten days vs. 14 days antibiotic therapy in culture-proven neonatal sepsis. J Trop Pediatr. 2010;56(6):433–5.
74. Manual of childhood infections: the blue book. 4th ed. New York: Oxford University Press; 2016.
75. Gordon SM, Srinivasan L, Harris MC. Neonatal meningitis: overcoming challenges in diagnosis, prognosis, and treatment with omics. Front Pediatr. 2017;5:139. https://doi.org/10.3389/fped.2017.00139.
76. Zaidi AKM, Tikmani SS, Warraich HJ, Darmstadt GL, Bhutta ZA, Sultana S, et al. Community-based treatment of serious bacterial infections in newborns and young infants: a randomized controlled trial assessing three antibiotic regimens. Pediatr Infect Dis J. 2012;31(7):667–72.
77. Brocklehurst P, Farrell B, King A, Juszczak E, Darlow B, Haque K, et al. Treatment of neonatal sepsis with intravenous immune globulin. N Engl J Med. 2011;365(13):1201–11.
78. DeJonge M, Burchfield D, Bloom B, Duenas M, Walker W, Polak M, et al. Clinical trial of safety and efficacy of IHN-A21 for the prevention of nosocomial staphylococcal bloodstream infection in premature infants. J Pediatr. 2007;151(3).
79. Bilgin K, Yaramiş A, Haspolat K, Ali Taş M, Günbey S, Derman O. A randomized trial of granulocyte-macrophage colony-stimulating factor in neonates with sepsis and neutropenia. Pediatrics. 2001;107(1):36–41.
80. Aktaş D, Demirel B, Gürsoy T, Ovali F. A randomized case-controlled study of recombinant human granulocyte colony stimulating factor for the treatment of sepsis in preterm neutropenic infants. Pediatr Neonatol. 2015;56(3):171–5.
81. Pammi M, Haque KN. Pentoxifylline for treatment of sepsis and necrotizing enterocolitis in neonates. Cochrane Database Syst Rev. 2015;(3):CD004205. https://doi.org/10.1002/14651858.CD004205.pub3.

82. Hamilcikan S, Can E, Büke Ö, Polat C, Özcan E. Pentoxifylline and pentaglobin adjuvant therapies for neonatal nosocomial sepsis in neonates less than 1500g weight. J Pak Med Assoc. 2017;67(10):1482–6.

83. Zhang G-Q, Hu H-J, Liu C-Y, Shakya S, Li Z-Y. Probiotics for preventing late-onset sepsis in preterm neonates. Medicine. 2016;95(8):e2581.

84. Manzoni P, Rinaldi M, Cattani S, Pugni L, Romeo MG, Messner H, et al. Bovine lactoferrin supplementation for prevention of late-onset sepsis in very low-birth-weight neonates: a randomized trial. JAMA. 2009;302(13):1421–8.

85. Underwood MA, German JB, Lebrilla CB, Mills DA. Bifidobacterium longum subspecies infantis: champion colonizer of the infant gut. Pediatr Res. 2015;77:229–35.

86. Legrand D. Overview of lactoferrin as a natural immune modulator. J Pediatr. 2016;173S:S10–5.

87. The ELFIN Investigators Group. Enteral lactoferrin supplemementation for very preterm infants: a randomized placebo-controlled trial. Lancet. 2019;393:423–33.

88. Ochoa T, Zegarra J, Cam L, Llanos R, Pezo A, Cruz K, et al. Randomised trial of lactoferrin for prevention of sepsis in peruvian neonates less than 2500g. Pediatr Infect Dis J. 2015;34:571–6.

Chapter 30
Withholding and Withdrawing Life-Sustaining Treatment

Marlyse F. Haward and Annie Janvier

Introduction

The hospice movement, championed by Dame Cicely Saunders, originated after a series of surveys in the mid-twentieth century uncovered tremendous suffering endured by patients dying from terminal diseases [1]. The movement inspired the development of care models for patients with life-limiting conditions worldwide, incorporating within its framework principles and practices of palliative care. Although palliative care goals focus on improving quality of life during life threatening illnesses even if trajectories do not result in death, these common historical origins likely contribute to illusions that 'palliative care' exists exclusively within the spectrum of 'hospice care' [2, 3].

While hospice and palliative care models were maturing in adult medicine, in paediatrics, concerns for the dying infant and child surfaced, prompted by controversies from the Baby Doe 'Rules', emergence of 'do not resuscitate orders' and increased attention to family centred care and shared decision making [4–6]. Baby Doe, an infant with a trachea-oesophageal fistula and trisomy 21, attracted national attention in the United States when the parents declined life-saving surgery. Although the infant died prior to arbitration, society had to grapple with questions related to quality of life, best interests of children, disability rights and limits of parental and societal authority.

M. F. Haward (✉)
Division of Neonatology, Department of Pediatrics, Albert Einstein College of Medicine, Children's Hospital at Montefiore, Bronx, NY, USA
e-mail: mhaward@montefiore.org

A. Janvier
Université de Montréal, Montréal, QC, Canada

CHU Sainte-Justine, Montréal, QC, Canada

© Springer Nature Switzerland AG 2020
E. M. Boyle, J. Cusack (eds.), *Emerging Topics and Controversies in Neonatology*, https://doi.org/10.1007/978-3-030-28829-7_30

A second case, baby Jane Doe with spina bifida, challenged these assumptions in the US Supreme court [7]. Concurrently, landmark publications exposed practices surrounding death in the neonatal intensive care unit (NICU) introducing tensions between sanctity of life and quality of life for critically ill infants, some with disability [8, 9] as neonatal leaders explored the roles neonatologists played in managing death and caring for families [10, 11].

As early as 1982, Whitfield and colleagues recognised the need for a 'hospice program' ('the family room') within their NICU and provided a 10-week course in hospice care for NICU staff [11]. Views of quality of life, futility and neonatal pain management evolved and care strategies began to encompass spirituality, cultural competence, bereavement, communication strategies and family support [12]. The neonatal intensive care unit presented itself as a complex clinical realm in which life and death decisions disrupted world views of parenthood and expectations of pregnancy.

Support from professional societies [13–15] prioritise early integration of palliative care in disease trajectories for patients with serious life-threatening illnesses. Currently, in the neonatal intensive care unit, palliative care approaches are recommended not only for infants who become critically ill after birth but also for those diagnosed in-utero.

Withdrawal of life-sustaining interventions has become the primary mode of death in the NICU, bringing debates about quality of life to the forefront [3, 16–18]. These trends suggest that neonatologists are adept in supporting early integration of palliative care in disease trajectories. On the other hand, surveys often reveal that some providers are reluctant to engage parents in these conversations [19, 20].

This chapter will explore potential barriers impeding the integration of palliative care in neonatology, contemplate what defines 'good' palliative care including communication practices, consider optimal delivery models for palliative care and illustrate how parental input can drive the field of neonatal palliative care forward.

Terminology and Biases

Inconsistent terminology or misperceptions perpetuate provider and patient/parent biases by artificially segregating palliative and curative therapies. 'Palliative care' is often erroneously considered synonymous with 'end of life care' or 'hospice care' [2, 3, 21].

In addition to concise goals of paediatric palliative care, the American Academy of Pediatrics (AAP) extends the definition to encompass informed decision making, care/team coordination and emphasises that palliative care is appropriate even under circumstances when 'cure' remains possible [14]. Conversely, 'end of life' care and 'hospice' are generally presented to families after curative therapies have failed and death is anticipated.

Despite this clear distinction, the term 'palliative care' often engenders negative feelings for providers and parents when compared with alternative terms such as 'supportive care' or 'complex care' [21–23].

Clinical behaviour seems to reinforce these associations as providers are reluctant to engage in conversations about palliative care until death becomes 'certain' [24, 25], insinuating a sequential, mutually exclusive model of care rather than an integrative one. Providers report they are less likely to seek consultations from services called 'palliative care' rather than 'supportive care' precisely due to the inherent negativity associated with the term 'palliative' [22]. Likewise, patients themselves view 'supportive care' more favourably than 'palliative care' in terms of understanding, impressions and perceived needs despite identical services rendered [26]. These *a priori* impressions compounded by a continued lack of discrimination between terms in practice and research, contribute not only to difficulty in generalising research findings but impedes strategies aimed to shift mindsets [2, 19, 27].

Curriculums incorporated into medical and graduate school training [28], symposiums and core competencies established by work groups [29] have attempted to detach the 'death' label from palliative care. Yet, these efforts often fail until terminology is changed. Harvard Medical School and the Dana Farber Institute have met success in transitioning to alternative names, the Pediatric Advanced Care Team, who frame their mission as providing "healing, comfort and quality of life—to the care of children with serious illness and their families" [30] while others, using 'supportive care', have seen a rise in inpatient and outpatient referrals [31].

However, is new terminology sufficient in permanently changing culture or are other barriers too powerful? Barriers cited in paediatric literature include availability of services/ resources, time, training/ knowledge, communication, and emotional toil [12, 25, 32, 33]. While the first few impediments have demonstrated improvement [19], overly optimistic beliefs for cures and trying not to appear as 'giving up' may not be straightforward beliefs to reconcile.

Cognitive biases often have deep roots hindering change even in the face of evidence. For example, empirical multi-centre evidence has already demonstrated the benefits of palliative care, most notably the ability to prolong survival by improving quality of life for patients [34]. Contrary to providers' fears [33], providing detailed, timely and complete information even under circumstances of dismal prognoses fosters hope regardless of whether such information is emotionally distressing [35–37].

It is also generally accepted that as parents begin to understand diagnoses more fully they are able to 're-frame' hope towards more realistic goals [38]. Yet, despite this evidence, providers still exhibit reluctance in seeking palliative care consultations due to the emotional labour exhibited both internally (within themselves in accepting treatment failure) and externally (explaining this approach to families) [24, 33, 39, 40]. As such, attention to strategies designed to overcome underlying biases, such as optimising defaults, may be important considerations.

'Good' Palliative Care: Multi-Dimensional and Integrative

'Good' palliative care is inherently multi-dimensional. While it can broadly be divided into infant focused care, family focused care and staff support and education, elements within each domain influence one another. Infant focused care includes pharmacologic and non-pharmacologic multi-sensory strategies for pain management, reduction of painful stimuli, quality of life measures and personalised decisions regarding care.

Family focused care includes care for the family with regards to emotional health, parental bonding, psychological, social and spiritual support. It includes bereavement care and grief counselling regardless of the infant's clinical prognosis, as parents experience loss even when their infant survives with a life-altering condition [41].

Staff support includes ongoing multi-disciplinary professional educational initiatives, robust training opportunities and mental health support for staff, such as debriefings, informed by parental and staff experiences.

These dimensions often intersect and complement one another. For example, pathologic parental long-term grief has been correlated with perceptions of inadequate symptom relief when children are dying [42, 43]. In neonatology, parental perceptions of infant pain are further complicated by indirect measurement tools for non-verbal patients which can appear imprecise [44].

However, by providing strong anticipatory communication parental expectations can be managed and anxiety diminished. In addition, non-pharmacologic symptom relief such as holding and suckling, can offer comfort to both the neonate and the parent.

In other instances, these dimensions intersect and oppose one another. For example, debate has raged in the literature about professional obligations in resuscitation attempts deemed futile, yet requested by parents. Under these circumstances, principles related to bests interests and care of the infant clash with palliative care principles for parental support.

Experts have argued that for some families a 'slow' or 'symbolic' resuscitation attempt can be beneficial in which resuscitative efforts are intentionally limited or performed ineffectively [45]. They argue that if families clearly understand that resuscitative efforts are unlikely to be successful and death is inevitable but cannot agree to forgo resuscitation, a 'slow' response could be ethically permissible [46].

Conversely, others argue that 'slow' resuscitation attempts are deceptive as they inherently deliver sub-optimal medical care. However, these experts argue that since the definition of 'full' resuscitation is ambiguous, and evidence is lacking regarding 'adequate trials' of resuscitation, a 'slow' resuscitative response may be appropriate under limited circumstances [45, 47]. Indeed, a significant portion of deaths in the NICU occur without CPR or DNR orders but in the presence of a trusted provider. This continuity, proximity, and trust or in other words 'loyalty' between the parent and provider facilitates 'appropriate' care at the end of the baby's life [47].

Unfortunately for each of these domains, while principles guiding palliative care are well developed, relatively little empirical evidence exists to determine best practices or a standard of care in the neonatal population [4, 5, 12, 48]. Much of the available evidence reviews single centre outcomes or focuses on one facet of care through commentaries and professional opinions [5].

One study evaluating multi-cultural practices reveals variability in practices irrespective of DNR orders [18]. Other investigations rely on indirect measures, such as presence of DNR orders, as a proxy for 'quality care' [49]. Although consensus-based single centre protocols have demonstrated benefits for all infants when palliative care consultation services are available in the NICU, only a few institutions have adopted protocols guiding management [40, 48–51].

Lack of empirical research, and paucity of formalised guidelines, provides unique opportunities to re-frame outcomes along parent driven measures. Traditional outcome data and assessments of 'quality' of care focuses on biomedical aspects of care determined by physicians. These measures however are not always aligned with what matters most to parents. For example, parents value communication highest when rating the quality of care delivered [42, 52].

Single interactions or statements with providers-positive or negative- can have lasting impacts on parent's ability to cope with the death of a child [38, 53] regardless of the quality of 'medical' care the child received. Provider mind-sets when assisting in the child's end of life are more important to parents than the 'location' of care [50]. Therefore, utilising outcome measures such as 'location of care' or 'presence of a DNR in the chart' to determine the quality of care delivered when determining best practices may be misleading. Rather, recognising the multi-faceted view of palliative care and including perspectives of parents in determining outcome driven research is critical to inform best practice guidelines.

Optimal Delivery Models: Personalisation, Proximity and Trust

Prior to the recognition of palliative care as a board-certified specialty in 2006, the primary provider coordinated patient care while addressing the family's psychological and emotional needs, including under circumstances when cure was no longer deemed probable [54]. As demand for services and availability of specialists trained in palliative care increased, institutions shifted towards consultative models. A review in 2012 of US based children's hospitals, indicated that 50% had distinct paediatric palliative care programs. However, significant variability existed amongst these programs especially with regards to weekend coverage and staff expertise [55].

In neonatology, current approaches vary between primary "inclusive" models led by neonatologists and consultative models [12, 49, 50, 56–58] initiated when goals of care transition. Consultative models are led by members who may or may not possess expertise in perinatal/ neonatal medicine while primary models often rely on neonatologists. Some leaders in the field advocate for the primary model due to the rapidly expanding realm of prenatal diagnostic capabilities contributing to medical complexity and clinical ambiguity [12]. We concur for reasons related to trust, proximity and continuity of care.

In the trajectory of any life-threatening illness, the rapport between providers and parents is paramount. Typically, when a diagnosis is made, energy is spent on understanding and attacking the ailment with an armamentarium of therapies in hopes a cure will soon follow. While second opinions may be sought and various plans considered, successful therapeutic alliances require trust; trust that providers are genuinely on the child's 'team' and trust that the parent(s) is (are) acting as a 'good parent(s)' [59].

This trust develops and is reinforced over time. As therapies gradually fail, and conditions worsen, 'good parent' attributes may become less obvious to providers, manifesting as 'heuristic' type decisions building on subtle patterns of behaviour [59, 60].

The stories parents create for themselves and subsequently tell their friends and family must resonate with these beliefs about being 'good parents' or 'having no regrets' [38]. Trust reinforces this reassurance which can subsequently help transition goals under less contentious / stressful conditions. For parents faced with diagnoses prenatally, they are thrust into grief precipitously and must integrate knowledge, manage emotions, align values and beliefs quickly before the birth of the infant.

They are presented complex medical information as they absorb the shock of the diagnosis and grieve a 'normal' pregnancy [61, 62]. Antenatal palliative care principles can be beneficial when prenatal diagnoses present with diagnostic certainty, prognostic certainty or significantly burdensome treatment according to best interest principles [57]. Comprehensive care depends on cooperation between neonatologists, obstetricians, genetic counsellors, other specialists involved in the care (cardiology, nephrology, etc.) and nurses. Under these circumstances, parents may choose to pursue termination, expectant management or induction of labour with care plans individualised based on their values [57]. For some parents, in-utero palliative care alternatives may be more acceptable than termination of pregnancy.

Primary models led by neonatologists may be better able to balance "being with" and "doing to" healing paradigms both antenatally and postnatally. "Being with" has been described as emotional, cognitive and spiritual support for patients and families, while "doing to" encompasses expert knowledge directed at relieving symptoms [41].

Contrary to other disease processes in paediatrics, a neonatal death can occur within a relatively short life-time span, making team transitions seem more pronounced or rushed. The vast majority of neonatal deaths occur in NICUs. On the other hand, neonatal deaths can also occur later in the course of a neonatal intensive care stay. Either way, the initial interaction is with the neonatologist. In the NICU, there is no ambiguity which specialty is coordinating care regardless of how many others are involved. In addition, parents have reported increased emotional fragility when care is fragmented, and continuity of care is disrupted [12, 42, 63] and no evidence exists indicating dissatisfaction with primary models led by neonatologists.

Therefore, while preferred models may be influenced by nuances of local culture, practical constraints, or resource availability [12, 64], we argue that the motivation in selecting a model should depend on the ability to build and maintain trust through continuity of care which occurs most naturally in the primary model.

'Primary model' recommendations should incorporate multi-disciplinary input and consist of formalised protocols. Formalising models and protocols have been shown to ameliorate the setting in which death occurs, peri-death interventions, advanced care planning, family meetings and emotional support for families and staff [40, 49, 65]. Primary models require training in palliative care principles for all neonatologists in training or disciplines in which death is not an uncommon occurrence. Team leaders should possess expertise in both medical facts and palliative principles and be present throughout the course of an illness. The same team who counsels the parents about the stress of having an infant in the NICU, who places the child on an oscillator or tries one last intervention in an effort to oxygenate, should also be the one providing comfort to the patient and the family as the infant takes their last gasp and be the one following up with the parents after death.

Team continuity, proximity and trust may be interpreted as 'loyalty' by parents which in turn can help decrease long term pathological grief as parents try to live with their story. We recommend reserving transitions to palliative care specialty teams for infants who are discharged from the NICU with life limiting conditions.

Communication: Broadening Concepts

Good communication is the cornerstone of quality medical care and highly valued by parents and patients. 'Clear, compassionate and forthright discussions' are considered critical elements in palliative care, endorsed by professional societies [14]. Recognition of 'lethal' language leading to self-fulfilling prophecies and 'framing' prognoses impacting choice underscores the influence language can have on outcomes [66, 67]. However, good communication does not only correlate with the semantics of word choice, the delivery of information and ensuring accurate understanding. It includes skills related to non-verbal behaviours and intuitions regarding personalised decision-making preferences [68, 69]. Paradigms, such as SOBPIE, have been developed to assist neonatologists in counselling parents paying particular attention to the parental experience within this broader concept of 'communication'. The SOBPIE approach assesses the **s**ituation, acknowledges **o**pinions, options and **b**iases, practices **b**asic human politeness, considers the **p**arents perspective, personalises **i**nformation while considering the myriad of **e**motions that complicate these encounters [70]. These recommendations are especially important in palliative care.

A primary goal of communication is to enable decision making. Processes of decision making however vary between individuals and depend upon specific qualities of decisions; end of life decisions, often influenced by emotions, may follow more affective decisional processes whereas simple therapeutic decisions, with decreased emotional burden, may follow more rational choice models. Understanding these nuances is critical for compassionate, effective communication. For example, while debate lingers about the necessity to challenge parental optimistic beliefs recognition that decisions often rely on emotional interpretations of facts and values broadens the concept of communication.

Understanding which outcomes matter to parents, and guiding conversations to meet those needs, helps parents maintain 'storylines' in sync with their beliefs and can facilitate timely decision making. Conversely, confrontational bedside exchanges focused on clarifying what is or is not realistic potentially makes families believe they need to "fight" for the right to preserve hope detracting from the 'job' of decision making. In these circumstances, acknowledging a parent's optimism, sharing in their hope with phrases such as *we also wish she gets better but in the next 24 h we will focus on how the lungs respond to…*" can help re-frame conversations and goals in a more collaborative manner. This broader vision, beyond accuracy and comprehension, to include emotional perspectives and recognise varied decisional processes, facilitates delivery of quality palliative care.

Broader visions in communication and personalised decision-making models permit parental individuality to drive partnerships central to palliative care. While shared-decision making has been touted as a gold standard in paediatrics, it has critical limitations. First, shared decision making presumes sharing; all parents want participation in decision making and all parents utilise similar, rational decisional strategies. Second, physician assumptions drive shared decision making; pre-determined information deemed necessary for informed decisions is structured by physicians. However, parental decision-making styles are anything but homogenous; not all parents benefit from the same approach nor the same information. Not all parents want to share these decisions. Some parents want the medical team to decide. Thus, practicing personalised decision making enables a broader vision of communication, respects decision making heterogeneity while building relationships based on the needs of parents [69].

Listening to Parents: Redefining Goals

Listening to parental perspectives on palliative care are transforming mindsets and redefining outcomes for medicine and society. Historically, debates about care for disabled children, boundaries of technology and definitions of futility originated in the NICU and overflowed into society inciting public debates.

More recently, however, these revolutions of mindsets are being driven by evidence stemming from parental perspectives and pushing inwards into the medical literature and community. Most illustrative of this shift, is the evidence stemming from parental perspectives on trisomy 13 and 18, redefining outcome measures. Parental hopes to meet their children, include them in the family, keep them happy and free from suffering has not only prompted some physicians to consider alternative care plans, including surgical interventions, but has changed the conversation about what can and should be considered 'reasonable' outcomes.

Prompting part of this evolution is the underrecognised capacity for resiliency and adjustment families often show as well as the gains palliative care has demonstrated enabling quality of life in the face of life-shortening conditions [71]. Retrospective perspectives from parents who experienced end of life care for their infants cite the importance of being able to fulfill their roles as parents [72–75]. Some highlight the physical barriers to feeling like they are parents, such as holding the baby during the early phases of the NICU hospitalisation.

This profound desire for direct contact becomes complicated by hesitation and intense fear for some during the dying process. Gentle yet strong encouragement by providers to hold their infant was found to be helpful [74]. They also remark on the importance of being listened to by staff, feeling respected, balancing regret with peace in their decisions and being provided with various sources of support including spiritual, bereavement and palliative care services throughout the disease trajectory [72, 73].

Others identify the importance of faith and trust in the staff, promoted by empathetic providers and continuity of care [73]. Meetings with providers after death helped validate their decisions [73], with some parents calling for more continuity after death [75]. Focusing on family involvement, such as siblings, was also suggested helpful with long term family adjustment [73]. Questionnaires developed to measure parental experiences with end of life care have been developed and can assist in further exploring these and other parent driven outcome measures of quality care. In these explorations, while the practical aspects of care (or 'doing to') were considered satisfactory by parents, the actual in hospital experience and follow up care (or 'being with') needed improvement [76].

Summary: The Last Chapter

The juxtaposition of birth and death has always co-existed in the NICU but how parents write or re-write this story can have a lasting impact on their long-term mental health. Loyalty of physician-parent alliances built through continuity, proximity and trust and delivered through primary models can help facilitate resiliency and adjustment for those who are 'left behind'. Attention to subtle cognitive biases present in both providers and parents with strategies designed to overcome these biases can help integrate palliative care principles earlier in disease trajectories. Broader concepts of communication emphasising personalisation delivered without crushing hope can have beneficial effects on long term adjustment and grief for parents [53]. Prioritising personalised decisional processes helps to ensure that partnerships are congruent with parental needs. Collecting evidence of parental perspectives to redefine outcomes and incorporating parental opinion in the construction of best practices can help align palliative care principles of 'being with' with 'doing to' paradigms for patient care.

References

1. Saunders C. The evolution of palliative care. J R Soc Med. 2001;94:430–2.
2. Meghani SH. A concept analysis of palliative care in the United States. J Adv Nurs. 2004;46(2):152–61.
3. Kang TI, Munson D, Hwang J, Feudtner C. Integration of palliative care into the care of children with serious illness. Pediatr Rev. 2014;35(8):318–26.
4. Warrick C, Perera L, Murdock E, Nicholl RM. Guidance for withdrawal and withholding of intensive care as part of neonatal end of life care. Br Med Bull. 2011;98:99–113.
5. Balaguer A, Martin-Ancel A, Ortigoza-Escobar D, Escribano J, Argemi J. The model of palliative care in the perinatal setting; a review of the literature. BMC Pediatr. 2012;12(25):1–7.
6. Feudtner C, Nathanson P. Pediatric palliative care and pediatric medical ethics: opportunities and challenges. Pediatrics. 2014;133:S1–7.
7. Kopelman LM. Are the 21-year-old baby doe rules misunderstood or mistaken? Pediatrics. 2005;115(3):797–802.
8. Duff RS, Campbell AG. Moral and ethical dilemmas in the special-care nursery. N Engl J Med. 1973;289:890–4.
9. Duff R, Campbell A. On deciding the care of severely handicapped or dying persons: with particular reference to infants. Pediatrics. 1976;57(4):487–93.
10. Silverman WA. A hospice setting for humane neonatal death. Pediatrics. 1982;69(2):239.
11. Whitfield JM, Siegel RE, Glicken AD, Harmon RJ, Powers LK, Goldson EJ. The application of hospice concepts to neonatal care. Am J Dis Child. 1982;136:421–4.
12. Carter BS. Pediatric palliative care in infants and neonates. Children. 2018;5(21):1–9.
13. American Academy of Pediatrics Committee on Fetus and Newborn. Noninitiation or withdrawal of intensive care for high-risk newborns. Pediatrics. 2007;119(2):401–3.
14. American Academy of Pediatrics Section on Hospice and Palliative Medicine and Committee on Hospital Care. Pediatric palliative care and hospice care commitments, guidelines, and recommendations. Pediatrics. 2013;132(5):966–72.
15. Royal College of Paediatrics And Child Health. Withholding or withdrawing life sustaining treatment in children: a framework for practice. In: Withholding or withdrawing life sustaining treatment in children: a framework for practice. 2nd edn. 2004. https://councilfordisabledchildren.org.uk/sites/default/files/field/attachemnt/Withholding%26withdrawing_treatment.pdf. Accessed 8 Jun 2018.
16. Weiner J, Sharma J, Lantos J, Kilbride H. How infants die in the neonatal intensive care unit. Arch Pediatr Adolesc Med. 2011;165(7):630–4.
17. Wall SN, Partridge JC. Death in the intensive care nursery: physician practice of withdrawing and withholding life support. Pediatrics. 1997;99(1):64–70.
18. Verhagen AA, Janvier A, Leuthner SR, Andrews B, Lagatta J, Bos AF, Meadow W. Categorizing neonatal deaths: a cross-cultural study in the United States, Canada, and The Netherlands. J Pediatr. 2010;156:33–7.
19. Cortezzo DE, Sanders MR, Brownell E, Moss K. Neonatologists perspective of palliative and end of life care in neonatal intensive care units. J Perinatol. 2013;33:731–5.
20. Boss RD, Hutton N, Donohue PK, Arnold RM. Neonatologist training to guide family decision making for critically ill infants. Arch Pediatr Adolesc Med. 2009;163(9):783–8.
21. Boldt AM, Yusuf F, Himelstein BP. Perceptions of the term palliative care. J Palliat Med. 2006;9(5):1128–36.
22. Katz NM. The term 'supportive care' is preferable to 'palliative care' for consults in the cardiothoracic intensive care unit. J Thorac Cardiovasc Surg. 2018;155(5):2030–1.
23. Fadul N, Elsayem A, Palmer L, Del Fabbro E, Swint K, Li Z, et al. Supportive verses palliative care: what's in a name? Cancer. 2009;115:2013–21.
24. Davies B, Sehring S, Partridge JC, Cooper BA, Hughes A, Philip JC, et al. Barriers to palliative care for children: perceptions of pediatric health care providers. Pediatrics. 2008;121(2):282–8.

25. Thompson LA, Knapp C, Madden V, Shenkman E. Pediatricians' perceptions of and preferred timing for pediatric palliative care. Pediatrics. 2009;123(5):e777–82.
26. Maciasz RM, Arnold R, Chu E, Park SY, White DB, Borgenheimer L, et al. Does it matter what you call it? A randomized trial of language used to describe palliative care services. Support Care Cancer. 2013;21(12):1–9.
27. Miyashita M, Hirai K, Morita T, Sanjo M, Uchitomi Y. Barriers to referral to inpatient palliative care units in Japan: a qualitative survey with content analysis. Support Care Cancer. 2008;16:217–22.
28. Horowitz R, Gramling R, Quill T. Palliative care education in U.S. medical schools. Med Educ. 2014;48:59–66.
29. Morrison L, Opatik Scott J, Block S, American Board of Hospice and Palliative Medicine Competencies Work Group. Developing initial competency-based outcomes for the hospice and palliative medicine subspecialist. Phase I of the Hospice and Palliative Medicine Competencies Project. J Palliat Med. 2007;10:313–30.
30. Dana-Farber Cancer Institute: Pediatric Advanced Care Team. 2018. https://www.dana-farber.org/pediatric-advanced-care-team/. Accessed 20 Aug 2018.
31. Dalal S, Palla S, Hui D, Nguyen L, Chacko R, Lia Z, et al. Association between a name change from palliative to supportive care and the timing of patient referrals at a comprehensive cancer center. Oncologist. 2011;16:105–11.
32. Marc-Aurele K, English NK. Primary palliative care in neonatal intensive care. Semin Perinatol. 2017;41:133–9.
33. Knapp C, Thompson L. Factors associated with perceived barriers to pediatric palliative care a survey of pediatricians in Florida and California. Palliat Med. 2011;26(3):268–74.
34. Feudtner C, Kang TI, Hexem KR, Friedrichsdorf SJ, Osenga K, Siden H, et al. Pediatric palliative care patients: a prospective multicenter cohort study. Pediatrics. 2011;127(6):1094–101.
35. Mack JW, Wolfe J, Cook F, Grier HE, Cleary PD, Weeks JC. Hope and prognostic disclosure. J Clin Oncol. 2007;25(35):5636–42.
36. Mack JW, Wolfe J, Grier HE, Cleary PD, Weeks JC. Communication about prognosis between parents and physicians of children with cancer parent preferences and the impact of prognostic information. J Clin Oncol. 2006;24(33):5265–70.
37. Mack JW, Wolfe J, Cook F, Grier HE, Cleary PD, Weeks JC. Understanding of prognosis among parents of children with cancer. Parental optimism and the parent physician interaction. J Clin Oncol. 2007;25(11):1357–62.
38. Cote-Arsenault D, Denney-Koelsch E. "Have no regrets": parents' experiences and developmental tasks in pregnancy with a lethal fetal diagnosis. Soc Sci Med. 2016;154:100–9.
39. Szymczak JE, Schall T, Hill DL, Walter JK, Parikh S, DiDomenico C, Feudtner C. Pediatric oncology providers perceptions of palliative care service: the influence of emotional esteem and emotional labor. J Pain Symptom Manage. 2018;55(5):1260–8.
40. Pierucci RL, Kirby RS, Leuthner SR. End of life care for neonates and infants: the experience and effects of a palliative care consultation service. Pediatrics. 2001;108(3):653–60.
41. Milstein J. A paradigm of integrative care: healing with curing throughout life, "being with" and "doing to". J Perinatol. 2005;25(9):563–8.
42. Van der Geest IM, Darlington AE, Streng IC, Michiels EMC, Pieters R, van den Heuvel-Eibrink MM. Parents experiences of pediatric palliative care and the impact on long term parental grief. J Pain Symptom Manage. 2014;47(6):1043–53.
43. Kreicbergs U, Valdimarsdóttir U, Onelöv E, Björk O, Steineck G, Henter JI. Care-related distress: a nationwide study of parents who lost their child to cancer. J Clin Oncol. 2005;23(36):9162–71.
44. Carter BS, Jones PM. Evidence-Based comfort care for neonates towards the end of life. Semin Fetal Neonatal Med. 2013;18:88–92.
45. Frader J, Kodish E, Lantos JD. Ethics rounds—symbolic resuscitation, medical futility, and parental rights. Pediatrics. 2010;126:769.

46. Lantos JD, Meadow WL. Should the "slow code" be resuscitated? Am J Bioeth. 2011;11(11): 8–12.
47. Janvier A, Barrington K. What is an appropriate code? Am J Bioeth. 2011;11(11):18–20.
48. Uthaya S, Mancini A, Beardsley C, Wood D, Ranmal R, Modi N. Managing palliation in the neonatal unit. Arch Dis Child Fetal Neonatal Ed. 2014;99(5):F349–52.
49. Younge N, Smith PB, Goldberg RN, Brandon DH, Simmons C, Cotton CM, Bidegain M. Impact of a palliative care program on end of life care in a neonatal intensive care unit. J Perinatol. 2015;35(3):218–22.
50. Caitlin A, Carter B. Creation of neonatal end of life palliative care protocol. J Perinatol. 2002;22:184–95.
51. Haug S, Farooqi S, Wilson CG, Hopper A, Oei G, Carter B. Survey on Neonatal end of life comfort care guidelines across America. J Pain Symptom Manage. 2018;55:979–84.
52. Widger K, Picot C. Parent's perceptions of the quality of pediatric and perinatal end of life care. Pediatr Nurs. 2008;34(1):53–8.
53. Melin-Johannson C, Axelsson I, Grundberg MJ, Hallqvist F. When a child dies: parents experience of palliative care an integrative literature review. J Pediatr Nurs. 2014;29:660–9.
54. Himelstein BP, Hilden JM, Boldt AM, Weissman D. Pediatric palliative care. N Engl J Med. 2004;350:1752–62.
55. Feudtner C, Womer J, Augustin R, Remke S, Wolfe J, Friebert S, Weissman D. Pediatric palliative care programs in children's hospitals: a cross sectional national survey. Pediatrics. 2013;132(6):1063–70.
56. Leuthner S. Fetal palliative care. Clin Perinatol. 2004;31:649–65.
57. Leuthner S, Jones EL. Fetal concerns program. A model for perinatal palliative care. MCN: Am J Matern Child Nurs. 2007;32(5):272–8.
58. Carter BS, Bhatia J. Comfort/ palliative care guidelines for neonatal practice development and implementation in an academic medical center. J Perinatol. 2001;21:279–83.
59. Feudtner C, Walter JK, Faeber JA, Hill DL, Carroll KW, Mollen CJ, et al. Good parent beliefs of parents of seriously ill children. JAMA Pediatr. 2015;169(1):39–47.
60. Feudtner C, Carroll KW, Hexem KR, Silverman J, Kang T, Kazak AE. Parental hopeful patterns of thinking, emotions and pediatric palliative care decision making. Arch Pediatr Adolesc Med. 2010;164(9):831–9.
61. Gaucher N, Nadeau S, Barbier A, Janvier A, Payot A. Personalized antenatal consultations for preterm labor: responding to mothers' expectations. J Pediatr. 2016;178:130–4.
62. Payot A, Gendron S, Lefebvre F, Doucet H. Deciding to resuscitate extremely premature babies: how do parents and neonatologists engage in the decision? Soc Sci Med. 2007;64(7):1487–500.
63. Cacciatore J, Thieleman K, Lieber AS, Blood C, Goldman R. The long road to farewell: the needs of families with dying children. Omega (Westport). 2017. https://doi.org/10.1177/0030222817697418. [Epub ahead of print].
64. Quill TE, Abernethy AP. Generalist plus specialist palliative care- creating a more sustainable model. N Engl J Med. 2013;368(13):1173–5.
65. Janvier A, Meadow W, Leuthner S, Andrews B, Lagatta J, Bos A, Lane L, Verhagen AAE. Whom are we comforting? An analysis of comfort medications delivered to dying neonates. J Pediatr. 2011;159:206–10.
66. Wilkenson D, Crespigny L, Xafis V. Ethical language and decision making for prenatally diagnosed lethal malformations. Semin Fetal Neonatal Med. 2014;19:306–11.
67. Haward MF, Murphy RO, Lorenz JM. Message framing and neonatal decisions. Pediatrics. 2008;122(1):109–18.
68. Haward MF, Janvier A, Lorenz JM, Fischhoff B. Counseling parents at risk of delivery of an extremely premature infant: differing strategies. AJOB Empir Bioeth. 2017;8(4):243–52.
69. Haward MF, Gaucher N, Payot A, Robson K, Janvier A. Personalized decision making: practical recommendations for antenatal counseling for fragile neonates. Clin Perinatol. 2017;44(2):429–45.
70. Janvier A, Barrington K, Farlow B. Communication with parents concerning withholding or withdrawing of life-sustaining interventions in neonatology. Semin Perinatol. 2014;38(1):38–46.

71. Janvier A, Farlow B, Barrington K. Parental Hopes, Interventions, and Survival of neonates with trisomy 13 and trisomy 18. Am J Med Genet C Semin Med Genet. 2016;172C:279–87.
72. Currie E, Christian BJ, Hinds PS, Perna SJ, Robinson C, Day S, Meneses K. Parent perspectives of neonatal intensive care at the end-of-life. J Pediatr Nurs. 2016;31:478–89.
73. Brosig CL, Pierucci RL, Kupst MJ, Leuthner SR. Infant end-of-life care: the parents' perspective. J Perinatol. 2007;27:510–6.
74. Abraham A, Hendricks MJ. "You can only give warmth to your baby when it's too late": parents' bonding with their extremely preterm and dying child. Qual Health Res. 2017;27(14):2100–15.
75. Cortezza DE, Sanders MR, Brownell EA, Moss K. End-of-life care in the neonatal intensive care unit: experiences of staff and parents. Am J Perinatol. 2015;32:713–72.
76. Williams C, Cairnie J, Fines V, Patey C, Schwarzer K, Aylward J, et al. Construction of a parent-derived questionnaire to measure end-of-life care after withdrawal of life-sustaining treatment in the neonatal intensive care unit. Pediatrics. 2009;123:e87–95.

Chapter 31
Effective Training in Neonatal Medicine

Adam Bonfield and Jonathan Cusack

Simulation Based Training

Teaching healthcare professionals and students through simulated experiences has rightly grown in popularity, partly as a result of an increased focus on patient safety and a recognition of the need for continuing professional development for neonatal staff [5–7]. Simulation-based education (SBE) has been described as "situations that mimic problems, events, or conditions that arise in professional encounters" [8].

Simulators used in neonatal medicine can be grouped according to their complexity:

- Low fidelity—these might be used to teach basic clinical skills, for example intravenous cannulation, or nasogastric tube insertion [9]
- Medium fidelity—these might be used to deliver simple scenarios on a national life support course
- High fidelity—these mannequins provide more information to learners and are useful to deliver complex scenarios looking at team-working and decision making.

Some useful areas of neonatal teaching have traditionally not been considered as 'simulation' but use exactly the same principles: for instance using actors to deliver standardised communication training and to help learners develop the skills to have difficult conversations with families [10].

A. Bonfield
University Hospitals of Leicester NHS Trust, Leicester, UK
e-mail: ab798@le.ac.uk

J. Cusack (✉)
Leicester Neonatal Service, University Hospitals of Leicester NHS Trust,
Leicester Royal Infirmary, Leicester Medical School, Leicester, UK
e-mail: jonathan.cusack@uhl-tr.nhs.uk

The fidelity of a simulation does not just relate to the equipment used: placing a mannequin in a real clinical environment can add a significant amount of realism.

In-Situ Simulation

In-situ or 'point of care' simulation training is the delivery of a simulation session within a real clinical environment. There are major benefits for learners, facilitators and organisations in delivering sessions to teams using the same tools and equipment that they use in their normal working day [11].

Figure 31.1 demonstrates a multidisciplinary team that work together undergoing a simulation training session on the neonatal unit 'in situ.'

In situ simulation helps to increase the authenticity of the session, which is an important feature of adult learning. Teams behave in a realistic way because they are working in an environment that is familiar to them [12].

From an educator's perspective, in-situ simulation helps to increase the authenticity of the learning experience because the learners are within their familiar clinical environment [12]. However, delivering simulation in a real clinical environment brings its own challenges. Simulators and computers may need to be moved around and this can be challenging, particularly in simulations that involve multiple locations (for example neonatal transport). Wires and cable may decrease the level of

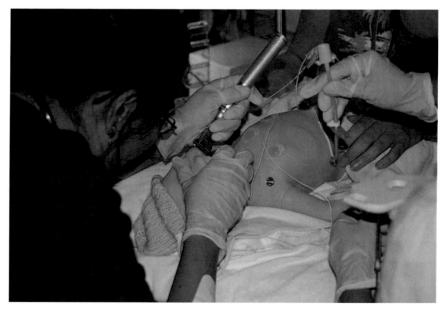

Fig. 31.1 Team training photograph. A team undergoing simulation training in the real clinical environment (used with permission)

realism, although there is some improvement in this with the increasing use of wireless compact simulators.

Clinical environments are not necessarily planned and built with the delivery of education sessions in mind. This needs to be considered when designing sessions. For example, it is important to make sure that there is an appropriate 'safe' space in which to carry out the debrief [13]. There must also be enough clinical staff on duty to ensure that patient care can safely continue and that training sessions do not adversely affect patient care [11]. There needs to be a degree of flexibility and planning in conducting in situ simulation sessions.

From the learner's perspective, in situ simulation is underpinned by a learning theory known as 'situativity theory', according to which learners benefit from the learning being delivered in in the correct context in the clinical environment [14]. Rather than have the trainees go to a simulation centre and expect them to transfer the learning *to* the clinical environment, it takes the simulation to the trainees and allows the learning to emerge *from* the clinical environment.

However, there are associated risks.

The clinical environment is complex, and this can be detrimental to trainees' learning. There is a vast amount of information that has to be assimilated by trainees and this can lead to 'cognitive overload' [15], which may be detrimental to learning. Simulation facilitators need to be aware of this. One technique is to focus learning onto one or two important points.

Another consideration is the learner's psychological safety. The principle of psychological safety is comprised of a number of factors, but at the heart of it, is the learner feeling free to undertake tasks without fear of negative consequences, such as a threat to self-image [16]. In situ simulation can threaten an individual's psychological safety in a number of ways: a learner may feel under increased scrutiny from their colleagues or they may feel burdened by their other clinical work. This can lead to learner disengagement and may even build resentment to the learning opportunity [17]. Suggestions to mitigate threats to psychological safety include the use of a pre-simulation brief where expectations and trust between educators and learners can be established.

Further practical guidance can be found in Table 31.1.

Table 31.1 Psychological safety issues and practical considerations

Psychological safety issue	Practical guidance
Threat to self-image	Only those taking part in the simulation and faculty are present
	If video recording the session, ensure adequate safeguards to what happens with the footage
High burden of clinical work	Ensure adequate cover of clinical tasks during simulation with flexible use of neonatal unit staff
	Hand pager to other colleagues
Fear of failure	Pre-brief before the scenario setting ground rules.
	Debrief after the scenario

Finally, at the institutional level, delivering simulation with real teams in their usual working area is helpful in uncovering team deficiencies [18]. This is particularly useful, as often, teams working on the neonatal unit comprise medical staff that rotate, and staff from different backgrounds such as surgeons, midwives, nursing and medical staff.

Simulation has the ability to move beyond team training to, arguably, its most useful quality; identifying latent threats to safety within the unit environment [13]. In our unit, we have identified and resolved a number of problems through our simulation program: confusing written instructions for drawing up resuscitation drugs; equipment that was mounted out of the eye line of a team leader during emergency intubation; and wall mounted resuscitation devices that could not be reached by short nursing staff! The importance of in situ simulation is increasingly being recognised and has the opportunity to provide some of the richest sources of learning for clinical teams.

Improving Fidelity

The fidelity or 'realism' of a simulation is much more than the complexity of the mannequin being used. The physical fidelity of the mannequin is important, but it is also useful to consider the surrounding environment, and the psychological fidelity.

Clinical teams respond to alarm sounds that they recognise, medical charts and records that look familiar to them. Low fidelity mannequins can be made to look surprisingly realistic, and can be used in complex scenarios by thinking about the surrounding environment and equipment [19, 20].

In situ simulation can increase psychological fidelity and encourage teams to 'buy in' and psychologically invest in the simulation. This has been shown to be an important factor in the transfer of learning [21].

Neonatal specific studies have demonstrated that high fidelity simulation can improve certain skills measured by the time to intubation [22] and team-working behaviours [23]. Studies to date have failed to show a statistically significant difference between high and low fidelity simulation in other modalities such as speed of completing a resuscitation.

Rapid Cycle Deliberate Practice

Deliberate practice is an evolving area in neonatal simulation. This is based around the concept that expertise in practical skills is generated through repeated practice of specific tasks, particularly tasks that the trainee is unable to do well [24, 25]. It has been extensively used in different domains, from military combat evaluation to motorsport pit stops, and has started to be used within medical simulation as 'Rapid Cycle Deliberate Practice' (RCDP) [26]. Within medicine, there are three key principles to RCDP:

1. Maximising the time spent in deliberate practice
2. Faculty providing expert solutions to common problems
3. Fostering psychological safety for the learner

This works best when a specific part of a well-defined skill is repeated multiple times with immediate feedback being given after each cycle to improve performance [27]. This is similar to how muscle memory is developed when learning a musical instrument. Learners are given multiple opportunities to perform the same skill.

They are given instant feedback and suggestions on their performance, and are then requested to "pause, rewind 10 s and try it again" until they reach a level of mastery [26].

This training technique has been utilised in simulated neonatal resuscitation scenarios, demonstrating improvement in learning related to positive pressure ventilation, emergency umbilical vessel catheterisation, administration of intravenous medication, and infant lumbar puncture [28].

We have used this is in repeatedly practising the process of quickly moving a neonate out of the incubator into an ideal position for intubation. Staff often identify issues with familiarisation with the incubator and monitoring equipment, and often change the way that team members are positioned to maximise their efficiency. In this way, the time to successful intubation can be significantly reduced.

Rapid cycle deliberate practice has been used to develop a surgical handover protocol through the observation of Formula 1 teams [29], in which members of the team have clearly defined tasks that are practised meticulously to improve outcomes.

RCDP is an emerging tool in simulation. Further research is planned, looking at learners retention of skills and the translation to real clinical behaviours [30].

It is useful to know, when planning training programs, that deliberate practice is a popular training method for new trainees, whereas more experienced learners may prefer more a in depth realistic simulation experience [31].

Debriefing Techniques

It is widely regarded that the most significant part of a clinical simulation is the debrief following the scenario. This is consistently rated by participants as the most important part of a simulation session [8, 32], yet a poorly conducted debrief can be destructive to learning [33]. Many models of debriefing have been described, and we will seek to highlight some of these. There are some key points that should be observed with any debrief:

1. Facilitators running a debrief should be trained educators [34]
2. Debriefing should not be too formulaic [35]; whilst there are very useful models of debriefing, asking the same type of question repeatedly can be frustrating for learners
3. Debriefing should focus on why an individual or team behaved in a particular way, rather than providing a list of errors [36]

Table 31.2 Pendleton rules

Check the learner is ready for feedback and clarify factual points
The learner comments on what went well and why
The group discusses what went well and why
The learner comments on what went less well and why and how it could be improved
The whole group discuss what went less well and why and how it could be done differently

Commonly used debriefing models and techniques that have been used in neonatal simulation training are discussed below.

Pendleton Debriefing [37]. This style of debriefing was previously used extensively in courses run by the Resuscitation Council, UK.

The process is outlined in Table 31.2.

The advantages of Pendleton's rules are that this approach is relatively easy to teach to facilitators, there is a focus on positive aspects of the simulation and this style of debrief can foster a constructive reflective process. However, experienced learners can find this model frustrating, as their personal learning agenda may be overlooked and they can find that the inflexibility of the model limits the time for constructive criticism [38]. Medical and nursing staff often want to discuss errors made and forcing them into an artificial conversation can be counterproductive.

Plus Delta

This style of debrief has been particularly popular in the United States and was adapted from the aviation industry [39]. The 'plus' refers to things that went well during a scenario and behaviours that should be repeated, whereas the 'delta' column focuses on aspects requiring change. Teams are encouraged to discuss both areas and to suggest ways to implement changes.

Advocacy with Enquiry

This style of debriefing has become increasingly popular over the last decade, and involves observing a team action or behaviour (advocacy) and then questioning the reason behind this observation (enquiry) [36]. From an educational perspective, this is important because we want to know *why* a participant behaved in a particular way, also known as the 'frame'. An example is shown in Fig. 31.2.

In this example, the facilitator notes that there was a delay in removing a blocked endotracheal tube, leading to hypoxia and bradycardia (the action leading to a result).

Fig. 31.2 Example of
advocacy with enquiry

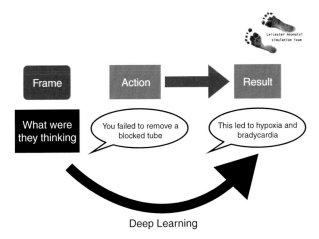

Deep Learning

From an educational perspective, the important thing is to find out *why* the team behaved in this way. There may be a range of reasons relating to practical skill levels, perceived hierarchy or communication issues and the debrief is designed to explore these with learners. The facilitator does not actually 'know' what the trainee was thinking and needs to explore this carefully to find out.

The advantage of this type of debrief is that it the reason behind actions becomes more transparent and it focuses on what an individual can practically do to change the outcome in the real world. In the example above, communication techniques could be explored, such as using individuals' names, giving specific instructions, the concept of a communication through the team leader, and communication receipts.

Narrative Debrief

This style of debrief originated as a therapeutic process in the military, allowing members of a team to come together and reconstruct events to develop meaning [40]. In medical simulation, the facilitator goes through the events that happened in chronological order, and asks participants to describe what they were thinking, and to provide a narrative as to why they behaved as they did. This has benefit in that questions are usually perceived to be less threatening than other styles of debrief. Narrative style questions are often as useful way to start a debrief.

Video Debriefing

Video debriefing is the use of recorded footage of the simulation to show trainees what had happened during the scenario. It was once thought to be the 'gold standard' of debriefing feedback [32], as it enabled events to be shown exactly as they occurred. However, recent studies have demonstrated a mixed picture. Video may distract from the learning objectives, result in less time for verbal feedback, and can provoke high levels of anxiety [32, 41, 42].

One meta-analysis also showed that multimedia aids, such as video, did not improve debriefing effectiveness [43].The authors concluded that the design of the simulation was more important than the media methods used. However, this does not mean that the use of video is never helpful, but rather that the design of the simulation is the factor of greater importance.

Gather, Analyse, Summarise (GAS)

There are a number of structured debriefing tools designed to improve the consistency of debriefing. One of these tools is 'GAS' which splits the debrief into three discrete sections; Gather, Analyse and Summarise [44].

During the 'gather' phase, the instructor questions and listens to the participants to ascertain how they think and feel about the simulated experience and to consider gaps that may exist.

This information is the used to fuel the discussion in the analysis and summary phases.

The 'analyse' phase is where participants are expected to reflect on actions taken and the consequences of these actions. A variety of resources might be used during this process to provide an accurate account of the simulation, such as video or a record of events. Finally, the 'summarise' phase enables a review of critical lessons learnt in order to clearly highlight these points.

The optimal way to conduct a simulation debrief is to have a range of debriefing styles and tools available and this has been described as the 'blended approach' [35]. This approach is useful and recognises that individuals learn in different ways, avoiding an over formulaic approach to discussions.

Debriefing: Moving from the Simulation Session to the Real World

We have described some of the research looking into simulation-based training and the best way to debrief teams after a simulated scenario. There is now an increasing focus on how this should be taken into the clinical area to be used after real clinical events [45]. Post event debriefing has mainly been applied to major clinical events such as resuscitation; however there is an argument that the scope of post event debriefing should be broadened to enhance learning and patient safety [45].

Medicine lags behind other high risk industries in how we analyse and learn from mistakes. It can be particularly useful to carry out a 'hot debrief' immediately after a real critical event [46]. Techniques used in simulation debriefing can be particularly helpful.

A method that has been adapted from military debriefing is the 'After Action Review'. We use a modified version on our neonatal intensive care unit following significant clinical events: (Fig. 31.3)

The key points in this method are:

1. An opportunity to 'decompress' following a stressful event
2. An exploration of what should have happened in an ideal resuscitation
3. An exploration of what did happen
4. Identification of practical things that can be done to 'close the gap'

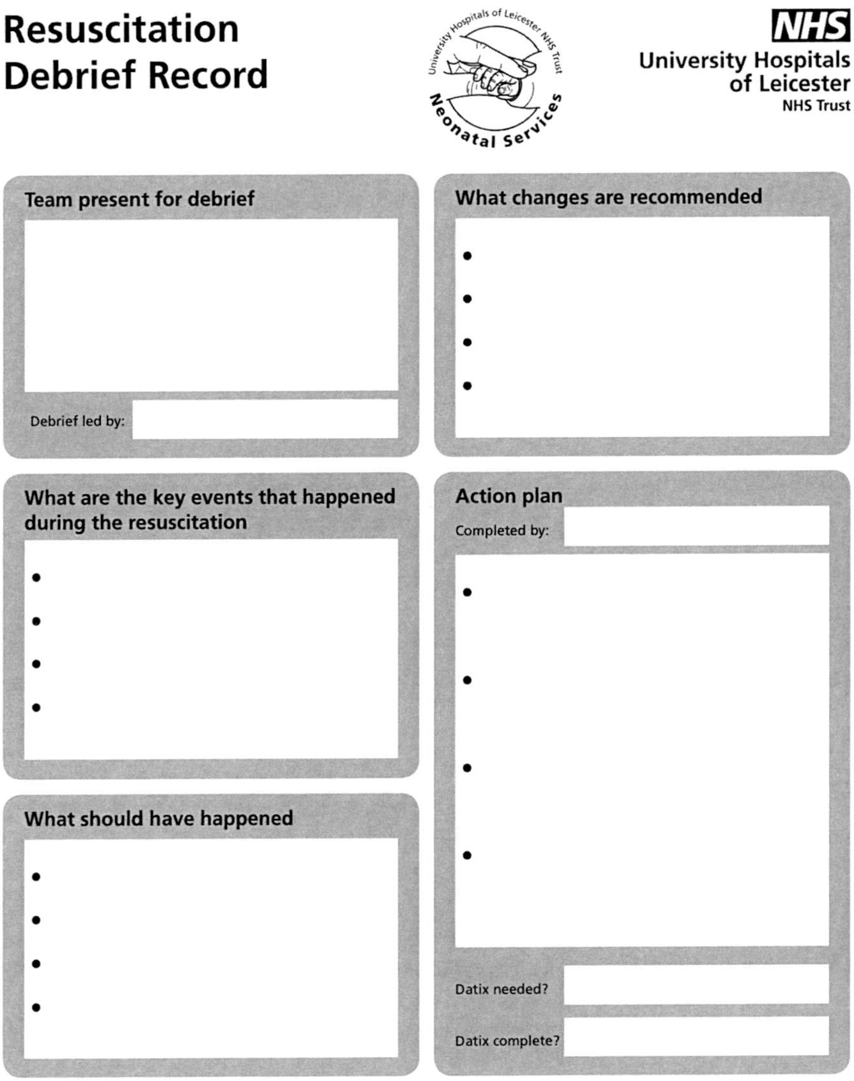

Resuscitation Debrief Record

University Hospitals of Leicester NHS Trust — Neonatal Services

NHS
University Hospitals
of Leicester
NHS Trust

Team present for debrief

Debrief led by:

What changes are recommended

-
-
-
-

What are the key events that happened during the resuscitation

-
-
-
-

Action plan

Completed by:

-
-
-
-

Datix needed?

Datix complete?

What should have happened

-
-
-
-

Fig. 31.3 Example of a resuscitation debriefing record

Maintaining Simulation Standards

It is important that simulation sessions are delivered to a high, but also to a consistent standard. It can be helpful for teams of educators to work together and to regularly seek feedback.

The GMC in the UK, now recommend that educational activity should be formally reviewed at appraisals for doctors [47]. There are a number of tools that can be used to assess the standard of simulation debriefing. The London Deanery has produced a simple tool, the Objective Structured Assessment of Debriefing [48], which allows educators to score each other and provides a basis for discussion and continuing professional development. The Centre for Medical Simulation at Harvard [49] have a similar but more in depth tool and has been shown to improve the quality of debriefing [50]. These tools allow an objective assessment of the quality of a debrief and can be useful to develop faculty skills.

Technology Enhanced Learning: What Does the Future Hold?

Over the last few decades, technology has advanced rapidly and has become more accessible, leading to significant changes in the ways we deliver education. Examples of this include the use of e-learning, Web 2.0 technologies [51] such as wikis, social media, mobile apps, and simulation. These technologies have increasing interactivity and user participation and are ideal for teaching and learning.

Neonatal simulators have become more user friendly and more portable. Recent developments include mannequins with much more realistic features which will continue to aid with the fidelity of simulations and allow the learners to suspend disbelief with greater ease (Fig. 31.4).

There have been developments in technology to allow simulators to provide immediate reproducible feedback on performance, particularly for practical skills. It has been shown that CPR performance can be improved by a visual feedback of rate, depth and quality of compressions when using biofeedback devices [52]. UK neonatal resuscitation courses have now included the use of 'mask leak' equipment to improve the practice of face mask ventilation by providing biofeedback to participants whilst they deliver ventilation breaths [53].

Whilst biofeedback has been shown to improve performance on task trainers, an important consideration is whether it could it be used during real resuscitations. Devices that measure mask leak and CPR performance during real resuscitation are under development and have huge potential. In the same way that debriefing is being transferred from simulation to real clinical practice, transferring biofeedback mechanisms into the clinical world provides the opportunity for immediate feedback even as one is performing the task. This has the potential to improve the quality of care given, as the care is delivered, rather than reflecting on a resuscitation after it has finished.

Simulation equipment continues to improve. One area that is being increasing developed is that of 'haptics' and this is an area of growing interest and develop-

Fig. 31.4 Mannequin
demonstrating increasing
realism (with permission
Lifecast®)

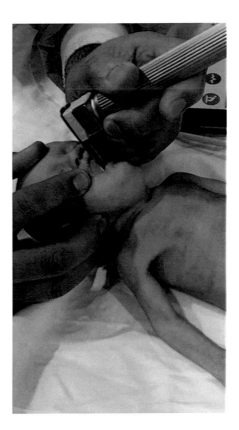

ment. Haptic feedback refers to the tactile stimulation that is felt when performing a particular skill [54]. This has been key in areas such as laparoscopic and orthopaedic surgery [55, 56].

Current research on using haptics in skills such as neonatal intubation is ongoing with inconclusive results so far [57]. Nonetheless, as this technology improves and becomes more available, we may see an increased uptake of its use when teaching neonatal clinical skills and the development of more realistic task trainers. Augmented and virtual reality have been extensively used in other industries, and are likely to be increasingly used in neonatal simulation, although such technologies may be limited by high costs.

We need to match the technological developments with advances in teaching practice. Whilst there are many studies looking at neonatal simulation, none has shown conclusively that the implementation of a simulation program on its own, has improved patient outcome. There is, however, a huge potential for technology enhanced learning to improve the outcome for babies. There is increasing evidence that it is possible to demonstrate improved clinical outcomes following the development of training programs [58]. It is important that future developments in technology run parallel with developments in education so that they can work together to improve patient outcome.

References

1. Wiese A, Kilty C, Bergin C, Flood P, Fu N, Horgan M, Higgins A, Maher B, O'Kane G, Prihodova L, Slattery D. Protocol for a realist review of workplace learning in postgraduate medical education and training. Syst Rev. 2017;6(1):10.
2. Asch DA, Bilimoria KY, Desai SV. Resident duty hours and medical education policy—raising the evidence bar. N Engl J Med. 2017;376(18):1704–6.
3. Dyer C, Cohen D. How should doctors use e-portfolios in the wake of the Bawa-Garba case? BMJ. 2018;360:k572.
4. Sandars J, Patel RS, Goh PS, Kokatailo PK, Lafferty N. The importance of educational theories for facilitating learning when using technology in medical education. Med Teach. 2015;37(11):1039–42.
5. Ker J, Bradley P. Simulation in medical education. In: Understanding medical education: evidence, theory and practice. 2013. p. 175–92.
6. Okuda Y, Bryson EO, DeMaria S Jr, Jacobson L, Quinones J, Shen B, Levine AI. The utility of simulation in medical education: what is the evidence? Mt Sinai J Med. 2009;76(4):330–43.
7. Gaba DM. The future vision of simulation in health care. Qual Saf Health Care. 2004;13(Suppl 1):i2–i10.
8. Barry Issenberg S, McGaghie WC, Petrusa ER, Lee Gordon D, Scalese RJ. Features and uses of high-fidelity medical simulations that lead to effective learning: a BEME systematic review. Med Teach. 2005;27(1):10–28.
9. Good ML. Patient simulation for training basic and advanced clinical skills. Med Educ. 2003;37:14–21.
10. Wong AH, Tiyyagura GK, Dodington JM, Hawkins B, Hersey D, Auerbach MA. Facilitating tough conversations: using an innovative simulation-primed qualitative inquiry in pediatric research. Acad Pediatr. 2017;17:807–13.
11. Patterson MD, Blike GT, Nadkarni VM. In situ simulation: challenges and results. In: Advances in patient safety: new directions and alternative approaches (Vol. 3: performance and tools). Agency for Healthcare Research and Quality (US). 2008.
12. Sørensen JL, Van der Vleuten C, Lindschou J, Gluud C, Østergaard D, LeBlanc V, Johansen M, Ekelund K, Albrechtsen CK, Pedersen BW, Kjærgaard H. 'In situ simulation 'versus' off site simulation' in obstetric emergencies and their effect on knowledge, safety attitudes, team performance, stress, and motivation: study protocol for a randomized controlled trial. Trials. 2013;14(1):220.
13. Schofield L, Welfare E, Mercer S. In-situ simulation. Trauma. 2017. https://doi.org/10.1177/1460408617711729.
14. Durning SJ, Artino AR. Situativity theory: a perspective on how participants and the environment can interact: AMEE Guide no. 52. Med Teach. 2011;33(3):188–99.
15. Norman G, Dore K, Grierson L. The minimal relationship between simulation fidelity and transfer of learning. Med Educ. 2012;46(7):636–47.
16. Schepers J, de Jong A, Wetzels M, de Ruyter K. Psychological safety and social support in groupware adoption: a multi-level assessment in education. Comput Educ. 2008;51(2):757–75.
17. Rudolph JW, Raemer DB, Simon R. Establishing a safe container for learning in simulation: the role of the presimulation briefing. Simul Healthc. 2014;9(6):339–49.
18. Mercer SJ, Wimlett S. In-situ simulation. Bull R Coll Anaesthet. 2012;76:28–30.
19. Maran NJ, Glavin RJ. Low-to high-fidelity simulation—a continuum of medical education? Med Educ. 2003;37:22–8.
20. Curran V, Fleet L, White S, Bessell C, Deshpandey A, Drover A, Hayward M, Valcour J. A randomized controlled study of manikin simulator fidelity on neonatal resuscitation program learning outcomes. Adv Health Sci Educ. 2015;20(1):205–18.

21. Brydges R, Carnahan H, Rose D, Rose L, Dubrowski A. Coordinating progressive levels of simulation fidelity to maximize educational benefit. Acad Med. 2010;85(5):806–12.
22. Finan E, Bismilla Z, Campbell C, Leblanc V, Jefferies A, Whyte HE. Improved procedural performance following a simulation training session may not be transferable to the clinical environment. J Perinatol. 2012;32(7):539–44.
23. Thomas EJ, Williams AL, Reichman EF, Lasky RE, Crandell S, Taggart WR. Team training in the neonatal resuscitation program for interns: teamwork and quality of resuscitations. Pediatrics. 2010;125(3):539–46.
24. Ericsson KA, Krampe RT, Tesch-Römer C. The role of deliberate practice in the acquisition of expert performance. Psychol Rev. 1993;100(3):363–406.
25. Ericsson KA, Prietula MJ, Cokely ET. The making of an expert. Harv Bus Rev. 2007;85(7/8):114.
26. Hunt EA, Duval-Arnould JM, Nelson-McMillan KL, Bradshaw JH, Diener-West M, Perretta JS, Shilkofski NA. Pediatric resident resuscitation skills improve after "rapid cycle deliberate practice" training. Resuscitation. 2014;85(7):945–51.
27. Ericsson KA. Deliberate practice and the acquisition and maintenance of expert performance in medicine and related domains. Acad Med. 2004;79(10):S70–81.
28. Sawyer T, Sierocka-Castaneda A, Chan D, Berg B, Lustik M, Thompson M. Deliberate practice using simulation improves neonatal resuscitation performance. Simul Healthc. 2011;6(6):327–36.
29. Catchpole KR, De Leval MR, Mcewan A, Pigott N, Elliott MJ, Mcquillan A, Macdonald C, Goldman AJ. Patient handover from surgery to intensive care: using Formula 1 pit-stop and aviation models to improve safety and quality. Pediatr Anesth. 2007;17(5):470–8.
30. Taras J, Everett T. Rapid cycle deliberate practice in medical education—a systematic review. Cureus. 2017;9(4):e1180.
31. Rapid cycle deliberate practice compared with immersive simulation and standard debriefing for neonatal simulation-based education. J Paediatr Child Health. 2017;53:45–5. https://doi.org/10.1111/jpc.13494_128.
32. Levett-Jones T, Lapkin S. A systematic review of the effectiveness of simulation debriefing in health professional education. Nurse Educ Today. 2014;34(6):e58–63.
33. Grant VJ, Robinson T, Catena H, Eppich W, Cheng A. Difficult debriefing situations: a toolbox for simulation educators. Med Teach. 2018;40(7):703–12.
34. Jewkes F, Phillips B. Resuscitation training of paediatricians. Arch Dis Child. 2003;88(2):118–21.
35. Eppich W, Cheng A. Promoting Excellence and Reflective Learning in Simulation (PEARLS): development and rationale for a blended approach to health care simulation debriefing. Simul Healthc. 2015;10(2):106–15.
36. Rudolph JW, Simon R, Dufresne RL, Raemer DB. There is no such thing as non-judgmental debriefing: a theory and method for debriefing with good judgment. Simul Healthc. 2006;1:49–55.
37. Pendleton D. The consultation: an approach to learning and teaching (Oxford General Practice Series). 1984.
38. Wood D. Formative assessment. In: Swanwick T, editor. Understanding medical education: evidence, theory and practice. 2nd ed. Chichester: Wiley-Blackwell; 2014.
39. Gardner R. Introduction to debriefing. In: Seminars in perinatology. Vol. 37, No. 3. WB Saunders; 2013. p. 166–74.
40. Fanning RM, Gaba DM. The role of debriefing in simulation-based learning. Simul Healthc. 2007;2(2):115–25.
41. Chronister C, Brown D. Comparison of simulation debriefing methods. Clin Simul Nurs. 2012;8(7):e281–8.
42. Lindon-Morris E, Laidlaw A. Anxiety and self-awareness in video feedback. Clin Teach. 2014;11(3):174–8.

43. Tannenbaum SI, Cerasoli CP. Do team and individual debriefs enhance performance? A meta-analysis. Hum Factors. 2013;55(1):231–45.
44. Phrampus PE, O'Donnell JM. Debriefing using a structured and supported approach. In: The comprehensive textbook of healthcare simulation. New York: Springer; 2013. p. 73–84.
45. Eppich WJ, Mullan PC, Brett-Fleegler M, Cheng A. "Let's talk about it": translating lessons from health care simulation to clinical event debriefings and coaching conversations. Clin Pediatr Emerg Med. 2016;17(3):200–11.
46. Shore H. After compression, time for decompression: debriefing after significant clinical events. Infant. 2014;10(4):117–9.
47. General Medical Council (Great Britain). Tomorrow's doctors: outcomes and standards for undergraduate medical education. GMC. 2009.
48. https://www.imperial.ac.uk/patient-safety-translational-research-centre/education/training-materials-for-use-in-research-and-clinical-practice/the-observational-structured/. Accessed 1 Sept 2018.
49. https://harvardmedsim.org/debriefing-assessment-for-simulation-in-healthcare-dash/. Accessed 1 Sept 2018.
50. Simon R, Raemer DB, Rudolph JW. Debriefing assessment for simulation in healthcare (DASH)© rater's handbook. Boston: Center for Medical Simulation. 2010. https://harvard-medsim.org/wp-content/uploads/2017/01/DASH.handbook.2010.Final.Rev.2.pdf.   English, French, German, Japanese, Spanish.
51. https://whatis.techtarget.com/definition/Web-20-or-Web-2. Accessed 1 Sept 2018.
52. Kong S, Shin S, Song K, et al. Effect of instructor's real-time feedback using QCPR-classroom device during layperson cardiopulmonary resuscitation (CPR) training on quality of CPR performances: a prospective cluster-randomised trial. BMJ Open. 2018;8. https://doi.org/10.1136/bmjopen-2018-EMS.25.
53. Wood FE, Morley CJ, Dawson JA, Kamlin COF, Owen LS, Donath S, Davis PG. Improved techniques reduce face mask leak during simulated neonatal resuscitation: study 2. Arch Dis Child Fetal Neonatal Ed. 2008;93(3):F230–4.
54. Botden SM, Torab F, Buzink SN, Jakimowicz JJ. The importance of haptic feedback in laparoscopic suturing training and the additive value of virtual reality simulation. Surg Endosc. 2008;22(5):1214–22.
55. Panait L, Akkary E, Bell RL, Roberts KE, Dudrick SJ, Duffy AJ. The role of haptic feedback in laparoscopic simulation training. J Surg Res. 2009;156(2):312–6.
56. Thawani JP, Ramayya AG, Abdullah KG, Hudgins E, Vaughan K, Piazza M, Madsen PJ, Buch V, Grady MS. Resident simulation training in endoscopic endonasal surgery utilizing haptic feedback technology. J Clin Neurosci. 2016;34:112–6.
57. Agarwal A, Leviter J, Mannarino C, Levit O, Johnston L, Auerbach M. Is a haptic simulation interface more effective than computer mouse-based interface for neonatal intubation skills training? BMJ Simul Technol Enhanc Learn. 2015;1(1):5–11.
58. Draycott TJ, Crofts JF, Ash JP, Wilson LV, Yard E, Sibanda T, Whitelaw A. Improving neonatal outcome through practical shoulder dystocia training. Obstet Gynecol. 2008;112(1):14–20.

Chapter 32
Genomics for the Neonatologist

Richard Hastings and Abhijit Dixit

Introduction

Congenital malformations and genetic disorders are the leading cause of death in both children and the neonatal population. A retrospective assessment of cause of death in a US children's hospital showed that malformations and genetic disorders were the cause in 34.4% of children. When the neonatal population was examined, the figure was 63.9% [1]. There are several thousand different genetic disorders and the clinical features of these conditions can be variable, making diagnosis challenging. Traditional genetic diagnosis is a hypothesis-driven stepwise approach which may start with a clinical assessment followed by chromosome analysis (previously by karyotype but more recently by chromosomal microarray) with the next step being specific gene or gene panel testing. This approach can take several months before results are reported. The use of next-generation sequencing (NGS) is changing the diagnostic approach in these conditions and an understanding of the strengths, pitfalls and ethical challenges in these methods is essential for the twenty-first Century neonatologist.

R. Hastings
Department of Paediatrics, Sherwood Forest Hospitals, Sutton-in-Ashfield, UK
e-mail: rhastings@nhs.net

A. Dixit (✉)
Department of Clinical Genetics, Nottingham University Hospitals, Nottingham, UK
e-mail: abhijit.dixit@nuh.nhs.uk

© Springer Nature Switzerland AG 2020
E. M. Boyle, J. Cusack (eds.), *Emerging Topics and Controversies in Neonatology*, https://doi.org/10.1007/978-3-030-28829-7_32

Important Concepts

The genetic code of the human genome is composed of four deoxyribonucleotides. Adenine (A) pairs with thymine (T), and guanine (G) pairs with cytosine (C) in the double-stranded DNA molecule. There are around three billion nucleotides in the entire human genetic code, and this is termed the genome. Within the 20,000 genes of the human genome, there are coding regions (exons) and non-coding regions (introns). Additionally, there is a large amount of non-coding material between genes so that only about 1.5% of the human genome is comprised of exons—and termed the exome. Genes are transcribed into messenger RNA with triplet nucleotide combinations (codons) corresponding to individual amino acids within the translated protein. The function of the remaining 98.5% of the genome is not fully understood but there are important regulatory regions within these sequences.

Within the three billion nucleotides of the human genome, there are approximately four million single nucleotide variants (SNVs) as compared to the 'standard' sequence. The vast majority of these variants are benign and contribute to the normal phenotypic variation seen between individuals. A small percentage of these variants are pathogenic (formerly called mutations) and can affect cellular function in a number of ways. For example, nonsense variants are single nucleotide changes that convert an amino acid codon into a termination codon, resulting in the translated protein being truncated. A missense variant changes the codon from one amino acid to a different amino acid. This may, or may not, have a significant impact on the function of the encoded protein.

Genomic Testing

A traditional clinical genetics approach involves a clinical evaluation which guides genetic testing. A particular presentation may implicate pathogenic variants in one or a small group of genes. For example, assessing a floppy baby may prompt testing for common trisomies, Prader Willi syndrome, congenital myotonic dystrophy and spinal muscular atrophy, depending on the associated phenotypic features. If these tests are reported as normal, further testing for more rare conditions may be undertaken. There are several limitations to this approach. Firstly, genetic conditions may not always present in a typical fashion [2]. Secondly, this approach relies on the skill of the neonatologist, paediatrician, or clinical geneticist. Thirdly, in many instances this method can take a long time to reach a diagnosis, often at great expense.

One type of genomic testing that many neonatologists will be familiar with is chromosomal microarray analysis. This technique using hybridisation of thousands of probes spaced out across the genome to identify where regions have been lost or duplicated. The resolution of this technique is nearly 1000-fold higher than karyotyping. Like whole genome sequencing, chromosomal microarray is a genotype driven approach: the results of the test are related to the phenotype of the baby rather than the phenotype directing specific gene testing.

The dramatic fall in the cost of next generation sequencing (NGS) has led to the emergence of whole exome sequencing (WES) and whole genome sequencing (WGS) as frontline tools on the neonatal intensive care unit. WES uses hybridisation techniques to select and then sequence only the exons. WGS allows sequencing of the majority of the three billion base pairs of the human genome. WES has the benefit that analysis of the resultant sequencing data is simpler, but hybridisation techniques are prone to selection bias and WES may miss variants which are identified by WGS.

Diagnostics

Perhaps the most exciting area of genomic research on the neonatal unit is in the area of diagnostics. It is estimated that 3% of babies are born with a congenital anomaly and the relative risk for this is doubled in certain ethnic groups [3]. A Canadian study examined almost 20,000 consecutive neonatal unit admissions and found that 13% of these babies had one or more congenital anomalies [4]. These anomalies are a predictor of both mortality and length of stay on NICU [5]. Genetic conditions are also the leading cause of death in the neonatal population [1]. Early diagnosis of a genetic condition has the potential to direct management for that condition such as guiding drug therapy or suggesting a specialised diet [6, 7]. In conditions that are known to be severely life-limiting, a diagnosis can direct management towards palliative care. The option for early palliation can provide relief to babies and their families as well as reduce the burden of long-term care on the healthcare system.

Diagnostic Yield

Several studies have highlighted the efficacy of NGS in the diagnosis of genetic disorders on the neonatal unit. Many of the studies described in Table 32.1 include older population groups but also examine neonatal patients. In one study 20 babies were recruited from two neonatal units who had approximately 2000 admissions during the study period (i.e. 1 in 100 admissions; [8]). These babies were selected both retrospectively and prospectively. They received a review by the clinical genetics or metabolic teams at these hospitals and had to have one of the following features: a congenital malformation; dysmorphic features, neurological impairment, abnormal growth parameters or clinical features of a metabolic condition. This team used a gene panel containing almost 5000 genes which have a known association with a human disease phenotype—in effect a very large gene panel. The NGS approach provided a molecular diagnosis in 40% of the patients in this study. This compared with a 10% diagnostic rate using standard care pathways [8].

Table 32.1 Summary of studies using next generation sequencing for diagnostic purposes

Study description	NGS methodology	Patient group	n	Diagnostic yield	Percentage with change in management[a]	Average time to diagnosis	Year and Reference
Retrospective and prospective recruitment of babies with suspected genetic diseases	5000 gene panel associated with clinical phenotypes	'Newborns'	20	40%	38%	15 weeks	2016 [8]
Prospective study of consecutive patients referred to clinical genetics service with suspected genetic condition	WES	All ages, 49% <5 years of age	814	26%	–	–	2014 [9]
Retrospective analysis of patients referred to clinical diagnostic laboratory	WES	Age not specified	7374	28%	–	–	2017 [10]
Prospective patients referred to clinical diagnostic laboratory	WES	1 month to 59 years. 14% < 12 months of age	1000	31%	–	–	2017 [11]
Retrospective observational study of patients referred to clinical diagnostic laboratory	WES	Mean age 6 years. 45% < 5 years of age including 11 fetal samples	2000	25%	19%	–	2014 [12]
Retrospective analysis of babies referred for exome sequencing	WES	<100 days of age, median of 28 days	278	37% (51% in trio-exomes)	52% (72% in seriously ill babies)	51 days (13 days for seriously ill babies)	2017 [7]
Prospective recruitment of infants with suspected genetic conditions	WES	<2 years of age	80	58%	33%	134 days	2016 [13]
Retrospective comparison of WGS with standard genetic testing on NICU/PICU in babies with suspected genetic disease	WGS	<4 months of age	35	57%	65%	23 days	2015 [6]

Prospective recruitment from sub-specialty paediatric clinics	WGS	Children <18 years of age	103	41%	–	–	2018 [14]
Prospective analysis of children referred to genetics service	WGS	Mean age of 5 years, 25% < 1 year of age	100	34%	–	–	2016 [15]
Retrospective study on infants where a genetic disorder was possible	WGS	Median age of 62 days. 71% in ICU	42	43%	72%	50 h	2018 [16]

aPercentage of those patients in whom a molecular diagnosis has been made

Several studies have used WES rather than large gene panels. The diagnostic yields in these studies range from 25 to 37% (see Table 32.1). A recent WES study which examined infants in the first 100 days of life recruited 278 babies with a mean age of 28.5 days, 68% of whom were being treated on NICU. A molecular diagnosis was obtained in 37% of infants [7]. Sequencing of Trio-exomes (analysis of the baby and both parents) had even higher diagnostic rates at 51%.

WGS is now commonly being employed on the intensive care unit. One retrospective study examined infants under 4 months of age admitted to either PICU or NICU. These babies were a selected group who were felt likely to have a genetic condition. During the study period 35 families were selected from a total of 2400 admissions. Of the 35 babies, 20 (57%) received a diagnosis using WGS compared with 3 (9%) using the standard approach [6]. Other studies have shown similar diagnostic rates using standard genetic testing [13].

Effect on Management

Identifying a genetic disease in itself can be important, not least for the family, but the main benefit of a diagnosis is in directing clinical management. The majority of studies that examine this aspect are undertaken on the intensive care unit where benefits of a diagnosis are expected to be highest. Of those studies on PICU/NICU, the percentage of patients who had their management changed in response to receiving a diagnosis ranged from 38 to 72% (see Table 32.1).

It is likely that careful selection has a significant impact on this figure—patients who are selected because they are critically ill and are thought to have a genetic disease, receive the most benefit from a diagnosis. In one study examining babies <100 days of age, a molecular diagnosis affected the management of 52% of those given a diagnosis.

This included 35% of babies in whom there was an informed redirection of care (including palliation and withdrawal of support). A further 51% of babies benefitted from a new sub-specialty review (which had not previously been considered). For example, one baby had a previously unrecognised aortic stenosis. A dietary or medication change was initiated in 13% and a major procedure was performed as a result of the diagnosis in 9% of babies. Of those who did not receive a diagnosis with WES, 88% underwent chromosomal microarray analysis but no additional diagnoses were made [7]. Another study looking at babies of a similar age group showed a WGS diagnosis to have immediate clinical usefulness in 65% of babies including a strongly favourable change in management in 20% and initiation of palliation in 30% [6].

Time to Reporting

Sequencing technology and interpretation pipelines are improving such that WGS data can now be reported in a very short period of time. In 2012, Saunders et al. made molecular diagnoses in samples that had previously been analysed using standard genetic testing. They reported WGS results in 50 h [17]. In 2015, another US group showed they are able to report provisional results in critically ill neonates in as little as 26 h [18]. Both of these studies were small pilots designed to improve on the sequencing and interpretation pipelines. A larger study from 2018 examined 42 babies with a median age at enrolment of 62 days and in seven children who were critically ill they were able to provide sequencing and interpretation in less than 48 h. The remaining 35 children received a reported WGS in 5 days. Rapid WGS produced diagnoses in 43% of patients compared with 10% of babies in whom standard genetic testing was employed [16].

Costs

The introduction of NGS approaches is also likely to be more cost-effective than traditional phenotype-driven genetic testing. Stark and colleagues recruited patients of less than 2 years of age with suspected genetic diseases (multiple congenital anomalies, skeletal dysplasias, neurometabolic conditions) and showed that the average cost per diagnosis using standard genetic testing was AU$27,050. This compared with AU$5047 using WES [19]. Not only was WES less expensive, it was also more effective with a diagnostic rate 3-times higher than standard approaches.

There is also evidence for cost benefit on the neonatal unit. Farnaes and colleagues performed a cost analysis on six babies who received a genetic diagnosis using WGS. They used the Delphi method to produce a consensus view of an international panel of paediatricians. The consensus was that in these six patients, WGS improved the care of the infants and reduced healthcare costs by at least US$800,000. When the cost of WGS of all 42 babies in this study was considered there was still a conservatively estimated net reduction of inpatient costs of US$128,000 [16].

There is not currently enough evidence to confirm the economic benefits of WGS on the neonatal unit. A systematic review that examined the cost-effectiveness of WES and WGS in 36 studies across wide clinical settings reported that the current economic evidence for using WGS and WES as a frontline test is lacking [20]. However, it is very likely that as the infrastructure for WGS becomes embedded into healthcare systems such as the NHS, the costs of WGS will continue to fall.

Although in a resource-limited healthcare system cost savings are important, clearly clinical outcomes are paramount. As shown above, early diagnosis of a genetic disorder can affect outcomes for babies. There is also good evidence to suggest that late diagnosis adversely affects parents' ability to cope with the diagnosis of a child with severe disability and that parents have particular problems coping with an uncertain future [21, 22].

At the time of writing, a prospective trial called NICUSeq evaluating the efficacy of WGS compared with standard care is ongoing [23]. This study aims to enrol 330 babies who will be randomised to either clinical whole genome sequencing or standard care. Both trial arms will actually undergo WGS but the clinical WGS arm will have a result within 15 days whereas the control arm will undergo standard care for

60 days at which point the WGS result will be provided. The primary outcome of the trial is whether the intervention results in a change in management. A change is defined as a condition-specific management or supportive intervention or initiation of palliative care.

Microbiology

Late onset neonatal sepsis is a common problem on NICU and rapid diagnosis of sepsis would be a major step forward in neonatal care. The current gold standard test for sepsis, the blood culture, has poor sensitivity and there is a significant reporting delay. Decisions regarding antibiotic treatment are often made based on blood culture results but inadequate sample volumes mean that falsely negative results are common [24]. Molecular techniques (PCR) to identify bacterial species have been in development for many years [25–28]. In 2017, a Cochrane systematic review was performed to advise on the use of molecular assays for diagnosing sepsis in neonates [29]. This review included 35 studies and showed a mean sensitivity of 0.9 and specificity of 0.93. The authors' conclusions were that "Molecular assays have the advantage of producing rapid results and may perform well as add-on tests". It is hoped that as these techniques are developed further, they will allow the rapid identification of organisms and guide treatment before the second antibiotic dose is due.

Challenges for WGS on the Neonatal Unit

There are a number of complex ethical and practical considerations applicable to the use of genomic diagnostic tests on the neonatal unit.

Interpretation of Variants

Given that there are four million variants in the average human genome, WGS can pose significant difficulties in analysis and interpretation to classify variants as pathogenic or benign. Guidelines produced by the American College of Medical Genetics and Genomics (ACMG) are commonly used to classify whether a variant is benign, likely benign, likely pathogenic or pathogenic. These guidelines categorise variants using 28 different criteria [30]. The following are examples of criteria suggesting a variant is pathogenic:

- There is a known pathogenic variant causing the same amino acid change.
- This is a *de novo* variant (not seen in either parent) in a patient with disease in whom there is no family history of disease (maternity and paternity must be confirmed).

- The variant is located within an important functional domain of the protein.
- The variant is not seen in databases of control (healthy) genomes.
- The variant causes truncation of the translated protein because it results in a premature stop codon.
- A different missense variant affecting the same amino acid has previously been described.

Computer algorithms are also often employed to help categorise variants. These algorithms use factors such as whether an affected amino acid is conserved amongst different species or if an amino acid is changed to a structurally similar amino acid or not.

Sometimes, despite using all available bioinformatics data, a variant cannot be classified as benign or pathogenic and is termed a variant of uncertain significance (VUS). It is important to understand though, that analysis of a genetic variant is an iterative process. Analysis of a variant at a particular time may result in its classification as a VUS. However, as time passes there is likely to be new phenotypic information (as the child grows), emerging laboratory or database evidence and perhaps further family history as genetic testing is extended to other family members. This new evidence may result in re-classification of the variant.

Incidental Findings

An incidental finding is a pathogenic variant that is not responsible for the patient's presenting problem but might have implications for the patient's future and/or for the wider family. For example, if a baby has WGS for an undiagnosed metabolic disorder but is found to have a pathogenic BRCA1 variant (associated with a significantly elevated risk of breast and ovarian cancer). The return of incidental findings to families is a hot topic and recommendations in this area are still evolving. The ACMG had published explicit recommendations in 2013 suggesting that a subset of potential incidental genomic findings from 56 genes should be reported by the laboratory to the ordering clinician when WES or WGS is performed for *any* indication [31]. These genes were selected based on substantial clinical evidence that pathogenic variants result in a high likelihood of severe disease that is preventable if identified before symptoms occur. These initial recommendations did not offer the choice to patients of opting out of receiving the incidental findings but after a survey of the ACMG membership, revised recommendations were published in 2015, offering the patient or parents of a child the choice of opting out from receiving such results [32]. European recommendations are less prescriptive, suggesting that a protocol has to be in place to give guidance on the reporting of unsolicited findings from WGS [33]. It is possible for a laboratory to perform WES or WGS but analyse only a subset of relevant genes. This will result in minimal loss of diagnostic rate and reduces the chances of incidental findings.

Prognostic Uncertainty

The use of genomic technologies has resulted in the identification of novel genetic disorders [34] and redefined the clinical spectrum of well-known disorders by removing ascertainment bias in identifying patients suitable for testing [35]. The standard paradigm of genetic disorders being recognised due to characteristic clinical features is no longer applicable. Genomic technology advances have necessitated 'reverse phenotyping' in many scenarios in which the novel genetic basis of a disorder is identified before the natural history is well-understood. This inevitably leads to difficulties in providing prognostic information to families and this is particularly relevant in the context of the neonatologist's practice as the patient is often not yet old enough to manifest even the standard clinical features.

Rationing of Healthcare

Early diagnosis of a serious genetic disease can cause difficult ethical situations. For example, WGS may identify that a child is at risk of a severe neurocognitive disorder. If this child is seriously ill requiring high levels of support, when is it appropriate to limit care to reduce the suffering of a baby who may have a life-limiting condition or is expected to have a poor quality of life? Will knowing a genetic diagnosis prejudice a child against having further costly healthcare input? Should a child with a serious genetic disorder be listed for an organ transplant? In some developed countries, there is already rationing of precious healthcare resources such as organ recipients in cases of genetic disorders. For example, there is evidence that children with trisomy 21 have fewer referrals made for heart transplants and bone marrow transplants [36].

In 2009 in the US, 43% of organ transplantation services were found to 'always' or 'usually' use neurodevelopmental delay of the child to help guide their transplant listing decisions [37].

Consent

Given the difficulties in variant interpretation, and the possibility of incidental findings and prognostic uncertainty, it is no surprise that obtaining consent for WGS can be challenging. As with any consent process, the clinician speaking with parents should understand the reason for the test, the benefits of getting a diagnosis and the potential consequences of data received from WGS. A systematic review of published work on informed consent has been used to propose a minimum set of information that should be included on a consent form for WGS [38]:

- The scope of the test.
- A description of the test process.

- The expected benefits.
- Possible risks or complications.
- The voluntary nature of the test.
- Permission to withdraw consent at any point.
- Possible alternative diagnostic tests.
- Description of safeguards to confidentiality.
- How samples are stored and possible future use of the samples.
- How incidental findings are handled and the rights of the patient/family to know these.

The British Society for Genetic Medicine has also given advice on genetic testing in children. In particular they advise that one should be very cautious when genetic testing is primarily predictive of illness or impairment in the future [39]. In the majority of cases testing should be delayed until the child is old enough to decide for themselves when, or whether, to be tested.

Newborn Screening

Most genetics professionals believe that NGS will be a part of the newborn screening (NBS) programme in the future [40]. Similarly, surveys show that parents are also interested in this technology [41]. Several studies have shown the feasibility of using the dried heel prick blood spot for NGS [42, 43], though technical challenges such as overcoming heterogeneity of NGS read depth remain [44]. Little is known about how NGS would perform as a large-scale predictive screening test but studies are ongoing [45]. It is likely that NGS will initially be used to complement current NBS tests but there will be an inevitable temptation to expand the programme to examine other parts of the genome with further ethical questions such as who has access to the data and when can it be used.

As large-scale genome sequencing projects mature and embed within healthcare systems one can imagine the integration of WGS with NBS to allow the widespread use of genomic data to help in the diagnosis and personalisation of medicine for the future population.

References

1. Stevenson DA, Carey JC. Contribution of malformations and genetic disorders to mortality in a children's hospital. Am J Med Genet A. 2004;126A(4):393–7.
2. Petrikin JE, Willig LK, Smith LD, Kingsmore SF. Rapid whole genome sequencing and precision neonatology. Semin Perinatol. 2015;39(8):623–31.
3. Sheridan E, Wright J, Small N, Corry PC, Oddie S, Whibley C, et al. Risk factors for congenital anomaly in a multiethnic birth cohort: an analysis of the Born in Bradford study. Lancet. 2013;382(9901):1350–9.

4. Synnes AR, Berry M, Jones H, Pendray M, Stewart S, Lee SK, et al. Infants with congenital anomalies admitted to neonatal intensive care units. Am J Perinatol. 2004;21(4):199–207.

5. Berry MA, Shah PS, Brouillette RT, Hellmann J. Predictors of mortality and length of stay for neonates admitted to children's hospital neonatal intensive care units. J Perinatol. 2008;28(4):297–302.

6. Willig LK, Petrikin JE, Smith LD, Saunders CJ, Thiffault I, Miller NA, et al. Whole-genome sequencing for identification of Mendelian disorders in critically ill infants: a retrospective analysis of diagnostic and clinical findings. Lancet Respir Med. 2015;3(5):377–87.

7. Meng L, Pammi M, Saronwala A, Magoulas P, Ghazi AR, Vetrini F, et al. Use of exome sequencing for infants in intensive care units: ascertainment of severe single-gene disorders and effect on medical management. JAMA Pediatr. 2017;171(12):e173438.

8. Daoud H, Luco SM, Li R, Bareke E, Beaulieu C, Jarinova O, et al. Next-generation sequencing for diagnosis of rare diseases in the neonatal intensive care unit. CMAJ. 2016;188(11):E254–60.

9. Lee H, Deignan JL, Dorrani N, Strom SP, Kantarci S, Quintero-Rivera F, et al. Clinical exome sequencing for genetic identification of rare Mendelian disorders. JAMA. 2014;312(18):1880–7.

10. Posey JE, Harel T, Liu P, Rosenfeld JA, James RA, Coban Akdemir ZH, et al. Resolution of disease phenotypes resulting from multilocus genomic variation. N Engl J Med. 2017;376(1):21–31.

11. Trujillano D, Bertoli-Avella AM, Kumar Kandaswamy K, Weiss ME, Köster J, Marais A, et al. Clinical exome sequencing: results from 2819 samples reflecting 1000 families. Eur J Hum Genet. 2017;25(2):176–82.

12. Yang Y, Muzny DM, Xia F, Niu Z, Person R, Ding Y, et al. Molecular findings among patients referred for clinical whole-exome sequencing. JAMA. 2014;312(18):1870–9.

13. Stark Z, Tan TY, Chong B, Brett GR, Yap P, Walsh M, et al. A prospective evaluation of whole-exome sequencing as a first-tier molecular test in infants with suspected monogenic disorders. Genet Med. 2016;18(11):1090–6.

14. Lionel AC, Costain G, Monfared N, Walker S, Reuter MS, Hosseini SM, et al. Improved diagnostic yield compared with targeted gene sequencing panels suggests a role for whole-genome sequencing as a first-tier genetic test. Genet Med. 2018;20(4):435–43.

15. Stavropoulos DJ, Merico D, Jobling R, Bowdin S, Monfared N, Thiruvahindrapuram B, et al. Whole genome sequencing expands diagnostic utility and improves clinical management in pediatric medicine. NPJ Genom Med. 2016;1:15012.

16. Farnaes L, Hildreth A, Sweeney NM, Clark MM, Chowdhury S, Nahas S, et al. Rapid whole-genome sequencing decreases infant morbidity and cost of hospitalization. NPJ Genom Med. 2018;3:10.

17. Saunders CJ, Miller NA, Soden SE, Dinwiddie DL, Noll A, Alnadi NA, et al. Rapid whole-genome sequencing for genetic disease diagnosis in neonatal intensive care units. Sci Transl Med. 2012;4(154):154ra135.

18. Miller NA, Farrow EG, Gibson M, Willig LK, Twist G, Yoo B, et al. A 26-hour system of highly sensitive whole genome sequencing for emergency management of genetic diseases. Genome Med. 2015;7:100.

19. Stark Z, Schofield D, Alam K, Wilson W, Mupfeki N, Macciocca I, et al. Prospective comparison of the cost-effectiveness of clinical whole-exome sequencing with that of usual care overwhelmingly supports early use and reimbursement. Genet Med. 2017;19(8):867–74.

20. Schwarze K, Buchanan J, Taylor JC, Wordsworth S. Are whole-exome and whole-genome sequencing approaches cost-effective? A systematic review of the literature. Genet Med. 2018;20(10):1122–30.

21. Graungaard AH, Skov L. Why do we need a diagnosis? A qualitative study of parents' experiences, coping and needs, when the newborn child is severely disabled. Child Care Health Dev. 2007;33(3):296–307.

22. Taanila A, Syrjälä L, Kokkonen J, Järvelin M-R. Coping of parents with physically and/or intellectually disabled children. Child Care Health Dev. 2002;28(1):73–86.

23. NICUSeq: a trial to evaluate the clinical utility of human whole genome sequencing (WGS) compared to standard of care in acute care neonates and infants—full text view—ClinicalTrials.gov [Internet]. [Cited 2018 Nov 25]. https://clinicaltrials.gov/ct2/show/NCT03290469.

24. Connell TG, Rele M, Cowley D, Buttery JP, Curtis N. How reliable is a negative blood culture result? Volume of blood submitted for culture in routine practice in a children's hospital. Pediatrics. 2007;119(5):891–6.

25. McCabe KM, Khan G, Zhang YH, Mason EO, McCabe ER. Amplification of bacterial DNA using highly conserved sequences: automated analysis and potential for molecular triage of sepsis. Pediatrics. 1995;95(2):165–9.

26. Jordan JA, Durso MB. Real-time polymerase chain reaction for detecting bacterial DNA directly from blood of neonates being evaluated for sepsis. J Mol Diagn. 2005;7(5):575–81.

27. Pammi M, Flores A, Leeflang M, Versalovic J. Molecular assays in the diagnosis of neonatal sepsis: a systematic review and meta-analysis. Pediatrics. 2011;128(4):e973–85.

28. Su G, Fu Z, Hu L, Wang Y, Zhao Z, Yang W. 16S ribosomal ribonucleic acid gene polymerase chain reaction in the diagnosis of bloodstream infections: a systematic review and meta-analysis. PLoS One. 2015;10(5):e0127195.

29. Pammi M, Flores A, Versalovic J, Leeflang MM. Molecular assays for the diagnosis of sepsis in neonates. Cochrane Database Syst Rev. 2017;2:CD011926.

30. Richards S, Aziz N, Bale S, Bick D, Das S, Gastier-Foster J, et al. Standards and guidelines for the interpretation of sequence variants: a joint consensus recommendation of the American College of Medical Genetics and Genomics and the Association for Molecular Pathology. Genet Med. 2015;17(5):405–24.

31. Green RC, Berg JS, Grody WW, Kalia SS, Korf BR, Martin CL, et al. ACMG recommendations for reporting of incidental findings in clinical exome and genome sequencing. Genet Med. 2013;15(7):565–74.

32. ACMG Board of Directors. ACMG policy statement: updated recommendations regarding analysis and reporting of secondary findings in clinical genome-scale sequencing. Genet Med. 2015;17(1):68–9.

33. Matthijs G, Souche E, Alders M, Corveleyn A, Eck S, Feenstra I, et al. Guidelines for diagnostic next-generation sequencing. Eur J Hum Genet. 2016;24(1):2–5.

34. Deciphering Developmental Disorders Study. Prevalence and architecture of de novo mutations in developmental disorders. Nature. 2017;542(7642):433–8.

35. van der Sluijs EPJ, Jansen S, Vergano SA, Adachi-Fukuda M, Alanay Y, AlKindy A, et al. The ARID1B spectrum in 143 patients: from nonsyndromic intellectual disability to Coffin-Siris syndrome. Genet Med. 2019;21(6):1295–307.

36. Leonard H, Eastham K, Dark J. Heart and heart-lung transplantation in Down's syndrome. BMJ. 2000;320(7238):816–7.

37. Richards CT, Crawley LM, Magnus D. Use of neurodevelopmental delay in pediatric solid organ transplant listing decisions: inconsistencies in standards across major pediatric transplant centers. Pediatr Transplant. 2009;13(7):843–50.

38. Ayuso C, Millán JM, Mancheño M, Dal-Ré R. Informed consent for whole-genome sequencing studies in the clinical setting. Proposed recommendations on essential content and process. Eur J Hum Genet. 2013;21(10):1054–9.

39. British Society for Genetic Medicine [Internet]. [Cited 2018 Oct 31]. http://www.bsgm.org.uk/.

40. Ulm E, Feero WG, Dineen R, Charrow J, Wicklund C. Genetics professionals' opinions of whole-genome sequencing in the newborn period. J Genet Couns. 2015;24(3):452–63.

41. Goldenberg AJ, Dodson DS, Davis MM, Tarini BA. Parents' interest in whole-genome sequencing of newborns. Genet Med. 2014;16(1):78–84.

42. Hollegaard MV, Grauholm J, Nielsen R, Grove J, Mandrup S, Hougaard DM. Archived neonatal dried blood spot samples can be used for accurate whole genome and exome-targeted next-generation sequencing. Mol Genet Metab. 2013;110(1–2):65–72.

43. Poulsen JB, Lescai F, Grove J, Bækvad-Hansen M, Christiansen M, Hagen CM, et al. High-quality exome sequencing of whole-genome amplified neonatal dried blood spot DNA. PLoS One. 2016;11(4):e0153253.

44. Boemer F, Fasquelle C, d'Otreppe S, Josse C, Dideberg V, Segers K, et al. A next-generation newborn screening pilot study: NGS on dried blood spots detects causal mutations in patients with inherited metabolic diseases. Sci Rep. 2017;7(1):17641.

45. Berg JS, Agrawal PB, Bailey DB, Beggs AH, Brenner SE, Brower AM, et al. Newborn sequencing in genomic medicine and public health. Pediatrics. 2017;139(2):e20162252.

Chapter 33
Research in the Newborn Period

Kamini Yadav and Elaine M. Boyle

Introduction

In the twenty-first century, it is imperative that policies and practices in neonatal and perinatal medicine are informed by evidence from high quality research and this is fundamental to improving neonatal outcomes. Evidence based interventions, such as the administration of antenatal corticosteroids, antenatal magnesium sulphate and surfactant, to name but a few, have transformed outcomes in preterm and sick term neonates with a life-long benefit disproportionate to their cost. At the same time, practices based on poor evidence may have potentially life-long adverse consequences. Clinicians and researchers now face the challenge of maintaining the trajectory of improvements in neonatal care and outcomes by pushing the boundaries of knowledge, through well conducted research, underpinned by a range of research approaches, from preclinical to large scale multicentre, randomised controlled trials (RCT). As research funding is a limited resource, this can be achieved only by coordination and collaboration of research efforts globally, identifying research priorities in collaboration with parents and families and finding novel ways to answer research questions. In this chapter, we focus on two key issues in neonatal research: Informed consent and outcome measures in neonatal research and briefly discuss some of the other more general challenges in delivering research in our smallest patients.

K. Yadav
University Hospitals of Leicester NHS Trust, Leicester, UK
e-mail: kamini.yadav@uhl-tr.nhs.uk

E. M. Boyle (✉)
Department of Health Sciences, University of Leicester, Leicester, UK
e-mail: eb124@le.ac.uk

© Springer Nature Switzerland AG 2020
E. M. Boyle, J. Cusack (eds.), *Emerging Topics and Controversies in Neonatology*, https://doi.org/10.1007/978-3-030-28829-7_33

Informed Consent

The Nuremburg Code, created in 1947, is one of several foundational documents that influence principles of good clinical practice. It marks one of the great advances in clinical research history and underpins the ethics of medical research aimed to protect human subjects. The Code states that consent should be voluntary, that participants should have sufficient understanding of the subject matter and must be able to reserve the rights to end their participation in the study at any time, without penalty. The Declaration of Helsinki, first set out in 1964 and subsequently updated several times, further emphasises that the fundamental moral responsibility of physicians conducting research is to respect research participants and their right to make informed decisions regarding participation, both initially and during the course of the research. The physician's primary responsibility is to the patient or the research volunteer and, while there is always a need for research, the subject's welfare must take precedence over the interests of science and society. Keeping these principles in mind, we approach the subject of consent in neonatal research. As neonates lack competency to consent for research participation, recruitment of neonates to clinical trials requires informed consent from parents. However, obtaining valid consent from parents during the antenatal, intrapartum or postpartum period may be compromised by situational incapacity due to maternal illness, stress of labour, influence of medications, and worries about their unborn/newborn child's illness and chances of survival. This raises questions regarding validity of consent, understanding the role of parents in giving and withholding consent, and different approaches to seeking consent and parental views.

Parental Role and Responsibility for Providing Consent

Informed consent in neonatology is the result of a conglomerate of events and interactions between the clinicians in charge of the study and the parents authorising their infant's participation. While a neonate is not yet autonomous, the parents are the best surrogate or proxy decision makers as they can be assumed to be acting to protect and promote their child's best interest. Obtaining parental consent also respects parental autonomy and parents' rights to make decisions for their child. In neonatal research, it is important to consider consent as a case of family decision making, as parents have to take responsibility for their decision and also bear the consequences of such decisions as some social scientists and philosophers would say [1]. However, parents should not be solely burdened with the responsibility of thinking about their child's best interest. It is a joint responsibility of the researcher and the ethical review process to act in the neonate's best interest; the needs of society and/or science should never take precedence. Some would suggest that parental consent in neonatal research is a misnomer. What it actually implies is parental permission or authorisation for their child to participate in a study [2].

Validity of Informed Consent

Voluntariness

A major impediment to valid consent is the potential situation of desperation and fear in which the parents find themselves, following admission of their baby to a neonatal intensive care unit (NICU). Free will of a parent may not be easy to assess in situations where they are vulnerable. The clinician or the researcher may be seen as a figure of authority or power, to whom they might find it difficult to refuse research participation. Parents may find it difficult to believe that there is clinical equipoise and the enthusiasm of the clinician or researcher for one line of treatment, or simply for the project itself, may influence information giving and place pressure on parents to make a particular decision. In addition, they might feel that they have a moral obligation to the clinicians, researchers, neonatal unit and society as a whole. Both their emotional status and the risk of being influenced by their baby's clinician may affect on the voluntariness of their consent through psychological coercion. In the Magpie trial, some women relied on the confidence they had in the recruiting clinician, trusting that he or she would not expose them or their babies to anything risky [3]. The Euricon study showed that only 10% of the parents appeared to have problems with the voluntariness of their consent while 55% of neonatologists had concerns in this area on behalf of parents [4].

Information and Understanding

Testing of parental understanding of research study is not easy. Helping parents understand the difficult concepts of randomisation and clinical equipoise can be challenging. Anecdotally, a common problem is parents thinking that they are being asked to choose one of the therapies being compared and they may ask the clinician for advice about that choice. This suggests a lack of understanding of the study information and its purpose. Two factors that have an impact on parental understanding are time limitations and language barriers, which have an effect on the amount and the quality of information that is given. Levene et al. pointed out that recruitment to urgent trials was higher as compared to non-urgent trials and it is suggested that this is a result of poor understanding [5]. They also contested that the process of obtaining informed consent was merely an elaborate clinician ritual, which would be invalid if lack of parental understanding was later proved, even if the consent form was signed. Due to the lack of understanding, parents may have therapeutic misconception and believe that the trial intervention is superior to standard treatment. They may incorrectly believe that taking part in the trial will directly benefit their baby or that their baby would receive better care [6, 7]. These issues can be addressed by ensuring that trained professionals provide both verbal and written information to parents about the study, its risk and benefits, in clear lay terms, avoiding medical jargon, followed up by provision of opportunities to ask questions before obtaining parental consent. Validity of informed consent could be further increased by discussion about the study and their child's participation during follow-up consultation. However, there is some evidence to suggest that short parent information leaflets may be preferable, rather than very large amounts of information at this time that may confuse and decrease understanding of important research concepts [8].

Competence

Following admission of their baby to NICU, parents are overwhelmed with emotions of stress, anxiety, fear, loss of control and uncertainty about the future, compounded by maternal illness, maternal medications, cultural beliefs and language barriers [9]. This can adversely affect their understanding and decision making. The Griffiths report suggested that, under the stressful conditions in which parents find themselves, it can never be assumed that consent is valid [9, 10]. Ballard et al. reported that only 3% of parents who signed the consent forms during the NEOPAIN (NEurologic Outcomes and Pre-emptive Analgesia in Neonates) trial truly met the criteria for consent validity on follow-up review [6]. Similarly, Mason et al. showed that, of the 200 parents who provided consent, 70% had difficulty in one or more areas of consent process [4]. Harth and Thong reported that nearly 20% of parents did not remember whether they had consented to their child entering the study 18 months after enrolment [11].

Different Forms of Consent

Prospective Consent

Prospective informed, written consent remains the gold standard in neonatal research. This involves provision of study information in a face-to-face consultation and a patient information leaflet by a clinician who is trained in Good Clinical Practice for research (GCP), and competent in the consent process for the trial. It should avoid medical jargon, and provide information in a language understood by parents with help of a competent interpreter if required, allowing parents time to digest the information and ask questions. However, this may not always be possible, especially in research studies that fall into the "emergency" category, where treatment may be needed immediately, for example, in resuscitation studies or where potentially life-saving intervention is urgently needed. In some cases, however, some time may be available before the intervention, for example, in trials of therapeutic hypothermia in hypoxic ischaemic encephalopathy or extracorporeal membrane oxygenation therapy. Other ways of addressing the need for obtaining consent have been proposed and used, as discussed below.

Waiver of Consent

It has been suggested that there are many scenarios in neonatal clinical research, such as trials in the emergency category, when informed consent could be waived [12–15]. This approach could be used in situations where no standard of care exists and different approaches are used in different centres. Provisional verbal assent could be obtained, which would enable clinicians to randomise to different therapies without parental informed consent. For this approach, extensive patient and public involvement during the study design stage and robust assessment by the ethics committee would be of paramount importance. Although this is reasonable from a clinical perspective, in many situations it might be difficult to justify from regulatory and ethical viewpoint. The aim of the consent waiver process should be to make research possible for the benefit of the patients, not to make research easier for researchers.

Antenatal Notification and Consent

Antenatal notification has been found to be popular with parents [16] as it allows them to obtain information about intended research studies during the antenatal period, with completion of the consent process only if they reach the eligibility criteria [17]. Such a consent process is ideal for intrapartum or emergency/urgent category neonatal research studies. Advantages of this method are allowing parents to obtain information in a stress-free environment, giving them extra time to consider and reflect on the study information and come to a decision, aiding understanding and alleviating stress and anxiety, which has been reported by many parents when giving consent was time-critical [18, 19]. Many clinical trials relating to clamping or milking of the umbilical cord used antenatal consent process before birth [16]. Although popular, such a consent process poses logistic challenges to deliver the study information in the antenatal period [13, 20]. It may place unnecessary burden on those that would not be eligible [15, 21] and risk lack of parental engagement, as they may assume that they may not reach eligibility [21]. These could be addressed by good communication during the antenatal information-giving process.

Deferred, Retrospective or Continuing Consent

Snowdon et al. interviewed the parents of 21 infants who were enrolled in the Extra Corporeal Membrane Oxygenation trial. They found that some were unsure whether their babies were in the trial or not [22]. This raises questions regarding the validity of informed consent. Researchers have proposed that deferred/retrospective or continuing consent may help address this issue [14]. In this case, randomisation is carried out at the clinician's discretion, according to criteria that have been made explicit during ethical review of the protocol, followed by the request for parental informed consent at a later stage, when they are able to understand the information and make an informed decision. If time permits, initial verbal assent may be sought. In the UK and approximately half of the European Union member states, clinical trials legislation amendments have been introduced to enable children under 16 years to be entered into a trial without prior informed consent when treatment is urgent, prospective consent is not possible and appropriate ethical approval has been obtained in advance [23–25]. Allmark et al. reported that the continuing consent process improved consent validity and parents found the follow-up consultation following the initial consent process useful [9, 26]. In research studies where amniotic fluid, umbilical cord or cord blood samples need to be collected, deferred consent may be the only appropriate consent process, where samples are collected at the time of delivery but processed only if parental consent is obtained; otherwise collected samples are appropriately discarded. In spite of the benefits, objection to this method of consent is that parents are unware or have not consented to enrolment and if they later refuse consent then the trial intervention could constitute assault. At the same time full consent only provides permission to continue and is irrelevant if the trial intervention is a one-off treatment.

Zelen's Method of Consent

In this method, consent is obtained after randomisation only for the study participants who are going to receive the trial intervention. In other words, parents of neonates randomised to standard treatment arm will not be approached for informed consent. An argument for this method is that it avoids additional stress to parents which can arise from participating in the consent process or from knowing that their child is in the control group due to therapeutic misconception [26–29]. However, such a consent process assumes the scientific robustness of the study and best interest of the participant. It also raises questions regarding challenges to ensure adequate parental understanding of the study, as even though their child did not receive the trial intervention, their data would be collected for the study and follow-up may be required. Some believe that this method breaches the right to autonomy and really circumvents the consent requirement rather than addressing it [30]. Parents do not like this concept as they would prefer to know if their child was enrolled to any research study [4, 31].

Opt-out

A contentious method of consent is the opt-out strategy. As the name suggests, neonates are enrolled to the study unless their parents have explicitly expressed their wish to opt out of the research. Advantages of such an approach are that it increases recruitment, the sample is more representative of the population assuring greater generalisation of the results, and it lessens the burden on parents [21] and clinicians [32]. There has been some success in adopting this method of recruitment for large observational studies in the UK. EUROPAIN (EUROpean Pain Audit In Neonates), was a prospective cohort study of the management of sedation and analgesia in patients in NICU. The approach of opt-out consent was used for this study, allowing the UK to recruit the highest number of babies of 18 European countries [33]. A similar opt-out strategy has also been used in the OptiPrem Study [34]. The WHEAT (WitHolding Enteral feeds Around packed red cell Transfusion to prevent NEC in preterm neonates) trial, currently recruiting in the UK, has had the approval of nine out of 12 Research Ethics Committee across the UK to use the "opt-out" method of consent, as both the care pathways being compared are part of standard UK practice [35]. Objections to such a process centre around the fact that the opt-out method may seem potentially coercive. Parents might find it difficult to approach the clinician caring for their baby to refuse research participation. There is concern that it might override the right to autonomy which is the cornerstone for informed consent and practical consideration of offering parents opt-out option in a timely manner before research participation may pose important ethical challenges [21].

Parental Views on Consent

Reasons for parental participation in research studies include societal benefits, personal benefits, perceived risk and perception of no harm. McCarthy et al. reviewed parental opinion of consent in neonatal research through parental questionnaire [7]. In 93% of cases, parents felt that their involvement in the consent process was essential. In emergency situations, 52% felt full prospective informed consent was necessary; however, almost 28% of parents felt pressure to consent. Similar findings regarding parental willingness to participate have been reported by others [4, 17, 36, 37]. Ayers et al. reported that the timing of recruitment was a concern to many [16]. Seventy-five percent of parents, in a review by McCarthy, preferred to be approached to discuss neonatal research studies antenatally, irrespective of study type [7] (McCarthy 2015). The main reason for participation in research studies was the altruistic principle to help improve care of future babies and advance medical knowledge [9, 38, 39]. It is likely that the extent of altruistic motivation varies depending on the extent that the trial can benefit participants. Parents expressed their wish that both parents should be involved in the research project [40]. In general, parents were happy to be involved in the consent process and were happy for their baby's participation.

Research Outcomes

Randomised controlled trials are central to evaluation of the efficacy of any new intervention or treatment. The influence of RCTs on change of clinical practice may not only depend on assessment of effectiveness, safety and cost effectiveness of treatment, but also on additional factors such as the importance of the research question for clinical practice and patients, the rigor of the study design, the authority of the research team and the ease of implementation of treatment under investigation. For neonatal trials, these considerations all apply, but change in practice is also likely to be informed by the strength and credibility of the findings. The choice of outcomes measured in clinical trials is an important factor of study design. The primary outcome has much invested in it as it solely indicates whether the trial provides evidence at an acceptable levels regarding the effectiveness of the treatment. In neonatal research, analysing all-cause mortality, although one of the most important outcomes, if considered in isolation could lead to spurious results if, for example, long-term outcomes are not taken into account. In more recent years, trials have combined mortality with other important non-fatal outcomes to produce a single composite outcome. Selection of individual components of the composite outcome is important; they must be associated with the primary objective of the trial, be biologically plausible and meaningful to patients and clinicians. Composite outcomes should be defined before the start of the trial, and the definition should be adhered to through the conduct and analysis of the study. Although using primary composite outcomes has become a popular choice for many reasons, it comes with some inherent risks and these need to be understood and acknowledged.

Advantages of Using Primary Composite Outcome

Statistical Efficiency

The most popular motivation for using composite outcomes is statistical efficiency. Using composite outcomes comprising of a number of contributing outcomes may allow adequate accrual of events resulting in smaller sample size and/or shorter follow-up. This also helps trials to answer important clinical questions in a timely fashion. For example, the sample size for a study to have a 90% power to find a significant relative risk of 0.65 at 0.05 significance level, with a 20% event rate would be 1600 patients, while only 800 patients with 40% event rate.

Financial Benefit

Securing funding for clinical trials is extremely competitive with some specialities attracting more research grants as compared to others. It has become increasingly more difficult to conduct trials due to competition for limited resources. One of the important components of research design is to evaluate how the trial could be conducted more efficiently. Using composite outcomes improves statistical efficiency thereby answering the research question with a smaller trial which would help to make the trial financially feasible.

Importance of Individual Outcomes to Clinicians and Patients

The different components of composite outcomes may be of equal importance to clinicians and patients and are judged to be of equal value for evaluating the efficacy and effectiveness of treatment under investigation. For example, all-cause mortality and severe neurodevelopmental delay beyond 2 years are common individual components of composite outcome in neonatal trials, both of equal importance. The use of a composite outcome may help the investigators to capture multiple aspects of the treatment effect and avoid the challenge of making arbitrary choice between a number of clinically important outcomes.

Disadvantages of Using Primary Composite Outcomes

Selection of Components of a Composite Outcome

Composite outcomes should combine components of similar clinical importance and patient benefit; they should be defined clearly in the trial protocol and the same definition used throughout the trial and its reporting. Death is commonly used in composite outcomes, but it provides the lowest event rates and smallest treatment effect. If the associated non-fatal composite has higher event rates it would skew the results to show benefit for the composite outcome, even when there is no effect on death or rather detrimental effect. Composite outcomes provide substantial opportunity for inconsistent and unclear reporting, post hoc changes to the composites, and 'cherry picking' of favourable outcomes or combinations of outcomes to show statistical significance. In addition to this, inclusion of clinician chosen outcomes in the composite, such as duration of hospital stay, although important, for a patient it is far less important than the risk of death and there is a risk of bias in non-blinded trials. A survey showed that the inclusion of a clinician driven outcome was predictive of a statistically significant result for the primary composite outcome (odds ratio 2.24 (95% confidence interval 1.15–4.34), P = 0.02) [41].

Reporting of Composite Outcomes

There is a substantial risk associated with reporting of composite outcome in which the benefits may by falsely attributed to all the components of composite outcome. For example, a beneficial effect of a treatment on one individual component of the composite outcome may skew the composite outcome in favour of the treatment. If inadequately reported there is a risk that the authors may imply or the readers may infer beneficial effect on all the individual components of the composite outcome.

Secondly, even if there is no statistically significant difference in the composite outcomes between the intervention and the control arm, the individual components of the composite outcome could have been affected in opposite ways, keeping the composite outcome the same while the individual outcomes may reach clinical or statistical significance. For example, the SUPPORT oxygen targeting trial had a composite outcome of "death or severe retinopathy". The composite outcome was not significantly different between the low-oxygen and the high-oxygen saturation groups, and if the individual components were not reported separately, this would have led to misinterpretation that low oxygen saturation did not pose any higher risk. However, the authors had done three analyses and shown that the constituent outcomes had not moved in the same direction, with death being higher and retinopathy being lower with the lower saturation targets [42].

Contribution of Each Individual Component of the Composite Outcome

It is also important to consider the weight of each component outcome. Analysis of the composite outcomes is done by a count of events or assigning a score based on individual outcomes. The most common type of score is a binary score where patients with one or more events score 1, and score 0 for none. Such an approach makes an assumption that each composite is of equal importance.

Clinical Interpretation

Poor or unclear reporting may result in difficulty with interpretation of the results of the trial where a composite outcome is used. In particular, there might be limited evidence of benefit on the most important outcome such as mortality or long term neurodevelopmental outcome. The study is powered for the composite, but not individual outcomes so it may further raise questions on the robustness of the outcome data of the individual outcomes.

General Challenges in Delivering Research in the Neonatal Population

A number of challenges exist when attempting to conduct high quality, robust research in the neonatal population. Large numbers of research participants need to be recruited over a reasonable period of time for a RCT to successfully deliver robust, generalisable results that can then translate into evidence-based practice in a timely way. However, particularly when considering the extremely preterm group, numbers of babies are small, with extremely preterm births numbering around 2000 per annum in the UK. This means that trials can take a number of years to complete, and can be expensive to fund for this reason. During the course of a long trial recruitment period, other advances in treatment may be developed and introduced, which may either hinder recruitment, or render the results less important. It is possible that this may make the funding of neonatal trials less attractive to granting bodies than, for example, a study of cardiovascular disease or diabetes in adults, where there is a large number of potential research participants available.

Neonates are a heterogeneous group, with varying gestational ages, birth weights, and changes over time that occur as they mature. This further diminishes the pool of potential research participants if research studies employ strict inclusion or exclusion criteria for research. Size, gestation at birth and postnatal age also influence neonatal physiology in terms of handing of drugs, with changing pharmacokinetic and pharmacodynamics parameters complicating the delivery of drug trials.

Parents of vulnerable or sick newborn infants may, understandably, be cautious about subjecting their child to medications, devices or treatments that have not been fully tested. This can make recruitment challenging in the first days of life, and this concern is heightened if compounded by maternal ill health post delivery. Most couples wish to make the decision enrolling their baby in research as a couple, so maternal illness may rule out participation.

For research that is occurring around the time of delivery, the logistics of having necessary staff and resources in place can be challenging, as timing of births is often unpredictable, and the condition or needs of babies cannot always be anticipated prior to birth. Selection bias can therefore be a problem, if only anticipated births or babies with antenatally diagnosed conditions can reliably be included in studies requiring early intervention.

Conclusion

The delivery of high quality neonatal research is not without it challenges, and here we have focused in detail on two of the contentious areas around research practice in the neonatal period. However, neonatology is a relatively young specialty, and many of the practices that have become commonplace have not yet been subjected to rigorous investigation through well-designed randomised controlled trials or detailed observation. A very large number of drugs that are in regular use in the newborn population are currently used "off label", extrapolating from data available for older children; there is an urgent need for proper evaluation in the neonatal population. New devices are constantly being developed that require testing to ensure safety, efficacy and cost-effectiveness. It is therefore imperative that, despite the challenges involved, neonatal research is seen as a priority in order to enable the delivery of safe, evidence-based care to babies at this crucial time of life.

References

1. McDonnell K. Volunteering children. Proc Am Cathol Philos Assoc. 1990;63:182–92.
2. Kodish E. Informed consent for pediatric research: is it really possible? J Pediatr. 2003;142(2):89–90.
3. Smyth RM, Jacoby A, Elbourne D. Deciding to join a perinatal randomised controlled trial: experiences and views of pregnant women enroled in the Magpie Trial. Midwifery. 2012;28(4):E478–85.
4. Mason SA, Allmark PJ. Obtaining informed consent to neonatal randomised controlled trials: interviews with parents and clinicians in the Euricon study. Lancet. 2000;356(9247):2045–51.

5. Levene M, Wright I, Griffiths G. Is informed consent in neonatal randomised controlled trials ritual? Lancet. 1996;347(8999):475.
6. Ballard HO, et al. Neonatal research and the validity of informed consent obtained in the perinatal period. J Perinatol. 2004;24(7):409–15.
7. McCarthy KN, et al. Parental opinion of consent in neonatal research. Arch Dis Child Fetal Neonatal Ed. 2019;104(4):F409–14.
8. Freer Y, et al. More information, less understanding: a randomized study on consent issues in neonatal research. Pediatrics. 2009;123(5):1301–5.
9. McKechnie L, Gill AB. Consent for neonatal research. Arch Dis Child Fetal Neonatal Ed. 2006;91(5):F374–6.
10. Report of a review of the research framework in North Staffordshire Hospital NHS Trust (Griffiths Report). Leeds: NHS Executive; 2000.
11. Harth SC, Thong YH. Sociodemographic and motivational characteristics of parents who volunteer their children for clinical research: a controlled study. BMJ. 1990;300(6736):1372–5.
12. Amin SB, McDermott MP, Shamoo AE. Clinical trials of drugs used off-label in neonates: ethical issues and alternative study designs. Account Res. 2008;15(3):168–87.
13. Boyle RJ, McIntosh N. Ethical considerations in neonatal resuscitation: clinical and research issues. Semin Neonatol. 2001;6(3):261–9.
14. Brierley J, Larcher V. Emergency research in children: options for ethical recruitment. J Med Ethics. 2011;37(7):429–32.
15. Vain NE, et al. Oropharyngeal and nasopharyngeal suctioning of meconium-stained neonates before delivery of their shoulders: multicentre, randomised controlled trial. Lancet. 2004;364(9434):597–602.
16. Ayers S, et al. Parents report positive experiences about enrolling babies in a cord-related clinical trial before birth. Acta Paediatr. 2015;104(4):e164–70.
17. Burgess E, et al. Consent for clinical research in the neonatal intensive care unit: a retrospective survey and a prospective study. Arch Dis Child Fetal Neonatal Ed. 2003;88(4):F280–5; discussion F285–6.
18. Jansen-van der Weide MC, et al. Clinical trial decisions in difficult circumstances: parental consent under time pressure. Pediatrics. 2015;136(4):e983–92.
19. Lockwood CJ, Kuczynski E. Markers of risk for preterm delivery. J Perinat Med. 1999;27(1):5–20.
20. Cuttini M. Intrapartum prevention of meconium aspiration syndrome. Lancet. 2004;364(9434):560–1.
21. Lantos JD. The "inclusion benefit" in clinical trials. J Pediatr. 1999;134(2):130–1.
22. Snowdon C, Garcia J, Elbourne D. Making sense of randomization; responses of parents of critically ill babies to random allocation of treatment in a clinical trial. Soc Sci Med. 1997;45(9):1337–55.
23. Iwanowski P, et al. Informed consent for clinical trials in acute coronary syndromes and stroke following the European Clinical Trials Directive: investigators' experiences and attitudes. Trials. 2008;9:45.
24. Kompanje EJ, et al. Medical research in emergency research in the European Union member states: tensions between theory and practice. Intensive Care Med. 2014;40(4):496–503.
25. European Commission. Directive 2001/20/EC of the European Parliament and of the Council of 4 April 2001 on the approximation of the laws, regulations and administrative provisions of the member states relating to the implementation of good clinical practice in the conduct of clinical trials on medicinal products for human use. Off J Eur Commun. 2001;34–44. https://ec.europa.eu/health/sites/health/files/files/eudralex/vol-1/dir_2001_20/dir_2001_20_en.pdf. Accessed 16 September 2019.
26. Allmark P, Mason S. Improving the quality of consent to randomised controlled trials by using continuous consent and clinician training in the consent process. J Med Ethics. 2006;32(8):439–43.
27. Braunholtz DA. A note on Zelen randomization: attitudes of parents participating in a neonatal clinical trial. Control Clin Trials. 1999;20(6):569–72.

28. Megone C, et al. The ethical issues regarding consent to clinical trials with pre-term or sick neonates: a systematic review (framework synthesis) of the analytical (theoretical/philosophical) research. Trials. 2016;17(1):443.
29. Worrall J. Evidence and ethics in medicine. Perspect Biol Med. 2008;51(3):418–31.
30. Silverman WA, Altman DG. Patients' preferences and randomised trials. Lancet. 1996;347(8995):171–4.
31. Snowdon C, Elbourne D, Garcia J. Zelen randomization: attitudes of parents participating in a neonatal clinical trial. Control Clin Trials. 1999;20(2):149–71.
32. Mason S. Obtaining informed consent for neonatal randomised controlled trials—an "elaborate ritual"? Arch Dis Child Fetal Neonatal Ed. 1997;76(3):F143–5.
33. Carbajal R, et al. Sedation and analgesia practices in neonatal intensive care units (EUROPAIN): results from a prospective cohort study. Lancet Respir Med. 2015;3(10):796–812.
34. OPTI-Prem: optimising neonatal service provision for preterm babies born between 27 and 31 weeks of gestation in England (OPTI-Prem). ClinicalTrials.gov. Identifier: NCT02994849. 2018.
35. Gale C, et al. Research ethics committee decision-making in relation to an efficient neonatal trial. Arch Dis Child Fetal Neonatal Ed. 2017;102(4):F291–8.
36. Cartwright K, et al. Parents' perceptions of their infants' participation in randomized controlled trials. J Obstet Gynecol Neonatal Nurs. 2011;40(5):555–65.
37. Morley CJ, et al. What do parents think about enrolling their premature babies in several research studies? Arch Dis Child Fetal Neonatal Ed. 2005;90(3):F225–8.
38. McCann SK, Campbell MK, Entwistle VA. Reasons for participating in randomised controlled trials: conditional altruism and considerations for self. Trials. 2010;11:31.
39. Truong TH, et al. Altruism among participants in cancer clinical trials. Clin Trials. 2011;8(5):616–23.
40. Korotchikova I, et al. Presence of both parents during consent process in non-therapeutic neonatal research increases positive response. Acta Paediatr. 2010;99(10):1484–8.
41. Freemantle N, Calvert MJ. Interpreting composite outcomes in trials. BMJ. 2010;341:c3529.
42. SUPPORT Study Group of the Eunice Kennedy Shriver NICHD Neonatal Research Network, et al. Target ranges of oxygen saturation in extremely preterm infants. N Engl J Med. 2010;362(21):1959–69.

Chapter 34
Parent Perspectives of Neonatal Intensive Care

Samantha Batt-Rawden

Initial Birth

In almost all of the experiences that were collated, parents, particularly mothers, devoted a considerable time discussing the initial birth of their child. For parents of a premature baby, or one who requires an admission to a neonatal intensive care unit (NICU), many describe grieving the loss of the birth experience that they had so hoped for.

The sensitivity with which this was handled by different hospitals and neonatal units seemed to vary. In some cases, mothers with an extremely premature or critically unwell child were placed in an open bay with mothers of healthy babies, which many described as an intensely painful experience. Several parents described gratitude, and in some cases overwhelming relief, after being offered a side room, especially if their partners were also able to stay on site.

Also acknowledged was the pain of seeing celebrations on the ward around them of the healthy babies that had been born, and not having a similar reception of their premature or critically unwell child in the NICU. Understandably, it was felt strongly by all NICU parents that each baby's entry to the world should be celebrated, even if it was much earlier, or not in the way they expected. Those who had received cards or balloons and congratulations from NICU staff were incredibly grateful for this, and many have kept these cherished tokens.

S. Batt-Rawden (✉)
Air Ambulance Kent Surrey Sussex, Rochester, UK
e-mail: samantha.batt-rawden@nhs.net

© Springer Nature Switzerland AG 2020
E. M. Boyle, J. Cusack (eds.), *Emerging Topics and Controversies in Neonatology*, https://doi.org/10.1007/978-3-030-28829-7_34

Early Days

Should it be appropriate, and should there be time, parents are immensely grateful for the opportunity to visit the NICU prior to their baby's birth and to meet the neonatal team. Those that were able to do this felt more prepared for the journey that awaited them, and for seeing their child receiving organ support.

For those mothers with ongoing maternal complications requiring extended admission to hospital it often seemed that there was little or no communication between NICU and maternity ward staff. It was therefore common for mothers to describe receiving little support whilst on a postnatal ward, should their baby have taken a turn for the worse. Equally, it was common that mothers described missing out their own postnatal care, such as having inadequate pain relief after a Caesarean section, as they did not wish to leave their baby's side. Those hospitals who offered postnatal care and checks to mothers on the neonatal unit were praised.

Many parents, mothers in particular, described the pain of not being able to hold their baby. For mothers of the most premature or critically unwell neonates, this period extended to several weeks. Where it is not possible to facilitate early skin-to-skin, the reasons for this should be explained to the parents.

Communication

For parents, examples of exemplary, as well as poor communication formed powerful memories of their child's time in the NICU. A common theme was that small gestures and compassionate communication made a real difference to parents, at what many describe as the most difficult time in their lives. One such example was that parents often equated how much a clinician cared by whether they knew the child's, and the parents' names.

Universally mentioned by parents when collating responses for this chapter was the gratitude that parents had towards neonatal teams, when parents were included in their daily ward rounds. In fact, many parents plan their visits to the NICU around ward rounds. After several weeks some parents, familiar with the numbers and trends of their baby were invited to present their child on the ward round. For many this made the parents feel an important part of the team.

A common theme was having and being involved in making a plan for the child. Although parents acknowledged that the clinical situation can change as often as hour to hour, that knowing an overall plan for a day or week, was helpful and grounding. Parents were grateful to be invited to multi-disciplinary meetings and found this to be very useful. Having a lead or named consultant for a neonate who was able to provide a holistic view of their child's trajectory and ongoing treatment was very much appreciated by parents.

Psychological Care

Universally praised was the pastoral care provided by NICUs which is a marker of the compassion and skill required to enter neonatology. However, it is certainly true that many parents felt so well supported on the NICU, that it was very difficult once their child was medically fit for discharge. Many units recognised this and provided counselling or access to psychological support staff. Parents who had had psychological input prior to discharge felt more prepared, and were aware of the prevalence and signs of post-traumatic stress disorder (PTSD), as well as where to seek help if required.

Parents were very aware of what goes on around them in the NICU. After spending such a long time surrounded by monitors, many developed a grasp for the numbers, and knew what each alarm meant. It is also certainly true of most neonatal units that cots are closer together compared to an adult ICU. As such, parents-particularly mothers-spent a lot of time together. It is common that lifelong friendships are formed in NICUs, and that parents will have an in-depth knowledge of the medical issues of those babies who are not their own!

As such, it can be extremely distressing when an emergency, a deterioration, or a death occurs in neonatal intensive care; for the staff, for the parents of the child, and for those witnessing the event. Rightly, much energy is directed at supporting the parents of the child involved, and the way staff looked after families at their most difficult times on the unit was universally praised. However, the other parents did not receive any such support. As a result, many describe PTSD symptoms, not for things that happened to their own child, but to other babies, particularly of parents to whom they had grown close.

Visitors

In the case of a regional tertiary unit, it may be that a baby is admitted to hospital miles away from home. This puts a significant strain on families. It may be the case that one parent is living on site in charity-provided accommodation, thus isolated from the support of a partner or family and friends. Having a baby in neonatal intensive care is especially challenging for families who have other small children to care for at home. Visiting rules varied from unit to unit; however flexible policies enabling parents to be able to access the support of their friends and families significantly contributed to their wellbeing during their child's admission. This was especially true for families of other small children if siblings were permitted to visit.

Parents of Non-premature Babies

Those parents of babies who were requiring neonatal intensive care for reasons other than prematurity often felt they had less support. The reasons for this are unclear, but many parents mentioned that the majority of the literature available to parents was geared towards prematurity.

Breastfeeding and Expressing

A range of views were given regarding breast feeding and expressing breast milk. For many, expressing milk became somewhat of a mission, with some mothers feeling that this was the only thing they could do to help their child. Thus, it was common for mothers to feel like a failure should their milk supply not keep up with their baby's feeding regime. Mothers are required to express between 6 and 8 times a day, and are encouraged to wake up at least once overnight to express. This takes a significant toll on mothers who are often also on the NICU most of the day, and it can be a source of undue stress. Mothers very much appreciated support with their expressing, particularly those with a lower milk supply.

Mothers who could not express enough milk must be supported and encouraged. The possibility of donor milk may be offered; however it is important that infant formula is offered in a non-judgmental manner.

Transfers

Transfers are a source of huge stress for parents. Often, a baby may spend several weeks or months in one NICU before returning to a unit nearer to home, or before transfer to a specialist centre for specialist care. Thus, parents become accustomed to the culture of one unit, and become close to the staff. Different centres have different approaches to a number of things which can throw a family out of balance. Examples include differing visitor policies; one unit may have allowed a sibling to visit, however following a transfer they may no longer be able to. In smaller centres there may be less input from clinicians which may leave a family used to daily ward rounds feeling adrift.

The transfer itself can be very frightening for parents. Specialist retrieval services were unanimously praised for explaining the process to the parents, and for allowing a parent to accompany their baby.

Discharge

When a baby is ready for discharge home it is a cause for celebration. However, for parents this can be a daunting prospect. This is particularly true in the case of first time parents, as looking after their child in a heavily supported environment of a NICU is all they have ever known. As such, parents should be involved as much as possible in discharge planning. The opportunity to "room in"—that is, for one parent or preferably both to stay in a private room on the neonatal unit with their child—helps make the process easier. Early involvement in their child's care, such as changing, bathing and administering feeds helps build confidence in parents that they will be able to look after their child independently once they reach home.

Taking a baby home from the NICU is often just the first step in a long journey for a family, particularly those whose children have ongoing complications from their prematurity or critical illness. It is common that parents are bombarded with appointments on discharge, often several in a week, which can leave already sleep deprived parents exhausted and in need of support. Many families will have used any paternity leave they were entitled to at the time of their child's birth, and thus the early days at home can be even more of a challenge.

In particular, for those vulnerable premature neonates with chronic lung disease who may be discharged on home oxygen, parents described feeling isolated at home due to the need to keep their child away from crowded areas. A source of stress for many was the need to explain to well-meaning families, visitors and well-wishers the need to stay away should a potential visitor be ill. Thus, neonatal units who were able to give this advice or written information to extended family were very much appreciated.

Many parents talked in detail about the emotional toll of returning home with their baby. For some, the reality and trauma of what they had experienced on NICU did not come to the surface for several months after discharge. Trigger points included the initial discharge, mothers returning to work, and the child's first birthday. Those who were counselled by NICU staff to expect this, and to be vigilant for symptoms of anxiety, depression and PTSD felt more able to recognise these symptoms when they occurred, and knew where to access help and support.

Index